New Frontiers in Geriatric Medicine

New Frontiers in Geriatric Medicine

Edited by Roger Simpson

hayle
medical

New York

Hayle Medical,
750 Third Avenue, 9ᵗʰ Floor,
New York, NY 10017, USA

Visit us on the World Wide Web at:
www.haylemedical.com

ISBN: 978-1-63241-506-6

Trademark Notice: Registered trademark of products or corporate names are used only for explanation and identification without intent to infringe.

Cataloging-in-Publication Data

New frontiers in geriatric medicine / edited by Roger Simpson.
    p. cm.
Includes bibliographical references and index.
ISBN 978-1-63241-506-6
1. Geriatrics. 2. Older people--Diseases. 3. Older people--Health and hygiene. I. Simpson, Roger.
RC952.5 .N49 2018
618.97--dc23

Table of Contents

Preface

In my initial years as a student, I used to run to the library at every possible instance to grab a book and learn something new. Books were my primary source of knowledge and I would not have come such a long way without all that I learnt from them. Thus, when I was approached to edit this book; I became understandably nostalgic. It was an absolute honor to be considered worthy of guiding the current generation as well as those to come. I put all my knowledge and hard work into making this book most beneficial for its readers.

Geriatrics refers to the medical practice of providing special health care to elderly people. It includes studies related to prevention, diagnosis and treatment of diseases and disorders affecting the older individuals. The common diseases studied under this field are heart disease, Parkinson's disease, arthritis, high cholesterol, dementia, etc. This book aims to shed light on some of the unexplored aspects of geriatrics and the recent researches in this field. The various advancements in geriatric medicine are glanced at and their applications as well as therapeutic effects are looked at. It is a vital tool for all researching and studying this field.

I wish to thank my publisher for supporting me at every step. I would also like to thank all the authors who have contributed their researches in this book. I hope this book will be a valuable contribution to the progress of the field.

Editor

Trajectories in Glycemic Control over Time Are Associated with Cognitive Performance in Elderly Subjects with Type 2 Diabetes

Ramit Ravona-Springer[1]*, Anthony Heymann[2], James Schmeidler[3], Erin Moshier[4], James Godbold[4], Mary Sano[3], Derek Leroith[5], Sterling Johnson[6], Rachel Preiss[7], Keren Koifman[1], Hadas Hoffman[7], Jeremy M. Silverman[3], Michal Schnaider Beeri[3,8]

1 Memory clinic, Sheba Medical Center, Tel Hashomer, Ramat Gan, Israel, 2 Department of Family Medicine, University of Tel Aviv, Tel Aviv, Israel, 3 Department of Psychiatry, Icahn School of Medicine at Mount Sinai, New York, United States of America, 4 Department of Preventive Medicine, Icahn School of Medicine at Mount Sinai, New York, United States of America, 5 Department of Medicine, Icahn School of Medicine at Mount Sinai, New York, United States of America, 6 Geriatric Research Education and Clinical Center, Madison VA Hospital and Alzheimer's Disease Research Center, Department of Medicine, University of Wisconsin, WI, United States of America, 7 Maccabi Health Services, Tel Aviv, Israel, 8 The Joseph Sagol Neuroscience Center, Sheba Medical Center, Ramat Gan, Israel

Abstract

Objective: To study the relationships of long-term trajectories of glycemic control with cognitive performance in cognitively normal elderly with type 2 diabetes (T2D).

Methods: Subjects (n = 835) pertain to a diabetes registry (DR) established in 1998 with an average of 18 HbA1c measurements per subject, permitting identification of distinctive trajectory groups of HbA1c and examining their association with cognitive function in five domains: episodic memory, semantic categorization, attention/working memory, executive function, and overall cognition. Analyses of covariance compared cognitive function among the trajectory groups adjusting for sociodemographic, cardiovascular, diabetes-related covariates and depression.

Results: Subjects averaged 72.8 years of age. Six trajectories of HbA1c were identified, characterized by HbA1c level at entry into the DR (Higher/Lower), and trend over time (Stable/Decreasing/Increasing). Both groups with a trajectory of decreasing HbA1c levels had high HbA1c levels at entry into the DR (9.2%, 10.7%), and high, though decreasing, HbA1c levels over time. They had the worst cognitive performance, particularly in overall cognition ($p<0.02$) and semantic categorization ($p<0.01$), followed by that of subjects whose HbA1c at entry into the DR was relatively high (7.2%, 7.8%) and increased over time. Subjects with stable HbA1c over time had the lowest HbA1c levels at entry (6.0%, 6.8%) and performed best in cognitive tests.

Conclusion: Glycemic control trajectories, which better reflect chronicity of T2D than a single HbA1c measurement, predict cognitive performance. A trajectory of stable HbA1c levels over time is associated with better cognitive function.

Editor: Stephen D. Ginsberg, Nathan Kline Institute and New York University School of Medicine, United States of America

Funding: This study was supported by the American Federation for Aging Research (AFAR), Young investigator award 2011 and NIRG-11-205083 Alzheimer's Association, 2012 to RRS, NIA grant R01 AG034087 to MSB, NIA-AG02219 (VH), the Helen Bader Foundation and the Irma T. Hirschl Scholar Award as well as the Leroy Schecter Foundation Award to MSB. National Institute of Aging grant P01-AG02219, a Merit Award to JMS from the United States Department of Veterans Affairs; Berkman Charitable Trust. The funders have no role in study design, data collection and analysis, decision to publish, or presentation of the manuscript.

Competing Interests: The authors have declared that no competing interests exist.

* E-mail: ramit.ravona@sheba.health.gov.il

Introduction

Type 2 diabetes (T2D) is one of the most common chronic diseases worldwide and is associated with an increased risk for cognitive decline and dementia [1,2]. Chronic hyperglycemia and alterations of cellular homeostasis, characteristic of T2D, lead to diffuse vascular damage and multi-organ dysfunction [3]. Hyperglycemia is a key determinant of both macrovascular (e.g. myocardial infarction, stroke) and microvascular (e.g. retinopathy) complications of T2D, and there is extensive evidence showing that both acute and chronic hyperglycemia are deleterious [4,5,6]. Hemoglobin A1c (HbA1c) levels (the gold standard measurement

of glycemic control), even in non-diabetic individuals [7], are associated with cognitive performance [8,9] and brain volume [10,11]. Based on the beneficial effect of good glycemic control in preventing other diabetes complications [12], it is clinically reasonable to strive for an optimal level of glycemic control [13] in order to mitigate or perhaps prevent cognitive decline and dementia [13]. Good glycemic control has been demonstrated by some [14,15] to be associated with better cognitive function even in non-T2D individuals [16]. However, strict glycemic control achieved by anti-diabetic medications has been shown to increase risk for morbidity and mortality in some T2D subjects [17] and therefore cannot be homogenously applied. It is therefore relevant and useful as an initial approach to study the association of trajectories in glycemic control over time–reflecting long-term T2D processes rather than glycemic control at a certain period in time, with cognition. Such an approach may form a basis for identification of T2D subjects in which achievement of good glycemic control may be safe and efficacious as a means for dementia prevention.

Studies on the relationship of other cardiovascular risk factors (e.g blood pressure and weight) and dementia have demonstrated that trends over time–not only mean levels–were associated with increased risk for dementia [18,19,20]. Trends in glycemic control among T2D subjects, as reflected in trajectories of repeated HbA1c measurements over years, were associated with mortality [21]. However, to the best of our knowledge, the relationship of such trajectories with cognitive function has not been studied. The present study examined the relationship of empirically developed trajectories of HbA1c levels over time and cognitive function in a cognitively normal cohort of elderly T2D subjects participating in the Israel Diabetes and Cognitive Decline (IDCD) study, a longitudinal investigation of the relationship of long-term T2D characteristics with cognitive decline.

Results

Description of the Sample

There were 1288 subjects who passed the preliminary screening, expressed interest in participating, were approached by a study physician and signed informed consent. Of them, 282 (21.1%) were excluded from the study due to incompatibility with eligibility criteria (based on physician assessment) and 109 (8.5%) refused to continue their participation in the study, so 897 subjects remained active participants. The study consists of 835 subjects who had complete data on sociodemographic, cardiovascular, and diabetes-related covariates as well as GDS score and had at least 2 HbA1c measurements. Table 1 describes the sample characteristics and compares the HbA1c trend categories using analysis of variance for continuous outcomes, and Pearson's chi square for dichotomous outcomes. The mean age at entry into the IDCD was 72.75 (4.63) years, with a majority of males (60%). The average levels of total, HDL, and LDL cholesterol, diastolic blood pressure, and GFR were consistent with the general elderly population in this age range. Systolic blood pressure was higher than in the general population but similar to that observed in other T2D samples [22]. Most subjects were treated with oral anti-diabetic medications (79%), 1% were treated with insulin only, 9% were treated with a combined therapy of oral anti-diabetic medications and insulin and 11% were controlled by diet only. The mean number of HbA1c measurements per subject was 17.9 (SD = 9.6). Mean duration of inclusion in the DR was 8.70 (2.64) years, mean HbA1c levels at entry into the DR and at follow up were 6.95% (1.32) and 6.96% (1.01) respectively.

The PROC TRAJ analysis identified six trajectories, with each characterized by (1) the HbA1c level at entry into the DR (intercept), and (2) the trend over time in the registry (figure 1). Three types of trends (stable, increasing and decreasing) in HbA1c over time were observed, and within each type there were two groups with nearly parallel trends but with different intercepts (HbA1c levels at entry to the Registry). For convenience purposes, the groups are referred to by (1) whether it has a Higher or Lower intercept within each type of trend (the terms higher and lower were used for descriptive purposes rather than for clinical purposes, in order to differentiate, within each trend in HbA1c, those who entered with a relatively higher from those who entered

with a relatively lower HbA1c into the DR), and (2) the type of trend in HbA1c over time, either Stable, Increasing or Decreasing. Groups differed in number of years in the DR (longest duration for the groups whose HbA1c decreased, followed by the groups whose HbA1c increased and finally by the groups that remained stable); HbA1c levels at baseline was highest for the groups whose HbA1c decreased, followed by the groups whose HbA1c increased and lowest for the groups that remained stable; mean HbA1c during follow up was highest for the Higher Decreasing and Higher Increasing groups and lowest for the two groups that remained stable. Differences were found for anti-diabetic medications use such that the Higher Decreasing group had the lowest use of oral anti-diabetics only and the highest use of both oral anti-diabetics and insulin. Additional differences were observed for age at entry into the IDCD, LDL cholesterol, and diastolic blood pressure.

The Association of HbA1c Trajectories with Cognitive Function

The overall models were significant for overall cognition, semantic categorization, and executive functions (see Table 2). For descriptive purposes, Table 3 presents comparisons among the different trajectories. Mean overall cognitive z-score was significantly lower in the Higher Decreasing group compared to all other groups except Higher Increasing- in which the difference approached significance. Similarly, for semantic categorization, mean z-scores were lower for the Higher Decreasing group compared to all other groups (approaching significance for the Lower Decreasing group). The Lower Decreasing group had poorer z-scores than the other groups except for the Higher Increasing group. Scores for executive function were lower for Higher Decreasing compared to all other groups except the Higher Increasing group which by itself had poorer function compared to the two stable groups. The mean z-score for the Lower Increasing group was significantly lower than that of the Lower Stable group and approached significance compared to the Higher Stable group (tables 2 and 3). Finally, no significant differences were observed among groups in the episodic memory and attention/working memory domains.

After applying the Bonferroni-Holms step down correction to account for multiple comparisons, the following pairwise comparisons remained significant: for overall cognition, the comparison of the Higher Decreasing group to the Lower stable group (p = 0.0021) and to the Higher Stable group (p = 0.0029), for semantic categorization, the comparison of the Higher Decreasing group to the Lower Increasing group (p = 0.0031) and for executive function, the comparison of the Higher Decreasing group with the Lower Stable group (0.0015).

A secondary analysis demonstrated that higher mean HbA1c was associated with lower scores in overall cognitive score (p = 0.01) and executive functions (p = 0.0003) and with a trend for lower scores in semantic categorization (p = 0.06). Higher standard deviation in HbA1c was associated with lower scores in executive function (p = 0.025) and a trend towards lower scores in overall cognitive score (p = 0.07).

Exclusion of the handful of cases in which there was a gap between the CDR score and the MMSE scores did not affect the results.

Discussion

The present study demonstrated that among elderly T2D subjects, the trajectories of glycemic control over time were associated with cognitive functioning in the cognitive domains of semantic categorization, executive function and overall cognition.

Table 1. Characteristics of the sample by HbA1c* Trajectory group.

Variable	Lower Stable*	Higher Stable*	Lower Increasing	Higher Increasing	Lower Decreasing	Higher Decreasing	Total	p-value
	N = 227	N = 365	N = 123	N = 46	N = 59	N = 15	N = 835	
Years in Diabetes Registry	8.35 (2.58)	8.35 (2.81)	9.36 (2.32)	8.88 (2.57)	10.13 (1.7)	10.95 (0.56)	8.70 (2.64)	<0.0001
HbA1c at entry into Diabetes Registry	5.96 (0.67)	6.84 (0.94)	7.26 (0.84)	7.76 (0.95)	9.19 (1.4)	10.73 (0.97)	6.95 (1.32)	<0.0001
Mean HbA1c During Follow-Up	6.01 (0.28)	6.70 (0.23)	7.45 (0.23)	8.35 (0.34)	7.61 (0.36)	9.22 (0.45)	6.82 (0.77)	<0.0001
Current age	72.99 (4.75)	72.91 (4.66)	72.52 (4.46)	70.78 (4.16)	73.63 (4.48)	69.73 (3.35)	72.75 (4.63)	0.0027
Education (years)	13.43 (3.47)	13.21 (3.71)	13.12 (3.18)	12.59 (2.8)	12.75 (2.71)	12.00 (2.80)	13.17 (3.45)	0.3857
HDL*	48.39 (11.24)	48.06 (10.68)	47.93 (11.58)	43.97 (8.35)	46.73 (9.44)	44.98 (11.8)	47.76 (10.82)	0.1427
LDL*	102.15 (19.12)	103.69 (19.82)	98.38 (19.22)	97.84 (27.38)	95.56 (14.46)	93.89 (22.7)	101.42 (19.9)	0.0050
Total cholesterol	179.65 (24.69)	182.69 (25.96)	180.14 (23.61)	182.28 (28.45)	172.31 (18.34)	167.58 (27.52)	180.46 (25.12)	0.0184
Systolic BP*	133.4 (8.86)	134.88 (9.11)	135.45 (9.42)	137.70 (9.98)	135.38 (12.04)	133.99 (8.01)	134.74 (9.39)	0.0659
Diastolic BP	76.85 (4.74)	77.40 (4.81)	76.90 (4.52)	77.52 (4.66)	75.15 (5.84)	76.18 (5.54)	77.00 (4.85)	0.0319
GFR*	80.38 (23.87)	81.71 (27.13)	79.33 (25.98)	83.31 (32.5)	77.82 (25.73)	91.43 (24.42)	80.99 (26.29)	0.4852
GDS*	1.00 [0-9]	1.00 [0-11]	2.00 [0-9]	2.00 [0-10]	1.00 [0-14]	1.00 [0-9]	1.00 [0-14]	0.3249
Diabetes medication group								
Oral antidiabetic Only	164 (72%)	324 (89%)	103 (84%)	25 (54%)	45 (76%)	2 (13%)	663 (79%)	<0.0001
Insulin Only	3 (1%)	2 (1%)	2 (2%)	1 (2%)	1 (2%)	0 (0%)	9 (1%)	
Insulin+Oral antidiabetic	3 (1%)	6 (2%)	17 (14%)	20 (43%)	13 (22%)	12 (80%)	71 (9%)	
None	57 (25%)	33 (9%)	1 (1%)	0 (0%)	0 (0%)	1 (7%)	92 (11%)	

*HbA1c = hemoglobin A1c, HDL = High density lipoprotein, LDL = low density lipoprotein, GFR = glomerular filtration rate, GDS = geriatric depression scale.

```
┌─────────────────────────┐
│ Screening for eligible  │
│ subjects on the MHS     │
│ diabetes registry       │
└─────────────────────────┘
     │
     ↓
   ┌──────────────────────────┐
   │ MHS sends letters to     │
   │ primary care physicians  │
   │ + phone calls to         │
   │ potential subjects and   │
   │ further screening n=1402 │
   └──────────────────────────┘
        │
        ↓
      ┌──────────────────────────┐
      │ Passed preliminary       │          ⟹  Refused physician's
      │ screening, were referred │             visit n=55
      │ to study physicians      │
      │ n= 1203                  │
      └──────────────────────────┘
           │
           ↓
         ┌──────────────────────────┐     Excluded from the study due to
         │ Physician visit: IC,     │     incompatibility with inclusion
         │ neurological, medical,   │ ⟹   criteria n=181 (164 with
         │ geriatric and            │     cognitive impairment, 2 with
         │ nutritional assessment+  │     PD*, 7 without informant, 8
         │ bloods n=1148            │     other)
         └──────────────────────────┘     Refused to continue participation
              │                           n=70
              ↓
            ┌──────────────────────────┐
            │ Neuropsychologist visit: │
            │ cognitive assessment     │
            │ n=897                    │
            └──────────────────────────┘
                 │
                 ↓
               ┌──────────────────────────┐
               │ Consensus conference to  │
               │ determine eligibility    │
               │ n=897                    │
               └──────────────────────────┘
```

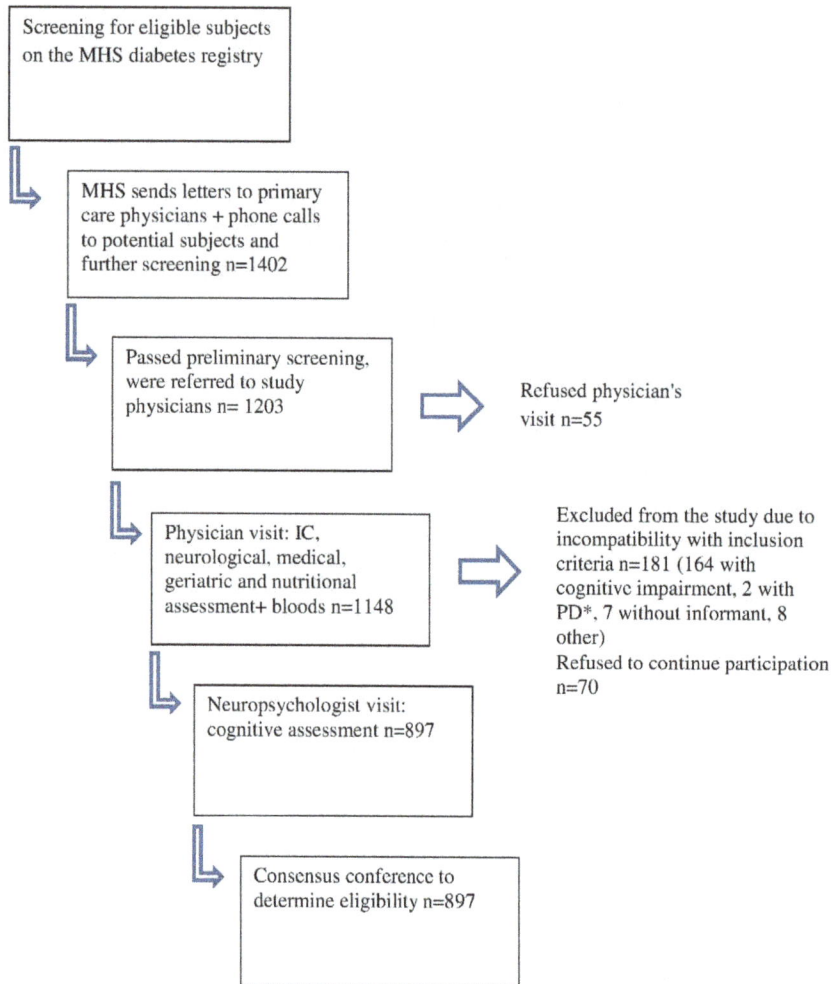

Figure 1. Trajectories in HbA1c levels. Groups: 1=lower Stable, 2=Higher Stable, 3=Lower Increasing, 4=Higher Increasing, 5=Lower Decreasing, 6=Higher Decreasing.

Subjects with a trajectory of decreasing HbA1c levels over the years, were characterized by very high (mean = 10.73%) or high (mean 9.19%) HbA1c levels at entry into the DR, and high, though decreasing, HbA1c levels over their T2D course. These subjects had the poorest cognitive performance. Their performance was followed by that of subjects whose HbA1c at entry into the DR was relatively high (mean = 7.76) and increased over time. Subjects with stable HbA1c throughout the years, had the lowest HbA1c levels at all times and performed best in cognitive tests. These analyses were adjusted for sociodemographic, cardiovascular, and T2D-related variables. Trajectories in HbA1c over time were not associated with episodic memory or attention/working memory. Importantly, the trajectories were not defined a-priori and were not based on clinical cutoffs but were rather empirical. Following correction of the analysis for multiple comparisons, the comparison between the most extreme trajectories remained significant in overall cognition, semantic categorization and executive functions. Examining trajectories in HbA1c as predictors of T2D outcomes is advantageous since they describe better the natural history of T2D, with varying degrees of glycemic control over time [23]. In contrast to variability around the mean, the trajectories capture the true course of T2D through a combination of its inherent components (baseline HbA1c, overall slope of the trajectory, the mean, the end levels etc), rather than each component separately, thus allowing detection of subgroups of change in HbA1c that follow a distinct course.

To the best of our knowledge, this is the first study to investigate the association of trajectories in glycemic control over time with cognitive functioning. Most studies reporting on the association of T2D and glycemic control with cognitive outcomes (or cognitive related outcomes such as brain volume), used diagnosis of T2D or degree of glycemic control at entry as predictors, as opposed to glycemic control over time.

The decrease in HbA1c levels over time in subjects with very high HbA1c at baseline, suggests that these subjects were treated with anti-diabetes medications as clinically warranted. Indeed, they had the highest percentage of use of both hypoglycemic medications and insulin. Nevertheless, these subjects failed to reach the clinically acceptable goals of HbA1c despite treatment, and were thus at higher risk for the detrimental effects of chronic hyperglycemia on cognition [24]. The trajectories observed suggest that these subjects suffer from a more "aggressive" course of T2D, possibly underlying the poorer cognitive functioning in this group. Alternatively, the anti-diabetic treatments may have exposed these subjects to an increased risk for hypoglycemic episodes [25] and to the implications of the latter on cognition

Table 2. Cognitive scores (Z scores) in groups of subjects defined by HbA1c at entry into the Diabetes Registry and trend over time in the registry*.

Group	Z score overall cognitive function	Standard Error	Pr>|t|	Overall P-value
Overall cognitive score				
Lower Stable (n = 232)	1.39	0.79	0.0789	
Higher Stable (n = 371)	1.13	0.76	0.1366	
Lower Increasing (n = 124)	0.72	0.88	0.4142	
Higher Increasing (n = 47)	−0.76	1.20	0.5273	0.0479
Lower Decreasing (n = 61)	−0.03	1.11	0.9765	
Higher Decreasing (n = 15)	−4.93	2.00	0.0140	
Episodic memory				
Lower Stable (n = 232)	0.16	0.24	0.4943	
Higher Stable (n = 371)	0.25	0.23	0.2674	
Lower Increasing (n = 124)	0.16	0.26	0.5511	
Higher Increasing (n = 47)	−0.59	0.36	0.1032	0.3275
Lower Decreasing (n = 61)	0.25	0.33	0.4422	
Higher Decreasing (n = 15)	−0.13	0.60	0.8304	
Semantic categorization				
Lower Stable (n = 232)	0.16	0.24	0.4875	
Higher Stable (n = 371)	0.10	0.23	0.6547	
Lower Increasing (n = 124)	0.19	0.27	0.4803	
Higher Increasing (n = 47)	−0.02	0.36	0.9535	0.0252
Lower Decreasing (n = 61)	−0.52	0.33	0.1152	
Higher Decreasing (n = 15)	−1.63	0.60	0.0066	
Attention/working memory				
Lower Stable (n = 232)	0.04	0.23	0.8551	
Higher Stable (n = 371)	−0.18	0.22	0.3948	
Lower Increasing (n = 124)	0.05	0.25	0.8573	
Higher Increasing (n = 47)	0.09	0.34	0.8004	0.2848
Lower Decreasing (n = 61)	−0.09	0.32	0.7766	
Higher Decreasing (n = 15)	−1.10	0.57	0.0568	
Executive function				
Lower Stable (n = 232)	0.88	0.29	0.0021	0.0069
Higher Stable (n = 371)	0.62	0.27	0.0241	
Lower Increasing (n = 124)	0.12	0.32	0.7137	
Higher Increasing (n = 47)	−0.26	0.44	0.5498	
Lower Decreasing (n = 61)	0.33	0.40	0.4130	
Higher Decreasing (n = 15)	−1.48	0.73	0.0418	

*Analysis of covariance to estimate and compare mean z-scores in the different cognitive domains among the trajectory groups, adjusting for sociodemographic, cardiovascular, diabetes-related covariates (years in the DR and anti-diabetic medications), and GDS score.

[26]. The analysis was adjusted for sociodemographic (age, sex, and years of education), cardiovascular (glomerular filtration rate calculated by the MDRD formula, total cholesterol, HDL, LDL, diastolic and systolic blood pressure), T2D related factors (estimated duration of T2D and diabetes medications) and depression (based on GDS score). Nevertheless, we cannot rule out the possibility that an overall higher severity of T2D in the two groups with decreasing HbA1c over time, contributed to their poorer cognitive function.

It is important to note the differences between the two groups with a trajectory of decrease in HbA1c over time; both had high HbA1c levels throughout their follow up in the DR, however, the group with the lower levels (Lower Decreasing) performed better in overall cognition and executive function than the group with the highest levels (Higher Decreasing). These differences suggest that cognitive function in T2D may be better preserved when aiming towards lower HbA1c levels, even without achieving optimal glycemic control. Trajectories in HbA1c levels over time were associated with cognitive decline even in non-diabetic, non-demented elderly subjects [16] suggesting that long-term peripheral glucose levels per se, not only in the context of T2D, may be associated with biological mechanisms for neuronal dysfunction/neurodegeneration and subsequent cognitive compromise. This hypothesis is further supported by studies showing a negative

Table 3. Comparisons between cognitive scores in groups of subjects defined by HbA1c at entry into the Diabetes Registry and trend over time in the registry.

Overall cognitive score

	Lower Stable	Higher Stable	Lower Increasing	Higher Increasing	Lower Decreasing	Higher Decreasing
Lower Stable		0.6680	0.4191	0.0852	0.1845	**0.0021**
Higher Stable			0.5890	0.1143	0.2543	**0.0029**
Lower Increasing				0.2374	0.4977	**0.0059**
Higher Increasing					0.6075	0.0508
Lower Decreasing						**0.0213**

Episodic memory

	Lower Stable	Higher Stable	Lower Increasing	Higher Increasing	Lower Decreasing	Higher Decreasing
Lower Stable		0.6207	0.9893	0.0451	0.7692	0.6373
Higher Stable			0.6768	0.0192	0.9895	0.5327
Lower Increasing				0.0476	0.7708	0.6405
Higher Increasing					0.0473	0.4729
Lower Decreasing						0.5465

Semantic categorization

	Lower Stable	Higher Stable	Lower Increasing	Higher Increasing	Lower Decreasing	Higher Decreasing
Lower Stable		0.7303	0.9248	0.6202	**0.0320**	**0.0036**
Higher Stable			0.7011	0.7324	**0.0403**	**0.0045**
Lower Increasing				0.5798	**0.0334**	**0.0031**
Higher Increasing					0.2363	**0.0118**
Lower Decreasing						0.0817

Attention/working memory

	Lower Stable	Higher Stable	Lower Increasing	Higher Increasing	Lower Decreasing	Higher Decreasing
Lower Stable		0.1944	0.9853	0.8978	0.6678	0.0538
Higher Stable			0.2826	0.4274	0.7462	0.1184
Lower Increasing				0.9080	0.6707	0.0524
Higher Increasing					0.6622	0.0536
Lower Decreasing						0.0994

Executive function

	Lower Stable	Higher Stable	Lower Increasing	Higher Increasing	Lower Decreasing	Higher Decreasing
Lower Stable		0.2306	**0.0103**	**0.0115**	0.1526	**0.0015**
Higher Stable			0.0642	**0.0422**	0.4305	**0.0045**
Lower Increasing				0.4054	0.6008	**0.0317**
Higher Increasing					0.2508	0.1153
Lower Decreasing						**0.0190**

association between HbA1c levels (within the normal range in non-demented non-diabetic individuals) and brain volume at 6 years follow up [10].

A trajectory of increasing HbA1c levels over time has previously been demonstrated to be associated with increased mortality in a dose-response manner in a cohort of 8,812 T2D subjects, with a mean follow up duration of 4.5 years [21]. Consistent with that, the present results show that the groups with increasing HbA1c over time had poorer cognitive performance compared to subjects with stable HbA1c levels over time.

The groups that performed best on cognition were those with stable and relatively low HbA1c levels over the course of the disease. Findings regarding the role of glycemic control in prevention of other T2D complications are heterogeneous, with results varying by study population, outcome and type of intervention [27]. In the ACCORD study, higher levels of HbA1c at entry were associated with lower cognitive performance (based on the Digit Symbol Substitution Test-DSST) at <45 days afterwards [8]. Interestingly, in the 40-months follow up phase of the ACCORD study, the intensive treatment arm (aiming for HbA1c less than 6.0%) was associated with greater total brain volume but not with DSST score, compared to standard treatment (aiming for HbA1c between 7% and 7.9%) [11]. The authors concluded that such results, combined with the increased mortality in the intensive care group and the non-significant effects on other ACCORD outcomes, do not support the use of intensive therapy to reduce the adverse effects of T2D on the brain. A departure from some disease-state homeostasis by enforcing too strict glycemic control was hypothesized to render some subjects to hypoglycemic episodes or other conditions with negative consequences on cognition. The present results suggest that stabilization of glycemic control over many years may be advantageous.

Despite lower cognitive function in some domains, the subjects participating in the IDCD were all broadly within cognitive normal limits. Previous studies have demonstrated that people with normal, albeit lower range of cognitive function, are at higher risk of developing cognitive decline and dementia [28]. The numerous HbA1c assessments available for the IDCD cohort, enabled detection of trajectories in glycemic control that are particularly deleterious, suggesting target T2D subjects who are at higher risk for lower cognitive function and for future incident dementia and thus candidates for evolving therapies to maintain or slow cognitive decline.

The HbA1c trends were measured from several years before the cognitive assessment, and the cognitive outcomes were all within the normal range, suggesting that glycemic control affects cognition rather than an incipient dementing process affecting glycemic control. However, this study is observational and at this point only cross-sectional cognitive data is available. Thus causality should not be inferred; we cannot rule out the possibility that poor, albeit normal, cognitive performance is associated with poor self-care, leading to high HbA1c levels. When longitudinal cognitive follow-ups become available, evaluations of the relationships of patterns of glycemic control with cognitive decline, and incident MCI and dementia will elucidate the direction of the relationship between glycemic control and cognition. Examination of the association, within each trajectory group, of each trajectory component (the mean HbA1c, standard deviation in HbA1c and change in HbA1c), to assess their unique contribution to cognition was not possible. Such an examination would require at least three different slopes (trend patterns) at each different baseline HbA1c, along with at least 2 different standard deviations (e.g. lower and higher) around each of the slopes at each baseline HbA1c. This would permit a variety of scenarios such as high baseline HbA1c, negative slope, low standard deviation, etc. However, the trajectories that we found are empirical, reflecting the true reality of our sample, and converged to 6 trajectories, which do not cover all the spectrum of trajectories to, theoretically, enable such an examination. This is a limitation of an observational study, but, a randomized trial where patients with high initial HbA1c levels were treated/not treated to decrease it, would be unethical. We nevertheless, performed, on the full sample, secondary analyses examining the relationships of mean and standard deviation of HbA1c with the cognitive outcomes and found that higher mean and standard deviation in HbA1c measurements over time were associated with lower scores in overall cognitive score and in executive functions, consistent with the trajectories results. Brain imaging was not performed in this study, thus limiting our ability to evaluate the contribution of cerebrovascular abnormalities to the association of trends in glycemic control with cognition. This is

particularly relevant both because T2D is a vascular disease, but also because trajectories of HbA1c were not associated with episodic memory, suggesting non AD-related mechanisms. Entry into the DR, rather than time of T2D diagnosis, which was not available to us, is referred to as "baseline". Although women are slightly under-represented in the study, sex was one of the covariates in the comparison of groups. Israel has a strong family oriented culture, so a major role in grand- parenting was the primary reason of refusal by women to participate in the study.

Additional strengths of this study include the large sample, validated T2D diagnosis for each subject, an average of 18 HbA1c measurements permitting investigation of trajectories of HbA1c over time, strong validity for risk factor levels and medical diagnosis, and a thorough cognitive evaluation.

Methods

Ethics Statement

The study was approved by the IRB committees of the Sheba Medical Center, Israel, the Maccabi Health Services (MHS), Israel and the Icahn School of Medicine at Mount Sinai, NY. Informed consent was signed by all study participants.

Population

This study consisted of elderly (≥65 years old) T2D subjects in the IDCD, a collaboration between the Icahn School of Medicine at Mount Sinai, NY, the Sheba Medical Center, Israel, and the Maccabi Health Services (MHS), Israel. Detailed methods have been presented [29]. IDCD subjects were randomly selected from the approximately 11,000 T2D individuals aged ≥65 years that are in the Diabetes Registry (DR) of the MHS, the second largest HMO in Israel. The MHS DR is an integral part of the MHS Electronic Patient Record system, which was established in 1998 to facilitate disease management and to improve treatment. The DR has collected detailed laboratory, medication, and diagnoses information since 1998 [30]. The present analysis assesses the relationship of long term trajectories in HbA1c, since the subject's entry into the MHS DR diabetes registry (the earliest time was 1998, when the diabetes registry was established) until the IDCD baseline cognitive evaluation (2010–2011).

Any of the following criteria should be met in order to be included in the MHS DR: 1) HbA1c >7.25%, 2) Glucose > 200 mg/dl on two exams more than three months apart, 3) purchase of anti-diabetic medication twice within three months supported by a HbA1c >6.5% or Glucose >125 mg/dl within half a year, 4) diagnosis of T2D (ICD9 code) by a general practitioner, internist, endocrinologist, ophthalmologist, or T2D advisor, supported by a HbA1c >6.5% or Glucose >125 mg/dl within half a year. These criteria have been validated by twenty physicians in MHS against their own practice records [30]. Additionally, age specific prevalence rates were similar to those of a DR of another large HMO in Israel[28].

Eligibility Criteria for the IDCD

(1) In the MHS DR, i.e. diagnosed with T2D (2) lives in the central area of Israel (near Tel Aviv), (3) 65 years of age or above, (4) cognitively normal (not suffering from dementia or MCI) at entry into the IDCD (based on a multidisciplinary consensus conference), (5) two or more HbA1c measurements in the DR, (6) has an informant, and (7) speaks Hebrew fluently. Potential subjects were excluded if they had an ICD code for dementia or its subtypes, treatment with prescribed cholinesterase inhibitors, or had a major psychiatric or neurological condition (such as

schizophrenia, stroke or Parkinson's disease) that could affect cognitive performance.

IDCD Subjects' Recruitment Process (Figure 2)

An algorithm including the eligibility criteria that were available in the MHS Electronic Patient Record was used to randomly select the subjects. After random selection of subjects, letters were sent by MHS to the primary care physicians, asking for permission to contact each patient regarding the study. If the doctor agreed, a letter was sent to the patient briefly describing the study and saying he or she would be contacted by phone in the following two weeks. The study coordinator then called the patient and invited participation in the study, after determining fluency in Hebrew and that there was an informant willing to provide information about the subject's health. The social structure of Israel is such that most elderly individuals live with or near their extended family, so few are excluded for this reason. A second informant was sought to be a replacement if necessary. Subjects were assessed in two phases, typically at their residence, or at the Sheba Medical Center memory clinic, according to their preference. In the first meeting, a study physician obtained signed informed consent; performed medical, neurological, geriatric and nutritional (Food Frequency Questionnaire- FFQ) assessments; and drew blood for inflammatory markers (Il-6, CRP), and haptoglobin and ApoE genotypes. The second meeting, conducted within two weeks after the physician's assessment, involved a neuropsychologist administering to the subject a cognitive battery, and both to the subject and an informant questionnaires for cognitive and functional impairment, and for depression and behavioral disturbances characteristic of dementia.

Cognitive Assessment

The present analysis examined the association between long term trends in glycemic control (using all HbA1c measurements present in the subjects' DR from their entry into the registry until IDCD initiation) with cognitive outcomes based on cognitive assessment that was performed at entry into the IDCD (baseline cognitive assessment). The cognitive assessment includes the scales and neuropsychological tests described below and takes approximately 2 hours to be administered. The study is ongoing and follow-up cognitive assessments have recently begun and do not enable, at this phase, report of the association of trajectories of glycemic control and changes in cognition over time.

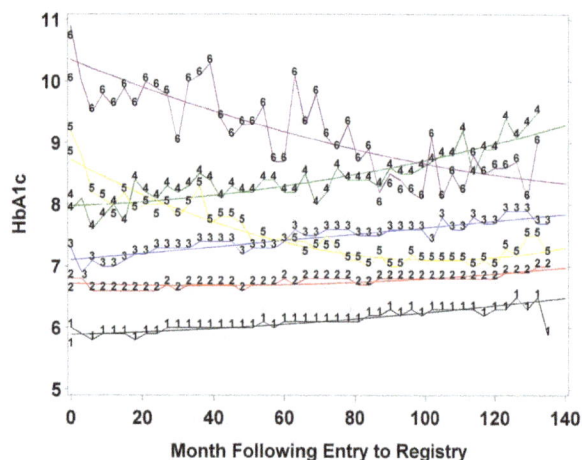

Figure 2. Study flow chart.

Clinical Dementia Rating (CDR) scale. This scale assesses, through an interview with the subject and an informant, the severity of cognitive and functional impairment in 6 domains: memory, orientation, judgment and problem solving, community affairs, home and hobbies and personal care. A score of 0 represents normal cognition (an inclusion criteria for the IDCD study), 0.5 represents questionable dementia, and scores of 1 through 3 reflect increasing severity of dementia [31,32].

Mini Mental State Exam (MMSE). This questionnaire assesses orientation, concentration, memory, praxis and language [33]. Maximal score is 30.

Geriatric Depression Scale (GDS). This is a self-report scale designed to be simple to administer and not to require the skills of a trained interviewer. The original instrument is a 30-item questionnaire developed for the assessment of depressive symptoms in older people [34]. The answers have a yes/no format. In the present study, the short version of the scale (composed of 15 items), was administered [35].

Neuropsychological battery. A thorough neuropsychological battery that characterizes the breadth of cognitive functions is administered. The battery is administered by experienced and certified interviewers which are blind to the diabetes related data. The neuropsychological evaluation is the basis for the outcome measures described below and includes the following tests:

(1) Word List Memory [36]- This is a free recall memory test that assesses learning ability for new verbal information.

(2) Similarities. This is a subtest from the Wechsler Adult Intelligence Scale-Revised. The test measures abstract thinking by asking the subject to state how pairs of words (e.g., egg/seed) are alike [37].

(3) Letter fluency [38]: In three one-minute trials, this test of phonemic fluency assesses the ability to name as many words as possible beginning with three Hebrew letters-beit, gimel, shin [39].

(4) Digit Span [40]: This is a subtest of the WAIS-III. The Digit Forward section assesses attention by reading sequences of digits to the subject for immediate verbatim repetition. Then the Digit Backwards section consists of sequences to be repeated in reverse order.

(5) Diamond Cancellation Test: This test is used to assess vigilance and speeded attention. It requires subjects to identify target stimuli (diamonds) randomly interspersed among distractor stimuli on a sheet of 8.5-by-11 paper.

(6) Trail Making Test [41]: The Trails tests measure timed attention, mental flexibility and sequencing. Part A entails connecting randomly ordered numbers by drawing a line in sequence. Part B entails connecting numbers and letters in alternating order (i.e. 1, A, 2, B, etc.).

(7) Digit-symbol substitution test (DSST) [37]: this test consists of nine digit-symbol pairs followed by a list of digits. Under each digit the subject should write down the corresponding symbol as fast as possible. The number of correct symbols within 90 is measured.

Multidisciplinary consensus conference: All the information obtained from the scales and the neuropsychological battery was discussed by a multidisciplinary consensus conference (in which a neuropsychologist and a physician expert in diagnosis of dementia-psychiatrist, neurologist or geriatrician, were mandatory participants) in order to ensure normal cognition, which is an inclusion criterion for the study. Normal cognition was defined as a clinical dementia rating scale (CDR) score = 0 (no dementia) and the score of the MMSE test (based on norms for age and education) corroborated by the multidisciplinary consensus conference. There were a handful of cases with gaps between the CDR and the MMSE scores. In such cases we based our decision on the CDR score which more closely reflects the effect of cognitive decline on everyday functional abilities, a decline which is required for the formal diagnosis of dementia.

Outcome Measures

A factor analysis with varimax rotation of the comprehensive neuropsychological battery of the IDCD subjects was used to identify cognitive domains in this study. Four domains were identified. For each domain, a summary was calculated as the sum of z-scores (test scores transformed to mean zero and standard deviation one, reversed if necessary for positive values to indicate good cognition) of tests with high loadings: episodic memory (immediate and delayed recall, and recognition word list), semantic categorization [39] (letter and category fluency, and similarities), attention/working memory (diamond cancellation test, digit span forward and backward), and executive functions (Trails making A and B and the DSST). Finally, an overall cognition measure was calculated by summing the four domain summaries.

Confounding Variables

Sociodemographic factors (age, sex, and years of education) were collected at entry into the IDCD. Cardiovascular covariates (glomerular filtration rate calculated by the MDRD formula, total cholesterol, HDL, LDL, diastolic and systolic blood pressure) were defined as means of all measurements available in the DR. Diabetes-related covariates were the estimated duration of T2D (based on time in the DR) and diabetes medications (which was categorized as oral anti-diabetic medications only, insulin only, combination of oral anti-diabetic and insulin and no medication). Since depression has been associated both with T2D [42], degree of glycemic control [43], risk for T2D- related complications [44] and with dementia [45], we also included the geriatric depression scale (GDS) score as a potential confounder. HbA1c levels at entry

into the DR were defined as the third HbA1c recorded in the registry after excluding the first two HbA1c measurements, since these might reflect instability of glycemic control prior to diagnosis of T2D and treatment initiation.

Statistical Analyses [46]

We identified distinctive trajectory groups of HbA1c using a SAS macro named PROC TRAJ [46]. This approach applies a multinomial modeling strategy to identify relatively homogenous clusters of developmental trajectories within a sample population, that is, the modeling strategy allows for the emergence of more than two trajectories. Trajectory parameters are derived by latent class analysis using maximum likelihood estimation. In particular, the distinctive trajectories of HbA1c were derived by modeling HbA1c as a function of the number of years in the DR. Quadratic curves were used to model the trends over time. The number of trajectories was determined using the guidelines suggested by Jones et al [46]. The output of PROC TRAJ includes the equations for the different trajectories along with the assignment of each patient to one of the trajectory groups. This group assignment was then used in an analysis of covariance to estimate and compare mean cognitive domain z-scores among the trajectory groups while adjusting for sociodemographic, cardiovascular, diabetes-related covariates (years in the DR and anti-diabetic medications), and GDS score.

In order to provide analyses that are comparable with those of other studies [47], we assessed the relationships of mean and standard deviations of HbA1c with cognitive function in secondary analyses, using the GLM procedure.

Author Contributions

Conceived and designed the experiments: RMS AH DL MSB. Performed the experiments: RMS AH MSB. Analyzed the data: RMS MSB. Wrote the paper: RMS. Contributed to the discussion: AH MS DL SJ JMS. Performed statistical analysis: JS EM JG. Reviewed the manuscript: JS EM MS DL SJ JMS JG. Searched the Data: RP KK HH. Supervised the manuscript write up: MSB.

References

1. Ahtiluoto S, Polvikoski T, Peltonen M, Solomon A, Tuomilehto J, et al. (2010) Diabetes, Alzheimer disease, and vascular dementia: a population-based neuropathologic study. Neurology 75: 1195–1202.
2. Schnaider Beeri M, Goldbourt U, Silverman JM, Noy S, Schmeidler J, et al. (2004) Diabetes mellitus in midlife and the risk of dementia three decades later. Neurology 63: 1902–1907.
3. Mokini Z, Chiarelli F (2006) The molecular basis of diabetic microangiopathy. Pediatr Endocrinol Rev 4: 138–152.
4. Milicevic Z, Raz I, Beattie SD, Campaigne BN, Sarwat S, et al. (2008) Natural history of cardiovascular disease in patients with diabetes: role of hyperglycemia. Diabetes Care 31 Suppl 2: S155–160.
5. Nathan DM, Cleary PA, Backlund JY, Genuth SM, Lachin JM, et al. (2005) Intensive diabetes treatment and cardiovascular disease in patients with type 1 diabetes. N Engl J Med 353: 2643–2653.
6. Stratton IM, Adler AI, Neil HA, Matthews DR, Manley SE, et al. (2000) Association of glycaemia with macrovascular and microvascular complications of type 2 diabetes (UKPDS 35): prospective observational study. BMJ 321: 405–412.
7. Crane PK, Walker R, Larson EB (2013) Glucose levels and risk of dementia. N Engl J Med 369: 1863–1864.
8. Cukierman-Yaffe T, Gerstein HC, Williamson JD, Lazar RM, Lovato L, et al. (2009) Relationship between baseline glycemic control and cognitive function in individuals with type 2 diabetes and other cardiovascular risk factors: the action to control cardiovascular risk in diabetes-memory in diabetes (ACCORD-MIND) trial. Diabetes Care 32: 221–226.
9. Christman AL, Matsushita K, Gottesman RF, Mosley T, Alonso A, et al. (2011) Glycated haemoglobin and cognitive decline: the Atherosclerosis Risk in Communities (ARIC) study. Diabetologia 54: 1645–1652.
10. Enzinger C, Fazekas F, Matthews PM, Ropele S, Schmidt H, et al. (2005) Risk factors for progression of brain atrophy in aging: six-year follow-up of normal subjects. Neurology 64: 1704–1711.
11. Launer LJ, Miller ME, Williamson JD, Lazar RM, Gerstein HC, et al. (2011) Effects of intensive glucose lowering on brain structure and function in people with type 2 diabetes (ACCORD MIND): a randomised open-label substudy. Lancet Neurol 10: 969–977.
12. American Diabetes A (2010) Diagnosis and classification of diabetes mellitus. Diabetes Care 33 Suppl 1: S62–S69.
13. Gerstein HC, Miller ME, Byington RP, Goff DC, Jr., Bigger JT, et al. (2008) Effects of intensive glucose lowering in type 2 diabetes. N Engl J Med 358: 2545–2559.
14. Zhong Y, Zhang XY, Miao Y, Zhu JH, Yan H, et al. (2012) The relationship between glucose excursion and cognitive function in aged type 2 diabetes patients. Biomed Environ Sci 25: 1–7.
15. Cooray G, Nilsson E, Wahlin A, Laukka EJ, Brismar K, et al. (2011) Effects of intensified metabolic control on CNS function in type 2 diabetes. Psychoneuroendocrinology 36: 77–86.
16. Ravona-Springer R, Moshier E, Schmeidler J, Godbold J, Akrivos J, et al. (2012) Changes in glycemic control are associated with changes in cognition in non-diabetic elderly. J Alzheimers Dis 30: 299–309.
17. Kishore P, Kim SH, Crandall JP (2012) Glycemic control and cardiovascular disease: what's a doctor to do? Curr Diab Rep 12: 255–264.
18. Bellelli G, Pezzini A, Bianchetti A, Trabucchi M (2002) Increased blood pressure variability may be associated with cognitive decline in hypertensive elderly subjects with no dementia. Arch Intern Med 162: 483–484.
19. Chen YC, Chen TF, Yip PK, Hu CY, Chu YM, et al. (2010) Body mass index (BMI) at an early age and the risk of dementia. Arch Gerontol Geriatr 50 Suppl 1: S48–52.

20. Stewart R, Masaki K, Xue QL, Peila R, Petrovitch H, et al. (2005) A 32-year prospective study of change in body weight and incident dementia: the Honolulu-Asia Aging Study. Arch Neurol 62: 55–60.

21. Gebregziabher M, Egede LE, Lynch CP, Echols C, Zhao Y (2010) Effect of trajectories of glycemic control on mortality in type 2 diabetes: a semiparametric joint modeling approach. Am J Epidemiol 171: 1090–1098.

22. Rajala U, Laakso M, Paivansalo M, Suramo I, Keinanen-Kiukaanniemi S (2005) Blood pressure and atherosclerotic plaques in carotid, aortic and femoral arteries in elderly Finns with diabetes mellitus or impaired glucose tolerance. J Hum Hypertens 19: 85–91.

23. (1995) U.K. prospective diabetes study 16. Overview of 6 years' therapy of type II diabetes: a progressive disease. U.K. Prospective Diabetes Study Group. Diabetes 44: 1249–1258.

24. Manschot SM, Biessels GJ, de Valk H, Algra A, Rutten GE, et al. (2007) Metabolic and vascular determinants of impaired cognitive performance and abnormalities on brain magnetic resonance imaging in patients with type 2 diabetes. Diabetologia 50: 2388–2397.

25. Ahren B (2013) Avoiding hypoglycemia: a key to success for glucose-lowering therapy in type 2 diabetes. Vasc Health Risk Manag 9: 155–163.

26. Yaffe K, Falvey CM, Hamilton N, Harris TB, Simonsick EM, et al. (2013) Association between hypoglycemia and dementia in a biracial cohort of older adults with diabetes mellitus. JAMA Intern Med 173: 1300–1306.

27. Andersson C, van Gaal L, Caterson ID, Weeke P, James WP, et al. (2012) Relationship between HbA1c levels and risk of cardiovascular adverse outcomes and all-cause mortality in overweight and obese cardiovascular high-risk women and men with type 2 diabetes. Diabetologia 55: 2348–2355.

28. Blacker D, Lee H, Muzikansky A, Martin EC, Tanzi R, et al. (2007) Neuropsychological measures in normal individuals that predict subsequent cognitive decline. Arch Neurol 64: 862–871.

29. Ravona-Springer R, Heymann A, Schmeidler J, Guerrero-Berroa E, Sano M, et al. (2013) Haptoglobin 1-1 genotype is associated with poorer cognitive functioning in the elderly with type 2 diabetes. Diabetes Care 36: 3139–3145.

30. Heymann AD, Chodick G, Halkin H, Karasik A, Shalev V, et al. (2006) The implementation of managed care for diabetes using medical informatics in a large Preferred Provider Organization. Diabetes Res Clin Pract 71: 290–298.

31. Fillenbaum GG, Peterson B, Morris JC (1996) Estimating the validity of the clinical Dementia Rating Scale: the CERAD experience. Consortium to Establish a Registry for Alzheimer's Disease. Aging (Milano) 8: 379–385.

32. Hughes CP, Berg L, Danziger WL, Coben LA, Martin RL (1982) A new clinical scale for the staging of dementia. Br J Psychiatry 140: 566–572.

33. Folstein MF, Folstein SE, McHugh PR (1975) "Mini-mental state". A practical method for grading the cognitive state of patients for the clinician. JPsychiatrRes 12: 189–198.

34. Yesavage JA, Brink TL, Rose TL, Lum O, Huang V, et al. (1982) Development and validation of a geriatric depression screening scale: a preliminary report. J Psychiatr Res 17: 37–49.

35. Conradsson M, Rosendahl E, Littbrand H, Gustafson Y, Olofsson B, et al. (2013) Usefulness of the Geriatric Depression Scale 15-item version among very old people with and without cognitive impairment. Aging Ment Health 17: 638–645.

36. Welsh KA, Butters N, Mohs RC, Beekly D, Edland S, et al. (1994) The Consortium to Establish a Registry for Alzheimer's Disease (CERAD). Part V. A normative study of the neuropsychological battery. Neurology 44: 609–614.

37. Wechsler D (1981) Wechsler Adult Intelligence Scale-Revised Manual. San Antonio: The Psychological Corporation.

38. Spreen O, Benton AL (1977) Neurosensory Center Comprehensive Examination for Aphasia: Manual of instructions (NCCEA) (rev. ed.). Victoria, BC: University of Victoria.

39. Fernaeus SE, Almkvist O (1998) Word production: dissociation of two retrieval modes of semantic memory across time. J Clin Exp Neuropsychol 20: 137–143.

40. Wechsler D (1987) Wechsler Memory Scale-Revised Manual. San Antonio: The Psychological Corporation.

41. Reitan RM (1955) The relation of the trail making test to organic brain damage. J Consult Psychol 19: 393–394.

42. Ali S, Stone MA, Peters JL, Davies MJ, Khunti K (2006) The prevalence of co-morbid depression in adults with Type 2 diabetes: a systematic review and meta-analysis. Diabet Med 23: 1165–1173.

43. Lustman PJ, Anderson RJ, Freedland KE, de Groot M, Carney RM, et al. (2000) Depression and poor glycemic control: a meta-analytic review of the literature. Diabetes Care 23: 934–942.

44. Lin EH, Rutter CM, Katon W, Heckbert SR, Ciechanowski P, et al. (2010) Depression and advanced complications of diabetes: a prospective cohort study. Diabetes Care 33: 264–269.

45. Ownby RL, Crocco E, Acevedo A, John V, Loewenstein D (2006) Depression and risk for Alzheimer disease: systematic review, meta-analysis, and metaregression analysis. ArchGenPsychiatry 63: 530–538.

46. Jones B, Nagin D, K R (2001) A SAS procedure based on mixture models for estimating developmental trajectories.. Social Methods Res 29.

47. Yaffe K, Falvey C, Hamilton N, Schwartz AV, Simonsick EM, et al. (2012) Diabetes, glucose control, and 9-year cognitive decline among older adults without dementia. Arch Neurol 69: 1170–1175.

## 2

Shear Modulus Estimation on *Vastus Intermedius* of Elderly and Young Females over the Entire Range of Isometric Contraction

Cong-Zhi Wang[1,2,3]*, **Tian-Jie Li**[2], **Yong-Ping Zheng**[2]*

1 Paul C. Lauterbur Research Center for Biomedical Imaging, Institute of Biomedical and Health Engineering, Shenzhen Institutes of Advanced Technology, Chinese Academy of Sciences, Shenzhen, China, **2** Interdisciplinary Division of Biomedical Engineering, the Hong Kong Polytechnic University, Hong Kong, China, **3** Beijing Center for Mathematics and Information Interdisciplinary Sciences, Beijing, China

Abstract

Elderly people often suffer from sarcopenia in their lower extremities, which gives rise to the increased susceptibility of fall. Comparing the mechanical properties of the knee extensor/flexors on elderly and young subjects is helpful in understanding the underlying mechanisms of the muscle aging process. However, although the stiffness of skeletal muscle has been proved to be positively correlated to its non-fatiguing contraction intensity by some existing methods, this conclusion has not been verified above 50% maximum voluntary contraction (MVC) due to the limitation of their measurement range. In this study, a vibro-ultrasound system was set up to achieve a considerably larger measurement range on muscle stiffness estimation. Its feasibility was verified on self-made silicone phantoms by comparing with the mechanical indentation method. The system was then used to assess the stiffness of *vastus intermedius* (VI), one of the knee extensors, on 10 healthy elderly female subjects (56.7±4.9 yr) and 10 healthy young female subjects (27.6±5.0 yr). The VI stiffness in its action direction was confirmed to be positively correlated to the % MVC level ($R^2 = 0.999$) over the entire range of isometric contraction, i.e. from 0% MVC (relaxed state) to 100% MVC. Furthermore, it was shown that there was no significant difference between the mean VI shear modulus of the elderly and young subjects in a relaxed state ($p > 0.1$). However, when performing step isometric contraction, the VI stiffness of young female subjects was found to be larger than that of elderly participants ($p < 0.001$), especially at the relatively higher contraction levels. The results expanded our knowledge on the mechanical property of the elderly's skeletal muscle and its relationship with intensity of active contraction. Furthermore, the vibro-ultrasound system has a potential to become a powerful tool for investigating the elderly's muscle diseases.

Editor: Miklos S. Kellermayer, Semmelweis University, Hungary

Funding: This study was supported by the Research Grant Council of Hong Kong (PolyU 5331/06E), Hong Kong Innovation and Technology Fund (UI213), and the National Natural Science Found of China (11228411). The funders had no role in study design, data collection and analysis, decision to publish, or preparation of the manuscript.

Competing Interests: The authors have declared that no competing interests exist.

* Email: cz.wang@siat.ac.cn (CZW); ypzheng@ieee.org (YPZ)

Introduction

Sarcopenia refers to the degenerative decline of muscle strength in the elderly [1]. It will significantly increase their risk of sudden falls and dramatically impact on their quality of life [2,3]. As the population of elderly people continues to escalate, sarcopenia carries more burdens of public health care and social services. To reveal the process and mechanism of this disease, some studies have focused on the morphological change of skeletal muscle caused by age. Muscle features including size, fascicle length and pennation angle have been extensively investigated [4–7]. Moreover, some other studies applied biomedicine methods on elderly patients to investigate the fiber atrophy on different fiber types [8,9] and the phenomenon of "metabolic dysregulation", such as impaired oxidative defense and decreased mitochondrial function [10,11].

Besides these studies, mechanical properties, especially the stiffness of skeletal muscle, have also attracted broad research interest. Skeletal muscle stiffness has been verified to contribute significantly to action efficiency [12,13], hence its quantification measurement in vivo can help to improve the understanding of functional changes in muscle. Several experimental techniques including "quick release" and "sinusoidal perturbations" were developed to study the global mechanical properties of musculo-tendinous and musculoarticular complexes, but the various components of these complexes cannot be differentiated [14,15]. Furthermore, indentation devices, such as myotonometer [16,17] and Tissue Ultrasound Palpation System (TUPS) [18,19] have been developed to assess the muscle stiffness locally. Although these devices have acceptable reliability, muscle stiffness at different depths cannot be fully distinguished and the stiffness in muscle action direction cannot be obtained.

In the last two decades, elastography, the technology for noninvasively measuring or imaging the mechanical characteristics of soft tissue, has been rapidly evolving and applied in many clinical areas, such as the diagnosis of liver fibrosis and breast cancer [20]. Several quantitative elastography methods based on shear wave velocity estimation have also been proposed to quantify the elastic modulus of a single muscle. In a simple model of pure elastic, locally homogeneous and isotropic material, its shear modulus μ is related to the shear wave velocity c_s propagating in it via the following equation:

$$\mu = \rho c_s^2 \qquad (1)$$

where ρ is the mass density of the material. Although the assumptions of this model are not fully satisfied for skeletal muscle, they are generally assumed to yield an acceptable estimation of muscle stiffness and widely used by many methods [21–25].

In sonoelastography, tissues were stimulated with a low-frequency (10 to 1000 Hz) mechanical vibration. The induced tissue movement was measured by a Doppler instrument for obtaining the shear wave velocity [26,27]. Using this technique, Levinson et al. reported that the shear modulus of quadriceps femoris was positively correlated to the increasing load imposed on it [28]. However, the method requires a long acquisition time. When it is used on a muscle during high intensity contraction, the muscle will soon fatigue and the results will be different from those under normal condition. In transient elastography method, an ultrasound transducer was used as a piston-like vibrator to apply a pulsed excitation on the muscle, so the shear wave propagating perpendicularly to the muscle action direction could be studied [23]. This method has been used to assess the shear modulus of biceps brachii and gastrocnemius medius in the transverse direction [29,30]. However, since skeletal muscle is anisotropic, shear modulus in the muscle action direction is more important for muscle functional assessment. It has been reported that the shear modulus of biceps brachii in the muscle action direction was approximately 4 times larger than that in the perpendicular direction in a relaxed state and about 9 times larger during a low intensity isometric contraction [31]. Shear wave dispersion ultrasound vibrometry (SDUV) method can measure the muscle stiffness in its action direction [24]. It has been evaluated on animal muscles [32], but not on human muscle in vivo, since the results were not fully satisfactory. Acoustic radiation force induced by a focused ultrasound beam was used to generate a vibration source in the muscle and the propagation of shear wave was monitored by the detection beam. Shear wave velocity was then calculated from the time delay and distance between the two beams. This method has difficulty in generating decent waves in a deep muscle [33]. Another method named as supersonic shear imaging (SSI) has been reported to study the shear wave propagation in 2D plane [34]. After generating the shear wave within a tissue by acoustic radiation force, its propagation was monitored by a series of B-mode images at an ultra-high frame rate. SSI has been applied to study the stiffness of biceps brachii [35], lower leg muscles [36] and finger muscles [37]. However, the applied depth of SSI was also limited by the intensity of acoustic radiation force for safety consideration. In addition, it was reported that the measurement of SSI system would saturate at a shear modulus value of 266 kPa [37]. Therefore, the highest muscle contraction level in their study was only approximate 50% of maximum voluntary contraction (MVC) torque ("%MVC" is a generally used indicator for representing relative contraction intensity of muscle). Magnetic resonance elastography (MRE) is another technique which can visualize the propagation of shear wave excited by an external vibrator [25]. The wavelength can be measured from MRE images and then used to calculate shear wave velocity. In contrast to ultrasound, MRE has no limitation in penetration depth and can simultaneously provide images with high resolution. Many studies have been reported to assess muscle stiffness using MRE [38–41]. However, it requires very long

acquisition time (about 1–3 minutes for each measurement) which greatly limits its application on skeletal muscle, particularly during a high intensity contraction. The signal-to-noise ratio (SNR) of MRE images was reported to be significantly reduced when a high intensity muscle contraction was performed [42].

Based on these methods, many previous studies have reported the positive correlation between the muscle stiffness and the non-fatiguing muscle contraction intensity. However, rare studies have been performed to quantitatively assess the muscle stiffness of the elderly in relaxed and isometric contraction conditions. Domire et al. measured the stiffness of tibialis anterior muscle on 16 elderly females (mean age: 60 ± 7.2 yr) at a relaxed condition using MRE [43], and reported that the mean shear modulus was 10.0 ± 2.9 kPa and there was no significant relationship between age and the relaxed muscle stiffness. To our knowledge, all the methods mentioned above cannot cover the entire range of muscle contraction, i.e. from 0% to 100% MVC, due to the limitation of their measurement range. For example, it was reported that the satisfactory quantitative results could be only achieved under 20% MVC torque level using MRE [42], while the muscle stiffness was only assessed during a contraction equal to about 50% MVC level using SSI [37].

To fix this gap, a vibro-ultrasound system was developed in our study. It aims to characterize the skeletal muscle stiffness in the muscle action direction over the entire range of step isometric contraction. This method was then applied on the *vastus intermedius* (VI) to determine the relationship between the VI stiffness and the relative step isometric contraction level of knee extensors, and to evaluate the muscle stiffness difference between the elderly and young female subjects. The VI is one component of the quadriceps femoris muscle group which is shown in Fig. 1. It is crucial to the dynamic stability control for the elderly [2,3,44]. It is expected that this novel system can provide us a tool for muscle stiffness measurement under high intensity contraction. The results can help us to better understand the mechanism of sarcopenia, monitor its process on elderly sufferers, and provide useful information during their rehabilitation.

Materials and Methods

Ethics Statement

In this study, human subject ethical approval was sought from the Human Ethics Committee of the Hong Kong Polytechnic University, and all the subjects were explained with the experimental protocol and asked to sign on the informed consent form prior to the experiment.

Vibro-ultrasound System for Muscle Stiffness Measurement

The vibro-ultrasound system consisted of a mechanical vibrator, a programmable ultrasound scanner and a custom-made program for radio-frequency data acquisition. An electromagnetic vibrator (minishaker type 4810, Brüel & Kjær, Nærum, Denmark) which was driven by a power amplifier and controlled by a function generator was used to induce shear waves in the muscle. The vibrator impacted the muscle with a monochromatic low-frequency sinusoidal pulse. In general, the vibration frequency typically adopted in previous studies ranged from 90 to 150 Hz for skeletal muscle stiffness assessment [42,43]. In this study, 100 Hz frequency was selected to ensure a more reasonable comparison with those studies.

As demonstrated in Fig. 2 (left), shear waves with 10 cycles generated by the external vibrator propagated in the muscle action direction. An ultrasound linear array probe was placed along this

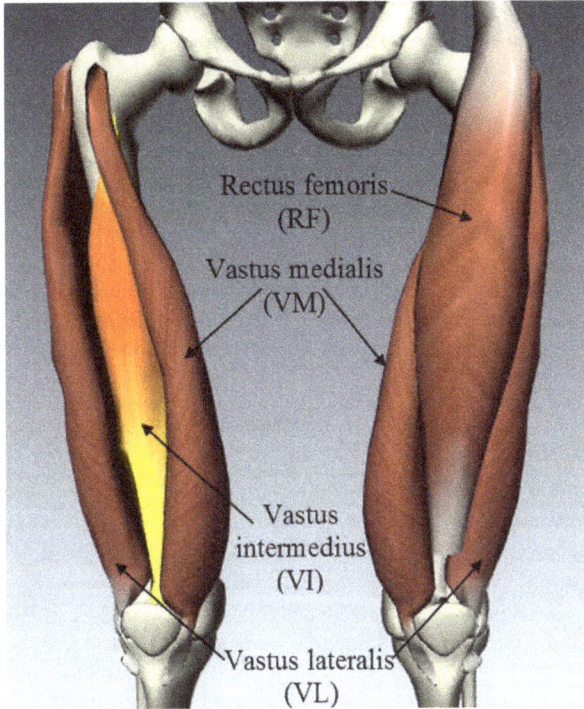

Figure 1. Anatomy of quadriceps femoris muscle group, which includes rectus femoris, vastus lateralis, vastus medialis and vastus intermedius. (Generated using the BioDigital Human Platform, BioDigital Systems, New York City, USA).

The ultrasound data acquisition system was developed based on a commercial ultrasound scanner SonixRP (Ultrasonix Medical Corp. Vancouver, Canada) with a 5–14 MHz linear array probe (driven by the central frequency 9.5 MHz), and its software developing kits applicable to Visual C++ (Microsoft Corporation, USA). A custom-designed ultrasound transmission and reception sequence was implemented. B-mode images were first acquired (with 256 scan lines corresponding to a 38 mm width) using a predefined penetration depth of 65 mm for helping position the probe at the expected place with a right orientation. For minimizing the anisotropic effects of wave propagation, a straight short push-bar was mounted on the piston of the vibrator and its position was carefully adjusted to guarantee the shear wave would propagate in the muscle action direction [29,45]. The repetition frequency of the two scan lines for monitoring was finally achieved as 4.6 kHz with the 65 mm penetration depth. Thus the upper limit of shear wave velocity measurement was theoretically 69 m/s, if assuming that the minimal detectable time delay corresponded to 1 frame interval. This value corresponded to a shear modulus of more than 4000 kPa. In addition, the vibrator and the scanner were synchronized by the external trigger. The sampling frequency of the radio-frequency signal was 40 MHz. For each measurement, the subject only needed to maintain the contraction for less than 4 seconds, then 10,000 frames of data were collected and transferred to a computer for further analysis.

The whole experimental setup also included a dynamometer. Isometric torque generated by the knee extensors was assessed using a HUMAC NORM rehabilitation system (Computer Sports Medicine, Inc., Stoughton, MA, USA), which included a specifically designed chair and a fixed dynamometer. The machine was set to the knee joint isolated movement pattern and isometric resistance mode. The knee joint angle can be set and fixed under this mode.

direction. At the proximal and distal positions, the tissue movements were monitored by two separated ultrasound scan lines. The distance between the two scan lines was Δr (in this study, 15 mm was used) and the time delay between the two detected waveforms was Δt. Then the wave velocity c_s could be calculated by:

Data Processing

All radio-frequency signals were processed off-line using a custom-developed program of Matlab (Version R2008, Math-Works, Inc., MA, USA). The main processing steps can be summarized as followings: 1) To arrange the ultrasound signals obtained at the proximal and distal locations into segments; 2) To obtain the transient time shifts of each segment between two consecutive frames; 3) To calculate the displacement waveforms

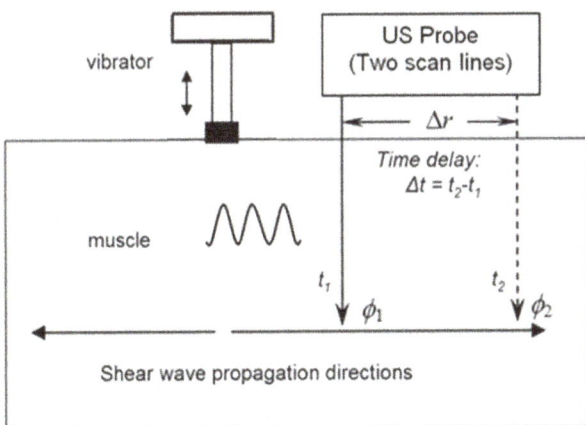

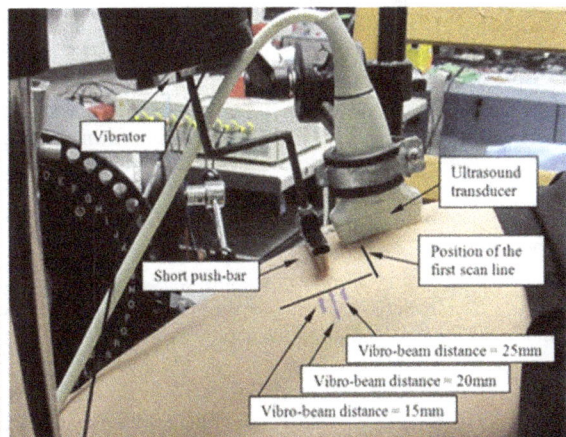

$$c_s = \Delta r / \Delta t \qquad (2)$$

Figure 2. Diagram of the vibro-ultrasound system for shear wave velocity measurement using two ultrasound scan lines (left) and the position of the ultrasound probe and the vibrator during the experiment on one human subject (right). The three positions of the vibrator used for the different vibro-beam distance test were also indicated.

using the transient time shifts and the speed of ultrasound in soft tissue; 4) To detect the peaks of the sinusoidal displacement waveforms; 5) To detect the time delay between each pair of the peaks obtained at the same depth; 6) To calculate the overall time delay between the two waveforms by averaging all the time delay values; 7) To calculate the shear wave velocity using its propagation time and distance.

The tissue displacement waveforms were determined by the normalized cross-correlation algorithm, which is also called the echo-tracking method and widely used in tissue displacement estimation [46,47]. The method was based on time shift estimation between two congruent segments in pairs of consecutive frames of radio-frequency signals. The time shift was caused by the tissue displacement along the axial direction of ultrasound beam and subsequently the change of travelling distance of the reflected echoes. A segment of reference signal from the initial frame was first defined, and then the most similar segment to this reference one in the subsequent frames was searched using the cross-correlation calculation. The temporal locations of the maximum value of the normalized cross-correlation function marked the time shift between the two segments. Then the tissue displacement was estimated by multiplying the time shift with the velocity of ultrasound. When the time shifts were tracked continuously, a displacement waveform could be correspondingly obtained.

The first frame signal was divided into segments each with 1 mm in depth and with 50% overlap. Each segment was treated as a reference segment and its movement was tracked frame by frame automatically using the cross-correlation method described above. Then the tissue displacement waveforms at certain depths were plotted with time for the distal and proximal locations, as shown in Fig. 3. Fig. 3(a) represents the tissue displacement waveform obtained at 0% MVC level (at rest), Fig. 3(b) at 50% MVC level, and Fig. 3(c) at 100% MVC level (corresponding to shear moduli of 9 kPa, 213 kPa, and 547 kPa). It can be observed that the time delay between the two waveforms became smaller when the contraction level increased, indicating that the shear wave moved faster. To measure this time delay, the peaks of the two displacement waveforms were detected using the zero-crossing points of their first-order derivatives, which were from greater-than-zero values to less-than-zero values. Then the positions of these peaks were plotted and used to determine the time delay values between the two waveforms. Shear wave consists of oscillations occurring perpendicular to the direction along its propagation. Since the shear wave fronts within the ROI were observed as straight lines perpendicular to the time axis, the shear wave propagation direction in VI muscle was confirmed to be perpendicular to the two ultrasound scan lines. That is why the shear wave velocity could be estimated by Δr and Δt using Eq. 2. Subsequently, Eq. 1 was used to calculate the shear modulus, with the generally used skeletal muscle density of 1000 kg/m^3 [29].

Feasibility Tests on Silicone Phantoms

To evaluate the feasibility of the vibro-ultrasound system, shear moduli of several custom-made silicone phantoms with different stiffness were assessed. Their stiffness was compared between the proposed method and the conventional indentation method.

Tissue-mimicking phantoms with a size of 100 mm×80 mm×20 mm were prepared for the experiment. The phantoms were made of addition-curing silicone rubbers RTV-2 (M4600 A/B, Wacker Chemicals Hong Kong Ltd., Hong Kong, China) and their stiffness was varied by adding silicone oil AK-35 (Wacker Chemicals Hong Kong Ltd., Hong Kong, China). The weight ratio between M4600A and AK-35 was selected as 1:0, 1:0.25, 1:0.5, 1:0.75 and 1:1, with a decreasing stiffness of

corresponding phantoms. The mixtures were then de-aerated in a vacuum cabinet until no more air bubbles were formed due to reduced air pressure. At last, the phantoms were heated at 60°C for several hours to increase the speed of curing. A total of ten phantoms were made (two for each concentration level).

The shear moduli of these phantoms were first assessed using indentation method with a material testing machine (Instron ASTM Method Set, Braintree, MA, USA). The diameter of the indenter a is 10 mm. The phantoms were compressed for 2 mm deformation with a rate of 0.5 mm/sec and then relaxed at the same deformation rate. During three cycles of compression-relaxation, the compression load P (N) and the deformation W (mm) values were collected. Then the Young's modulus E was calculated using the Eq. 3, which is based on the Hayes model for the elastic indentation problem of a thin elastic layer bonded to a rigid half-space with a rigid, frictionless cylindrical plane-ended indenter [48].

$$E = \frac{(1-\nu^2)}{2a\kappa(\nu,a/h)} \frac{P}{W} \tag{3}$$

where h is the tissue thickness, and κ is a scaling factor, which provides a theoretical correction for the finite thickness of the measured phantom and it depends on both the ratio a/h and the Poisson's ratio ν. The Poisson's ratio ν was defined as 0.5 in this study since the silicone phantom is nearly an incompressible material. Then the shear modulus μ of the phantoms could be calculated by the following equation:

$$\mu = \frac{E}{2(1+\nu)} = \frac{1}{3}E \tag{4}$$

The indentation tests were performed for 3 times on each of the phantoms. Then the stiffness of each phantom was assessed using the vibro-ultrasound system, also for 3 times. To reduce the influence from upper and lower boundaries, the phantom to be measured was placed between two blocks of elastic silicone layers with thickness of approximately 35 mm and shear modulus of approximately 100 kPa. The ROI was 10 mm thick and located in the middle portion of the phantom. All the measurements were performed at room temperature (25±1°C).

The shear moduli were averaged from the 3 measurements and the correlation between the results obtained by two methods were studied statistically. All the data were analyzed using SPSS Statistics (SPSS Inc. Chicago, IL, USA). Statistical significance was set at the 5% probability level.

Shear Wave Propagation Direction Validation Tests on Young Subjects

It should be confirmed that the shear wave propagates perpendicular to the ultrasound scan lines for the vibro-ultrasound system, so that its velocity can be estimated by a "time-to-flight" method. We assumed that the external disturbance can vibrate VI muscle fibers at different depths simultaneously and the induced shear wave propagates mainly in the muscle action direction. Otherwise, if the shear wave propagates as a spherical wave starting from the vibration source, it would reach the scan line with different propagation time at different depths. Thus when the distance between the two scan lines were fixed, different distance between the vibrator and the first scan line (in short "vibrator-beam distance") will lead to the different value of the measured shear wave velocity. Accordingly, the experiment was designed to verify whether the vibrator-beam distance would affect the measured shear wave velocity on human subjects.

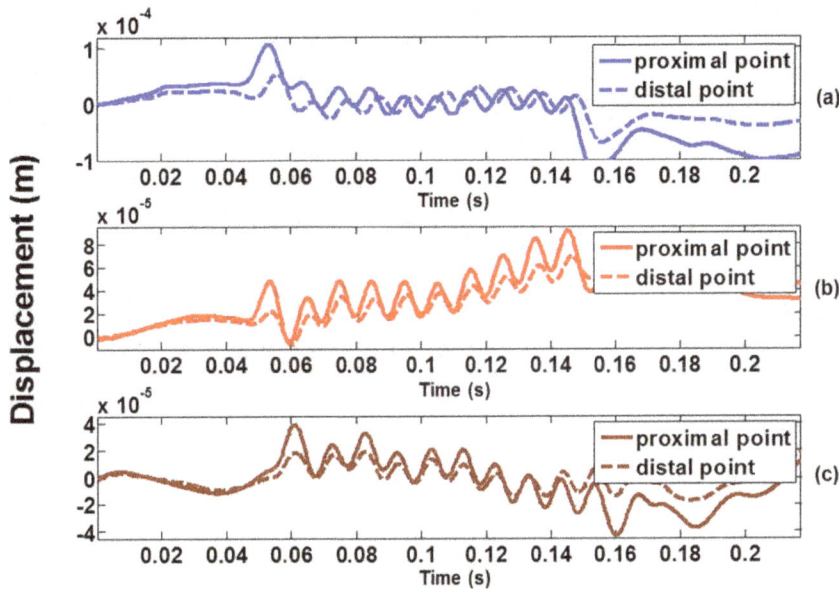

Figure 3. Typical tracking results of tissue displacement waveform of an elderly female human subject. (a) obtained under 0% MVC level (at rest), (b) 50% MVC level, and (c) 100% MVC level. The corresponding shear moduli for (a) to (c) were 9 kPa, 213 kPa, and 574 kPa. The solid line represents the tissue displacement waveforms detected at the proximal location, and the dashed line at the distal location, with reference to the vibration source.

Since this experiment was just to verify the feasibility of our approach, elderly subjects were not recruited this time. Ten healthy young subjects (8 males and 2 females, age: 30.7 ± 4.1 yr, height: 170.2 ± 10.7 cm, weight: 68.0 ± 14.4 kg) were included in this experiment. The subject was asked to sit on the chair with several straps restraining his/her waist and shoulders. A cuff was fastened around the right lower leg and fixed to the lever of the dynamometer. The axis of the lever was aligned with the supposed rotation axis of the right knee joint. With the guidance of B-mode images, the vibrator and the ultrasound probe were hung right above the middle part of the RF muscle belly with a predefined distance (if this distance was 10 mm, the vibrator-beam distance was approximately 20 mm), as shown in Fig. 2 (right). Ultrasound gel was applied between the ultrasound probe and the skin. The ultrasound probe was first adjusted to be aligned in the direction along the muscle fibers under the guidance of B-mode images (The muscle fibers could be seen as parallel straight lines in the images. If the ultrasound plane was at an angle to the fibers, the fibers would not be shown as clear lines). Then the straight short push-bar was adjusted to be perpendicular to the probe and muscle fibers also under the guidance of ultrasound images. Both the push-bar and the probe were then rigidly fixed. With the help of this push-bar, planar pattern shear wave would be generated at the expected depth and propagate in the direction of muscle action [40].

The experiment was performed at a 90° knee joint angle. First, the MVC torque was assessed as the highest torque value produced from three successive isometric contractions which were maintained for 5 seconds with about 30 seconds interval for rest. Next, the muscle stiffness was assessed at relaxed condition and at 20% MVC level, with three different vibrator-beam distances, i.e. 15 mm, 20 mm and 25 mm. For each measurement, the subject was asked to maintain the isometric contraction for approximately 4 seconds, and three repeated measurements were made under the same condition with 1 minute interval for rest.

The shear modulus was represented by the mean value of the three repeated measurements. The shear moduli of 10 subjects measured at different vibrator-beam distances were plotted using a linear correlation model, and then were analyzed using two-way repeated measure analyses of variance (ANOVA) to evaluate their differences. The normalized root mean squared deviation (NRMSD) among the results measured at different vibrator-beam distances was also calculated. The definition of NRMSD is as follows:

$$NRMSD(x_1, x_2) = \frac{\sqrt{\frac{\sum_{i=1}^{n}(x_{1,i} - x_{2,i})^2}{n}}}{x_{max} - x_{min}} \qquad (5)$$

$$x_1 = \{x_{1,1}, x_{1,2}, \cdots x_{1,n}\}; x_2 = \{x_{2,1}, x_{2,2}, \cdots x_{2,n}\}$$

where x_{max} and x_{min} are the maximal and minimal values among the observed results. NRMSD value is often expressed as a percentage, where lower values indicate less residual variance.

Muscle Stiffness Measurements on Elderly and Young Female Subjects

Ten healthy elderly female subjects (age: 56.7 ± 4.9 yr, height: 156.9 ± 5.6 cm, weight: 58.9 ± 8.4 kg) and ten healthy young female subjects (age: 27.6 ± 5.0 yr, height: 164.3 ± 4.4 cm, weight: 55.3 ± 4.0 kg) volunteered to participate in this part of the study. The experimental setup was almost the same as described in the above section, and all the recruited subjects were also explained with the experimental protocol and asked to sign on the informed consent form prior to the experiment. However, to make the elderly subjects more comfortable, the experiment was performed at a 60° knee joint angle, but not 90°. The distance between the vibrator and the probe was set to be approximately 10 mm. The MVC torque value was also assessed first. Next, the muscle stiffness was measured for three times at relaxed condition. Then the subject was asked to maintain isometric contraction at different MVC levels, from 10% to 100%, with an increase of 10% for each step. At each MVC level, three assessments were performed with about 1 minute interval for rest. The shear modulus of each individual subject was represented by the mean value obtained from the three repeated measurements. Therefore, a total of 660 (20 [subjects] ×11 [contraction levels: 0%–100% MVC] ×3 [three times]) measurements of VI shear modulus were performed by the same investigator. The intra-class correlation coefficient (ICC) was used to evaluate the intra-observer repeatability. The shear moduli measured at the same contraction level across the ten elderly subjects and ten young subjects were then averaged and used to investigate the relationship between muscle stiffness and relative isometric contraction levels (% MVC). To determine the pattern of this relationship, polynomial regression analyses by linear, quadratic and cubic models were performed for each individual, and the coefficients of determination (R^2) values of these models were compared using paired samples T-test. Since we found that the quadratic regression model had the best performance, the mean shear moduli across the ten subjects were then fitted with the relative isometric contraction levels (% MVC) using a quadratic regression model. To study the difference of the VI stiffness between elderly and young female subjects in a relaxed state and at different isometric contraction levels, two-way repeated measure analyses of variance (ANOVA) (Age [young and elder] × % MVC [0%–100%, 11 levels]) were used to analyze the measured shear modulus. Specially, the comparison of the VI shear modulus measured in a relaxed state (0% MVC) was first performed separately using one-way ANOVA method.

Results

Feasibility Tests on Silicone Phantoms

A good linear correlation was found between the results obtained by the indentation method and those measured using vibro-ultrasound system for the 10 silicone phantoms, with a regression of $y = 1.07x - 8.70$ and R^2 value of 0.989, as shown in Fig. 4. This demonstrated that the vibro-ultrasound system was feasible for measuring the stiffness of tissue-mimicking phantoms and could be used for monitoring the change of muscle stiffness in a large measurement range.

Shear Wave Propagation Direction Validation Tests on Young Subjects

Fig. 5 shows the comparison of the shear moduli of VI measured at different vibrator-beam distances. The R^2 value was 0.978 and 0.955 for the correlations between the results measured at 15 mm and 20 mm vibrator-beam distances and between those at 25 mm and 20 mm, respectively. There was no significant individual effect of vibrator-beam distance (p = 0.818). On the other hand, the individual effect of isometric contraction levels was significant (p<0.001). The NRMSD values were 5.6% and 6.5%, respectively. The results demonstrated that the measured muscle shear modulus would not be significantly influenced by the small variation of vibrator-beam distance. It also provided another evidence to support the assumption that in this study the pattern of shear wave was quite close to planar when it propagated in the muscle action direction of VI.

Muscle Stiffness Measurements on Elderly and Young Female Subjects

The overall ICC for the measured shear moduli on all female subjects was 0.994, suggesting a high degree of reproducibility of the measurements. The mean R^2 values of the polynomial

regression analyses by linear, quadratic and cubic models on the relationship of shear modulus vs. % MVC level were 0.932 ± 0.034, 0.995 ± 0.004 and 0.997 ± 0.003, respectively. The results of paired samples T-test indicated that there was no significant difference between the R^2 values of quadratic model and cubic model (p = 0.153). However, significant differences were found between the R^2 values of linear model and the other two models (both p<0.001). Thus the quadratic regression model was selected to correlate the mean shear moduli with the relative isometric contraction levels, as shown in Fig. 6. The result indicated that the VI stiffness of both elderly and young female subjects in the muscle action direction was positively correlated to the relative muscle activity intensity (% MVC) of the knee extensors over the entire range of step isometric contraction. The mean VI shear modulus of elderly and young female subjects in a relaxed state (0% MVC) was 12.8 ± 5.4 kPa and 9.5 ± 3.3 kPa, respectively. And results of the one-way ANOVA showed that for "Age" factor there was no significant effect on VI shear modulus (p = 0.106) in a relaxed state. For VI shear modulus measured under different step isometric contraction levels, results of the two-way ANOVA showed that the main effects for "Age" and "% MVC" factors on VI shear modulus were both significant. The estimated marginal mean value of VI shear modulus of the young female subjects was larger than that of the elderly participants (p< 0.001). Furthermore, the two-way interactions of the two factors were also significant (p = 0.01). With the increasing of "% MVC", differences between the VI shear modulus of young female subjects and that of elderly subjects also increased, which was also directly indicated in Fig. 6.

Discussion

Vibro-ultrasound Muscle Stiffness Measurement System

In this study, a vibro-ultrasound system was developed and applied for muscle stiffness assessment on the VI muscle of elderly female subjects. The good agreement between the results obtained on silicone phantoms by both our system and the conventional indentation method suggested that the system was feasible for tissue stiffness assessment in a large measurement range. Moreover, the high ICC value (0.994) of the measured shear moduli of VI muscle indicated that the measurement was highly repeatable.

The shear wave velocity was determined by the distance and the propagation time between the two ultrasound scan lines in our system. The relatively larger distance (15 mm) and higher frame rate (4600 frames/second) help to achieve a better measurement range of shear modulus comparing to the existing methods. In addition, since a mechanical vibrator was used, the amplitude of shear wave generated by our system (50–80 μm at the proximal scan line, and 20–50 μm at the distal scan line) was much larger than the method based on acoustic radiation force (generally less than 10 μm) [24]. Therefore, the effect of jitters on the displacement waveforms of our system would be much smaller in comparison with the acoustic radiation force based methods, and this would also help to improve the precision of our measurements.

However, there is still some uncertainty on the accuracy of the presented measurement results. On self-made phantoms, we only confirmed the accuracy of this system with the shear modulus up to about 350 kPa (for the hardest one, the measured shear modulus was 347.2 ± 22.3 kPa with our system and 327.5 ± 6.4 kPa with indentation method). To our knowledge, this value is 30% larger than the maximal measurement upper limit of the existing methods, i.e. 266 kPa for SSI system [37], but is still smaller compared to the reported results measured on the elderly and

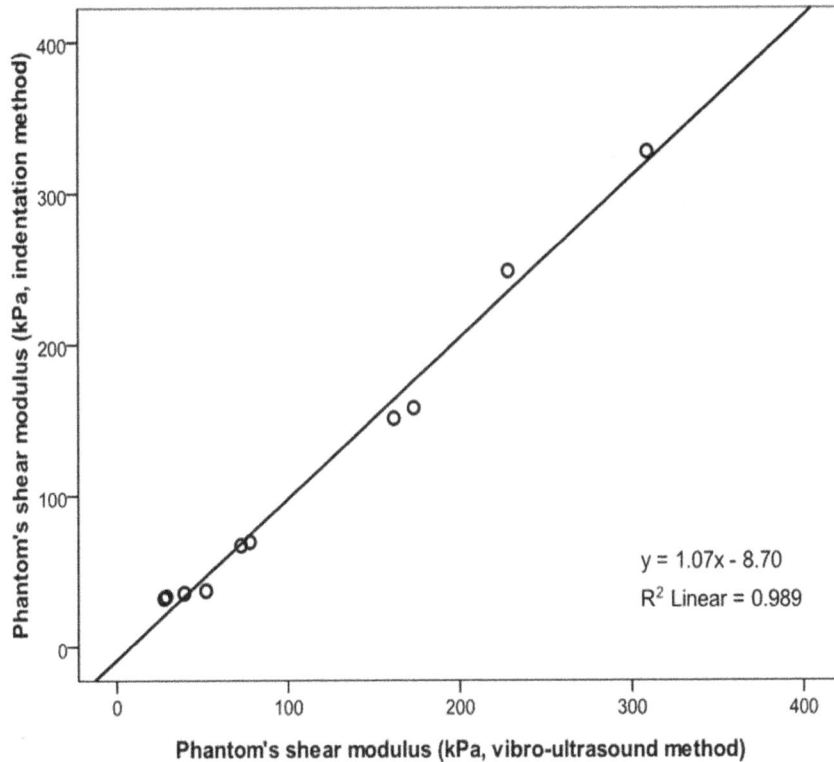

Figure 4. Correlation between the shear modulus values assessed by indentation method and the corresponding values measured by the vibro-ultrasound method.

young female subjects in this study (under 100% MVC level, the mean shear modulus of VI among ten elderly female subjects was 482.5 ± 189.6 kPa, the minimal and maximal values of individual were 148.1 ± 27.6 kPa and 1114.5 ± 151.4 kPa, respectively; and the mean shear modulus of VI among ten young female subjects was 877.5 ± 566.7 kPa, the minimal and maximal values of individual were 525.7 ± 56.9 kPa and 2454.9 ± 260.6 kPa, respectively). Although these results are theoretically credible, it is still uncertain whether they are equally accurate, since they are beyond the confirmed measurement range and the stiffness of silicone phantom can be hardly increased (for the hardest phantom, we did not add any silicone oil to soften it). Future studies should confirm this by finding other materials which can be used to make the phantom with higher stiffness.

In current method, a simple biomechanical model (Eq. 1) was adopted to calculate the shear modulus of tissue, assuming the tissue was pure elastic. While in some studies using SDUV and SSI, a more complicated model, Voigt model, has been used to estimate the shear modulus and shear viscosity simultaneously, based on the frequency-velocity dispersion curve. Some previous studies by Gennisson et al. and Deffieux et al. have reported that the shear wave velocity remained almost constant in the muscle action direction when the exciting frequency changed under both relax and isometric contraction conditions of *in vivo* muscle [31,49]. On the contrary, Chen et al. and Urban et al. found the velocity was frequency dependent [24,32]. The difference may be caused by their experimental designs. From another aspect, Gennisson and Deffieux conducted the measurement on human muscles *in vivo*, while Chen and Urban tested bovine and porcine muscles *in vitro*. In Chen's study, the bovine muscle was punched with a through hole at its center and a glass rod was glued in the hole throughout the thickness of the sample. Thus the structure of

muscle fibers was destructed and its mechanical properties should be different with that *in vivo*. In addition, it was shown in Urban's study that the shear modulus measured across muscle fibers (in transverse direction) was dependent on shear wave frequency, but that measured along muscle fibers (in the muscle action direction) was almost constant with the frequency increasing. This finding was consistent with those reported by Gennisson and Deffieux. Accordingly, the viscous effect can be neglected when a skeletal muscle is tested *in vivo* for its elasticity in the muscle action direction using shear wave propagation methods. Such a conclusion needs further verifying for different muscle groups under different physiological and pathological conditions.

The wave propagation pattern in skeletal muscle is another important factor which would affect the results and should be carefully studied and controlled. In our system, shear wave velocity was estimated by dividing the distance between the two scan lines with the corresponding wave propagating time. This required the wave front to be parallel to the two scan lines. If the wave front has a spherical or oblique plane surface, the distance used for calculation would theoretically be longer than the real length of the wave travelling path, resulting in overestimated shear modulus. To verify this issue, Sack et al. reconstructed the shear wave pattern under different conditions using *in vivo* MRE data collected on biceps brachii muscle [40]. In their results, planar wave pattern was observed when the external excitation was applied on muscle belly using a short push-bar, of which the orientation was kept to be vertical to the muscle fibers to minimize the anisotropic effects. In our study, the similar setup was used to facilitate the wave pattern be close to planar. Furthermore, the measured muscle shear modulus has been proved to be not significantly influenced by the small variation of vibrator-beam distance, which provided

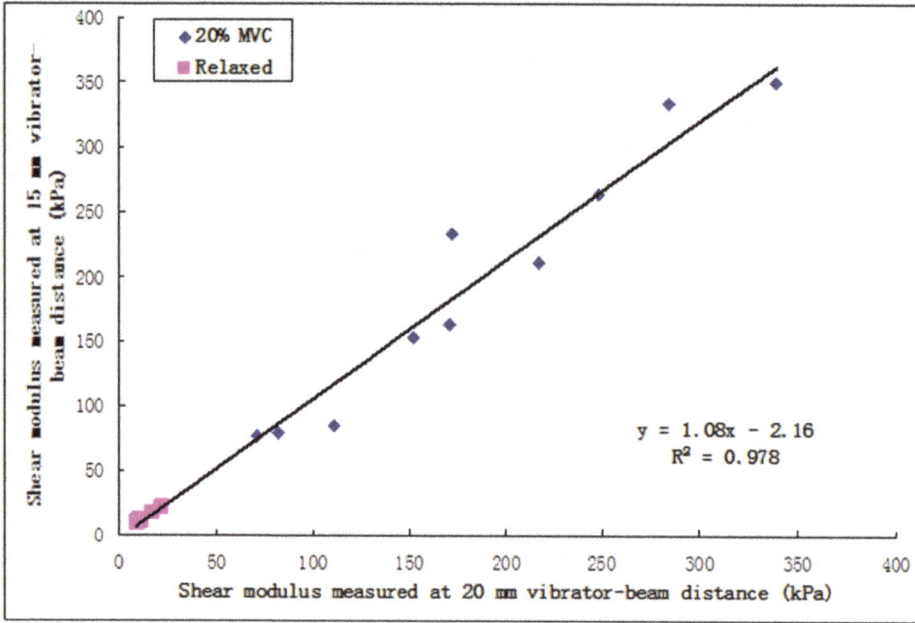

(a)

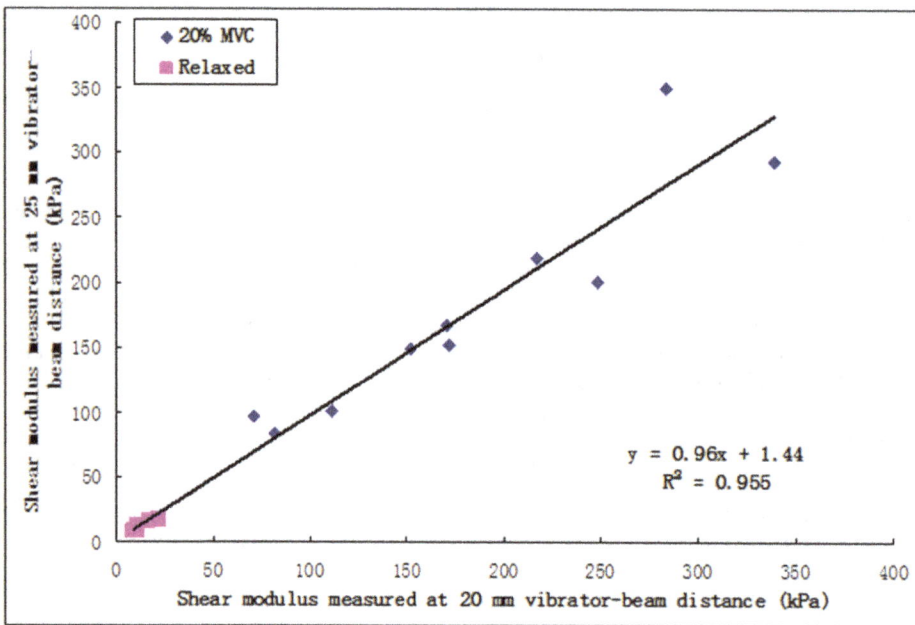

(b)

Figure 5. Comparison of the shear moduli between (a) 15 mm and 20 mm; and (b) 25 mm and 20 mm, revealed that the vibrator-beam distance appeared to affect very little on the measurement result of shear modulus.

another evidence to support the assumption of planar wave that propagating in the muscle action direction.

In this study, a mechanical vibrator was applied to generate shear waves in a deep muscle, VI, with enough amplitude and hence increase the SNR of the detected tissue displacements. Mechanical vibrator was generally considered to cause more wave reflection at the interface of different tissue layers, especially when there is complex bone-muscle geometry [50]. However, the VI has a large size, so plane shape and its muscle fibers are almost aligned along the same axis of muscle action direction (the pennation angle

is less than 10°) [51], the reflection phenomenon in wave propagation direction would be very small and not affect the results. In our pilot study, it was observed that the skin surface stress imposed by either the mechanical vibrator or ultrasound transducer would also influence the wave pattern by damping the vibration of underlying tissue. As a deep muscle like VI, such effect could be mostly avoided by fixing the vibrator and transducer rigidly to restrict the relative motion to the muscle.

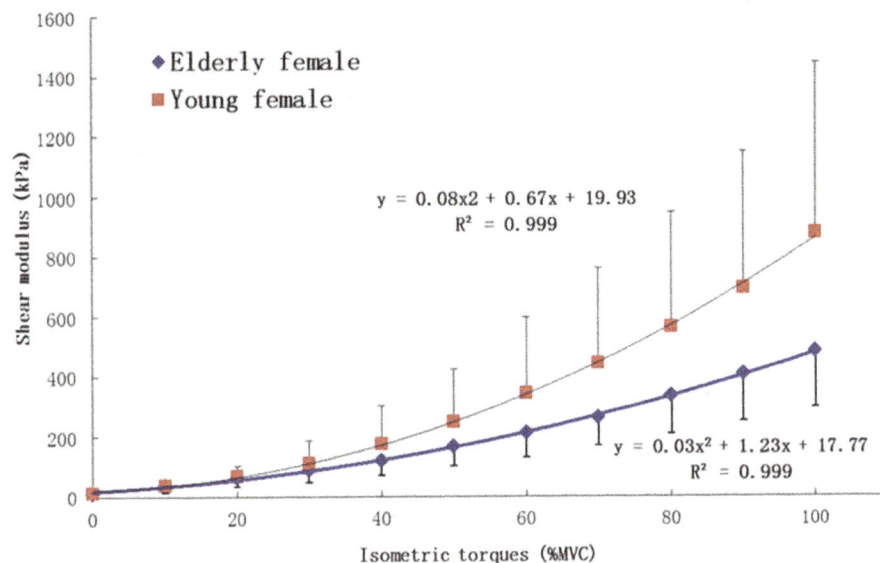

Figure 6. The averaged VI shear modulus of ten elderly healthy female subjects and that of ten young healthy female subjects, plotted with the different relative isometric contraction levels (% MVC torque). The error bar represents the standard deviation among the 10 subjects.

VI Stiffness of Elderly and Young Female Subjects in Relaxed Condition

In relaxed condition, the measured mean shear modulus of VI in ten elderly female subjects was 9.5±3.3 kPa and in ten young female subjects was 12.8±5.4 kPa. Although several methods have been used to estimate the shear modulus of skeletal muscle, few studies have been performed on elderly female subjects and even more few on the VI muscle. Domire et al. measured the stiffness of tibialis anterior muscle at a relaxed condition on 20 female subjects with an age range of 50 to 70 years using MRE [43]. They reported that there was no significant effect of age on the stiffness of relaxed muscle, which is in agreement with ours. Kot et al. measured the shear modulus of RF in relaxed condition on young healthy subjects (14 males and 6 females, mean age 26.4±3.5 yr) and the mean value was 12.78±3.56 kPa, which is almost in the same range of ours [52]. Bensamoun et al. measured the shear modulus of VL and *vastus medialis* (VM) in relaxed condition on young healthy subjects (4 males and 10 females, mean age 25.2±1.78) [38]. The mean values were 3.73±0.85 kPa and 3.91±1.15 kPa, which is smaller than ours. Besides the effects for different age ranges, the different stiffness observed in different muscles may also indicate that the propagation of shear waves is influenced by the muscle structure, such as muscle fiber orientation. The RF and VI, which are bipennate muscles, exhibit higher muscle stiffness than the VL and VM, in which the fiber orientation is unipennate [38]. In addition, these differences may be also related to the muscle volume, fiber type distribution, function or other specific characteristics of different muscles. Although it is difficult to compare these results directly, all these shear modulus values in relaxed condition fall into a similar range.

The results in relaxed condition may be also influenced by other factors. All the subjects were asked to fully relax their muscles during the tests, but they might have slightly contracted their muscles unconsciously. Since muscle stiffness is strongly influenced by the muscle contraction, this kind of slight tension might affect the measurement results. In addition, the momentary muscle stiffness might also change with their preceding usage before the measurements [41]. This was the reason that the subjects were asked not to participate in any strength or flexibility training one day before the measurement in our study.

Age Effect on VI Stiffness under Different Step Isometric Contraction Levels

Our results demonstrated that the stiffness of VI muscle in the muscle action direction was positively correlated to the relative muscle contraction level (% MVC torque) over the entire range of step isometric contraction for both elderly and young female subjects. Some previous studies have used different weight loads imposed on the muscle to represent different contraction levels, such as on the knee extensors [28] and on the elbow flexors [39]. Their results have also reported that the muscle stiffness was positively correlated to the increasing weight loads. However, using weight load as an indicator of isometric contraction intensity was not accurate enough, since the muscle strength was different among the subjects and the lever arm of force was not counted. In other studies, the % MVC torque has been used to represent the muscle activity intensity level. However, in these measurements, the muscle contraction ranges rarely reached 50% MVC torque level due to the upper measurement limitation of the methods they used. For example, on young healthy subjects, Bensamoun et al. measured the shear modulus of VL and VM at 10% and 20% MVC torque, and it was 6.11±1.15 kPa and 8.49±4.02 kPa for VL, while it was 4.83±1.68 kPa and 6.40±1.79 kPa for VM [38]. They concluded that the shear modulus of VL and VM both increased significantly with the increase of % MVC torque. Although it was difficult to compare the shear modulus they measured with ours due to the different muscles and different age ranges, our conclusion that the muscle stiffness increased with the increasing isometric contraction level was in good agreement with their finding.

In this study, it was also found that the relationship between the muscle stiffness and relative isometric contraction level could be better represented using a quadratic curve over the entire range of isometric contraction. This relationship was mostly reported to be linear in previous studies [28,39]. In their studies, the shear modulus was only measured under 3 or 5 different isometric contraction levels at low intensity range, which may explain why different correlation was observed in our study, since a small portion of the quadratic curve can be treated as being linear.

We also noticed that the standard deviations of the mean VI shear modulus values increased substantially with % MVC levels. We thought this mainly came from the differences of the individual muscle strength of the subjects. At lower % MVC levels, these differences were not obvious, and thus the differences of muscle stiffness among the subjects were also small. However, when performing high intensity contraction, the differences of the absolute torque values corresponding to the high % MVC levels became larger due to the individually different MVC torque.

We found that the mean VI shear modulus of the young female subjects was larger than that of the elderly participants, especially at the relatively higher step isometric contraction levels. Rare previous study has been reported on the age difference of muscle shear modulus under different step isometric contraction levels. Ochala et al. [31] measured the musculotendinous stiffness of plantar flexors at 20%, 40%, 60% and 80% MVC levels on young and elderly subjects. The results indicated that the musculotendinous stiffness of elderly subjects was smaller than that of young subjects measured at the same contraction level. Although musculotendinous stiffness can only reflect the global mechanical properties of musculotendinous complex, their results are still a valuable reference for ours. Further studies should be performed to reveal the internal relationship between the muscle morphology changes, the muscle fiber atrophy and the decreasing muscle stiffness in its aging process.

Although for the first time muscle stiffness over the entire range of isometric contraction was measured with a further verification of the correlation between muscle stiffness and % MVC torque, there are still some limitations in our study. The measurement range of current vibro-ultrasound system should be further improved for young and male subjects by increasing the frame rate of the ultrasound acquisition, and by accurately controlling the position, frequency and amplitude of the shear wave generated in the skeletal muscle. The gender, age and joint angle dependences of the muscle stiffness under different isometric contraction levels should be also studied. The pennation angle of VI muscle tested in this study is less than $10°$ [51] and roughly equal to the muscle action direction, so it is relatively easy to align the shear wave propagation direction along the muscle fiber direction. However, the pennation angles of other muscles may be very different. Further study is required to test the performance of the proposed system for the muscles with large pennation angle, so

other skeletal muscles can be also studied by the developed vibro-ultrasound system.

Our aim is to provide real-time muscle stiffness measurement simultaneously with some other signals, such as sonomyography (SMG) which are the sonographically detected signals of the architectural change of muscles [53], B mode ultrasound images, force or torque values, joint angle and surface EMG. Combining these signals into one system will help us further understand the function of skeletal muscles.

Conclusions

In this study, a vibro-ultrasound system was developed for skeletal muscle stiffness measurement. Feasibility test on silicone phantoms demonstrated that this system was capable of measuring the shear modulus of tissues. Then, this system was applied for *in vivo* tests on elderly and young female human subjects. For the first time, the relationship between the muscle stiffness of VI and the relative step isometric contraction level (% MVC torque) was studied over the entire range, i.e. from 0% to 100% MVC. A quadratic polynomial curve was found to well represent the correlation between the two parameters. These results provided additional information about the recruitment strategies of muscles under step isometric contraction, which needs to be further investigated. In addition, it has been shown that there was no significant difference between the mean VI shear modulus of the elderly and young female subjects in a relaxed state ($p>0.1$). However, when performing step isometric contraction, the VI stiffness of young female subjects was found to be larger than that of elderly participants ($p<0.001$), especially at the high contraction levels. The vibro-ultrasound system could be further improved and combined with other signals to provide better understanding of skeletal muscles.

Acknowledgments

The authors would like to thank the volunteers who participated in the study, Dr. Jingyi Guo for her support in data collection, and Sally Ding for her help in editing the manuscript.

Author Contributions

Conceived and designed the experiments: CZW YPZ. Performed the experiments: CZW TJL. Analyzed the data: CZW TJL YPZ. Contributed reagents/materials/analysis tools: CZW TJL. Wrote the paper: CZW YPZ.

References

1. Abernethy B, Mackinnon S, Kippers V, Hanrahan S, Pandy M (2005) The biophysical foundations of human movement. 2nd ed. Champaign, IL: Human Kinetics. 169–196.
2. Grabiner MD, Owings TM, Pavol MJ (2005) Lower extremity strength plays only a small role in determining the maximum recoverable lean angle in older adults. J Gerontol A Biol Sci Med Sci 60: M1447–M1450.
3. Karamanidis K, Arampatzis A, Mademli L (2008) Age-related deficit in dynamic stability control after forward falls is affected by muscle strength and tendon stiffness. J Electromyogr Kinesiol 18: 980–989.
4. Klein CS, Rice CL, Marsh GD (2001) Normalized force, activation, and coactivation in the arm muscles of young and elderly men. J Appl Physiol 91: 1341–1349.
5. Narici MV, Maganaris CN, Reeves ND, Capodaglio P (2003) Effect of aging on human muscle architecture. J Appl Physiol 95: 2229–2234.
6. Morse CI, Thom JM, Birch KM, Narici MV (2005) Changes in triceps surae muscle architecture with sarcopenia. Acta Physiol Scand 183: 291–298.
7. Narici MV, Maffulli N, Maganaris CN (2008) Ageing of human muscles and tendons. Disabil Rehabil 30: 1548–1554.
8. Larsson L, Sjodin B, Karlsson J (1978) Histochemical and biochemical changes in human skeletal muscle with age in sedentary males, age 22–65 years. Acta Physiol Scand 103: 31–39.
9. Lexell J, Henrikssonlarsen K, Winblad B, Sjostrom M (1983) Distribution of different fiber types in human skeletal-muscles - effects of aging studied in whole muscle cross-sections. Muscle Nerve 6: 588–595.
10. Giresi PG, Stevenson EJ, Theilhaber J, Koncarevic A, Parkington J, et al. (2005) Identification of a molecular signature of sarcopenia. Physiol Genomics 21: 253–263.
11. Dela F, Kjaer M (2006) Resistance training, insulin sensitivity and muscle function in the elderly. Essays Biochem 42: 75–88.
12. Fung YC (1993) Biomechanics, Mechanical Properties of Living Tissues. New York: Springer. 392–424.
13. Wilson GJ, Murphy AJ, Pryor JF (1994) Musculotendinous Stiffness - Its Relationship to Eccentric, Isometric, and Concentric Performance. J Appl Physiol 76: 2714–2719.
14. Brown SHM, McGill SA (2009) The intrinsic stiffness of the in vivo lumbar spine in response to quick releases: Implications for reflexive requirements. J Electromyogr Kinesiol 19: 727–736.
15. Ochala J, Valour D, Pousson M, Lambertz D, Van Hoecke J (2004) Gender differences in human muscle and joint mechanical properties during plantar flexion in elderly age. J Gerontol 59: 441–448.
16. Leonard CT, Deshner WP, Romo JW, Suoja ES, Fehrer SC, et al. (2003) Myotonometer intra- and interrater reliabilities. Arch Phys Med Rehabil 84: 928–932.

17. Murayama M, Nosaka K, Yoneda T, Minamitani K (2000) Changes in hardness of the human elbow flexor muscles after eccentric exercise. Eur J Appl Physiol 82: 361–367.

18. Zheng YP, Mak AFT, Qin L (1998). Load-indentation response of soft tissues with multi-layers. 10th Annual International Conference of the IEEE EMBS, Hong Kong, PR China.

19. Zheng YP, Mak AFT, Lue B (1999) Objective assessment of limb tissue elasticity: Development of a manual indentation procedure. J Rehabil Res Dev 36: 71–85.

20. Bamber J, Cosgrove D, Dietrich CF, Fromageau J, Bojunga J, et al. (2013) EFSUMB guidelines and recommendations on the clinical use of ultrasound elastography. Part 1: Basic principles and technology. Ultraschall Med. 34(2): 169–184.

21. Chino K, Akagi R, Dohi M, Fukashiro S, Takahashi H (2012) Reliability and Validity of Quantifying Absolute Muscle Hardness Using Ultrasound Elastography. PLoS One 7: e45764.

22. Leong HT, Ng GYF, Leung VYF, Fu SN (2013) Quantitative Estimation of Muscle Shear Elastic Modulus of the Upper Trapezius with Supersonic Shear Imaging during Arm Positioning. PLoS One 8: e67199.

23. Catheline S, Thomas JL, Wu F, Fink MA (1999) Diffraction field of a low frequency vibrator in soft tissues using transient elastography. IEEE Trans Ultrason Ferroelectr Freq Control 46: 1013–1019.

24. Chen SG, Urban MW, Pislaru C, Kinnick R, Zheng Y, et al. (2009) Shearwave Dispersion Ultrasound Vibrometry (SDUV) for Measuring Tissue Elasticity and Viscosity. IEEE Trans Ultrason Ferroelectr Freq Control 56: 55–62.

25. Muthupillai R, Lomas DJ, Rossman PJ, Greenleaf JF, Manduca A, et al. (1995) Magnetic-resonance elastography by direct visualization of propagating acoustic strain waves. Science 269: 1854–1857.

26. Hoyt K, Kneezel T, Castaneda B, Parker KJ (2008) Quantitative sonoelastography for the in vivo assessment of skeletal muscle viscoelasticity. Phys Med Biol 53: 4063–4080.

27. Parker KJ, Huang SR, Musulin RA, Lerner RM (1990) Tissue-response to mechanical vibrations for sonoelasticity imaging. Ultrasound Med Biol 16: 241–246.

28. Levinson SF, Shinagawa M, Sato T (1995) Sonoelastic determination of human skeletal-muscle elasticity. J Biomech 28: 1145–1154.

29. Gennisson JL, Cornu C, Catheline S, Fink M, Portero P (2005) Human muscle hardness assessment during incremental isometric contraction using transient elastography. J Biomech 38: 1543–1550.

30. Nordez A, Guevel A, Casari P, Catheline S, Cornu C (2009) Assessment of muscle hardness changes induced by a submaximal fatiguing isometric contraction. J Electromyogr Kinesiol 19: 484–491.

31. Gennisson JL, Deffieux T, Macé E, Montaldo G, Fink M, et al. (2010) Viscoelastic and anisotropic mechanical properties of in vivo muscle tissue assessed by supersonic shear imaging. Ultrasound Med Biol 36: 789–801.

32. Urban MW, Chen SG, Greenleaf JF (2009) Error in Estimates of Tissue Material Properties from Shear Wave Dispersion Ultrasound Vibrometry. IEEE Trans Ultrason Ferroelectr Freq Control 56: 748–758.

33. Chen SG, Urban MW, Greenleaf JF, Zheng Y, Yao AP (2008) Quantification of Liver Stiffness and Viscosity with SDUV: In Vivo Animal Study. 2008 IEEE Ultrasonics Symposium, Vols 1–4 and Appendix: 654–657.

34. Sandrin L, Tanter M, Catheline S, Fink M (2002) Shear modulus imaging with 2-D transient elastography. IEEE Trans Ultrason Ferroelectr Freq Control 49: 426–435.

35. Nordez A, Hug F (2010) Muscle shear elastic modulus measured using supersonic shear imaging is highly related to muscle activity level. J Appl Physiol 108: 1389–1394.

36. Shinohara M, Sabra K, Gennisson JL, Fink M, Tanter M (2010) Real-time visualization of muscle stiffness distribution with ultrasound shear wave imaging during muscle contraction. Muscle Nerve 42: 438–441.

37. Bouillard K, Nordez A, Hug F (2011) Estimation of Individual Muscle Force Using Elastography. PLoS ONE 6: e29261.

38. Bensamoun SF, Ringleb SI, Littrell L, Chen Q, Brennan M, et al. (2006) Determination of thigh muscle stiffness using magnetic resonance elastography. J Magn Reson Imaging 23: 242–247.

39. Dresner MA, Rose GH, Rossman PJ, Muthupillai R, Manduca A, et al. (2001) Magnetic resonance elastography of skeletal muscle. J Magn Reson Imaging 13: 269–276.

40. Sack I, Bernarding J, Braun J (2002) Analysis of wave patterns in MR elastography of skeletal muscle using coupled harmonic oscillator simulations. Magn Reson Imaging 20: 95–104.

41. Uffmann K, Maderwald S, Ajaj W, Galban CG, Mateiescu S, et al. (2004) In vivo elasticity measurements of extremity skeletal muscle with MR elastography. NMR Biomed 17: 181–190.

42. Bensamoun SF, Glaser KJ, Ringleb SI, Chen Q, Ehman RL, et al. (2008) Rapid magnetic resonance elastography of muscle using one-dimensional projection. J Magn Reson Imaging 27: 1083–1088.

43. Domire ZJ, McCullough MB, Chen QS, An KN (2009) Feasibility of Using Magnetic Resonance Elastography to Study the Effect of Aging on Shear Modulus of Skeletal Muscle. J Appl Biomech 25: 93–97.

44. Arampatzis A, Karamanidis K, Mademli L (2008) Deficits in the way to achieve balance related to mechanisms of dynamic stability control in the elderly. J Biomech 41: 1754–1761.

45. Kruse SA, Smith JA, Lawrence AJ, Dresner MA, Manduca A, et al. (2000) Tissue characterization using magnetic resonance elastography: preliminary results. Phys Med Biol 45: 1579–1590.

46. Cespedes I, Huang Y, Ophir J, Spratt S (1995) Methods for Estimation of Subsample Time Delays of Digitized Echo Signals. Ultrason Imaging 17: 142–171.

47. Wang CZ, Zheng YP (2010) Comparison between reflection-mode photoplethysmography and arterial diameter change detected by ultrasound at the region of radial artery. Blood Press Monit 15: 213–219.

48. Hayes WC, Herrmann G, Mockros LF, Keer LM (1972) A mathematical analysis for indentation tests of articular cartilage. J Biomech 5: 541–551.

49. Deffieux T, Montaldo G, Tanter M, Fink M (2009) Shear Wave Spectroscopy for In Vivo Quantification of Human Soft Tissues Visco-Elasticity. IEEE Trans Med Imaging 28: 313–322.

50. Heers G, Jenkyn T, Dresner MA, Klein MO, Basford JR, et al. (2003) Measurement of muscle activity with magnetic resonance elastography. Clin Biomech 18: 537–542.

51. Blazevich AJ, Gill ND, Zhou S (2006) Intra- and intermuscular variation in human quadriceps femoris architecture assessed in vivo. J Anat 209: 289–310.

52. Kot BCW, Zhang ZJ, Lee AWC, Leung VYF, Fu SN (2012) Elastic Modulus of Muscle and Tendon with Shear Wave Ultrasound Elastography: Variations with Different Technical Settings. PLoS One 7: e44348.

53. Zheng YP, Chan MMF, Shi J, Chen X, Huang QH (2006) Sonomyography: Monitoring morphological changes of forearm muscles in actions with the feasibility for the control of powered prosthesis. Med Eng Phys 28: 405–415.

## 3

Decreased Fixation Stability of the Preferred Retinal Location in Juvenile Macular Degeneration

Richard A. I. Bethlehem[1,4]*, Serge O. Dumoulin[1], Edwin S. Dalmaijer[1], Miranda Smit[1,2], Tos T. J. M. Berendschot[3], Tanja C. W. Nijboer[1,2], Stefan Van der Stigchel[1]

1 Experimental Psychology, Helmholtz Institute, Utrecht University, Utrecht, The Netherlands, 2 Rudolf Magnus Institute of Neuroscience and Centre of Excellence for Rehabilitation Medicine, University Medical Centre Utrecht and Rehabilitation Centre De Hoogstraat, Utrecht, The Netherlands, 3 University Eye Clinic Maastricht, Maastricht, The Netherlands, 4 Autism Research Centre, Department of Psychiatry, University of Cambridge, Cambridge, United Kingdom

Abstract

Macular degeneration is the main cause for diminished visual acuity in the elderly. The juvenile form of macular degeneration has equally detrimental consequences on foveal vision. To compensate for loss of foveal vision most patients with macular degeneration adopt an eccentric preferred retinal location that takes over tasks normally performed by the healthy fovea. It is unclear however, whether the preferred retinal locus also develops properties typical for foveal vision. Here, we investigated whether the fixation characteristics of the preferred retinal locus resemble those of the healthy fovea. For this purpose, we used the fixation-offset paradigm and tracked eye-position using a high spatial and temporal resolution infrared eye-tracker. The fixation-offset paradigm measures release from fixation under different fixation conditions and has been shown useful to distinguish between foveal and non-foveal fixation. We measured eye-movements in nine healthy age-matched controls and five patients with juvenile macular degeneration. In addition, we performed a simulation with the same task in a group of five healthy controls. Our results show that the preferred retinal locus does not adopt a foveal type of fixation but instead drifts further away from its original fixation and has overall increased fixation instability. Furthermore, the fixation instability is most pronounced in low frequency eye-movements representing a slow drift from fixation. We argue that the increased fixation instability cannot be attributed to fixation under an unnatural angle. Instead, diminished visual acuity in the periphery causes reduced oculomotor control and results in increased fixation instability.

Editor: Chris I. Baker, National Institute of Mental Health, United States of America

Funding: This research was funded by a grant from the Dutch MD-foundation to authors SD, TN, and SvS. The funders had no role in study design, data collection and analysis, decision to publish, or preparation of the manuscript.

Competing Interests: The authors have declared that no competing interests exist.

* E-mail: rb643@cam.ac.uk

Introduction

Juvenile macular degeneration (JMD) affects approximately 1 in 10.000 individuals [1]. Most often it is caused by mutations in the ABCA4 gene, which transcribes a large retina-specific protein, leading to Stargardt disease [2,3,4]. As a result patients commonly develop a central scotoma that involves the fovea. The resulting loss of foveal vision has a severe impact on patients visual acuity. Early research has shown that this can be accompanied by a shift in the oculomotor reference from the fovea to a nonfoveal locus [5]. Subsequently patients suffering from macular degeneration often adopt one or multiple preferred retinal loci (PRL) that can serve as a 'pseudo-fovea' [6,7]. This PRL is an eccentric location on the retina that is used for fixation in favor of the fovea. Crossland et al. [8] have shown that this PRL can develop within six months of visual loss onset and further research shows that the PRL location can remain relatively stable in people with age-related macular degeneration [9]. Additionally, strategies for developing a PRL appear to be slightly different for different causes of macular degeneration [10], with Stargardts disease being the more variable one. Apart from the obvious poorer resolution of the visual retina in the periphery, fixation with the PRL in patients with MD (Throughout this manuscript we use JMD to refer to juvenile macular degeneration, MD to refer to non-specific macular degeneration and AMD to refer to age-related macular degeneration) also tends to be unstable [11,12]. In healthy individuals fixation instability can be beneficial in the central retina because of a low tolerance for image motion [13,14]. As resolution decreases with higher velocity eye movements [14] fixation instability recovers some of this loss [13]. During stable fixation peripheral vision also tends to decrease (Troxler fading) and unstable fixation partially recovers this fading. As Deruaz et al point out this has led to the suggestion that increased fixation instability for people that use peripheral fixation (such as people with MD) might be equally beneficial [15]. However, Macedo et al. have showed that this is not necessarily the case for patients with MD using peripheral vision [16]. Specifically, Macedo and colleagues [16] showed that fixation instability does not reduce crowded or non-crowded visual acuity. Thus, in standard reading or acuity test this instability does not produce any net benefit for people with MD. At the same time, paradigms utilizing visual acuity types of tests might not be the best predictors in determining fixation patterns and rehabilitation outcomes in patients with macular degeneration [17].

Most studies to date have not explicitly focused on the juvenile form of macular degeneration but on age-related macular degeneration (AMD) [10,17,18,19,20,21,22,23,24]. AMD is the most common form and is considered to be the main cause of diminished visual acuity in the elderly [25]. One study has shown that in AMD training can significantly improve fixation stability [24]. It has also been shown that fixation stability can be strongly correlated with PRL eccentricity [23]. In addition, Tarita-Nistor et al. [21] have shown that patients with AMD generally have good ocular motor coordination and fixation control, but that this disappears when one eye is covered. In addition, it has been shown that fixation characteristics may differ between monocular and binocular viewing in patients with AMD when asked to fixate for relatively long time periods [26]. It is possible that the relative late onset of AMD compared to JMD allows for some sustaining of oculomotor control and that this is better during binocular viewing [21]. In the present study we will focus specifically on the ability to keep fixation steady for short periods during binocular viewing by individuals with JMD.

Most studies which have investigated fixation characteristics of patients with macular degeneration have used a microperimeter [18,19,23,24,27] to assess fixation stability of the PRL. This measure generally has a low temporal resolution (<25 Hz) and as a result partial saccades (start or end points) are often difficult to take into account, let alone remove from the data. Additionally, long fixation periods are often used (exceeding 10s) which might make it harder for participants to stay focused. In contrast, short fixation phases might give a more accurate account of fixation characteristics under ecologically important and valid conditions such as during reading, visual search, visual scene processing or even typing. These types of fixation phases generally fall well within a 150 to 450 ms. time-scale [28]. In addition, precisely these types of viewing conditions have been shown to be impaired in MD [11,29]. Infrared eye-trackers allow short but detailed recording at this high temporal resolution as well as detection of trials containing saccades that can subsequently be removed. Infrared eye-trackers have already shown high test-retest reliability and have been proven useful in the assessment of fixation characteristics when compared to standard Scanning Laser Ophthalmoscope (SLO) measurements [30]. Although Crossland and Rubin [30] show that the eye-tracker methodology tends to overestimate the fixation instability, they also argue that this overestimation might be caused by small compensatory eye-movements. These are a result of the fact that participants' heads were completely unrestrained during testing. In addition, because infrared eye-trackers can record at high temporal resolutions, the need for long fixation periods becomes unnecessary and paves the way for more ecologically valid ways of assessing fixation in patients with MD. Furthermore, they allow for more fine-grained analyses of eye-tracking data such as power spectral densities with high temporal resolution that can further elucidate underlying fixation characteristics [31].

In the present study we aim to investigate the fixation characteristics in a group of patients with JMD that have stable PRL's during a paradigm that can potentially distinguish between foveal and peripheral types of fixation using an infrared eye-tracker. To this end we adopted a fixation offset paradigm [32]. This paradigm includes a short fixation phase that covers the range of fixation times reported during various different types of viewing [28] without explicitly restraining the fixation characteristics by a specific cue. In this paradigm participants do not focus explicitly on a fixation cross but instead are shown fixation anchors at a distance of either $1°$ degree or $3°$. Machado and Rafal [32] have shown that in healthy controls the $1°$ condition represents a foveal specific type of fixation whereas the $3°$ does not. In the $1°$ condition, introducing a gap between target onset and fixation offset results in a decrease in saccade latencies which does not occur in the $3°$ condition [33]. Fendrich et al. [33] argue that the $1°$ anchor falls within foveal fixation and the gap-effect thus only occurs for foveal fixation. In a previous study we have shown that a central scotoma combined with peripheral viewing impairs search efficiency and that these results can be explained without the necessity of reorganisation in the visual system [29]. Since the JMD group will use their periphery for both the foveal as well as the peripheral fixation anchor conditions the difference in fixation stability should be minimal. For the control group we would expect a difference for foveal (1 degree condition) versus non-foveal (3 degree condition) fixation, whereby the non-foveal fixation may resemble the general fixation of the patient group more closely.

We hypothesize that patients with JMD will have greater overall fixation instability due the use of peripheral viewing when compared to controls. Based on our previous study [29] using a visual search paradigm we do not expect that the PRL will have adopted foveal fixation properties and thus we do not expect an effect of fixation anchor-size. In contrast, we expect healthy controls to have an overall more stable fixation pattern that is strongest in the foveal (1 degree) fixation condition. To assess this instability, we will first look at the number of intrusive saccades, defined as a saccade during a moment in the task where stable fixation is required. Second, as a measure of fixation instability we use a bivariate contour ellipse area (BCEA) [23,30,34,35] and the overall displacement during the course of the fixation period. Finally, to further investigate the nature of fixation in JMD we will analyze the power spectral densities [31]. To ensure that any fixation instability is not explained by an 'unnatural' position of the eye during eccentric viewing we also tested a simulated PRL version of this paradigm in healthy controls.

Methods

Ethics Statement

The ethical institutional review board of the University Medical Centre Utrecht approved this study, and all subjects gave written informed consent prior to participation. All study procedures have been conducted according to the principles expressed in the Declaration of Helsinki.

Participants

For this study, we recruited 10 patients with juvenile MD. Additionally, 10 healthy age-matched controls participated in the same paradigm and another 6 healthy controls were recruited for participation in a simulation version of this paradigm. The JMD participants had an official diagnosis of JMD (assessed by their own physician and confirmed by means of a questionnaire) and had no history of neurological and/or psychiatrical disorders or substance abuse. Controls had normal or corrected to normal acuity and had no history of neurological and/or psychiatrical disorders or substance abuse either. All participants received 20 euro and travel expenses for their participation.

Procedure, Stimuli and Design

Clinical characteristics of the JMD patients were verbally interrogated by means of a questionnaire, see Table 1. After filling out the questionnaire, the experimental procedure started. All measurements were conducted in a sound-attenuated, dimly lit room. Eye movements were recorded by an Eyelink1000 system (SR Research Ltd, Canada), an infrared video-based eye-tracker.

The dominant eye, which was verified with a visual alignment task [36], was monitored and analysed in all participants. The non-dominant eye was not occluded during the course of the experiment to allow for naturalistic viewing. Although no research to date has established a clear link between eye dominance as measured by an alignment task and the dominant eye for fixation, this was the least arbitrary way to determine which eye to track. The participants' heads were stabilized using a chin rest to control for compensatory head movements. We acknowledge that head stabilization may somewhat limit the ecological validity, but it was necessary to make full use of the eye trackers temporal and spatial specificity. The distance between monitor and chin rest was 57 cm. A nine-point grid calibration and subsequent validation procedure was utilized before the start of the experiment.

Scanning Laser Opthalmology

In order to gain information about fixation stability and absolute locus of the PRL, patients were invited for a separate Scanning Laser Ophthalmoscope measurement (SLO) at the University Eye Clinic Maastricht [37]. We used a custom build Scanning Laser Ophthalmoscope [37,38] to image the fundus and to present the stimulus. The subjects fixated on a red cross that was presented in the SLO. To determine the absolute location of the PRL at the retina and its stability, we acquired 60 SLO images per participant with the use of a frame grabber, having a 1 sec interval in between. Similarly as described in Reinhard et al. [39] we used an SLO that shows the fundus and the fixation cross simultaneously on a video monitor. Further analysis was done also similar as described in the Reinhard et al. paper [39]. We aligned the subsequent images and calculated the PRL and its movement. Images are shown in Figure 1. The fundus photographs show the location of this PRL over time.

Visual Field Test

In addition, we used a visual field test to confirm the absolute visual field defect. In the visual field test, one target at a time was shown and a fixation cross was used which remained on screen during presentation of the target. The target was a black $1.5°$ dot and could appear at 33 possible stimulus locations with a background luminance of 52.95 cd/m2. The target was presented for 1500 ms. The 33 locations were organised in five rows; three rows consisted of seven locations and two rows of six locations. The centre-to-centre distance, both within and between rows of each location had a visual angle of $5°$. Participants were instructed to remain fixated on the fixation cross and report, using the 'z' and '/' keys, whether they had seen a target or not. After their response a confirmation of their choice was presented on screen. Target present trials were mixed with 'catch' trials in which no target was

presented. All target locations were presented four times along with 16 catch trials, making for 148 trials in total [29]. The visual field defect has been incorporated in Figure 1. MD case number 6 was excluded based on converging evidence from both the SLO and visual field test that the fixation overlapped with the fovea. For MD 3 there was a technical issue with the visual field data, but the SLO showed clear use of a PRL.

Fixation Offset Paradigm

To test fixation characteristics we used a fixation-offset paradigm [32]. All trials started with a drift check to ensure the calibration was still accurate. Participants were instructed to fixate on an unmarked centre containing four eccentric anchors surrounding the *unmarked* centre (background luminance of 32.07 cd/m2). The unmarked centre served as the fixation point and was located at the centre of the display. The eccentric fixation anchors consisted of four black crosses $(0.64°×0.64°)$ and were presented on the corners of an unmarked square. The distance from the crosses to the centre of the screen was either $3°$ or $1°$. After a pseudo-random interval (between 550 and 950 ms.), a black target circle appeared (diameter of $1.43°$). See figure 2A for an overview. In the patient group the location of target dots was dependent of the scotomatous area (either left, right, above or below the eccentric fixation anchor) as target locations that fell within the scotoma, as assessed with a visual field test, were removed from the location possibilities. The eccentric anchors were the same as in the control group to minimize potentially biasing the fixation stability by using different fixation anchors. In the control group targets were presented in all four (left, right, above and below the fixation anchor) possible locations. Participants were instructed to fixate at the *unmarked* centre until the target dot appeared, and subsequently were to move their eyes as fast as possible to the target circle. The target display was presented for 1500 ms. Afterwards all objects were removed from the display. The experiment consisted of 240 experimental trials and 24 practice trials.

Fixation Offset Simulation Paradigm

To investigate whether any difference in fixation might be caused by an unnatural eye-position in the patient group we also conducted a separate simulation in healthy controls. In this adaptation a para-foveal fixation cross at $8°$ eccentricity is presented at the right side of the true fixation. This eccentric fixation is an offset of the eye-position as measured with the eye-tracker and is thus controlled by participants' eye-movement. Participants are instructed to move this alternative fixation point over a centrally located fixation cross, hold their fixation steady and press the spacebar. When this alternative fixation was stable

Table 1. Clinical characteristics of individual patients.

Patient	Gender	Official Diagnosis	Age (y)	Age onset (y)
MD1	F	Stargardt	33	23
MD2	F	Stargardt	29	12
MD3	M	X-Chromosal schisis*	48	congenital
MD4	M	Stargardt	47	gradual
MD5	M	Stargardt	23	6
MD6	F	Best's Disease	38	20

*X-chromosome-linked juvenile retino- schisis.

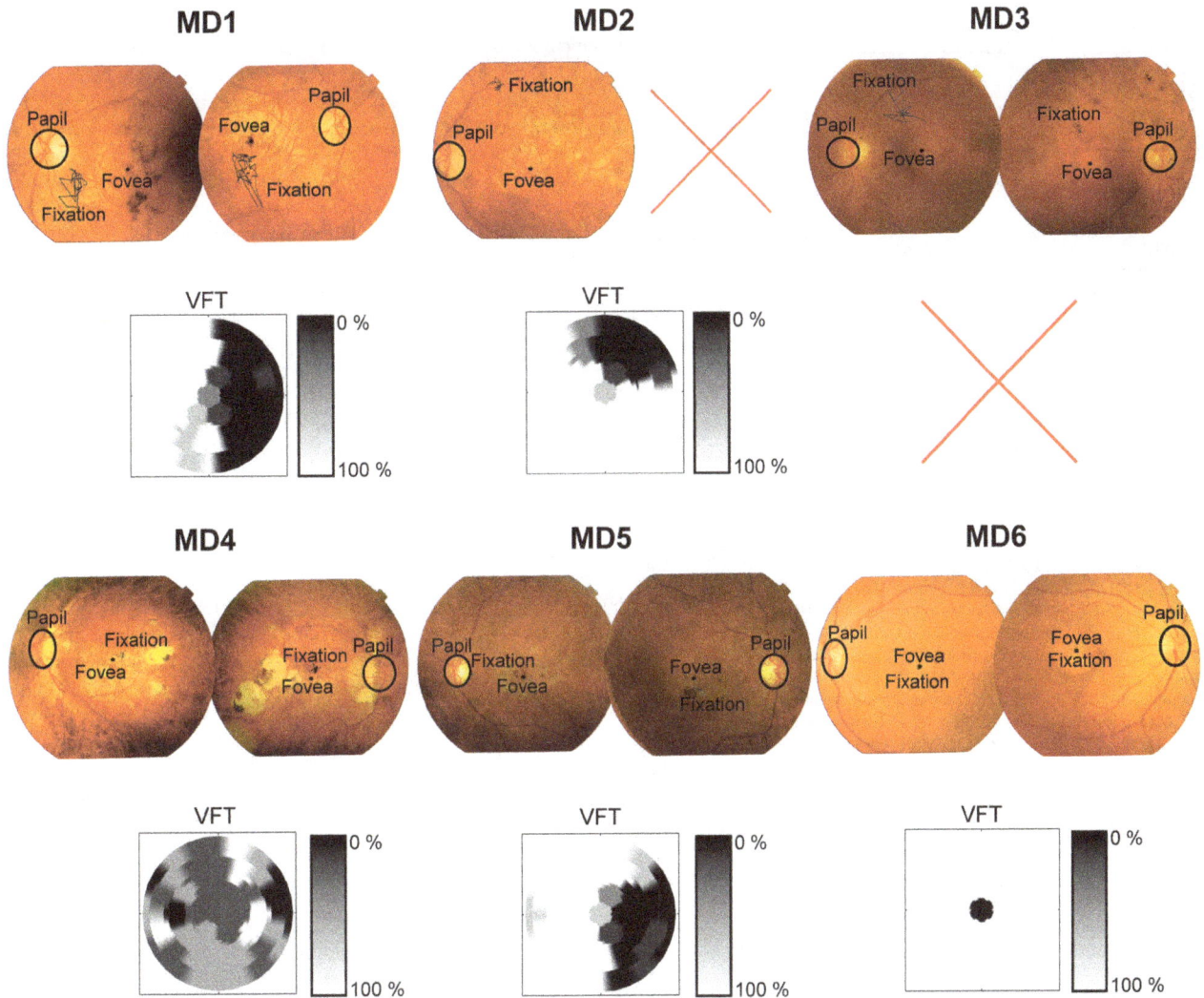

Figure 1. Scanning Laser Opthalmoscope photo's. SLO photographs of all JMD participants. Participant 6 (lower right) was excluded due to the evident overlap of fixation and fovea. Interpolated visual field task images are shown below each respective SLO image. These show the visual field defect (VFT) for an 18° by 18° degrees visual field. Dark areas represent the point in the visual field where there was a defect, white represent no defect (ranging from 0–100%). Because the VFT measurements are based on binocular viewing and the SLO images are from each eye separately they not always clearly translate to one another [21,26].

within 2° degrees of the central fixation cross the trial started by removal of the central fixation point. See figure 2B for a graphical overview. At the same time as the central fixation cross disappeared, fixation anchors were presented at either 1° or 3° degrees eccentricity from fixation. These were exactly the same as in the original paradigm and were presented for the same pseudorandom interval (550 ms-950 ms). After this a target was presented above, below or to the left of the true fixation and participants were instructed to move the eyes there as fast as possible and press the spacebar once they had done so. Size of the target dots, fixation crosses and fixation anchors as well as all luminance ratios was kept the same as in the original paradigm. This task was programmed using PyGaze [40]. We acknowledge that the simulation group cannot be considered the ideal comparison to the behaviour observed in the MD group. A gaze-contingent eccentric fixation anchor might not be the best reflection of the deficit that people with MD experience and an alternative might have been the use of a gaze-contingent artificial scotoma. However, we chose not to use a gaze-contingent artificial

scotoma because this would have provided the healthy participants of the simulation study with a strong cue (namely the border of the artificial scotoma) to be aligned with the eccentric fixation anchors. Furthermore, an artificial gaze-contingent scotoma is still always visible to a healthy control subject and is thus likely to affect the oculomotor programming. Also, healthy subjects might not necessarily deviate attention to a peripheral location when the artificial scotoma is visible. Instead they might simply attend to the borders of the artificial scotoma. We aimed to minimize these effects by using a gaze-contingent eccentric anchor instead.

Data Analysis

Our main question concerned the fixation behaviour with patients with JMD and a stable PRL in the absence of a clear fixation point. Therefore we focussed our analysis on the pseudo-random fixation phase at the start of each trial during which participants have to keep their fixation steady and within which the anchor points are presented on screen (Figure 2A).

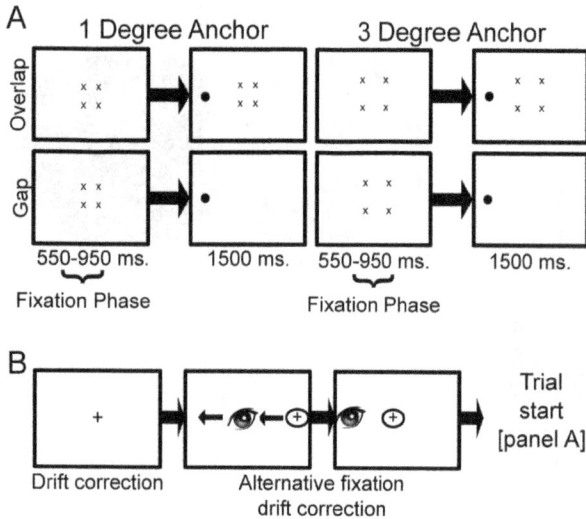

Figure 2. Paradigm overview. Panel A shows a schematic overview of the fixation-offset paradigm as used by Machado & Rafal [32]. After drift correction participants are instructed to keep a steady fixation within the four anchors. As soon as a target appears they are instructed to make an eye-movement to that target as fast as possible. Presently, we focussed on the fixation phase (before target presentation) of this paradigm. Panel B shows the adaptation used in the PRL simulation version of this paradigm. Prior to the normal trial procedure (but after drift correction), participants had to align a gaze-controlled alternate eccentric fixation point over a central fixation cross. This led them to use their peripheral vision to fixate on the central fixation cross before the start of the trial. In panel B the "eyeball" symbol represent the true fixation, the '+' sign represents the central fixation and the circled '+' sign represents the eccentric fixation point that was controlled by the participants eye movement. There was no minimum fixation time during alignment of the eccentric fixation point that participants had to maintain for the trial to start. However, should participants make a saccade directing the eccentric fixation to the central fixation cross and then press the spacebar, the subsequent saccade parser would have detected a saccade at trial start and the trial would have been removed from subsequent analysis.

Three main measures were taken during this period. First, we determined the number of saccades during the fixation phase (figure 2A). Thresholds for detecting the onset of a saccadic movement were an acceleration of $8000°/s2$ and a velocity of $30°/s$. These are the standard criteria used by SR Research's Eyelink systems to detect saccades. During this part of the task people are explicitly instructed to keep a steady fixation, thus we termed saccades during this period 'intrusive saccades' as opposed to the subsequent saccade made to the target after the fixation phase. Trials containing such 'intrusive saccades' were subsequently removed from further analysis and these trials are thus not included in any of the other reported measures. Second, we determined the total displacement of the fixation position at a single point in time as the distance between the original fixation and the position of the eye at target onset in degrees. The total displacement measure is potentially more sensitive to slow one-directional drift as opposed to fixation area. The rationale behind this measure was that if an eye movement (below saccade thresholds described above) would go in a single direction then the overall fixation instability, as determined by the BCEA, would be relatively small since this measure is largely determined by the standard deviation of eye-movement in x and y directions. Thus the total displacement might reflect a different type of fixation instability. Third, fixation stability was calculated using the

method of determining a bivariate contour ellipse area the methodology of which is extensive described elsewhere [23,30,34,35].

To investigate the nature of the instability we analysed the power spectral density (using a fast fourier transformation) of the time-courses of the displacement [31,41] of trials without saccades and blinks. The rationale behind this approach is that it might be more sensitive to detect a slow displacement drift as opposed to faster 'jerky' eye-movement instability that might be the result of reduced oculomotor control.

All measures were analysed using 2x3 mixed ANOVA with condition (1degree anchor vs. 3degree anchor) as within subjects factor and group (Control vs. MD vs. Simulation) as between subjects factor. Post-hoc t-tests (two-sided) were conducted using Bonferroni correction for multiple comparisons.

Apart from a diagnosis of JMD, inclusion criteria for the JMD group included a clear usage of a stable PRL as measured with the SLO and the ability to perform both a nine-grid calibration and validation on the Eyelink system prior to the start of the experiment. Four participants from the JMD group were unable to attend an SLO measurement and were thus excluded from the final analysed sample. In one case the PRL overlapped almost perfectly and was thus also excluded (MD6 in figure 1). If the number of valid trials, after removal of trials including an intrusive saccade, was more than 3 standard deviations away from the group mean, that subject was considered an extreme outlier. In the control and simulation group one extreme outlier on the intrusive saccade measure was excluded. In total our exclusion criteria thus led to a loss of 5 JMD participants, 1 control participant and 1 control participant performing the simulation experiment. The final analysed sample thus included 5 JMD participants (see Table 1 for clinical characteristics of the JMD group) and 9 controls matched for age and 5 controls participating in the simulation experiment. This relatively small number of JMD participants is not uncommon in the literature [16,24,29,42,43,44]. In addition all our results figures include individual data points showing that our results are consistent across patients and that the behaviour of nearly each patient deviates from the control group.

Results

Example eye-movement recordings and BCEA computation are shown in Figure 3. Figure 3 depicts three types of trials. The top trial (3A and 3B) is an example of a trial with an intrusive saccade. The scatterplot (3B) shows how an intrusive saccade influences the spread of the displacement and thus the BCEA and overall displacement. Intrusive saccades can greatly bias the displacement and fixation stability measures and therefore all trials that included intrusive saccades were removed from the remaining analysis. The two other trials show a 'normal' time-course (3C) and scatterplot (3D) of a healthy control and a time-course (3E) and scatterplot (3F) of a patient with JMD. In the scatterplots of the included trial types (3D and 3F) examples of a BCEA are shown.

Intrusive Saccades

We measured the amount of intrusive saccades, as defined above, during the fixation phase (figure 2A) of the fixation-offset paradigm. JMD patients made more intrusive saccades than both the control and simulation groups as is evident from a main effect of Group $F(2,16) = 46.243$, $p<0.001$ and Post-hoc tests: JMD> Control ($p<0.001$) and JMD>Simulation ($p<0.001$), see figure 4. There was no apparent Post-hoc difference between the control group and the simulation group. These results clearly show that

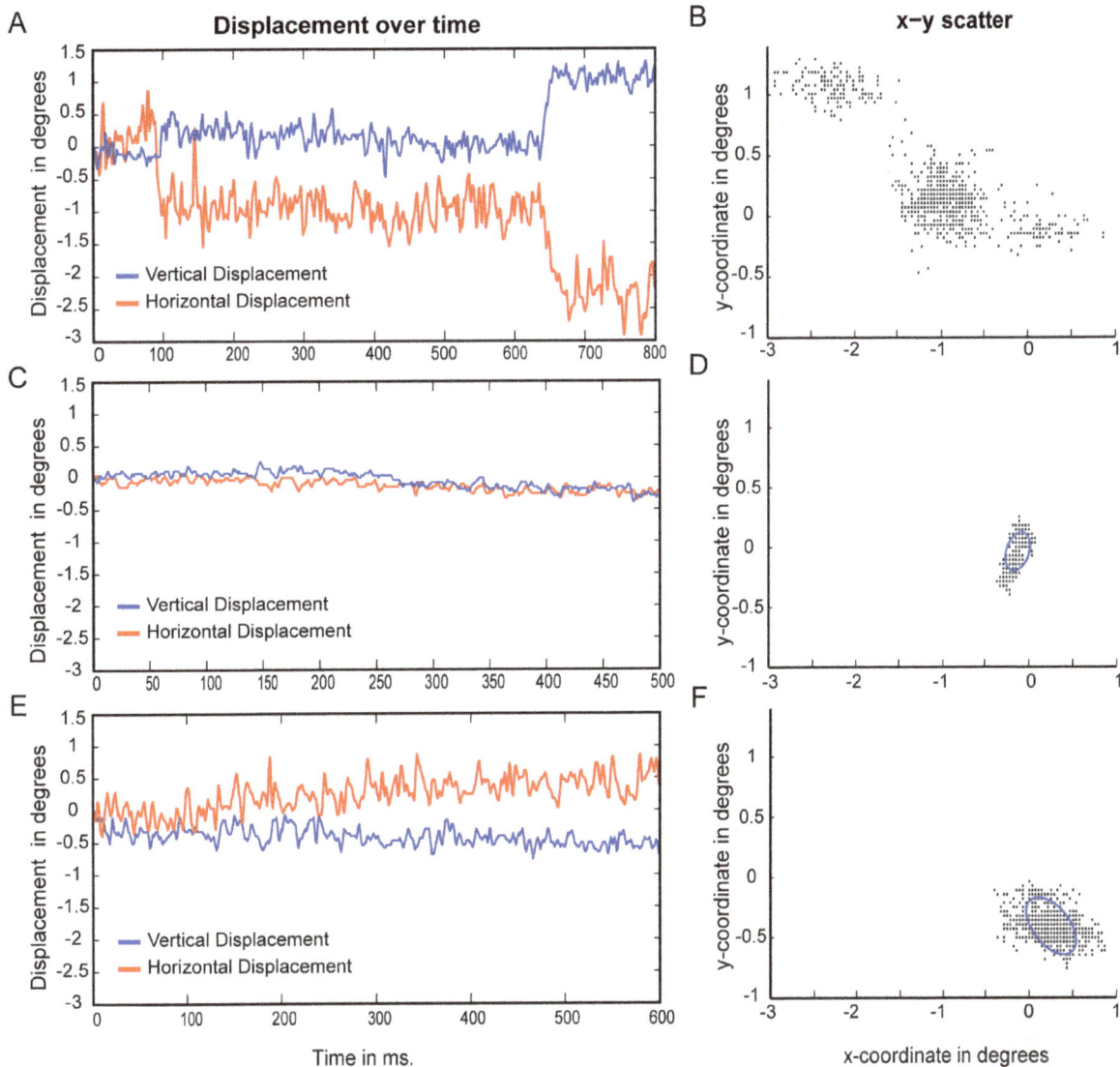

Figure 3. Time-course and scatterplot examples for different types of trials. Panels A, C and E show example time-courses of eye-position over time, lines indicate horizontal (red) and vertical (blue) displacement over time. The example time-courses illustrate measurement with (A) and without (C) an intrusive saccade in control subjects and a typical trial without saccades or blinks of a JMD patient (E). Panels B, D and F show the corresponding eye-positions across the entire measurement duration, indicating the effect of saccade and blinks on the displacement spread (Panel B). Displacement was summarized by the BCEA and examples are shown in blue circles in panels D and E. Only trials that did not include these intrusive saccades or blinks were included in the analysis of the BCEA, displacement and power spectral densities.

patients with JMD have difficulty in maintaining fixation even for a very short duration.

Our within subjects factor of fixation anchor-size also showed a main effect: $F(2,16) = 8.746$, $p = 0.009$. The interaction between the size of the fixation anchor and Group was not significant $F(2,16) = 3.373$, $p = 0.060$.

Displacement

Second, we measured the displacement between the start- and end-point of the eye at the onset of the fixation phase. Here, results show a main effect of Group $F(2,16) = 16.904$, $p<0.001$. This effect also seems to be mainly driven by the JMD group as Post-Hoc tests show: JMD>Control ($p<0.001$) and JMD>Simulation ($p<0.001$), see figure 5. There was no main effect of Anchorsize, nor an interaction effect on the total displacement. These results

confirm that patients with JMD have an unstable fixation pattern even when trials that contained saccades were removed from the analysis.

Fixation Stability

Third, we determined the total fixation area using a BCEA for all time-points during the fixation-phase of the fixation-offset paradigm (Figure 3D & F). The results show that fixation stability as measured with a bivariate contour ellipse during a short fixation phase was significantly different across the three groups $F(2,16) = 4.476$, $p = 0.029$, see figure 6. Post-hoc tests show that this effect is mainly caused by the JMD group: JMD>Control ($p = 0.047$) and that there was no significant effect for the JMD group compared to the simulation JMD>Simulation ($p = 0.059$). There was no main effect of Anchorsize, nor an interaction effect

Intrusive Saccades

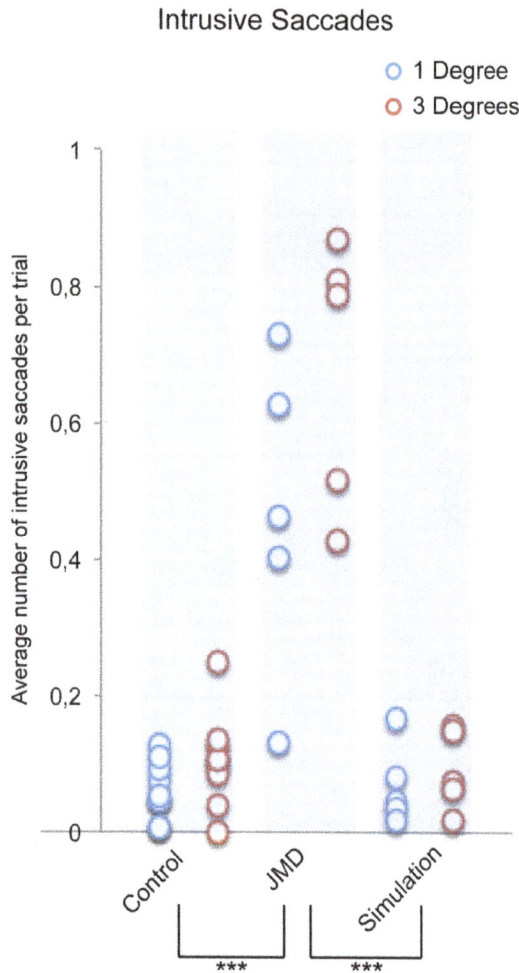

Displacement

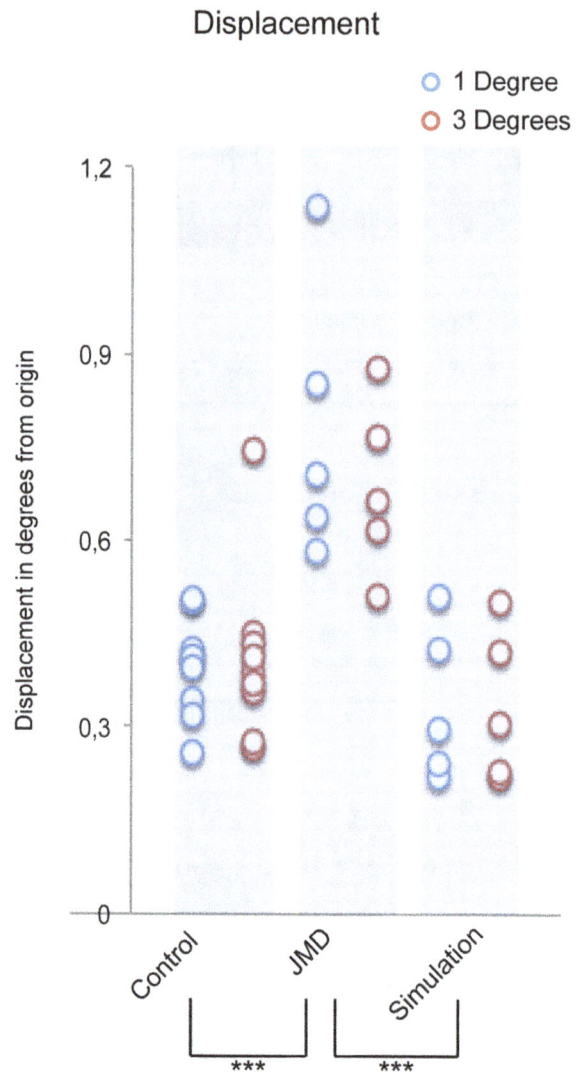

Figure 4. Number of intrusive saccades during fixation. The average number of intrusive saccades per trial are shown. Significant differences are marked: p<0.001 = ***, p<0.01 = ** & p<0.05 = *. This figure shows that the JMD group (1 degree [M: 0.47 SD: 0.23], 3 degrees [M: 0.68 SD: 0.20]) made significantly more intrusive saccades compared to healthy controls (1 degree [M: 0.06 SD: 0.04], 3 degrees [M: 0.11 SD: 0.07]) and controls performing the simulation (1 degree [M: 0.07 SD: 0.06], 3 degrees [M: 0.09 SD: 0.06]). It also shows that in the control group people made less intrusive saccade in the 1-degree condition.

Figure 5. Displacement during fixation. The start-to-end displacement in degrees of visual angle is shown. Significant differences are marked: p<0.001 = ***, p<0.01 = ** & p<0.05 = *. This figure shows that patients with JMD (1 degree [M: 0.78 SD: 0.22], 3 degrees [M: 0.69 SD: 0.14]) deviated more from their original fixation at the end of the fixation phase compared to controls in both the normal (1 degree [M: 0.40 SD: 0.08], 3 degrees [M: 0.41 SD: 0.14]) and simulation (1 degree [M: 0.34 SD: 0.12], 3 degrees [M: 0.34 SD: 0.12]) paradigm.

on the fixation stability. The results remained statistically significant even with the JMD outlier removed (main effect of Group $(F2,15) = 11.537$, $p = 0.001$ and Post-Hoc differences: JMD>Control, $p = 0.003$ and JMD>Simulation, $p = 0.001$). Again, these results show that patients with JMD have an unstable fixation that cannot directly be related to an unnatural eye-position.

Power Spectral Density

In order to measure the nature of the fixation instability we measured the power spectral density of the first 500 ms. of the fixation time-courses [31,41]. The results from our power spectral density analyses are plotted in figure 7. This analysis suggests that the difference in fixation stability reported above is primarily driven by low frequency eye-movements. Figure 7 shows that below 10 Hz all patients from the JMD group fall well outside the 95% confidence interval of the healthy control group. Although the saccade parser used in the present study did not explicitly

detect micro-saccades, low-frequency eye movements are often interpreted as slow variations in eye position such as drift [31,45]. These low frequency differences can thus not be attributed to potential contamination with high-frequency eye movements such as micro-saccades or tremors [46].

Discussion

The PRL in individuals with JMD exhibits unstable fixation patterns compared to fixation patterns of the healthy fovea. This instability is reflected in more intrusive saccades and decreased fixation stability. The decreased fixation stability is driven by slow variations in eye-position. The intrusive saccades measure we used in the present study might also reflect the fact that a decrease in visual acuity causes a deficit in terms of maintaining attention on

Fixation Stability

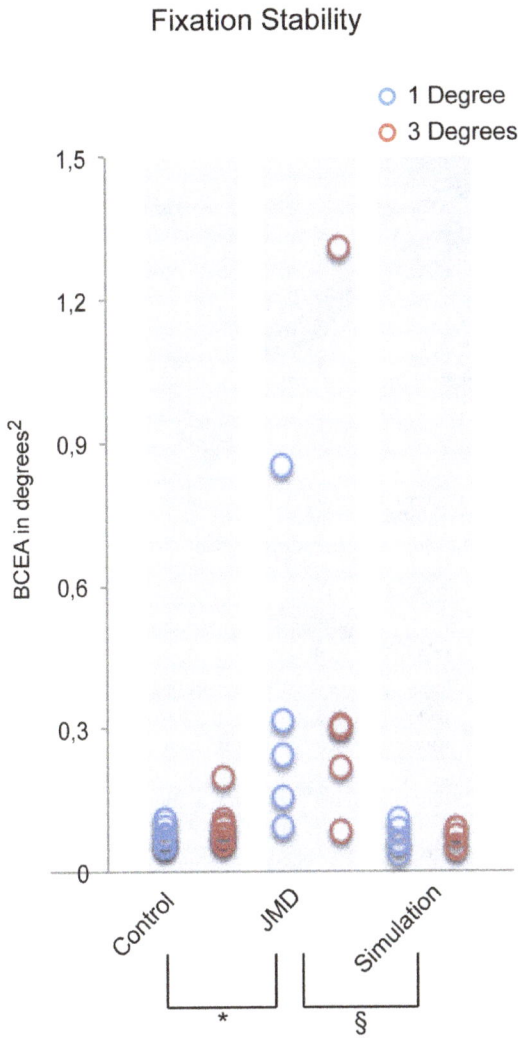

Figure 6. Fixation stability during fixation. The fixation stability in squared degrees as measured with a bivariate contour ellipse area (see figures 3B and 3D for an example). Significant differences are marked: p<0.001 = ***, p<0.01 = ** & p<0.05 = *. The "§" marks a trend. This figure shows that fixation was more unstable in the JMD group (1 degree [M: 0.33 SD: 0.20], 3 degrees [M: 0.44 SD: 0.49]) compared to the healthy control group (1 degree [M: 0.08 SD: 0.02], 3 degrees [M: 0.09 SD: 0.04]). The difference between the JMD group and the simulation group (1 degree [M: 0.07 SD: 0.03], 3 degrees [M: 0.07 SD: 0.02]) was not significant but a Bonferroni corrected p-value of 0.067 might be considered a trend.

the fixation stimulus. The decreased visual acuity might lead to uncertainty concerning the possible offset of the fixation cross, resulting in an increase in preliminary saccades away from the fixation stimulus, even though it is still physically present on the screen. Since all trials that contained such saccades were subsequently removed from further analysis this would not directly explain differences in fixation stability. Another potential cause for the detection of these saccades might have been a switch to a different PRL. Such a switch might be detected by the eye tracker as a rapid saccade, although it is unlikely that PRL switch will occur in such a short time-frame. If participants indeed switched to a different PRL the eye-tracker would have to be re-calibrated. Because it was calibrated for another PRL the drift check preceding each trial would fail after a PRL switch and would

only continue after re-calibrating for the new PRL. Since no re-calibration was needed we assume that the final analysed trials were all from the same PRL.

The simulation suggest that it is unlikely that the present results can be explained by the notion that during peripheral viewing the eye-muscles are in an unnatural position and are thus more prone to saccadic behavior back to a more natural position. The control group performing the simulation shows similar fixation characteristics as the group performing the normal paradigm. Consequently, they also show the same differences when compared with the JMD group performing the normal paradigm. This is in line with previous research using simulated scotomas that show intact oculomotor control during reading [47] as well as during visual search [48]. Thus it is unlikely that any differences in oculomotor control in the patient group can be ascribed to peripheral vision alone.

Recently, there is a debate about the degree of plasticity and stability in the human brain following retinal degeneration. This debate is centred on the observation that regions deprived of retinal input, such as the foveal projection zone, can still respond to visual stimulation. Some authors have argued that these signals reflect cortical reorganization [42,43,49] whereas others don't [29,44,50]. In the present study we found that in the control group fixation is more stable during presentation of foveal anchors (1 degree) compared to parafoveal anchors (3 degrees) as measured by the number of intrusive saccades. This increased stability was absent in both the JMD and the simulation group. Furthermore, the present results also show that peripheral fixation using a PRL is significantly more unstable in JMD patients compared to the simulation group. This indicates that the instability cannot be attributed to peripheral fixation alone. Thus even in the periphery where the PRL is located patients with JMD suffer from reduced fixation stability. This is in contrast to a previous study by White and Bedell [5] showing relatively stable fixation patterns in patients with bilateral macular disease. This study however used a much lower temporal resolution and might have been unable to accurately filter out intrusive saccades nor detect slow drift. Our results align with a more recent study that also showed decreased fixation stability in patients with JMD [51]. Given results from our previous study [29] it is likely that diminished visual acuity in the periphery contributes to this decreased fixational control. Although acuity was not measured in the present study, we assume that acuity diminishes at increased eccentricity for both controls and patients. With regards to plasticity, the behavioural eye-movement characteristics in the present study do not mimic the characteristics of the fovea when compared in a fixation-offset paradigm with foveal and parafoveal anchors. Therefore, the present results can be explained without the need for plasticity and instead be attributed to eccentric viewing with possible additional reduced visual acuity. We note, however, that current results might not extent to the non-dominant eye, as we only measured the oculomotor characteristics of the dominant eye Previous studies that focussed on AMD have shown that oculomotor control can differ between monocular and binocular viewing [21,26]. Interestingly and in contrast to the present study, in AMD oculomotor control seems to be relatively good during binocular viewing [21]. As stated before it is possible that the relative late onset of AMD might allow for some sustaining of oculomotor control. In the present study we did however not test the effects of monocular versus binocular viewing. Future studies investigating oculomotor control of the PRL in individuals with macular degeneration should therefore carefully control for acuity and test both eyes separately to make such a direct comparison possible.

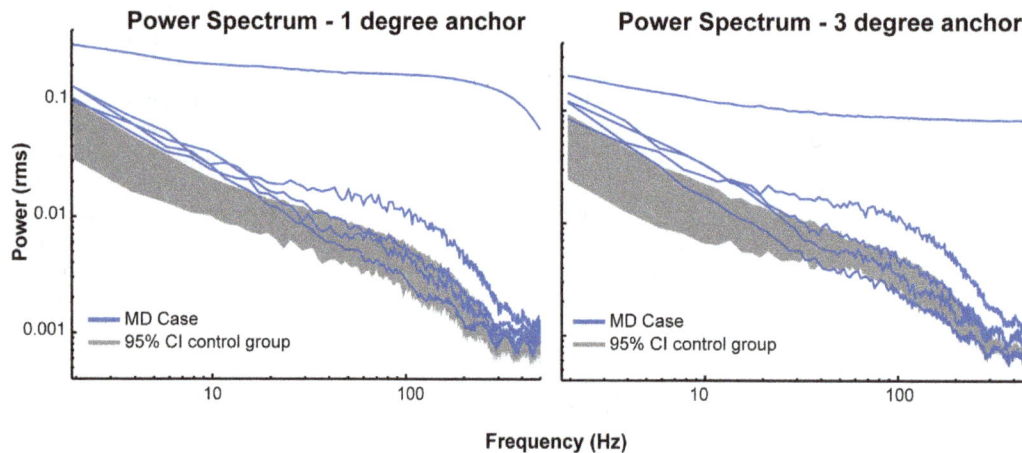

Figure 7. Power spectral density plots. Power spectral densities for the one and three degrees condition. The grey bars represent the 95% confidence interval (CI) of the control group mean. Each blue line represents one JMD patient. This figure shows that JMD patients had significant more power in the lower frequencies, indicating that low frequency eye-movements dominate the differences in displacement and fixation stability.

The differences in low-frequency eye-movements, interpreted as drift, provide another clue about the effect of macular degeneration on fixation characteristics. Under normal conditions drift is sometimes termed 'slow control' [52]. This refers to the balance between maintaining fixation on a certain object while allowing some eye-movements oscillation to prevent perceptual fading [13,45]. As such, it is possible that the increased power of these types of eye-oscillations in JMD reflects a compensatory mechanism for loss of visual acuity due to peripheral viewing. It is also possible that this increased drift is simply a result of decreased oculomotor control as drift can sometimes also be triggered by spontaneous activation of peripheral oculomotor mechanisms [45]. Because we also observed an increased number of intrusive saccades in the JMD group the latter explanation seems the most likely. This finding is further supported by early findings showing that especially slow eye-movements are normally controlled by the fovea [53], although this study investigated fixation during a fairly

long interval of 12 seconds and with considerably lower temporal resolution (<100 Hz).

In sum, our findings show a clear deficit in oculomotor control in patients with JMD during fixation. Given that we ruled out an unnatural eye-position as the cause for this instability we suggest that diminished peripheral acuity may be the most likely explanation. This may also be the factor underlying increased low-frequency drift. Perhaps, the adoption of a fixation stimulus that is scaled, such that is easier to see for the patients with JMD, might restore normal fixation behaviour.

Author Contributions

Conceived and designed the experiments: RB SD ED MS TB TN SvS. Performed the experiments: RB MS TB TN. Analyzed the data: RB SD MS TB SvS. Contributed reagents/materials/analysis tools: RB SD ED MS TB TN SvS. Wrote the paper: RB SD ED MS TB TN SvS.

References

1. Bither PP, Berns LA (1985) Stargardt's disease: A review of the literature. Journal of the American Optomology Association 59: 106–111.
2. Allikmets R (1997) A photoreceptor cell-specific ATP-binding transporter gene (ABCR) is mutated in recessive Stargardt macular dystrophy. Nature genetics 17: 122.
3. Allikmets R, Shroyer NF, Singh N, Seddon JM, Lewis RA, et al. (1997) Mutation of the Stargardt disease gene (ABCR) in age-related macular degeneration. Science 277: 1805–1807.
4. Koenekoop RK (2003) The gene for Stargardt disease, ABCA4, is a major retinal gene: a mini-review. Ophthalmic genetics 24: 75–80.
5. White JM, Bedell HE (1990) The oculomotor reference in humans with bilateral macular disease. Investigative ophthalmology & visual science 31: 1149–1161.
6. Crossland MD, Engel SA, Legge GE (2011) The preferred retinal locus in macular disease: toward a consensus definition. Retina 31: 2109–2114.
7. Greenstein VC, Santos RA, Tsang SH, Smith RT, Barile GR, et al. (2008) Preferred retinal locus in macular disease: characteristics and clinical implications. Retina 28: 1234–1240.
8. Crossland MD, Culham LE, Kabanarou SA, Rubin GS (2005) Preferred retinal locus development in patients with macular disease. Ophthalmology 112: 1579–1585.
9. Sunness JS, Applegate CA (2005) Long-term follow-up of fixation patterns in eyes with central scotomas from geographic atrophy that is associated with age-related macular degeneration. American journal of ophthalmology 140: 1085–1093.
10. Sunness JS, Applegate CA, Haselwood D, Rubin GS (1996) Fixation patterns and reading rates in eyes with central scotomas from advanced atrophic age-related macular degeneration and Stargardt disease. Ophthalmology 103: 1458–1466.
11. Crossland MD, Culham LE, Rubin GS (2004) Fixation stability and reading speed in patients with newly developed macular disease. Ophthalmic & physiological optics : the journal of the British College of Ophthalmic Opticians 24: 327–333.
12. Timberlake GT, Mainster MA, Peli E, Augliere RA, Essock EA, et al. (1986) Reading with a macular scotoma. I. Retinal location of scotoma and fixation area. Investigative ophthalmology & visual science 27: 1137–1147.
13. Martinez-Conde S, Macknik SL, Hubel DH (2004) The role of fixational eye movements in visual perception. Nature reviews Neuroscience 5: 229–240.
14. Morgan MJ, Benton S (1989) Motion-deblurring in human vision. Nature 340: 385–386.
15. Deruaz A, Matter M, Whatham AR, Goldschmidt M, Duret F, et al. (2004) Can fixation instability improve text perception during eccentric fixation in patients with central scotomas? The British journal of ophthalmology 88: 461–463.
16. Macedo AF, Crossland MD, Rubin GS (2011) Investigating unstable fixation in patients with macular disease. Investigative ophthalmology & visual science 52: 1275–1280.
17. Cacho I, Dickinson CM, Reeves BC, Harper RA (2007) Visual acuity and fixation characteristics in age-related macular degeneration. Optometry and vision science 84: 487–495.
18. Gonzalez EG, Tarita-Nistor L, Mandelcorn ED, Mandelcorn M, Steinbach MJ (2011) Fixation control before and after treatment for neovascular age-related macular degeneration. Investigative ophthalmology & visual science 52: 4208–4213.
19. Sivaprasad S, Pearce E, Chong V (2011) Quality of fixation in eyes with neovascular age-related macular degeneration treated with ranibizumab. Eye 25: 1612–1616.

20. Tarita-Nistor L, Brent MH, Steinbach MJ, Gonzalez EG (2011) Fixation stability during binocular viewing in patients with age-related macular degeneration. Investigative ophthalmology & visual science 52: 1887–1893.
21. Tarita-Nistor L, Brent MH, Steinbach MJ, Gonzalez EG (2012) Fixation patterns in maculopathy: from binocular to monocular viewing. Optometry and vision science 89: 277–287.
22. Tarita-Nistor L, Gonzalez EG, Markowitz SN, Steinbach MJ (2006) Binocular function in patients with age-related macular degeneration: a review. Canadian journal of ophthalmology Journal canadien d'ophtalmologie 41: 327–332.
23. Tarita-Nistor L, Gonzalez EG, Markowitz SN, Steinbach MJ (2008) Fixation characteristics of patients with macular degeneration recorded with the mp-1 microperimeter. Retina 28: 125–133.
24. Tarita-Nistor L, Gonzalez EG, Markowitz SN, Steinbach MJ (2009) Plasticity of fixation in patients with central vision loss. Visual neuroscience 26: 487–494.
25. Leibowitz HM, Krueger DE, Maunder LR, Milton RC, Kini MM, et al. (1980) The Framingham Eye Study monograph: An ophthalmological and epidemiological study of cataract, glaucoma, diabetic retinopathy, macular degeneration, and visual acuity in a general population of 2631 adults, 1973–1975. Survey of ophthalmology 24: 335–610.
26. Kabanarou SA, Crossland MD, Bellmann C, Rees A, Culham LE, et al. (2006) Gaze changes with binocular versus monocular viewing in age-related macular degeneration. Ophthalmology 113: 2251–2258.
27. Crossland MD, Crabb DP, Rubin GS (2011) Task-specific fixation behavior in macular disease. Investigative ophthalmology & visual science 52: 411–416.
28. Rayner K (1998) Eye movements in reading and information processing: 20 years of research. Psychological bulletin 124: 372–422.
29. Van der Stigchel S, Bethlehem RA, Klein BP, Berendschot TT, Nijboer TC, et al. (2013) Macular degeneration affects eye movement behavior during visual search. Frontiers in psychology 4: 579.
30. Crossland MD, Rubin GS (2002) The use of an infrared eyetracker to measure fixation stability. Optometry and vision science 79: 735–739.
31. Eizenman M, Hallett PE, Frecker RC (1985) Power spectra for ocular drift and tremor. Vision research 25: 1635–1640.
32. Machado L, Rafal RD (2000) Strategic control over saccadic eye movements: studies of the fixation offset effect. Perception & psychophysics 62: 1236–1242.
33. Fendrich R, Demirel S, Danziger S (1999) The oculomotor gap effect without a foveal fixation point. Vision research 39: 833–841.
34. Steinman RM (1965) Effect of Target Size, Luminance, and Color on Monocular Fixation. J Opt Soc Am 55: 1158–1164.
35. Timberlake GT, Sharma MK, Grose SA, Gobert DV, Gauch JM, et al. (2005) Retinal location of the preferred retinal locus relative to the fovea in scanning laser ophthalmoscope images. Optometry and vision science 82: 177–185.
36. Porac C, Coren S (1976) The dominant eye. Psychological bulletin 83: 880–897.
37. Ossewaarde-Van Norel J, van Den Biesen PR, van De Kraats J, Berendschot TT, van Norren D (2002) Comparison of fluorescence of sodium fluorescein in retinal angiography with measurements in vitro. J Biomed Opt 7: 190–198.
38. van Norren D, van de Kraats J (1989) Imaging retinal densitometry with a confocal Scanning Laser Ophthalmoscope. Vision research 29: 1825–1830.
39. Reinhard J, Messias A, Dietz K, Mackeben M, Lakmann R, et al. (2007) Quantifying fixation in patients with Stargardt disease. Vision research 47: 2076–2085.
40. Dalmaijer ES, Mathot S, Van der Stigchel S (2013) PyGaze: An open-source, cross-platform toolbox for minimal-effort programming of eyetracking experiments. Behavior research methods.
41. Findlay JM (1971) Frequency analysis of human involuntary eye movement. Kybernetik 8: 207–214.
42. Baker CI, Peli E, Knouf N, Kanwisher NG (2005) Reorganization of visual processing in macular degeneration. The Journal of neuroscience 25: 614–618.
43. Dilks DD, Baker CI, Peli E, Kanwisher N (2009) Reorganization of visual processing in macular degeneration is not specific to the "preferred retinal locus". The Journal of neuroscience 29: 2768–2773.
44. Masuda Y, Dumoulin SO, Nakadomari S, Wandell BA (2008) V1 projection zone signals in human macular degeneration depend on task, not stimulus. Cerebral cortex 18: 2483–2493.
45. Murakami I (2010) Eye movements during fixation as velocity noise in minimum motion detection. Japanese Psychological Research 52: 54–66.
46. Steinman RM, Cunitz RJ, Timberlake GT, Herman M (1967) Voluntary control of microsaccades during maintained monocular fixation. Science 155: 1577–1579.
47. Lingnau A, Schwarzbach J, Vorberg D (2008) Adaptive strategies for reading with a forced retinal location. Journal of vision 8: 6 1–18.
48. Lingnau A, Schwarzbach J, Vorberg D (2010) (Un-) coupling gaze and attention outside central vision. Journal of vision 10: 13.
49. Baker CI, Dilks DD, Peli E, Kanwisher N (2008) Reorganization of visual processing in macular degeneration: replication and clues about the role of foveal loss. Vision research 48: 1910–1919.
50. Baseler HA, Gouws A, Haak KV, Racey C, Crossland MD, et al. (2011) Large-scale remapping of visual cortex is absent in adult humans with macular degeneration. Nature neuroscience 14: 649–655.
51. Macedo AF, Nascimento SM, Gomes AO, Puga AT (2007) Fixation in patients with juvenile macular disease. Optometry and vision science : official publication of the American Academy of Optometry 84: 852–858.
52. Steinman RM, Haddad GM, Skavenski AA, Wyman D (1973) Miniature eye movement. Science 181: 810–819.
53. Whittaker SG, Budd J, Cummings RW (1988) Eccentric fixation with macular scotoma. Investigative ophthalmology & visual science 29: 268–278.

## 4

Mediating Effect of Social Support on the Association between Functional Disability and Psychological Distress in Older Adults in Rural China: Does Age Make a Difference?

Danjun Feng[1], Linqin Ji[2], Lingzhong Xu[3]*

1 School of Nursing, Shandong University, Jinan, China, **2** School of Psychology, Shandong Normal University, Jinan, China, **3** Department of Health Services Management and Maternal & Child Healthcare, Shandong University, Jinan, China

Abstract

This study aimed to determine the prevalence of psychological distress among elderly people in rural China. Moreover, the mediating effect of social support on the association between functional disability and psychological distress and whether this effect varies with age would be examined. A total of 741 elderly people aged 60–89 years from a rural area of Shandong Province, China participated in a cross-sectional survey. Their psychological distress, perceived social support, enacted social support, and functional disability were assessed through questionnaires. A total of 217 (29.3%) rural elderly people had psychological distress. The functional disability of people ≥75 years old had smaller total effects (0.18) on their psychological distress than in people <75 years old (0.30). Moreover, most of the effects of functional disability on psychological distress among the people ≥75 years old were indirect (0.12; 66.67% of total effects) through the mediating effect of social support especially perceived support, while the direct effect of functional disability was insignificant. In contrast, most of the effects of functional disability on psychological distress among the people <75 years old were direct (0.29; 96.67% of total effects), while the mediating effect of social support was insignificant. In conclusion, the total effect of functional disability, especially the direct effect, on psychological distress decreases sharply with age. The mediating effect of social support on the association between functional disability and psychological distress varies with age and is only found in people ≥75 years.

Editor: Robert Stewart, Institute of Psychiatry, United Kingdom

Funding: This study was supported by the Ministry of Education in China, Project of Humanities and Social Sciences (grant No. 10YJCXLX007). The URL of its website is http://www.sinoss.net/. The funders had no role in study design, data collection and analysis, decision to publish, or preparation of the manuscript.

Competing Interests: The authors have declared that no competing interests exist.

* Email: lzxu@sdu.edu.cn

Introduction

The results of the latest National Census in 2010 indicate that China has the largest elderly population in the world, with 117.6 million people aged 60 and over, representing 13.26% of the total population of China and more than 20% of the world's total elderly population. In addition, China is projected to age much faster than Western countries in the near future: about 25% of the total population will be aged 60 and over by 2030 [1].

China is a typical agricultural country, with 60% of the elderly population living in rural areas. Traditionally, there have been large gaps between urban and rural areas in China with respect to economic and social development. China has had one of the highest urban–rural income ratios worldwide until recently [2]. Elderly people residing in rural areas have a much lower education level than their urban counterparts. Moreover, less-educated elderly Chinese people have higher levels of distress than their better-educated counterparts [3]. Thus, rural-dwelling elderly people in China usually have lower socioeconomic status than urban elderly people, and these conditions increase the rates of mental disorders [4].

Psychological distress is a nonspecific negative psychological state that includes combined feelings of anxiety and depression. In addition to being significantly associated with mental disorders [5], psychological distress also affects a greater percentage of the population than mental disorders. Whilst several studies have investigated the prevalence of pure anxiety or depression in rural older Chinese adults [6,7], no study has assessed their prevalence of psychological distress. The present study aims to fill this knowledge gap.

Elderly people in rural China have a higher prevalence of functional disability than their urban counterparts [8]. Functional disability is among the most significant risk factors for psychological distress [9,10]. Nevertheless, The effects of functional disability on one's psychological distress may vary as a function of the time or age when functional disability developed. The time which does not conform to socially based expectations of normative timing may be viewed as being "early" or "late" from a life course perspective [11]. These norms are likely to exacerbate the stress induced by functional disability by increasing their undesirability for individuals at younger stages of late life [12]. On the contrary, a higher prevalence of functional disability among age peers may

Table 1. Prevalence of psychological distress according to sociodemographic variables.

Groups	n(%)	Psychological distress(≥16)(n,%)	p
Age group			
Younger elderly (<75)	609(82.2)	176(28.9)	
Older elderly (≥75)	132(17.8)	41(31.1)	>0.05
Gender			
Men	396(53.4)	91(23.0)	
Women	345(46.6)	126(36.5)	<0.001
Education level			
No school education	393(53.0)	140(35.6)	
Primary school	221(29.8)	50(22.6)	
High school and college	127(17.1)	27(21.3)	<0.001
Marital status			
Widowed/single	145(19.6)	54(37.2)	
Married	596(80.4)	163(27.3)	<0.05
Total	741(100.0)	217(29.3)	

result in a greater desensitization to these problems among the older elderly group [13].Therefore, the effects of functional disability on distress may decrease with aging. However, current empirical evidence is inconsistent. One study supported this viewpoint and reported that increasing age reduces the strength of the association between functional disability and depression [14]. Another study reported that functional disability has a stronger effect on distress in older age in some people [15]. There was also one study which reported that age moderates the relationship between functional disability and depression only among elderly with higher perceived social support [16]. Therefore, the role of social support should be taken into account when studying the moderating effect of age on the relationship between functional disability and psychological distress.

The moderating or buffering effect of social support on the relationship between stressors including functional disability and mental health is well studied and supported [17,18]. However, its mediating effect is less studied. Results regarding the mediating effect of social support on the relationship between stressors and mental health are inconsistent. Ensel and Lin propose 2 models of this mediating effect [19]. One is called the "counteractive model," which assumes that stressors mobilize social support that suppresses the effects of stressors on distress. The other is called the "deterioration model," which postulates that stressors exhaust social support and thus support cannot continuously suppress the effects of stressors on distress. One study tested these 2 competing models in a sample of African-American college students, and supported the deterioration model [20]. In contrast, another study partly supported the counteractive model [21]. They found that stress leads to increased social support; however, only one type of social support (i.e., practical help) significantly reduced distress among widows. Yange reports that functional disability, as a specific stressor, leads to both higher instrumental social support and lower perceived social support [10]. However, only perceived social support was found to significantly affect a person's depression; this suggests that different types of social support have

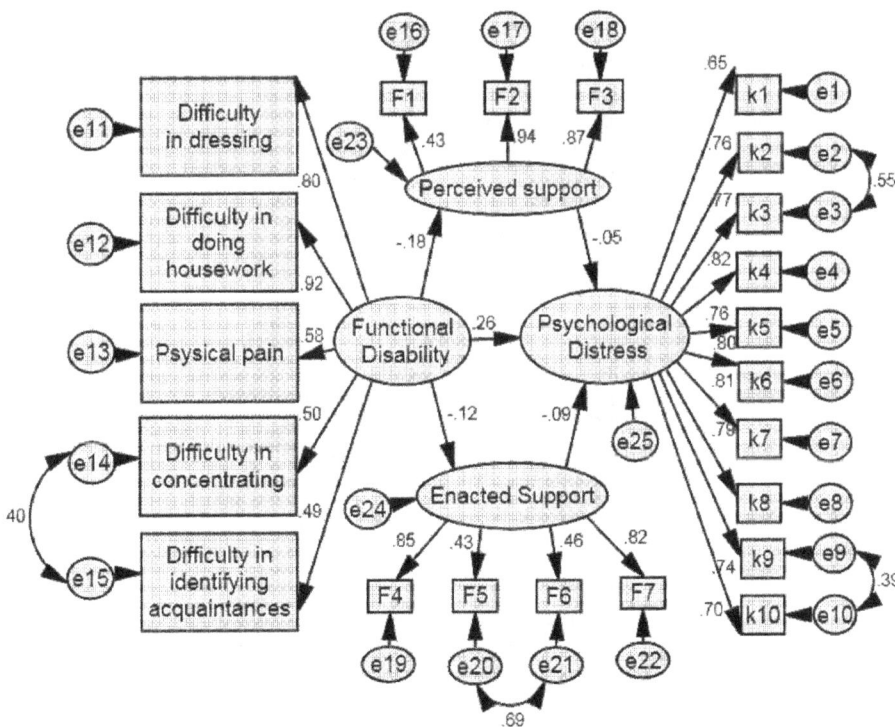

Figure 1. Results of SEM analysis among whole sample. All the coefficients are standardized. The path coefficient (−0.12) from functional disability to enacted support is significant at 0.01 level, that from enacted support (−0.09) to psychological distress are significant at 0.05 level, that from perceived support to psychological distress (−0.05) are not significant at 0.05 level and all other coefficients in the figure are significant at 0.001 level.

Table 2. Matrix of variables (means, standard deviations, ranges and correlations).

	M	SD	Range	1	2	3	4
1.Funtional disability	7.40	3.18	5.00–25.00	1			
2.Perceived social support	10.21	2.13	3.00–12.00	−0.14**	1		
3. Enacted social support	10.40	3.62	2.00–18.00	−0.12**	0.31**	1	
4.Psychological distress	14.67	6.68	10.00–44.00	0.29**	−0.14**	−0.13**	1

Note. **$p < 0.01$.

different mediating effects on the relationship between functional disability and psychological distress. Therefore, the present study also examined the mediating effects of 2 usual types of social support—perceived support and enacted support—on the association between functional disability and psychological distress, and whether these mediating effects vary by age among rural elderly Chinese.

Methods

Ethics Statement

Written informed consent was provided by all the participants, and the study was approved by the Ethics Committee of School of Public Health in Shandong University, P. R. China.

Participants

The participants were recruited from 3 counties in Dongying City, Shandong Province in Eastern China using 2-stage random sampling. In the first stage, 3 towns were randomly selected from each county for a total of 9 towns. By employing the same procedure, 3 villages from each town were sampled in the second stage. Finally, a total of 27 villages were sampled. All residents aged 60 and above in the sample villages were approached to be included in the study. As such subjects have great difficulties finishing the questionnaires independently because of their lower education level (only 17.1% have finished high school education), the investigators conducted face–to-face interviews using a structured questionnaire. A total of 741 valid questionnaires were obtained, representing an 87.18% response rate. The socio-demographic characteristics of the sample are presented in Table 1.

Measures

The Kessler 10 (K10) was used to assess nonspecific psychological distress. This instrument has previously exhibited excellent psychometric properties [5], and the Chinese version has also been proven to have good reliability and validity [22,23]. An example item is, "Have you often felt worn out without good reason in the past 30 days?" Responses are recorded on a 5-point scale ranging from 1 (never) to 5 (all the time); the total score is calculated by summing the responses. According to the Victorian Population Health Survey [24], scores >16 indicate moderate to serious psychological distress. The Cronbach's alpha of this instrument is 0.93.

Functional disability was assessed on the basis of 5 items reflecting difficulties in doing housework, dressing, physical pain, concentrating, and identifying acquaintances. An example item is, "Overall in the last 30 days, how much difficulty did you have with dressing yourself?" Responses were recorded on a 5-point scale ranging from 1 (none) to 5 (very much). The Cronbach's alpha of this instrument is 0.81.

Perceived social support was measured by 3 items inquiring about the participants' feelings about their relationships with friends, co-workers, and neighbors respectively. An example item is, "How do you feel about your relationships with your friends?" Responses were recorded on a 4-point scale ranging from 1 (never care for each other) to 4 (often care for each other). The Cronbach's alpha of this instrument is 0.74.

Enacted social support (i.e., support received from others) was measured by 4 items asking about the social support the participants have received. An example item is, "Where do you get financial assistance in emergencies?" Responses for these multiple-choice items included none, spouse, other family members, friends, relatives, workmates, employer, official or semi-

Table 3. Results for the direct and indirect effects of functional disability on psychological distress with social support as mediator.

Sample	n	Effects	Point estimate (%)	95% bias-corrected CI
Younger elderly	609	Direct effect	0.29(96.67)	(0.17, 040) ***
		Indirect effect	0.01(3.33)	(−0.00, 0.03)
		Total effect	0.30(100)	(0.18, 0.41) ***
Older elderly	132	Direct effect	0.06(33.33)	(−0.16, 0.27)
		Indirect effect	0.12(66.67)	(0.02, 0.27) *
		Total effect	0.18(100)	(0.00, 0.36) *
Whole sample	741	Direct effect	0.26(92.86)	(0.16, 0.37) ***
		Indirect effect	0.02(7.14)	(0.01, 0.05) *
		Total effect	0.28(100)	(0.18, 0.38) ***

Note. CI, confidence interval. Biased-corrected bootstrap with 2000 replications.
*p<0.05,
**p<0.01,
***p<0.001.

official agency, non-government organization, and others. These items were scored on the basis of the number of chosen sources of social support. The Cronbach's alpha of this instrument is 0.79.

Statistical analyses

Descriptive analyses were conducted to determine sociodemographic differences in the prevalence of psychological distress

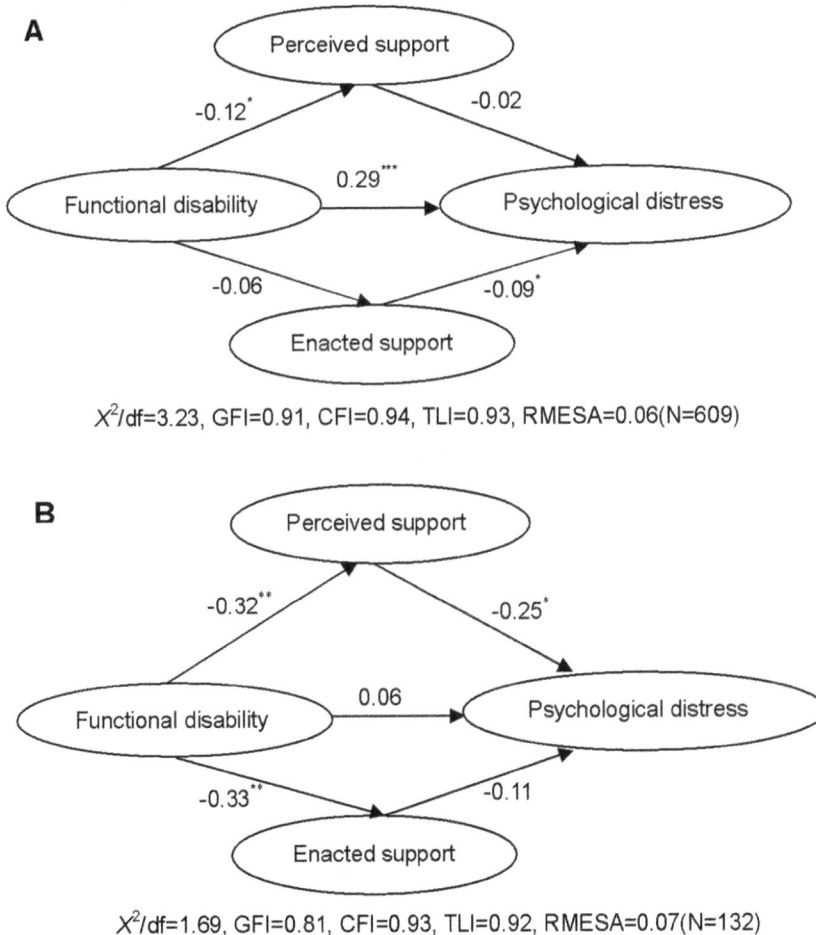

A

X^2/df=3.23, GFI=0.91, CFI=0.94, TLI=0.93, RMESA=0.06(N=609)

B

X^2/df=1.69, GFI=0.81, CFI=0.93, TLI=0.92, RMESA=0.07(N=132)

Figure 2. Results of SEM analysis among the people <75 years old (A) and the people ≥75 years old (B). All the coefficients in the figures are standardized. *p<0.05, **p<0.01,*** p<0.001.

Table 4. Goodness-of-fit statistics for the multiple group analysis.

Goodness-of-fit statistics	x^2(df)	P	Δx^2(df)	P	GFI	CFI	TLI	RMSEA
Model with no restrictions	985.61(400)	0			0.89	0.94	0.93	0.05
Model with restricted measurement weights	1024.08(418)	0	38.46(18)	<0.01	0.89	0.93	0.93	0.04
Model with restricted structural weights	1041.85(423)	0	17.77(5)	<0.01	0.89	0.93	0.93	0.04
Model with restricted structural covariance	1052.26(424)	0	10.42(1)	<0.001	0.88	0.93	0.93	0.05
Model with restricted structural residuals	1054.54(427)	0	2.28(3)	>0.05	0.88	0.93	0.93	0.05
Model with restricted measurement residuals	1199.71(453)	0	145.11(26)	<0.001	0.87	0.92	0.92	0.05

Note. GFI, goodness of fit index. CFI, comparative fit index. TLI, Tucker Lewis Index. RMSEA, root mean square error of approximation.

among elderly people in rural China. Then, Pearson product−moment correlations among functional disability, perceived social support, enacted social support, and psychological distress were calculated. All data were analyzed by SPSS version 18.0 (IBM Corporation, Armonk, NY, USA).

We also employed a structural equation modeling (SEM) approach with the bias-corrected bootstrap method (2,000 replicates) using AMOS version 18.0 (IBM Corporation, Armonk, NY, USA) to determine the influence of functional disability on psychological distress with social support as a mediator. SEM estimates both the direct and indirect effects a variable has on the outcome variables while simultaneously minimizing the effects of measurement error [25]. AMOS generates several indices to determine if the hypothesized model fits the observed data. The original method for assessing model fit is the χ^2 statistic. However, χ^2 is sensitive to sample size. Therefore, a normed χ^2chi-square (χ^2/df) was used to assess model fit; a good fit is indicated when $\chi^2/df<3$. Several other indices of model fit were also used in the analysis. the root mean square error of approximation(RMSEA)< 0.08 is acceptable and <0.05 is excellent. Goodness of Fit Index(GFI) should be >0.90 in a good-fitting model. Values of Comparative Fit Index (CFI) and the Tucker Lewis Index (TLI)> 0.90 are considered to indicate acceptable fit.

Finally, a multiple group analysis of SEM was conducted to test the invariance of the final model (see Figure 1) between participants divided into the younger and older elderly groups: <75 and ≥75 years, respectively. This analysis specifically imposes successive restrictions on the measurement weights, structural weights, structural covariance, structural residuals, and measurement residuals, forcing them to remain identical between the 2 age groups.

Results

The prevalence of psychological distress with respect to sociodemographic characteristics is shown in Table 1. A total of 29.3% of participants scored >16 on the K10, indicating moderate or serious psychological distress. Women (36.5%) reported higher psychological distress than men (23%; $\chi^2_{(1)} = 16.33$, $p<0.001$). Participants without any school education reported the highest psychological distress (35.6%). Married elderly (27.3%) had a lower prevalence of psychological distress than widowed or single participants (37.2%; $\chi^2_{(1)} = 5.51$, $p<0.05$). There was no significant association between age and the prevalence of psychological distress.

The correlations among functional disability, perceived social support, enacted social support, and psychological distress are presented in Table 2. Psychological distress was positively correlated with functional disability and inversely correlated with perceived social support and enacted social support.

The SEM analysis of the effect of functional disability on psychological distress with social support as a mediator among whole sample indicated that the data failed to support the theoretical model $(\chi^2/df=7.88$, $p<0.001$, RMSEA = 0.10, GFI = 0.83, CFI = 0.85, TLI = 0.83). In an attempt to develop a better-fitting model, post hoc modifications were performed with reference to the modification index. Several pairs of error terms were specifically correlated. As a result, the final model yielded a good fit of the data $(\chi^2/df = 3.56$, $p<0.001$, RMSEA = 0.06, GFI = 0.92, CFI = 0.94, TLI = 0.94). Functional disability had both, a significantly direct (0.26, $p<0.001$) and a minor but significant indirect (0.02, $p<0.05$) effect on psychological distress (Table 3 and Figure 1).

The multiple group analysis of SEM demonstrated that differences in goodness-of-fit statistics existed among the models with no restrictions, restricted measurement weights, restricted structural weights, and restricted structural covariance (see Table 4). This indicates that the relationships among functional disability, perceived social support, enacted social support, and psychological distress differ between the younger and older elderly groups. The results of SEM analyses of the effect of functional disability on psychological distress with social support as a mediator by age group (see Figure 2 and Table 3) demonstrated that functional disability exerted different effects on psychological distress via different paths in both groups. In general, functional disability had smaller total effects (0.18) on psychological distress in the older elderly group than the younger elderly group (0.30). In particular, most of the effects of functional disability on psychological distress among the elderly were indirect (0.12; 66.67% of total effects) for functional disability had a significant negative effect on both enacted support ($\beta = -0.33$, $p<0.01$) and perceived support ($\beta = -0.32$, $p<0.01$), with the latter leading to a significant decrease in psychological distress ($\beta = -0.25$, $p<0.05$). In contrast, although functional disability did not have a significant effect on enacted support ($\beta = -0.06$, $p>0.05$) and a significantly negative effect ($\beta = -0.12$, $p<0.05$) on perceived support, the latter had no significant effect ($\beta = -0.02$, $p>0.05$) on psychological distress. Hence, most of the effects of functional disability on psychological distress among the younger elderly group are direct (0.29; 96.67% of total effects), with the mediating effect of social support being insignificant.

Discussion

To our knowledge, this is the first study in China to report the prevalence of psychological distress among rural elderly using the K10. The rate of psychological distress (i.e., K10≥16) in the present study was 29.3%, which is equal to that reported in elderly Australian people (>65 years, including both rural and urban residents) [24].

Concordant with the literature [26], elderly women had a higher prevalence of psychological distress than elderly men. The elderly people with less education reported the highest psychological distress, which is also consistent with a previous report [3]. There was no difference in the prevalence of psychological distress among rural elderly people with respect to age, which is also consistent with a recent study in Japan [27].

Unsurprisingly, functional disability had a significantly positive effect on psychological distress in both age groups when the indirect effects mediated by social support were taken into account. However, if only the direct effect is considered, the influence of functional disability on psychological distress in the older elderly group became insignificant. Even taking into account the indirect effects mediated by social support, the psychological distress of the older elderly group was less influenced by functional disability than that in the younger elderly group. These results are concordant with a study in America that also found a decreasing relationship between functional disability and depression with increasing age [14].

The mediating effect of social support on the relationship between functional disability and psychological distress only existed in the older elderly group. The functional disability of the older elderly people led to significant decreases in both perceived support and enacted support; however, only perceived support exerted a significant protective effect on mental health. These results partly support the deterioration model. However, in the younger elderly group, functional disability only reduced perceived support, which did not significantly affect psychological distress. These results indicate that the mediating effect of social support on the relationship between functional disability and distress varies with age. Interestingly, the present results show increasing age is associated with greater damage to social support caused by functional disability. Moreover, in younger elderly people, enacted support appears to play a more important role in protecting mental health than perceived support. In contrast, in older elderly people, perceived support appears to play a more important role in protecting mental health than enacted support. Nevertheless, further studies are required to confirm these findings before drawing conclusions.

Four pairs of error terms were significantly correlated in the SEM analysis (see Figure 1). In general, correlations among error terms should be interpreted cautiously. However, this practice is acceptable when supported by a strong theoretical framework [28]. Both items K9 ("how often do you feel that nothing can interest you?") and K10 ("how often do you feel bored?") are related to depressive personality; therefore, the correlation of their error terms is theoretically reasonable.

The present study has some limitations. The first limitation is related to the study's methodology. Because of the study's cross-sectional design, the causal paths in the model are still based on hypothetical relationships. Hence, a longitudinal study is required to ascertain causal relationships among variables. Second, all participants in the present study were from Dongying City, Shandong Province. Therefore, the sample is not representative of other rural regions in China considering China's vast size. Thus, further research with participants from a wider range of regions is required to determine the generalizability of the results to elderly people from other rural areas in China. Furthermore, in the current study, the direct effect of functional disability on psychological distress may operate through some variables which have not been measured and future studies are needed to explore these variables.

In conclusion, the total effect—especially the direct effect—of functional disability on psychological distress decreases sharply with age. The mediating effect of social support on the association between functional disability and psychological distress varies with age and is only found in people aged ≥75 years.

Author Contributions

Conceived and designed the experiments: LX DF. Performed the experiments: DF. Analyzed the data: DF. Contributed reagents/materials/analysis tools: LX DF. Wrote the paper: DF LJ.

References

1. He W, Sengupta M, Zhang K, Guo P (2007) Health and health care of the older population in urban and rural China: 2000.Washington, DC: U.S Government Printing Office.

2. Sicular T, Ximing Y, Gustafsson B, Shi L (2007) The urban–rural income gap and inequality in China. Review Income Wealth 53: 93–126.

3. Ross CE, Zhang W (2008) Education and psychological distress among older Chinese. J Aging Health 20: 273–289.

4. Hudson C (2005) Socioeconomic status and mental illness: tests of the social causation and selection hypotheses. Am J Orthopsychiatry 75: 3–18.

5. Kessler RC, Barker PR, Colpe LJ, Epstein JF, Gfroerer JC, et al. (2003) Screening for serious mental illness in the general population. Arch Gen Psychiatry 60: 184–189.

6. Chen R, Wei L, Hu Z, Qin X, Copeland JRM, et al. (2005) Depression in older people in rural China. Arch Intern Med 165: 2019–2025.

7. Prina AM, Ferri CP, Guerra M, Brayne C, Prince M (2011) Prevalence of anxiety and its correlates among older adults in Latin America, India and China: cross-cultural study. Br J Psychiatry 199: 485–491.

8. Liu J, Chi I, Chen G, Song X, Zheng X (2009) Prevalence and correlates of functional disability in Chinese older adults. Geriatr Gerontol Int 9: 253–261.

9. Vaeroy H, Tanum L, Bruaset H, Morkrid L, Forre O (2005) Symptoms of depression and anxiety in functionally disabled rheumatic pain patients. Nord J Psychiatry 59: 109–113.

10. Yang Y (2006) How does functional disability affect depressive symptoms in late life? The role of perceived social support and psychological resources. J Health Soc Behav 47: 355–372.

11. Elder Jr GH, Johnson MK, Crosnoe R (2003) The emergence and development of life course theory. In: Mortimer JT, Shanahan MJ, editors. Handbook of the life course. New York: Kluwer Academic/Plenum. pp. 3–19.

12. Schieman S, Turner HA (1998) Age, disability, and the sense of mastery. J Health Soc Behav 39:169–186.

13. Jang Y, Poon LW, Martin P (2004) Individual differences in the effect of disease and disability on depressive symptoms: The role of age and subjective health. Int J Aging Hum Dev 59: 125–137.

14. Schnittker J (2005) Chronic illness and depressive symptoms in late life. Soc Sci Med 60: 13–23.

15. Jang Y, Borenstein AR, Chiriboga DA, Mortimer JA (2005) Depressive symptoms among African American and white older adults. J Gerontol B Psychol Sci Soc Sci 60B: P313–P319.

16. Bierman A, Statland D (2010) Timing, social support, and the effects of physical limitations on psychological distress in late life. J Gerontol B Psychol Sci Soc Sci 65B: 631–639.

17. Barrera M (1986) Distinction between social support concepts, measures, and models. Am J Community Psychol 14: 413–445.

18. Suttajit S, Punpuing S, Jirapramukpitak T, Tangchonlatip K, Darawuttimapra-korn N, et al. (2010) Impairment, disability, social support and depression among older parents in rural Thailand. Psychol Med 40: 1711–1721.

19. Ensel WM, Lin N (1991) The life stress paradigm and psychological distress. J Health Soc Behav 32: 321–341.

20. Prelow HM, Mosher CE, Bowman MA (2006) Perceived racial discrimination, social support, and psychological adjustment among African American college students. J Black Psychol 32: 442–454.

21. Miller NB, Smerglia VL, Gaudet DS, Kitson GC (1998) Stressful life events, social support, and the distress of widowed and divorced women: a counteractive model. J Fam Issues 19: 181–203.

22. Zhou C, Chu J, Wang T, Peng Q, He J, et al. (2008) Reliability and validity of 10-item Kessler scale (K10) Chinese version in evaluation of mental health status of Chinese population (in Chinese). Chin J Clin Psychol 16: 627–629.

23. Huang JP, Xia W, Sun CH, Zhang HY, Wu LJ (2009) Psychological distress and its correlates in Chinese adolescents. Aust N Z J Psychiatry 43:674–681.

24. Department of Human Services (2008) Victorian Population Health Survey 2007. Melbourne, Victoria: Department of Human Services.

25. Briere J, Hodges M, Godbout N (2010) Traumatic stress, affect dysregulation, and dysfunctional avoidance: a structural equation model. J Trauma Stress 23: 767–774.

26. Kuriyama S, Nakaya N, Ohmori-Matsuda K, Shimazu T, Kikuchi N, et al. (2009) Factors associated with psychological distress in a community-dwelling Japanese population: the Ohsaki cohort 2006 study. J Epidemiol 19: 294–302.

27. Hamano T, Yamasaki M, Fujisawa Y, Ito K, Nabika T, et al. (2011) Social capital and psychological distress of elderly in Japanese rural communities. Stress Health 27: 163–169.

28. Hooper D, Coughlan J, Mullen M (2008) Structural equation modelling guidelines for determining model fit. Electron J Bus Res Meth 6: 53–60.

## 5

Determinants of Receiving the Pandemic (H1N1) 2009 Vaccine and Intention to Receive the Seasonal Influenza Vaccine in Taiwan

Ta-Chien Chan[1], Yang-chih Fu[2], Da-Wei Wang[3], Jen-Hsiang Chuang[4,5]*

1 Research Center for Humanities and Social Sciences, Academia Sinica, Taipei, Taiwan, Republic of China, 2 Institute of Sociology, Academia Sinica, Taipei, Taiwan, Republic of China, 3 Institute of Information Science, Academia Sinica, Taipei, Taiwan, Republic of China, 4 Deputy Director-General's Office, Centers for Disease Control, Taipei, Taiwan, Republic of China, 5 Institute of Public Health, National Yang-Ming University, Taipei, Taiwan, Republic of China

Abstract

Objectives: The paper examines the factors associated with both receiving pandemic (H1N1) 2009 vaccines and individuals' intentions to get the next seasonal influenza vaccine in Taiwan.

Methods: We conducted a representative nationwide survey with in-person household interviews during April–July 2010. Multivariate logistic regression incorporated socio-demographic background, household characteristics, health status, behaviors, and perceptions of influenza and vaccination.

Results: We completed interviews with 1,954 respondents. Among those, 548 (28.0%) received the pandemic (H1N1) 2009 vaccination, and 469 (24.0%) intended to get the next seasonal influenza vaccine. Receipt of the H1N1 vaccine was more prevalent among schoolchildren, the elderly, those who had contact with more people in their daily lives, and those who had received influenza vaccinations in previous years. In comparison, the intention to receive the next seasonal influenza vaccine tended to be stronger among children, the elderly, and those who reported less healthy status or lived with children, who received a seasonal influenza vaccination before, and who worried more about a possible new pandemic.

Conclusions: Children, the elderly, and those who had gotten seasonal flu shots before in Taiwan were more likely to both receive a pandemic H1N1 vaccination and intend to receive a seasonal influenza vaccine.

Editor: Mohammed Alsharifi, The University of Adelaide, Australia

Funding: This work was supported in part by the grants DOH99-DC-1004 and DOH101-DC-1011 from the Centers for Disease Control, Ministry of Health and Welfare, Taiwan, Republic of China. The funders had no role in study design, data collection and analysis, decision to publish, or preparation of the manuscript.

Competing Interests: The authors have declared that no competing interests exist.

* Email: jhchuang@cdc.gov.tw

Introduction

Epidemic and pandemic influenza infections cause tremendous social impacts in addition to generating serious threats to the health and lives of the global population [1,2]. To reduce such threats and impacts, governments have implemented or promoted two primary public-health approaches to prevent and control influenza: a pharmaceutical approach such as vaccinations [3] and anti-viral drugs [4], and a non-pharmaceutical approach such as self-protective behavior [5] and social distancing [6]. As is the case with many other diseases, prevention always yields better outcomes than controlling the epidemic afterwards. Among current prevention policies, influenza vaccinations for children and the elderly have proven to be a highly cost-effective method to prevent people from getting severe influenza illnesses [7,8]. Other high-risk subpopulations, such as healthcare workers, poultry workers, and people with chronic diseases, are also among the priority groups to receive influenza vaccines.

Due to the limited budget for purchasing influenza vaccines and for other reasons, vaccination coverage rates vary widely across countries. According to surveys in 11 European countries during the 2007/08 influenza season [9], for example, coverage rates ranged from 9.5% to 28.7% among the general population, from 13.9% to 70.2% among the elderly, and from 4.2% to 19.3% among children. In the non-western countries that have implemented various policies related to prevention and control of influenza, the vaccine coverage rate has been a key issue, while policy-makers strive to keep a reasonable balance between effective coverage and cost-effectiveness.

In Taiwan, government-funded influenza vaccinations started in 1998, when the coverage rate among the elderly was only 9.9% [10]. As in many other countries, Taiwan's annual budget for purchasing the influenza vaccine is too limited to cover the whole population. The influenza vaccination policy in Taiwan has gradually expanded from high-risk populations to key spreaders to further reduce the number of cases and deaths. Therefore, the government announces the priority groups for vaccinations every year based on recommendations from the Advisory Committee on Immunization Practices (ACIP).

High-risk subpopulations have a chance to receive vaccinations free of charge beginning in October of each year. Because such

Table 3. Multivariate logistic regression for covariates of receiving pandemic (H1N1) 2009 vaccination.

Variables	Multivariate Analysis		
	Odds Ratio	95% CI	p-value
Age groups			
0–18	23.5	11.8–46.8	<0.001
19–35	1 (Reference)		
36–50	1.5	0.9–2.3	0.128
51–64	1.3	0.8–2.2	0.331
65 & older	2.2	1.2–4.0	0.007
Working status			
Pre-school	0.2	0.1–0.4	<0.001
Students	1.3	0.6–2.8	0.457
Work	1.0	0.6–1.5	0.973
Unemployed	1 (Reference)		
Previous vaccination against seasonal influenza	6.4	4.7–8.9	<0.001
Contact diary			
# people> = 10	1.4	1.0–1.8	0.043

Asking about Vaccination: Behaviors and Intentions

We asked our respondents both "Have you received a pandemic (H1N1) 2009 vaccination?" and "Will you receive a seasonal influenza vaccination this coming flu season?" The answer to the pandemic (H1N1) 2009 vaccination was simply either Yes or No. For the seasonal influenza vaccination, we pooled the original answers into a dichotomy, indicating the intention to receive the vaccination (including "definitely will" and "probably will") or not to receive the vaccination (including "probably will not," "definitely will not," and "don't know").

Socio-demographic and household characteristics

We used such socio-demographic variables as gender, age groups, education status, and work status as the adjusted confounders in the models. The classifications of age groups differed in the two analyses because the vaccination policy assigned different priority groups for the pandemic (H1N1) 2009 and regular seasonal influenza in Taiwan. The survey did not track household members' vaccination history. Nor did it ask these members about their intentions toward vaccination. As an alternative, we examined whether one's cohabitants included someone who belonged to a high-risk subpopulation or was a medical professional. In the analysis, we examine whether respondents' behaviors and intentions regarding influenza vaccination vary by the number of contacts, the percentage of bodily contacts, the number of household members, the numbers of children and the elderly, and whether someone in the household worked in the medical industry.

To compare high and low frequencies of the number of household members and contact number, and partly to simplify the analyses, we selected the median values as the thresholds. Variables used for the household included whether the number of household members was equal to or larger than 5 (median = 4), whether there was any household member with a medical background, and whether there was any household member under age 12 or over age 65. Furthermore, we constructed two measures from the contact diaries to indicate contact intensity: whether the number of contacts with people within the past 24

hours was equal to or larger than 10 (median = 9), and the percentage of bodily contacts among all contacts within 24 hours.

Health status, behaviors, and perceptions

We also took into account several other factors that might affect the behaviors of receiving and intentions to receive influenza vaccinations. The self-reported health condition reflected how respondents perceived their health condition in general. We recoded the answering categories, from 1 to 5, into: poor, fair, good, very good, and excellent, so that a higher score always indicates a better health condition. How often one went to public places (from 1 "almost never" to 5 "almost every day") serves as a proxy indicator of exposure to the influenza virus from human gatherings and environmental contamination. Watching intense political talk shows about the adverse effects of influenza vaccination may affect how one perceives the safety of vaccinations, which in turn may influence individuals' intentions and subsequent behaviors. Both the perception of the severity of the (H1N1) 2009 pandemic in Taiwan and the level of worry about a new pandemic serve as measurements of risk perception. Respondents' past experience of influenza vaccinations could also be an important factor: If respondents had received influenza vaccination at least once in the past five years, we coded their experience as 1, and those with no vaccination were coded as 0.

Statistical analysis

We first used Pearson's chi-square test to compare the categorical variables' frequency distributions, and the Wilcoxon rank-sum test to compare the continuous variables' medians in the two separate analyses, one about the pandemic (H1N1) 2009 vaccination, and the other about the intention to receive a seasonal influenza vaccination. Due to different age limits set for government-funded vaccination plans, we used age groups under age 18 in two ways (ages 0–10 and ages 0–18) when analyzing who received the pandemic H1N1 vaccination and who intended to get the seasonal influenza vaccine. For the pandemic (H1N1) 2009 vaccine, all children under age 18 belonged to the priority group for free vaccination (Table 1). For the seasonal influenza vaccine,

Table 4. Selected variables associated with intention to get seasonal influenza vaccines.

Variables	Do not intend to get vaccine		Intend to get vaccine		p-value
	n = 1,485		n = 469		
Gender, no.(%)					0.407
Male	764	(51.5)	231	(49.3)	
Female	721	(48.6)	238	(50.8)	
Age groups, no. (%)					<0.001
0–10	134	(9.0)	108	(23.0)	
11–18	180	(12.1)	62	(13.2)	
19–35	404	(27.2)	49	(10.5)	
36–50	353	(23.8)	60	(12.8)	
51–64	300	(20.2)	54	(11.5)	
65 & older	114	(7.7)	136	(29.0)	
Education, no. (%)					<0.001
Elementary	366	(24.7)	258	(55.0)	
High school	630	(42.5)	128	(27.3)	
College or higher	486	(32.8)	83	(17.7)	
Working status, no. (%)					<0.001
Pre-school	78	(5.3)	61	(13.0)	
Students	298	(20.1)	114	(24.3)	
Work	766	(51.6)	150	(32.0)	
Unemployed	342	(23.1)	144	(30.7)	
Self-reported health status, median (IQR)	3	(2–4)	2	(2–4)	0.055
Frequency of visiting public place, median (IQR)	4	(3–5)	4	(3–5)	0.964
Habit of watching political talk shows, no. (%)	485	(32.7)	124	(26.4)	0.011
Perception of severity of pandemic in 2009, median (IQR)	3	(2–3)	3	(2–3)	0.436
Level of worry about new pandemic, median (IQR)	3	(2–3)	3	(2–3)	0.005
Previous vaccination against seasonal influenza, no. (%)	194	(13.1)	357	(76.1)	<0.001
Household, no. (%)					
# members>=5	593	(39.9)	218	(46.5)	0.012
with med. background	130	(8.8)	57	(12.2)	0.029
someone under age 12	460	(31.0)	180	(38.4)	0.003
someone over age 65	395	(26.6)	162	(34.5)	0.001
Contact diary					
# people>=10, no. (%)	742	(50.3)	249	(53.3)	0.251
% bodily contact, median (IQR)	0.25	(0.1–0.8)	0.33	(0.1–0.7)	<0.001

IQR interquartile range (25th percentile–75th percentile).

only children under 10 (up to grade 4 schoolchildren) were on the priority list.

We selected the variables that had a p-value less than 0.2 for the stepwise multivariate logistic regression to determine the factors associated with receiving pandemic (H1N1) 2009 vaccines and the intention to get influenza shots in the next season and to estimate their adjusted odds ratios (AOR) with 95% confidence intervals (CI) as well. The selection criterion of p-value used for both the chi-square test and the Wilcoxon rank sum test served to filter out the variables unrelated to the dependent variables [25]. To assess the performance of the final multivariate model, we used the Hosmer-Lemeshow goodness-of-fit test and the area under the receiver operating characteristic (ROC) to measure calibration and discrimination, respectively. A two-sided p-value of less than 0.05 was considered statistically significant. All statistical analyses

were performed with Stata (StataCorp LP, College Station, TX). The summarized list of the variables and their responses in this study are shown in Table S1.

Results

The survey data of this study were collected during April–July 2010, immediately after the (H1N1) 2009 pandemic in Taiwan. We finished the survey with 1,954 cases of individual questionnaires and 1,943 24-hour contact diaries, at a response rate of 51%. There were 548 (28.0%) respondents having received pandemic (H1N1) 2009 vaccines and 469 (24.0%) persons classified as intending to get seasonal influenza vaccines in the next season, respectively.

Table 5. Multivariate logistic regression for covariates of intention to get seasonal influenza vaccines.

Variables	Multivariate Analysis		
	Odds Ratio	95% CI	p-value
Age groups			
0–10	2.4	1.5–4.0	0.001
11–18	1.4	0.8–2.3	0.208
19–35	1 (Reference)		
36–50	1.3	0.8–2.0	0.323
51–64	1.3	0.8–2.0	0.403
65 & older	3.0	1.8–4.9	<0.001
Self-reported health status	0.9	0.8–1.0	0.050
Level of worry about new pandemic	1.3	1.1–1.5	0.003
Previous vaccination against seasonal influenza	16.1	11.9–21.5	<0.001
Household			
someone under age 12	1.4	1.0–1.9	0.030

Factors on receiving a pandemic (H1N1) 2009 vaccination

The socio-demographic variables, such as age group, education, and working status, all turned out to be significant factors in distinguishing between those who received a pandemic (H1N1) 2009 vaccination and those who did not (all p<0.001, Table 2). The youngest age group (i.e., 0–18 years old) had the highest vaccination rate (65.7%; 318/484), because they were the priority groups, and all schoolchildren received school-based pandemic (H1N1) 2009 vaccination services. Respondents with better self-reported health condition, higher frequency of visiting public places, and higher risk perception of the 2009 pandemic and future pandemics were all more likely to receive a pandemic (H1N1) 2009 vaccination (details in Table S2). In contrast, respondents who had a habit of watching political talk shows were less likely to receive a pandemic (H1N1) 2009 vaccination. If respondents believed that the pandemic in 2009 was serious, or had the past experiences of getting seasonal influenza shots, they were also more likely to get the pandemic (H1N1) 2009 shot. In addition, higher percentages of receiving pandemic (H1N1) 2009 vaccinations prevailed among those who lived in a large household (with at least 5 members), who had contacts with more people (≥ 10 persons) during the past 24 hours, and who had more bodily contact with individuals out of these daily contacts.

In the final model of the multivariate logistic regression (Table 3), higher percentages of children (ages 0–18, AOR: 23.5; 95% CI: 11.8–46.8) and the elderly (AOR: 2.2; 95% CI: 1.2–4.0) received pandemic (H1N1) 2009 vaccination than adults ages 19–35 years. When we examine respondents' study or work statuses, pre-schoolers had the lowest probability of getting the pandemic (H1N1) 2009 vaccination (AOR: 0.2; 95% CI: 0.1–0.4). Respondents with past influenza vaccination experiences had more opportunities to get pandemic (H1N1) 2009 vaccinations (AOR: 6.4; 95% CI: 4.7–8.9). Respondents who had contact with more people (≥ 10 persons) in one day were more likely to prefer getting pandemic (H1N1) 2009 vaccines (AOR: 1.4; 95% CI: 1.0–1.8). The overall ROC of the model was 86.4%, and the results of the Hosmer-Lemeshow goodness-of-fit test showed that the data were well fitted by the model (p = 0.24).

Factors on the intention to receive seasonal influenza vaccines

Socio-demographic variables, such as age group, education, and working status, were all significant factors (p<0.001) affecting respondents' decisions to receive seasonal influenza vaccines (Table 4). The major groups with no intention to get seasonal influenza vaccines were adults, those having a high-school educational level, and workers. Respondents who watch political talk shows preferred not to receive seasonal influenza vaccines. If respondents perceived higher levels of worry about future pandemics or had previous experiences in receiving the seasonal influenza vaccination, they were willing to get a seasonal influenza vaccine in the coming influenza season. Regarding household characteristics, those in larger households (household members ≥ 5), households having members with a medical background, and those having members under age 12 or over 65 were more willing to receive seasonal influenza vaccines. Respondents with more bodily contacts in a single day were also more willing to receive seasonal influenza vaccines.

In the final model of the multivariate logistic regression (Table 5), children (ages 0–10 years, AOR: 2.4; 95% CI: 1.5–4.0) and the elderly (AOR: 3.0; 95% CI: 1.8–4.9) were more willing to get seasonal influenza vaccines than adults ages 19–35 years. Respondents who reported being healthier were less likely to get seasonal influenza vaccines (AOR: 0.9; 95% CI: 0.8–1.0). Those who worried the most about a new pandemic (AOR: 1.3; 95% CI: 1.1–1.5) and who had previously received a seasonal influenza vaccination (AOR: 16.1; 95% CI: 11.9–21.5) were more willing to get the next seasonal influenza vaccine. If someone in the household was under age 12, respondents were more likely to receive seasonal influenza vaccines (AOR: 1.4; 95% CI: 1.0–1.9). The overall ROC of the model was 85.1%, and the results of the Hosmer-Lemeshow goodness-of-fit test showed that the data were well fitted by the model (p = 0.81).

Discussion

In this study, we have explored the factors that influenced whether the general public received pandemic (H1N1) 2009 vaccinations and, at the same time, their intentions to get seasonal influenza vaccines in the coming influenza season. Most current surveys have separated the actual vaccination factors and intentions into different surveys [26,27], and thus the possibility of making comparisons between them is limited or unlikely. Furthermore, the percentage of those getting pandemic (H1N1) 2009 vaccines (28.0%) in this study was very close to the coverage rate (24.6%) reported by the IVIS. Although pandemic (H1N1) 2009 vaccinations covered a greater portion of the population than seasonal influenza vaccinations in Taiwan, our study showed that previous influenza vaccination experience [13,15,28], priority groups with government-funded vaccines (such as children and the elderly), and school-based vaccination programs played crucial roles in both receiving pandemic vaccinations and intention to receive vaccines.

One study on pandemic (H1N1) 2009 vaccination intention in Taiwan [16] showed that those who intended to get pandemic (H1N1) 2009 vaccines tended to be males, young adults (ages 18–24 years), the elderly, and those living in households with a mid-range monthly income (USD$ 1,667–3,333). It showed that 75.3% of the respondents ages 18–24 years, who were mostly college students, intended to get the pandemic (H1N1) vaccination. In comparison, respondents ages 25–44 had the weakest intentions to get the pandemic (H1N1) vaccination. According to the vaccination plan (the left column of Table 1), adults ages 19–24 years were one of the targeted groups (albeit among the last three) of government-funded pandemic (H1N1) vaccinations. Thus, the high intention within this group might be due to the promotion of free vaccinations.

The actual pandemic (H1N1) vaccination rate in the 19–35 age group, however, was only 9.27% (42 out of 453) in our study, which was the lowest vaccination rate among all age groups. The fact that few young adults got pandemic (H1N1) shots might be due to the passing of the pandemic peak (Nov. 22–Nov. 28, 2009) before they were eligible to get immunized [29]. A similarly low influenza vaccination rate among college students was also found in Hong Kong [30].

The previous study in Taiwan [16] also showed that those who intended to receive pandemic (H1N1) 2009 vaccines were more likely to perceive the pandemic as being more severe, to believe the H1N1 vaccine is more effective, and to foresee a lower barrier to receiving vaccinations in general. Unlike this previous study, gender was not a significant factor for receiving pandemic (H1N1) 2009 vaccines according to our findings. The elderly group and respondents who perceived higher pandemic risk, however, also had higher intention to receive seasonal influenza vaccines, which is similar to findings in Huang et al. for Taiwan [16] and Liao et al. for Hong Kong [31]. In other words, if respondents perceived their health status as good, they had lower intention to receive a seasonal influenza vaccine.

Compared with schoolchildren, pre-school children (ages ≤ 6 years) were found to have a lower pandemic (H1N1) vaccination rate. The possible reasons might be accessibility and concerns about vaccine safety. During the pandemic period, the vaccination campaign was implemented in all school settings (including elementary, middle, and high schools), which made the campaign more efficient and extensive. It was hard to reach pre-school children without parents' help, however. The other potential concern was the safety of the pandemic influenza vaccines for young children. One review study in Europe found that the vaccine effectiveness was moderate to good, and that the safety of non-adjuvanted trivalent inactivated influenza vaccines was excellent among children [32]. In addition, the vaccination among children was also a cost-effective approach for preventing influenza disease burden [33]. How to enhance pre-school

children's vaccination coverage rate will be an ongoing challenge for public-health workers.

There were some concerns related to the validity of the responses from the children under age 8. In our survey, we instructed the interviewers that "if the targeted respondents were under age 8, all interviews and records must be answered and taken by a parent or a guardian." So the information obtained under such circumstances refer to that received from the parent. In addition, because Taiwan's civil law stipulates that children under age 8 lack behavioral competence, the acceptance of vaccination must be decided by a parent or guardian.

We included all age groups in the analysis, because the priority groups for free influenza vaccinations were set mostly by age limits, and young children are often a top priority. To verify that the results were not altered by the inclusion of young children, we conducted a separate analysis on the respondents under age 8. There were 168 respondents in this subsample (i.e., ages 0–7, about 8.6% of the full sample). The results from the analysis of this subsample in terms of both receiving the pandemic (H1N1) 2009 vaccination and intention to get the seasonal influenza vaccine showed that only receipt of the previous seasonal influenza vaccination was a significant explanatory factor (for receiving the pandemic 2009 vaccination, odds ratio = 4.01, 95% CI: 1.8–9.2, p<.001; for intention to take the next seasonal influenza vaccine, odds ratio = 8.75, 95% CI: 3.6–21.5, p<.001). Because such results are identical to those from the full sample, the inclusion of young children under age 8 in the models did not distort the analysis.

From the viewpoint of vaccination policy, it was desirable to examine why some respondents received either the pandemic (H1N1) 2009 vaccine or past seasonal influenza vaccines but did not intend to receive the next seasonal influenza vaccine. To explore the possible reasons, we summarized the differences in the respondents' characteristics in Table S3. It was of interest to find that respondents ages 11–18 had the highest percentage of those deciding not to get seasonal influenza vaccination. A possible reason might be that this age group was not a routine priority group for the seasonal influenza vaccination. One study in the United States also found that vaccination rate decreased with age, with high-school students having the lowest vaccination rate and elementary schoolchildren having the highest rate [34]. Perceiving good health status and frequently visiting public places were two factors linked to the intention not to get the next seasonal influenza vaccination. However, 87.0% of respondents with both pandemic (H1N1) vaccination and previous seasonal influenza vaccination experience intended to get the next seasonal influenza vaccination.

People with more contacts were more likely to get pandemic (H1N1) 2009 vaccines. A direct explanation for this phenomenon was not found in previous literature. Indirect evidence from Europe, however, indicated that vaccination target populations, such as the elderly, healthcare workers, and people suffering with chronic illness, would like to get seasonal influenza vaccines because they do not want to infect their friends and family [35]. Similar observations were also found in our results (Table 4). If the number of household members was equal to or larger than 5, the household included a member with a medical background, or someone in the household was under age 12 or over age 65, individuals had higher intention to receive seasonal influenza vaccines.

One interesting finding from this study was the negative effect of the habit of watching political talk shows on either receipt of the pandemic (H1N1) 2009 vaccination or intention to receive a seasonal influenza vaccine. During the pandemic (H1N1) 2009 vaccination in November 2009, some negative discussions on the safety of the vaccine were featured on TV political talk shows every day. That might partially explain why those respondents were less likely to get a pandemic (H1N1) 2009 vaccine or had a lower intention to receive seasonal influenza vaccine. One study in Canada also found that having negative beliefs about the pandemic (H1N1) 2009 vaccine and deciding not to be vaccinated were highly correlated [36].

There were some limitations in this study. The study was initiated right after the 2009/10 flu season. The acceptance of pandemic (H1N1) 2009 vaccinations might not be the same as the acceptance of seasonal influenza vaccine, due to differing perceptions of disease risk. The pandemic (H1N1) 2009 vaccination rate approximated the official coverage rate among the whole population. Therefore, the representativeness of the data could be assured. In Taiwan, most government-funded influenza vaccines were targeted on the priority populations. Therefore, some socio-demographic factors, such as age or working status, were also highly related to the specific population. In future studies, understanding the factors affecting healthy adults' decisions to get influenza vaccinations at their own expense would be beneficial for health education.

Conclusions

To our knowledge, this was the first study to compare the factors of pandemic (H1N1) 2009 vaccination and intentions to receive seasonal influenza vaccine at the same time. Since children, the elderly, and those with previous vaccination experiences are more likely both to have received pandemic vaccines and to intend to receive seasonal influenza vaccines, the school-based vaccination program and government-funded vaccines for the priority groups play crucial roles for promoting influenza vaccination in Taiwan. Successful vaccination campaigns during annual influenza seasons will be strong support for promoting the acceptance and delivery of novel influenza vaccines during pandemic periods. Perceptions of pandemic or worries

about friends or family being infected are related to people's intention to receive influenza vaccinations. Thus, prompt and clear risk communication about an influenza epidemic or pandemic through mass media can help generate the correct perception of the disease among the public and enhance acceptance of the vaccine.

Supporting Information

Table S1 Summary of variables and response categories.

Table S2 The four ordinal variables associated with receipt of pandemic (H1N1) 2009 vaccination in Table 2.

Table S3 Differences in characteristics of the respondents who received influenza vaccination but decided not to get the next seasonal influenza vaccination. (A) Respondents who got pandemic (H1N1) influenza vaccination but decided not to get the next seasonal influenza vaccination (N = 548). (B) Respondents who got at least one seasonal influenza vaccination in the past five years but did not intend to get the next seasonal influenza vaccination (N = 551).

Acknowledgments

We thank Szu-Ying Lee for helping with data collection and analyses.

Author Contributions

Conceived and designed the experiments: YCF JHC. Performed the experiments: YCF. Analyzed the data: TCC DWW. Contributed reagents/materials/analysis tools: YCF JHC. Wrote the paper: TCC YCF DWW JHC.

References

1. Szucs TD, Nichol K, Meltzer M, Hak E, Chancelor J, et al. (2006) Economic and social impact of epidemic and pandemic influenza. Vaccine 24: 6776–6778.
2. Nair H, Brooks WA, Katz M, Roca A, Berkley JA, et al. (2011) Global burden of respiratory infections due to seasonal influenza in young children: a systematic review and meta-analysis. Lancet 378: 1917–1930.
3. Tricco AC, Chit A, Soobiah C, Hallett D, Meier G, et al. (2013) Comparing influenza vaccine efficacy against mismatched and matched strains: a systematic review and meta-analysis. BMC Medicine 11: 153.
4. Lugner AK, Mylius SD, Wallinga J (2010) Dynamic versus static models in cost-effectiveness analyses of anti-viral drug therapy to mitigate an influenza pandemic. Health Economics 19: 518–531.
5. Mao L (2011) Evaluating the combined effectiveness of influenza control strategies and human preventive behavior. PLoS One 6: e24706.
6. Shim E (2013) Optimal strategies of social distancing and vaccination against seasonal influenza. Mathematical Biosciences and Engineering 10: 1615–1634.
7. Nichol KL, Nordin JD, Nelson DB, Mullooly JP, Hak E (2007) Effectiveness of influenza vaccine in the community-dwelling elderly. New England Journal of Medicine 357: 1373–1381.
8. Tarride JE, Burke N, von Keyserlingk C, O'Reilly D, Xie F, et al. (2011) Intranasal live attenuated (Laiv) versus injectable inactivated (Tiv) influenza vaccine for children and adolescents: A Canadian cost effectiveness analysis. Value in Health 14: A119–A120.
9. Blank PR, Schwenkglenks M, Szucs TD (2009) Vaccination coverage rates in eleven European countries during two consecutive influenza seasons. Journal of Infection 58: 446–458.
10. Chan TC, Hsiao CK, Lee CC, Chiang PH, Kao CL, et al. (2010) The impact of matching vaccine strains and post-SARS public health efforts on reducing influenza-associated mortality among the elderly. PLoS One 5: e11317.
11. Lee CL, Chen TY, Chih YC, Chou SM, Chen CH, et al. (2013) The overview of government-funded influenza vaccination program during influenza season 2011–2012. Taiwan Epidemiology Bulletin 29: 252–259.
12. Plans-Rubio P (2012) The vaccination coverage required to establish herd immunity against influenza viruses. Preventive Medicine 55: 72–77.
13. Mok E, Yeung SH, Chan MF (2006) Prevalence of influenza vaccination and correlates of intention to be vaccinated among Hong Kong Chinese. Public Health Nurs 23: 506–515.
14. Sypsa V, Livanios T, Psichogiou M, Malliori M, Tsiodras S, et al. (2009) Public perceptions in relation to intention to receive pandemic influenza vaccination in a random population sample: evidence from a cross-sectional telephone survey. Euro Surveill 14: 19437.
15. Setbon M, Raude J (2010) Factors in vaccination intention against the pandemic influenza A/H1N1. Eur J Public Health 20: 490–494.
16. Huang JH, Miao YY, Kuo PC (2012) Pandemic influenza H1N1 vaccination intention: psychosocial determinants and implications from a national survey, Taiwan. Eur J Public Health 22: 796–801.
17. Brunson EK (2013) The impact of social networks on parents' vaccination decisions. Pediatrics 131: e1397–1404.
18. Mamelund SE, Riise Bergsaker MA (2011) Vaccine history, gender and influenza vaccination in a household context. Vaccine 29: 9441–9450.
19. Glass LM, Glass RJ (2008) Social contact networks for the spread of pandemic influenza in children and teenagers. BMC Public Health 8: 61.
20. Fu YC, Wang DW, Chuang JH (2012) Representative contact diaries for modeling the spread of infectious diseases in Taiwan. PLoS One 7: e45113.
21. Mossong J, Hens N, Jit M, Beutels P, Auranen K, et al. (2008) Social contacts and mixing patterns relevant to the spread of infectious diseases. PLoS Med 5: e74.
22. Read JM, Eames KT, Edmunds WJ (2008) Dynamic social networks and the implications for the spread of infectious disease. J R Soc Interface 5: 1001–1007.
23. Read JM, Edmunds WJ, Riley S, Lessler J, Cummings DA (2012) Close encounters of the infectious kind: methods to measure social mixing behaviour. Epidemiol Infect 140: 2117–2130.
24. Chang YH, Fu YC (2004) The evolution of the Taiwan Social Change Survey, Japanese General Social Survey. JGSS Symposium 2003: Birth of JGSS and Its Fruit: Social Surveys in Different Countries and Areas and JGSS. East Osaka City: Institute of Regional Studies, Osaka University of Commerce. 149–160.
25. Hosmer DW, Lemeshow S (2000) Model-building strategies and methods for logistic regression. Applied Logistic Regression. New York: Wiley. 95.

26. Brien S, Kwong JC, Buckeridge DL (2012) The determinants of 2009 pandemic A/H1N1 influenza vaccination: A systematic review. Vaccine 30: 1255–1264.

27. Nguyen T, Henningsen KH, Brehaut JC, Hoe E, Wilson K (2011) Acceptance of a pandemic influenza vaccine: a systematic review of surveys of the general public. Infect Drug Resist 4: 197–207.

28. Painter JE, Sales JM, Pazol K, Wingood GM, Windle M, et al. (2010) Psychosocial correlates of intention to receive an influenza vaccination among rural adolescents. Health Educ Res 25: 853–864.

29. Chuang JH, Huang AS, Huang WT, Liu MT, Chou JH, et al. (2012) Nationwide surveillance of influenza during the pandemic (2009–10) and post-pandemic (2010–11) periods in Taiwan. PLoS One 7: e36120.

30. Liao Q, Wong WS, Fielding R (2013) How do anticipated worry and regret predict seasonal influenza vaccination uptake among Chinese adults? Vaccine 31: 4084–4090.

31. Liao QY, Wong WS, Fielding R (2013) Comparison of different risk perception measures in predicting seasonal influenza vaccination among healthy Chinese adults in Hong Kong: A Prospective Longitudinal Study. PLoS One 8: e68019.

32. Heikkinen T, Heinonen S (2011) Effectiveness and safety of influenza vaccination in children: European perspective. Vaccine 29: 7529–7534.

33. Marchetti M, Kuhnel UM, Colombo GL, Esposito S, Principi N (2007) Cost-effectiveness of adjuvanted influenza vaccination of healthy children 6 to 60 months of age. Hum Vaccin 3: 14–22.

34. Carpenter LR, Lott J, Lawson BM, Hall S, Craig AS, et al. (2007) Mass distribution of free, intranasally administered influenza vaccine in a public school system. Pediatrics 120: e172–178.

35. Muller D, Szucs TD (2007) Influenza vaccination coverage rates in 5 European countries: a population-based cross-sectional analysis of the seasons 02/03, 03/04 and 04/05. Infection 35: 308–319.

36. Ashbaugh AR, Herbert CF, Saimon E, Azoulay N, Olivera-Figueroa L, et al. (2013) The decision to vaccinate or not during the H1N1 pandemic: selecting the lesser of two evils? PLoS One 8: e58852.

## 6

Socio-Economic Inequalities in the Prevalence of Multi-Morbidity among the Rural Elderly in Bargarh District of Odisha (India)

Pallavi Banjare, Jalandhar Pradhan*

Department of Humanities & Social Sciences, National Institute of Technology (NIT), Rourkela, Odisha, India

Abstract

Background: Multi-morbidity among elderly is increasingly recognized as a major public health challenge in most of the developing countries. However, information on the size of population suffering from multi-morbidity and socio-economic differentials of multi-morbidity is scarce. The objectives of this paper are twofold; first, to assess the prevalence of various chronic conditions and morbidity among rural elderly and second, to examine the socio-economic and demographic factors that have a significant effect on the morbidity.

Methods: A cross-sectional survey has been done using multi-stage random sampling procedure that was conducted among elderly (60+ years) in Bargarh District of Odisha during October 2011-February 2012. The survey was conducted among 310 respondents including 153 males and 157 females. Descriptive analyses were performed to assess the pattern of multi-morbidity. Logistic regression analyses were used to see the adjusted effect of various socio-economic and demographic covariates of multi-morbidity.

Results: The overall prevalence of multi-morbidity is 57% among rural elderly in Bargarh District of Odisha. The most common diseases in rural areas are: Arthritis, Chronic Obstructive Pulmonary Disease (COPD), High Blood Pressure and Cataract. Results from the logistic regression analyses show that age, state of economic independence and life style indicators are the most important measured predictors of multi-morbidity. Unlike earlier studies, wealth index and education have a marginal impact on multi-morbidity rate. Moreover, the occurrence of multi-morbidity is higher for elderly males compared to their female counterparts, though the difference is not significant.

Conclusion: The high prevalence of morbidity observed in the present study suggests that there is an urgent need to develop geriatric health care services in a developing country like India. Any effort to reorganize primary care for elderly people should also consider the high prevalence of multi-morbidity among rural elderly in India.

Editor: Sudha Chaturvedi, Wadsworth Center, United States of America

Funding: The authors report no current funding sources for this study.

Competing Interests: The authors have declared that no competing interests exist.

* E-mail: jpp_pradhan@yahoo.co.uk

Introduction

The world is moving towards population aging. It is projected that by the year 2020, there will be one billion elderly people (65+ years) in the world and 71% of whom will live in low-income countries [1]. Elderly population in India is approximately hundred million forming 10% of the total population [2,3]. The report by Integrated programs for older person in 2008 by the Ministry of Social Justice and Empowerment (Government of India 2008) reveals that the number of people in the 60+ age group in India will increase to 198 million by 2030 [4]. However, the progression of aging leads to loss of adaptive response towards stress and growing risk of age related diseases, resulting in progressive increase in age specific mortality. From morbidity point of view, at least 50% of the elderly in India have chronic diseases [2]. This implies that aging population will suffer from chronic medical conditions and the prevalence of multiple chronic conditions is expected to increase [5]. Many studies have been carried out on the prevalence of multi- morbidity in Europe [6,7,8], the Middle East [9], Australia [10], the United States [5,11,12], Bangladesh [13] and Canada [14,15,16]. However the available literature reveals limited studies on multi-morbidity amongst elderly people in developing countries. In Indian context few studies on prevalence of multi-morbidity have been conducted [17,18]. Multi-morbidity becomes progressively more common with age [19,20,21,22] and is associated with high mortality [23], reduced functional status [24,25], and increased use of both inpatient and ambulatory health care [5].

Although, the association between socioeconomic status and prevalence of individual chronic diseases is well established [26,27] few studies have examined the association between multi-morbidity and socio-economic status [20,21,28]. Another set of studies have investigated how diseases distribute or co-occur in the same individual. Several studies have used different approaches to address these issues [23,16]. A study conducted in Australia found that 85% of 70+ year elderly have multi-morbidity and the prevalence is higher among elderly with obesity, elderly female, elderly with low socioeconomic status, elderly living alone and less educated [20].

A nested case–control study of general practitioners in South Netherlands Community residents found that multi-morbidity was highly correlated with increasing age, low socioeconomic status, and those who had diseases prior to the study [29]. A small number of studies have identified the relationship between multi-morbidity, disability and functional decline. However, study among the Spanish elderly found out that multi-morbidity was associated with impaired functioning [30]. In contrast another study found that multi-morbidity was not associated with physical activity levels [31]. Landi et al. (2010) studied on Italians living in a community and concluded that multi-morbidity affected 4-year mortality, only if associated with disability [32]. A research on residential volunteers in Hong Kong concludes that depression prevalence was associated with the number of chronic conditions [33]. Walker. (2007) conducted a study on multi-morbidity with healthcare utilization and quality of life among Australian general population. He found that persons with 3 or more chronic conditions were more likely to feel distressed or pessimistic about their lives [20]. Wolff et al. (2002) concluded that increasing number of diseases increases hospitalizations, preventable complications, and expenditures [5].

Most of the available studies on multi-morbidity in India are disease specific and fail to provide comprehensive overview of wide range of diseases occurring among rural elderly. One of the studies in Chandigarh found that elderly female were more prone to morbidity [34,35]. Another study on multi-morbidity among elderly in Karnataka, found that the prevalence of multi-morbidity was equally distributed among both men and women [35]. A study conducted by Shankar et al., found that the common morbidity among Indian elderly is Arthritis with overall prevalence of 57.08%, followed by Cataract (48.33%), Hypertension (11.25%) [36]. But the prevalence of old age related morbidities have increased with advancing age. Variables like caste, literacy and socioeconomic status did not show significant association with the prevalence of multi-morbidity [36].

Looking at the growing concern on multi-morbidity in India, there is necessity of better understanding of the epidemiology of multi-morbidity to develop interventions to prevent it and align health care services more closely for the rural elderly patients' needs. So, an intensive study on multi-morbidity among rural elderly is necessary to address the multiple deprivation of health to reduce the health burden among elderly. The objectives of this paper are two fold; first, to assess the prevalence of various chronic conditions (ICD 10) and morbidity among rural elderly in Bargarh district of Odisha and second, to examine the socio-economic and demographic factors that have a significant effect on the morbidity.

Data and Methods

Ethics Statement

The study was conducted in Bargarh district of Odisha, India. The study aims to explore the familial setups, roles, health status and expectations of the elderly. Before collecting necessary information from selected elderly, following consent form was signed by the respective respondent:

"I am going to ask you some personal questions that some of the people find difficult to answer. Your answers are completely confidential, your name, will not be disclosed to anyone, and will never be used in connection with any of the information you tell me. You do not have to answer any questions that you do not feel comfortable, and you may withdraw from this interview at any time you want to. However, your answers to these questions will help us to understand the senior citizens situation. We would greatly appreciate your help in responding to this interview. Would you be willing to participate?"

If the respondent provided consent, an interview was conducted.

The study was approved by the Doctoral Research Committee (DRC) of National Institute of Technology, Rourkela, Odisha, India.

Sample Selection

A cross-sectional survey using multi-stage random sampling procedure was conducted among elderly (60+ years) in Bargarh District of Odisha during October 2011-February 2012. Selection of respondents involved three stages of sampling procedure. Block was selected at the first stage. Then village was selected at the second stage followed by selection of target respondents at the third stage. The targeted sample size was 320. Data were collected by face-to-face interviews with a pre-tested structured questionnaire. Ten respondents who were extremely frail could not respond to the questionnaires. So, finally 310 respondents were considered for analysis resulting in a response rate of 97%.

As per Census 2001, there are 12 blocks in Bargarh i.e. Bargarh, Barpali, Attabira, Bheden, Sohella, Bijepur, Padmpur, Gaisilet, Paikmal, Jharbandh, Ambabhona and Bhatli. Two blocks namely Sohella and Padmpur were selected randomly. Twenty respondents (10 Male and 10 Female) were selected from each village. So, 16 villages (10 from Sohela and 10 from Padampur) were selected to get the required number of respondents. Villages were selected using probability proportion to sample size (PPS). At the village level, a sampling framework was prepared separately for male and female respondents. A complete listing of the households in a selected village was done. During the listing in each household, all the members aged 60+ were listed. Each member's actual age and gender were noted. Accordingly, 10 Male and 10 Female elderly were selected randomly.

Dependent Variables

In this paper morbidity has been taken as dependent variable. In order to determine the occurrence of morbidities, respondents were asked, *"Has a doctor or nurse ever told you that you have any of the following ailments viz; Arthritis, Cerebral embolism, Stroke or Thrombosis, Angina or heart disease, Diabetes, Chronic lung disease, Asthma, Depression, High blood pressure, Alzheimer's disease, Cancer, Dementia, Liver or Gall bladder illness, Osteoporosis, Renal or Urinary tract infection, Cataract, Loss of all natural teeth, Accidental injury (in past one year), Injury due to fall (in the past one year), Skin disease, and Paralysis?".*

For descriptive analysis, we have categorized the prevalence of morbidity into four groups: 1) elderly having no morbidity, 2) elderly having one morbidity, 3) elderly having two morbidities & 4) elderly having three or more morbidity. Multi-morbidity is defined as those who are having 2 or more morbidities. For logistic regression, morbidity was recorded into binary form i.e. elderly having one or no morbidity was taken as '0' and one having 2 or more morbidity i.e. multi morbidity was taken as '1'.

Independent Variables

Various socio-economic and demographic factors are treated as independent variables namely a) Age (in five years age groups), b) Sex, c) Marital status, d) Education, e) Wealth quintile, f) Caste, g)

Table 1. Model design for logistic regression analysis.

Models	Model 1	Model 2	Model 3	Model 4
Variables	**Only demographic variables**	**Only Socio-economic variables**	**Only life style indicators**	**All independent covariates**
	• Age • Sex • Marital status	• Education • Wealth Index • Caste • State of economic dependence • Living arrangements	• Smoking • Consuming tobacco	• Age • Sex • Marital status • Education • Wealth Index • State of economic dependence • Living arrangements • Smoking • Consuming tobacco

State of economic dependence, h) Living arrangement, and i) Life style indicators.

The demographic variables which have been considered are: a) Sex divided into two categories (1. female 2. male), b) Age group (in five years group) divided into four categories (1. 60–65 years 2. 65–70 years 3. 70–75 years 4. 75+ years).

The role of marital status has been clearly demonstrated in the literature examining the relationship between marital status and health outcomes [39]. All of the various unmarried states (being single, never married, being separated/divorced and being widowed) have been associated with elevated mortality risks [40]. It has been proved that married people are better-off in health and suffer from less morbidity. In this study, marital status has been classified into two categories viz., 1) currently married, 2 widowed/divorced or separated. Educational qualification is divided into four categories - 1. No formal education, 2. Primary school and less completed 3. Primary school completed 4. Secondary school and above completed.

The questionnaire also has questions related to thirty three assets owned by households which were later converted into wealth quintile or wealth index. The wealth index is based on household assets and housing characteristics, such as (mattress, pressure cooker, chair, bed, table, electric fan, radio, black and white television, color television, sewing machine, mobile phone, any other phone, computer, refrigerator, watch, bicycle, motor-cycle, animal drawn cart, car, water pump, thresher, tractor and electricity). Using principal component analysis these assets and their characteristics were combined into a single variable. After ranking this variable from low to high, households were divided into five equal-sized groups namely - 1) Poorest (Q1) 2) Poorer (Q2) 3) Middle (Q3) 4) Richer (Q4) 5) Richest (Q5). Caste is divided based on caste schedule followed as per Government of India guidelines - 1. Scheduled Caste/Scheduled Tribe 2. Other Backward Caste 3. General. The state of economic dependence is divided into three categories 1. Not depending on others, 2. Partially dependent 3. Fully dependent.

Living arrangements refers to the type of family in which the elderly live, the headship they enjoy, the place they stay in and the people they stay with, the kind of relationship they maintain with their kith and kin, and the extent to which they adjust to the changing environment [37,38]. While dealing with the welfare of any specific group, it is important to study their pattern of living arrangement. There exists several living patterns for the elderly such as - living with the spouse, living with children, living with other relations and non-relations and living alone (as an inmate of old age homes). In this study living arrangement is categorized into four categories i.e. 1) living alone, 2) living with spouse/son/

daughter, 3) living with spouse and unmarried sons, 4) living with spouse and married son.

A report by US National Cancer Institute in 2002 reveals that the Asian people have been using tobacco in various forms since ages [41]. Moreover, the International Agency for Research on Cancer in 2007 [42] strongly expresses that SLT (smokeless tobacco) is common in Asian countries such as India, Pakistan and Bangladesh. The use of SLT varies by age, sex, ethnicity and socioeconomic status, both within and among countries [43]. A study by Accortt. et.al. (2002) concluded that use of tobacco as well as SLT leads to chronic heart diseases [44].

In this study, we have considered a set of variables as risk behaviors like i) Smoking (1. Yes 2. No), ii) Consumption of alcohol (1. Yes 2. No), iii) Chewing tobacco (1. Yes 2. No).

At first, descriptive analysis was done to assess the socio-economic differentials in the prevalence of multi-morbidity. Secondly, binary logistic regressions were carried out to explore factors responsible for the prevalence of multi-morbidity among rural elderly in Odisha.

Logistic regression can be used to predict a dependent variable on the basis of independents and to determine the per cent of variance in the dependent variable explained by the independents; to rank the relative importance of independents; to assess interaction effects; and to understand the impact of covariates. Logistic regression applies maximum likelihood estimation after transforming the dependent into a logit variable (the natural log of the odds of the dependent occurring or not). So, logistic regression estimates the probability of certain event whether occurring or not. The multiple logistic models can be noted as:

$$\ln\left(\frac{p}{1-p}\right) = \alpha + \beta_1 x_1 + \beta_2 x_2 + \beta_3 x_3 + \ldots \beta_i x_1 + e.$$

Where, p is the probability of occurrence of multi-morbidity, p $(y = 1)$; β_1, β_2, β_3,... β_i refers to the beta coefficients; x_1, x_2, x_3, ...x_i refers to the independent variables and e is the error term.

In all, four models have been applied with different categories of independent covariates (Table 1). SPSS V 20 is used to analyze the data. The survey data was analyzed using descriptive and logistic regression analysis.

Results

Socio-economic and Demographic Profiles of Respondents

Table 2 presents the sample characteristics of the studied population by selected socio-economic covariates. Out of the total

Table 2. Percentage distribution of respondents by selected socio-economic characteristics by Gender.

Covariates	%	N
Sex		
Male	49.4	153
Female	50.6	157
Age of the respondents		
60–65 Years	30.6	95
65–70 Years	35.5	110
70–75 Years	20	62
75 & Above	13.9	43
Marital Status		
Currently married	60.3	187
Widowed/Divorced or Separated	39.7	123
Education status of respondents		
No formal education	60.3	187
Less than primary	27.7	86
Primary school completed	7.4	23
Secondary school and above	4.5	14
Wealth quintile		
Poorest	19.7	61
Poorer	19.4	60
Middle	21	65
Richer	19.7	61
Richest	20.3	63
Caste		
General	11	34
Scheduled Caste/Scheduled Tribe	31.9	99
Other Backward Caste	57.1	177
State of economic dependence		
Not dependent	42.3	131
Fully dependent	11.3	35
Partially dependent	46.5	144
Living arrangements		
Living alone	7.7	24
Living with spouse/Son/Daughter	25.5	79
Living with Spouse and unmarried son	12.3	38
Living with Spouse and married son	54.5	169
BPL card holder		
Has the card	58.1	180
Risk Behaviors		
Smoking (Yes)	31	96
Consuming Alcohol (Yes)	4.19	13
Consuming Tobacco (Yes)	63.2	196
N		**310**

sample of 310 respondents, 153 are male and 157 are female. The married people comprise of 60.3% and widowed/divorced or separated comprise of 39.7% of the total sample. Study on Literacy or Education of the respondents' shows that about 60.3% have no formal education, followed by 27.7% who have completed primary education or less and only 4.5% have completed their secondary school and above. In State of Economic Dependence,

about 46.5% are partially dependent, followed by not dependent on others (42.3%) and 11.3% are fully dependent on their spouse, son or other relative. While analyzing Caste structure, Other Backward Caste have the highest share of 57.1%, followed by Scheduled Caste/Scheduled Tribe with 31.9% and General have 11% only. Elderly living with spouse and married son are the most with about 54.5%, followed by living with either spouse/son or

Table 3. Percent of respondents having selected morbidities by Gender.

Morbidities	Male (N = 153)	Female (N = 157)	Total (310)
Arthritis	50.9	54.7	52.9
Cerebral-embolism, stroke or Thrombosis	0.6	1.9	1.2
Heart disease	0.6	4.4	2.5
Diabetes	7.8	10.8	9.3
Chronic obstructive pulmonary disease	30.0	10.1	20.0
Asthma	9.1	10.1	9.6
Depression	7.1	4.4	5.8
High blood pressure	26.1	12.7	19.3
Alzheimer's disease	3.9	9.5	6.6
Cancer	0.0	1.9	0.9
Dementia	4.5	7.6	6.1
Liver or gall bladder illness	4.5	3.1	3.8
Osteoporosis	1.9	3.1	2.5
Renal or Urinary tract infection	9.1	3.8	6.4
Cataract	21.5	15.9	18.7
Loss of all natural teeth's	4.5	7.0	5.8
Accidental injury (in past one year)	11.7	6.3	9.0
Injury due to fall (in past one year)	3.9	2.5	3.2
Skin disease	6.5	7.0	6.6
Paralysis	8.4	4.4	6.4

daughter and elderly living alone are the least with only 7.7% share. About 58.1% of the population have Below Poverty Line card. About 63% of the respondents are consuming tobacco, 31% of them are used to smoking and a small proportion (4%) in drinking alcohol.

Prevalence of Morbidity by Gender

Table 3 presents percentage of respondents having selected morbidities by gender. The individuals were asked whether the doctor had ever told them that they might be having any of the above mentioned chronic diseases. To verify the responses, the test results/doctor's prescriptions/supporting documents were checked during the interview session. This table clearly shows that the most common disease in this rural setup is Arthritis with total 52.9% and it is slightly higher for females with 54.7% of the total sample.

A high prevalence of arthritis/joint pain in the current study especially among females was also reported in other studies [45], thus it reflects the hard life faced by women who never retire from household work unless totally disabled.

Next prevailing disease followed by Arthritis, with about 20% of the elderly reported was Chronic Obstructive Pulmonary Disease (COPD), with males having a higher share of 30% in comparison to females having just 10.1%. Globally, COPD is expected to rise to the 3rd position as a cause of death and at the 5th position as the cause of loss of disability adjusted life years (DALYs), according to the baseline projections made in the Global Burden of Disease Study (GBDS) by 2020 [46]. Tobacco smoking remains the most important risk factor identified as the cause of COPD and chronic respiratory morbidity [47]. Tobacco related mortality is estimated to be highest in India, China and other Asian countries [48].

Table 4. Prevalence of morbidity by age groups.

Number of morbidities	% of respondents by morbidity profile				
	Age group				
	60–65 years	65–70 years	70–75 years	75+years	Total
No morbidity	16.8	9.1	6.5	4.7	10.3
One morbidity	43.2	33.6	24.2	20.9	32.9
Two morbidity	17.9	28.2	35.5	30.2	26.8
Three or more morbidity	22.1	29.1	33.9	44.2	30.0
At least two morbidities (Multi-morbidity)	40.0	57.3	69.4	74.4	56.8
N	95	110	62	43	310

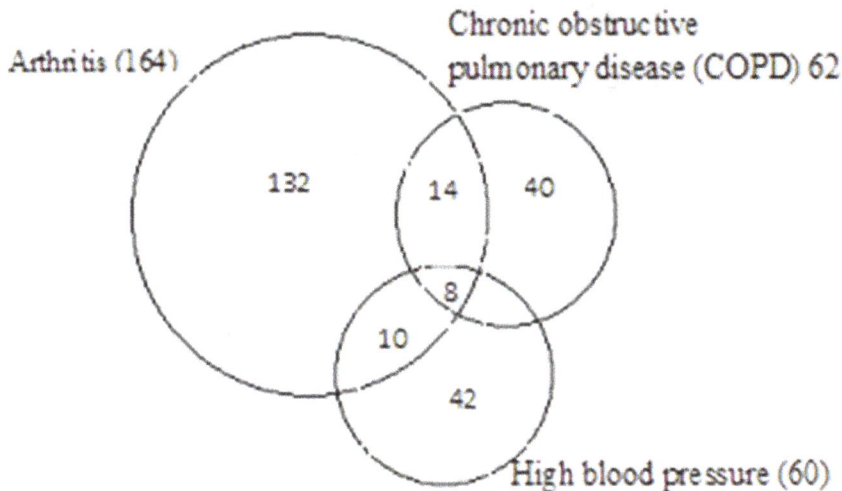

Figure 1. Venn diagram displaying the overlapping of multi-morbidity patterns in numbers related to the total population.

The third prevalent morbidity is High Blood Pressure or Hypertension. The result shows that about 19.35% of respondents are suffering from Hypertension. Studies from Karnataka and Kolkata have also reported that the prevalence of hypertension was about 30.5% and 40.5% respectively [49,50]. The difference in prevalence levels may be due to different geographical factors and may be due to differences in dietary pattern. Cataract is also one of the important morbidities present in the rural population in the studied villages i.e. 18.70%. It is more common in females compared to their male counterparts. Cataract is found to be more common in rural population, which may be due to increased exposure to ultraviolet radiation during long hours of work in open fields [51]. Eighty percent of this blindness is due to cataract alone [52]. Skin diseases, paralysis and accidental injury are also the other forms of morbidities occurring among rural elderly in Odisha.

While comparing the prevalence of disease amongst males and females, it shows that arthritis is more common among females than males, whereas chronic lung disease and high blood pressure are more common among males. Similarly, dementia and Alzheimer's disease are more common among females and cataract amongst males. For other diseases, both male and females shared similar patterns with slight variations.

Pattern of Multi-morbidity

The following Venn diagram (figure 1) shows the overlapping of major morbidities found among rural elderly in Odisha. The three common morbidities are arthritis (164), chronic obstructive pulmonary disease (62) and high blood pressure (60). Amongst 164 elderly people having arthritis about 62 (37%) are suffering from chronic obstructive pulmonary diseases, 60 (36%) are having high blood pressure and (8) 5% are having all the three morbidities.

Hence, the result shows that the occurrence of multi-morbidities is very common among our study population.

Prevalence of Multi-morbidity by Age Groups

Table 4 shows the relationship between age groups (60–65 years, 65–70 years, 70–75 years and 75+ years) and the intensity of morbidities. The occurrence of morbidities is classified into four groups - i) no morbidity, ii) having one morbidity, iii) having 2 morbidities and iv) having 3 or more morbidities. Multi-morbidity is defined as persons having two or more morbidities. Results from table 4 clearly suggest that, the rate of multi-morbidity increases with the increased age. The rate of multi-morbidity is 74% among 75+ year elderly compared to 40% for 60–65 years age group elderly. Another interesting finding of this study revealed that about 95% of the elderly (in the age group of 75+ years) have at least one morbidity.

Socio-economic Differentials in Multi-morbidity

As reviewed in earlier section, the rate of multi-morbidity varies with selected socio-economic and demographic covariates. Results from table 5 shows that the overall prevalence of multi-morbidity was 56.8% among rural elderly in Odisha, similar to what is frequently reported from many developed and developing nations e.g. 53.8% in Bangladesh [13], 55% in Swedish elderly [8], 75% in Australia [10], 65% in North America [11], although the criteria or definition were not identical in those studies. Unlike earlier studies the rate of multi-morbidities was higher for male compared to their female counterpart. This could be partly due to the response bias, as male are more open to disclose their disease experience compared to their female counterparts., Several recent studies revealed that the gender differences in multi-morbidity prevalence are marginal [54]. Many other studies on morbidity also found a strong positive relationship between age and multi-morbidity [55,10,11].

The relationship between economic status (measured in terms of wealth index) and occurrence of multi-morbidity is very weak. The prevalence of multi-morbidities by categories of educational status is identical, revealing the fact that occurrence of diseases are independent of education. Elderly belonging to Other Backward Caste (61%) are more prone to multi-morbidity compared to General Caste (58.8%) and Scheduled Caste/Scheduled Tribe (48.5%) elderly. State of economic independence is strongly associated with the rate of multi-morbidity. The multi-morbidity prevalence is about 71.4% for elderly who are fully dependent on others compared to elderly who are not dependent on others (48.1%). The disease prevalence is lower among elderly those who stay with their spouse and unmarried sons (42.1%) compared to their counterparts. As established in other studies, in this study too, life style indicators are positively associated with the occurrence of multi-morbidity.

Table 5. Multi-morbidity prevalence by selected socio-economic and demographic covariates.

Covariates	%	N
Sex		
Female	50.3	157
Male	63.4	153
Age of the respondents		
60–65 Years	40.0	95
65–70 Years	57.3	110
70–75 Years	69.4	62
75 Years & Above	74.4	43
Marital Status		
Currently married	57.8	187
Widowed/Divorced or Separated	55.3	123
Education status of respondents		
No formal education	56.7	187
Less than primary	57.0	86
Primary school completed	56.5	23
Secondary school and above	57.1	14
Wealth quintile		
Poorest	60.7	61
Poorer	53.3	60
Middle	52.3	65
Richer	63.9	61
Richest	54.0	63
Caste		
General	58.8	34
Scheduled Caste/Scheduled Tribe	48.5	99
Other Backward Caste	61.0	177
State of economic dependence		
Not dependent	48.1	131
Fully dependent	71.4	35
Partially dependent	61.1	144
Living arrangements		
Living alone	54.2	24
Living with spouse/Son/Daughter	59.5	79
Living with Spouse and unmarried son	42.1	38
Living with Spouse and married son	59.2	169
BPL card holder		
Yes	58.1	180
No	41.9	130
Smoking		
Yes	60.4	96
No	55.1	214
Consuming Tobacco		
Yes	60.7	196
No	50.0	114
N	**56.8**	**310**

Multivariate Logistic Regression Analysis

Since several of demographic, socio-economic and life style factors are interrelated, multivariate regression models of multi-morbidity are estimated to assess the independent effects of these factors on the occurrence of multi-morbidity, controlling for other

Table 6. Results of logistic regression analysis of factors associated with multi morbidity.

Variables	Model 1 OR (95% CI)	Model 2 OR (95% CI)	Model 3 OR (95% CI)	Model 4 OR (95% CI)
Sex				
Female	1.00			1.00
Male	1.39 (0.85–2.29)			1.68 (0.91–3.11)
Age				
60–65 years	1.00			1.00
65–70 years	2.04* (1.16–3.58)			2.33* (1.22–4.45)
70–75 years	3.43** (1.69–6.94)			4.91** (2.18–11.05)
75+years	4.27** (1.87–9.73)			4.65** (1.87–11.52)
Marital status				
Currently married	1.00			1.00
Widowed/Divorced or Separated	0.79 (0.47–0.133)			0.92 (0.47–1.78)
Wealth Index				
Poorest		1.00		1.00
Poorer		0.93 (0.43–2.02)		1.22 (0.52–2.84)
Middle		0.64 (0.28–1.47)		0.70 (0.28–1.72)
Richer		1.08 (0.47–2.46)		1.41 (0.57–3.48)
Richest		0.59 (0.24–1.43)		0.60 (0.23–1.54)
Education				
No formal education		1.00		1.00
Less than primary		1.22 (0.68–2.20)		1.38 (0.69–2.75)
Primary school completed		0.94 (0.37–2.39)		1.62 (0.54–4.89)
Secondary school and above		1.68 (0.49–5.75)		2.36 (0.54–10.35)
Caste				
General		1.00		1.00
Scheduled Caste/Scheduled Tribe		0.60 (0.25–1.42)		0.58 (0.22–1.54)
Other Backward Caste		1.02 (0.45–2.32)		0.891 (0.35–2.21)
State of Economic independence				
Not depending		1.00		1.00
Fully dependent		3.06* (1.29–7.24)		5.21** (1.99–13.60)
Partially dependent		2.05** (1.20–3.50)		3.02** (1.57–5.81)
Living arrangement				
Living alone		1.00		1.00
Living with spouse or son or daughter or anyone		1.44 (0.53–3.93)		1.35 (0.41–4.46)
Living with Spouse and unmarried son		0.64 (0.20–2.00)		0.40 (0.10–1.56)
Living with Spouse and married son		1.55 (0.57–4.20)		1.25 (0.40–3.86)
Smoking				
No			1.00	1.00
Yes			1.46* (0.87–2.46)	1.85* (0.98–3.50)
Chewing Tobacco				
No			1.00	1.00
Yes			1.72** (1.05–2.81)	2.82** (1.51–5.24)
Total				
Constant	−.481	−.183	−.185	−2.212

*significant at 5 per cent level;
**significant at 1 percent level.

predictors in the model. Table 6 presents the results of logistic regression analysis taking four models into consideration.

Results from Model 1 indicate that among demographic variables, age has a very large effect on the occurrence of multimorbidity. The prevalence of multi-morbidity increases steadily with age. The Odds Ratio (OR) of multi-morbidity prevalence is about 4.27 (CI: 1.87–9.73) times higher for elderly above 75 years compared to those in 60–65 years age group.

Model 2 assesses the cumulative impact of various socio-economic covariates on multi-morbidity. Results from the analysis shows that among socio-economic variables, only the state of economic independence has significant impact on multi-morbidity. The prevalence of multi-morbidity is significantly higher for the elderly who are dependent on others compared to their counterparts.

Life style indicators (smoking and chewing tobacco) have a significant effect on the occurrence of multi-morbidity (Model 3). The elderly consuming tobacco are 1.72 times more prone to morbidity than those who do not consume tobacco at all. Similarly, elderly who smoke regularly are about 1.46 times more prone to morbidity than those who do not smoke.

Finally, in Model 4 all variables are included to assess the adjusted effect of various demographic and socio-economic covariates on multi-morbidity.

Even after controlling all the covariates - like age and state of economic independence the life style indicators have retained their significant effect on the occurrence of multi-morbidity.

Conclusions

Given the increasing prevalence of multi-morbidity, understanding the socio-economic differentials in multi-morbidity among rural elderly is important to help national and sub-national health planners to address the issues in a broader perspective. The overall prevalence of multi-morbidity is 57% among rural elderly in Bargarh District of Odisha this fits well with the reporting range of multi-morbidity rates in elderly population [11,18,55,53,56]. The most common diseases in rural set-up are - Arthritis, COPD,

High Blood Pressure and Cataract. Results from the multivariate analysis show that age, state of economic independence and life style indicators are the most important measured predictors of multi-morbidity. Unlike earlier studies, wealth index and education have a marginal impact on multi-morbidity rate. Moreover, the occurrence of multi-morbidity is higher for male elderly compared to female counterparts though the difference is not significant.

The high prevalence of morbidity observed in the present study suggests that there is an urgent need to develop geriatric health care services in the developing country like India. Most of the developing countries like India are least prepared to meet the challenges of societies with rapid increase in ageing population [57]. The WHO has recently taken initiatives towards elderly-friendly primary healthcare and has introduced 'Age-Friendly Primary Health Care Centers Toolkit' aiming at improving the primary healthcare responses to older persons. Efforts should be made to educate the primary health care workers regarding explicit needs of the elderly and directions should be provided to make the primary health care management more open and friendly to the requirements of the elderly [58].

Since multi-morbidity may cause significant cognitive and functional consequences researcher and policy makers should work together to develop effective intervention strategies and programs to reduce the burden of multi-morbidity. Moreover, new health care model should be developed to meet the health care needs of elderly people with multi-morbidity in India.

Author Contributions

Conceived the study: PB JP. Wrote the first draft: PB. Edited the paper: JP. Performed statistical analysis: PB JP. Read and approved the final manuscript: PB JP.

References

1. Solomons NW, Flores R, Gillepsie S (2001) Health and nutrition: emerging and reemerging issues in developing countries. Journal of Health and Ageing 3: 3–6.
2. Bhatt R, Gandhvi MS, Sonaliya A, Nayak H (2011) An epidemiological study of the morbidity pattern among the elderly population in Ahmadabad, Gujarat. National Journal of Community Medicine 22: 233–236.
3. Bhattacharya P. (2005) Implications of an aging population in India: challenges and opportunities. Presented at the Living to 100 and Beyond. Symposium Sponsored by the Society of Actuaries.
4. Ministry of Social Justice & Empowerment. New Delhi (2008) Integrated program for older person's: A central sector scheme to improve the quality of life of older persons. New Delhi.
5. Wolff JL, Starfield B, Anderson G (2002) Prevalence, expenditures, and complications of multiple chronic conditions in the elderly. Archives of Internal Medicine 162: 2269–2276.
6. Uijen AA, van de Lisdonk EH (2008) Multi-morbidity in primary care: prevalence and trend over the last 20 years. European Journal of General Practice 1: 28–32.
7. Schram MT, Frijters D, van de Lisdonk EH, Ploemacher J, de Craen AJ, et al. (2008) Setting and registry characteristics affect the prevalence and nature of multi-morbidity in the elderly. Journal of Clinical Epidemiology 61: 1104–1112.
8. Marengoni A, Winblad B, Karp A, Fratiglioni L (2008) Prevalence of chronic diseases and multi-morbidity among the elderly population in Sweden. American Journal of Public Health 98: 1198–1200.
9. Fuchs Z, Blumstein T, Novikov I, Walter-Ginzburg A, Lyanders M (1998) Morbidity, co morbidity, and their association with disability among community-dwelling oldest-old in Israel. Journals of Gerontology Series A: Biological Sciences and Medical Sciences 53: 447–455.
10. Britt HC, Harrison CM, Miller GC, Knox SA (2008) Prevalence and patterns of multi morbidity in Australia. Medical Journal of Australia 189: 72–77.
11. Guralnik JM (1996) Assessing the impact of co-morbidity in the older population. Annals of Epidemiology 6: 76–80.
12. Hoffman C, Rice D, Sung HY (1996) Persons with chronic conditions, their prevalence and costs. Journal of the American Medical Association 276: 1473–1479.
13. Khanam MA, Streatfield PK, Kabir ZN, Qiu C, Cornelius C, et al. (2011) Prevalence and pattern of multi-morbidity among elderly people in rural Bangladesh: A cross-sectional study. Journal of Health, Population and Nutrition 4: 406–414.
14. Daveluy C, Pica L, Audet N, Courtemanche R, Lapointe F, et al. (2000) In Enquête sociale et de santé 1998 2nd edition. Québec: Institut de la statistique du Québec.
15. Rapoport J, Jacobs P, Bell NR, Klarenbach S (2004) Refining the measurement of the economic burden of chronic diseases in Canada. Journal of Chronic Diseases 25: 13–21.
16. Fortin M, Bravo G, Hudon C, Lapointe L, Dubois MF, et al. (2005) Psychological distress and multi-morbidity in primary care. Annals of Family Medicine 4: 417–422.
17. Joshi K, Kumar R, Avasthi A (2003) Morbidity profile and its relationship with disability and psychological distress among elderly people in northern India. International Journal of Epidemiology 32: 978–987.
18. Purty AJ, Bazroy J, Kar M, Vasudevan K, Veliath A, et al. (2006) Morbidity pattern among the elderly population in the rural area of Tamil Nadu, India. Turkish Journal of Medical Sciences 36: 45–50.
19. Akker M, Buntinx F, Metsemakers JF, Roos S, Knottnerus JA, et al. (1998) Multi morbidity in general practice: prevalence, incidence, and determinants of co-occurring chronic and recurrent diseases. Journal of Clinical Epidemiology 51: 367–375.
20. Walker AE. (2007) Multiple chronic diseases and quality of life: pattern emerging from large sample, Australia. Journal of Chronic Illness 3: 202–218.
21. Salisbury C, Johnson C, Purdy S, Valderas JM, Montgomery A, et al. (2011) Epidemiology and impact of multi-morbidity in primary care: A retrospective cohort study. The British Journal of General Practice 582: 12–21.
22. Barnett K, Mercer SW, Norbury M, Watt G, Wyke S, et al. (2012) Epidemiology of multi-morbidity and implications for health care, research, and medical education: a cross-sectional study. The Lancet 380: 37–43.
23. Gijsen R, Hoeymans N, Schellevis FG, Ruwaard D, Satariano WA, et al. (2001) Causes and consequences of co morbidity: A review. Journal of Clinical Epidemiology 54: 661–674.
24. Kadam U, Croft P (2007) Clinical multi-morbidity and physical function in older adults: a record and health status linkage study in general practice. The Journal of Family Practice 24: 412–419.

25. Fortin M, Dubois MF, Hudon C, Soubhi H, Almirall J, et al. (2007) Multi-morbidity and quality of life: A closer look. Journal of Clinical Epidemiology 5: 52–58.
26. Eachus J, Williams M, Chan P, Smith GD, Grainge M (1996): Deprivation and cause specific morbidity: Evidence from the Somerset and Avon survey of health. British Medical Journal 312: 287–292.
27. Marmot M (2005) Social determinants of health inequalities. Lancet 365: 1099–1104.
28. Mercer SW, Watt GCM (2007) The inverse care law: clinical primary care encounters in deprived and affluent areas of Scotland. Annals of Family Medicine 5: 503–510.
29. Akker VD, Buntinx F, Metsemakers JF, Knottnerus JA (2000) Marginal impact of psychosocial factors on multi-morbidity: Results of an explorative nested case-control study. Social Science and. Medicine 50: 1679–1693.
30. Loza E, Jover JA, Rodriguez L, Carmona L (2009) Multi-morbidity: prevalence, effect on quality of life and daily functioning, and variation of this effect when one condition is a rheumatic disease. Seminars in Arthritis and Rheumatism 38: 312–319.
31. Hudon C, Soubhi H, Fortin M (2008) Relationship between multi-morbidity and physical activity: Secondary analysis from Quebec health survey. Bio Med Central Public Health 8: 304–312.
32. Landi F, Liperoti R, Russo A, Capoluongo E, Barillaro C, et al. (2010) Disability, more than multi-morbidity, was predictive of mortality among older persons aged 80 years and older. Journal of Clinical Epidemiology 63: 752–759.
33. Wong SYS, Mercer SW, Woo J, Leung J (2008) The influence of multi-morbidity and self-reported socio-economic standing on the prevalence of depression in an elderly Hong Kong population. Bio Med Centarl Public Health 8: 119–124.
34. Swami HM, Bhatia B, Dutt R (2002) A community based study of morbidity profile among the elderly in Chandigarh, India. Bahrain Medical Bulletin 24: 13–16.
35. Shraddha K, Prashantha B, Prakash B (2012) Study on morbidity pattern among elderly in urban population of Mysore, Karnataka, India. International Journal of Medicine and Biomedical Research 13: 215–223.
36. Shankar R, Tondon J, Gambhir IS, Tripathi CB (2007) Health status of elderly population in rural area of Varanasi district. Indian Journal of Public Health 51: 56–58.
37. Palloni A (2001) Living arrangements of older persons. Population Bulletin of the United Nations 42: 54–110.
38. Rajan S, Mishra US, Sharma PS (1995) Living Arrangements among the Indian Elderly. Hong Kong Journal of Gerontology 9: 20–28.
39. Kiecolt-Glaser JK, Newton TL (2001) Marriage and health: his and hers. Psychological Bulletin 12: 472–503.
40. Manzoli L, Villari P, Pirone M, Boccia A (2007) Marital status and mortality in the elderly: A systematic review and meta-analysis. Journal of Social Science & Medicine 64: 77–94.
41. Roland M (2002) Smokeless tobacco fact sheets, Third International Conference on Smokeless Tobacco, Stockholm, Sweden.
42. Lyon F (2007) Smokeless Tobacco and Some Related Nitrosamines. International Agency for Research on Cancer France 89: 55–60.
43. Boffetta P, Hecht S, Gray N, Gupta P (2008) Smokeless tobacco and cancer. Lancet Oncology 9: 667–675.
44. Accortt N, Waterbor J, Beall C, Howard G (2002) Chronic Disease Mortality in a Cohort of Smokeless Tobacco Users. American Journal of Epidemiology 156: 730–737.
45. Khokhar A, Mehra M (2001) Life style and morbidity profile of geriatric population in an urban community of Delhi. Indian Journal of Medical Science 55: 609–615.
46. Murray CJL, Lopez AD (1997) Alternative projection of mortality and disability by cause 1990–2020: Global burden of disease study. Lancet 349: 1498–1504.
47. Jindal SK, Aggarwal AN, Chaudhry K, Chhabra SK, D'Souza GA, et al. (2006) Asthma Epidemiology Study Group. A multi-centric study on epidemiology of chronic obstructive pulmonary disease and its relationship with tobacco smoking and environmental tobacco smoke exposure. The Indian Journal of Chest Diseases and Allied Sciences 48: 23–27.
48. Mafranetra KN, Chuaychoo B, Dejsomritrutai W, Chierakul N, Nana A, et al. (2002) The prevalence and incidence of COPD among urban older persons of Bangkok Metropolis. Journal of Medical Association of Thailand 85: 1147–1155.
49. By Y, Mr NG, Ag U (2010) Prevalence, awareness, treatment, and control of hypertension in rural areas of Davanagere. Indian Journal of Community Medicine 35: 138–141.
50. Chinnakali P, Mohan B, Upadhyay RP, Singh AK, Srivastava R, et al. (2012) Hypertension in the elderly: Prevalence and Health seeking Behavior. North American Journal of Medical Sciences 4: 558–562.
51. Angra SK, Murthy GVS, Gupta SK, Angra V (1997) Cataract related blindness in India and its social implication. Indian Journal of Medical Research 106: 312–324.
52. Mohan M, Jose R (1992) National programs me for the control of blindness (NPCB). Ophthalmology section, Directorate General of Health Services, Ministry of Health and Family Welfare, Government of India: New Delhi: 80–100.
53. Schafer I, Leitner E, Schon G, Koller D, Hansen H et.al. (2010): Multi-morbidity Patterns in the Elderly: A New Approach of Disease Clustering Identifies Complex Interrelations between Chronic Conditions. PLOS ONE 5: 1–10.
54. Akker M, Buntinx F, Knottnerus JA (1996) Co-morbidity or multi-morbidity: what's in a name? A review of literature. European Journal of General Practice 2: 65–70.
55. Charlson ME, Pompei P, Ales KL, MacKenzie CR (1987) A new method of classifying prognostic co-morbidity in longitudinal studies: Development and validation. Journal of Chronic Diseases 40: 373–383.
56. Rana AM, Wahlin Å, Streatfield PK, Kabir ZN (2009) Association of bone and joint diseases with health-related quality of life among older people: a population based cross-sectional study in rural Bangladesh. Ageing Society journal 29: 727–743.
57. World Health Organization (2004) Towards age-friendly primary health care. Available: http://whqlibdoc.who.int/publications/2004/9241592184.pdf. Accessed 2014 May 15.
58. World Health Organization (2008) Age-friendly primary health care centers toolkit. Available: http://www.who.int/ageing/publications/AF_PHC_Centretoolkit.pdf. Accessed 2014 May 15.

## 7

Validation of a Pre-Coded Food Diary Used among 60–80 Year Old Men: Comparison of Self-Reported Energy Intake with Objectively Recorded Energy Expenditure

Tonje H. Stea[1]*, Lene F. Andersen[2], Gøran Paulsen[3], Ken J. Hetlelid[1], Hilde Lohne-Seiler[1], Svanhild Ådnanes[1], Thomas Bjørnsen[1], Svein Salvesen[1], Sveinung Berntsen[1]

1 Department of Public Health, Sport and Nutrition, University of Agder, Kristiansand, Norway, 2 Department of Nutrition, Institute of Basic Medical Sciences, University of Oslo, Oslo, Norway, 3 Department of Physical Performance, Norwegian School of Sport Sciences, Oslo, Norway

Abstract

Objective: To validate energy intake (EI) estimated from a pre-coded food diary (PFD) against energy expenditure (EE) measured with a valid physical activity monitor (SenseWear Pro₃ Armband) and to evaluate whether misreporting was associated with overweight/obesity in a group of elderly men.

Methods: Forty-seven healthy Norwegian men, 60–80 years old, completed the study. As this study was part of a larger intervention study, cross-sectional data were collected at both baseline and post-test. Participants recorded their food intake for four consecutive days using food diaries and wore SenseWear Pro₃ Armband (SWA) during the same period. Only participants with complete data sets at both baseline and post-test were included in the study.

Results: The group average EI was 17% lower at baseline and 18% lower at post-test compared to measured EE. Mean difference from Bland-Altman plot for EI and EE was −1.5 MJ/day (±1.96 SD: −7.0, 4.0 MJ/day) at baseline and −1.6 MJ/day (−6.6, 3.4 MJ/day) at post-test. The intraclass correlation coefficient (ICC) was 0.30 (95% CI: 0.02, 0.54, p = 0.018) at baseline and 0.34 (0.06, 0.57, p = 0.009) at post-test. Higher values of underreporting was shown among overweight/obese compared to normal weight participants at both baseline and post-test (p≤ 0.001), respectively.

Conclusions: The results indicate that the PFD could be a useful tool for estimating energy intake in normal weight elderly men. On the other hand, the PFD seems to be less suitable for estimating energy intake in overweight/obese elderly men.

Editor: Jung Eun Lee, Sookmyung Women's University, Republic of Korea

Funding: The present study was supported by grants from the Smartfish® company and Regional Research Founds, Agder [grant number 222933]. The funders had no role in study design, data collection and analysis, decision to publish, or preparation of the manuscript.

Competing Interests: The present study was supported by grants from the Smartfish® company and Regional Research Founds, Agder [grant number 222933]. The funders had no role in study design, data collection and analysis, decision to publish, or preparation of the manuscript.

* Email: tonje.h.stea@uia.no

Introduction

In European countries there is a growing elderly population, and it is predicted that the current 15% of the total population aged 65 or more years will increase to more than 25% by 2050 [1]. A similar growth rate of the elderly population is predicted in America and Australia [2,3]. As this is the fastest growing segment of the population, it becomes more apparent that investments in aging and health, including nutrition is essential. In several studies in older adults a relationship between dietary patterns and dietary quality and obesity-related health outcomes and mortality have been reported [4–7]. However, nutrition science is hampered by the fact that there is a questionable precision in most methods for dietary assessments [8–10].

A general finding in dietary studies is the tendency to underreport energy intake, and this is found both among children and adolescents [11,12], adults [13,14] as well as elderly [15,16]. In a study by Sharhar et al. [15] among high-functioning community-dwelling elderly, 70–79 years old, it was shown that underreporters had significantly higher body weight than the rest of the participants. A Danish cohort study, examining men at the mean ages of 20, 33, 44, and 49, has also shown that underreporting was more prevalent in obese men than those who were not obese [14].

In several studies energy expenditure (EE) has been estimated by the doubly labelled water (DLW) method to assess the possible disparity between EE and energy intake (EI), where EI is measured with either weighed or estimated methods [15,17]. The reason for using EE to validate EI is because there are no biochemical biomarkers of EI, so the methods of validation rest on the assumption that EI must be equal to EE when weight is stable [10]. Although the DLW method is clearly the most accurate method for measuring average EE, its use is limited in large groups because of its high cost, both for the labelled water, for the specialised equipment for the analysis and for the trained personnel [18]. Johannsen et al. [19] have reported that Sense-

Wear Pro$_3$ Armband (SWA; BodyMedia Inc., Pittsburg, PA, USA) register energy expenditure in healthy adults similar to or even more accurate than other available monitors during 14 days of monitoring. A reasonable level of concordance was demonstrated between SWA and DLW methods, both in the latter mentioned study (ICC = 0.63) and in another study (ICC = 0.46) for measuring daily EE in free-living adults during 10 days of monitoring [20]. Thus, comparison of different methods showed that SWA seemed to be a relatively inexpensive, practical and accurate monitor of EE.

The aim of the present study was to validate energy intake (EI) estimated from a pre-coded food diary (PFD) against energy expenditure (EE) measured with the SWA. Furthermore, to evaluate whether misreporting was associated with overweight/obesity in a group of Norwegian elderly men aged 60–80 years.

Subjects and Methods

Ethics Statement

The study has been approved by the Norwegian Regional Committee for Medical Ethics South-East C (2010/1352). This is an independent committee, appointed by the Norwegian Ministry of Education, IRB 00001870. Written informed consent was obtained from all the participants. The trial registration number was ACTRN12614000065695.

Subjects

Healthy men between 60–80 years old were invited to participate in the study and the participants were recruited in the south of Norway through advertisement in a local newspaper. A total of 200 men showed up at an open information meeting, and those who were healthy, non-smokers, did not use dietary supplements or any kind of medications that was likely to affect the results of the main study were invited to participate (n = 71). Medications to treat high cholesterol, blood pressure, migraine, and mild antidepressants were accepted. To ensure that the subjects were able to participate in the intervention study, a cardiologist at Sørlandet hospital, Kristiansand, conducted a medical screening before entering the study. Exclusion criteria included any overt disease, including COPD, cancer and heart disease. As a result of the health screening, 16 of the invited participants were excluded from the study. In addition, two subjects decided to drop out of the study due to personal circumstances. During the intervention, three more dropped out of the study due to a hip operation, a broken ankle and a biceps rupture, respectively. For analyzes, another three participants were excluded due to incomplete data sets. Thus, 47 participants completed the baseline study and the data sets were used in the analysis described in this report.

Design

This validation study is part of a larger double-blinded randomized placebo-controlled trial with aim to investigate whether supplementation with the antioxidants vitamin C and vitamin E may enhance adaptations to 12 weeks of strength training in terms of muscle growth and increase maximal strength in elderly men. The present study was initiated by the University of Agder in partnership with Norwegian School of Sports Science and Sørlandet hospital, Kristiansand.

Collection of data for the present study was carried out at two different occasions; in August (baseline) and December 2012 (post-test). The participants were given both written and oral instruction on how to fill out the PFD and how to use the SWA. It was emphasized that the participants should not change eating- and

activity patterns during the measurement period. Studies has confirmed that 3–5 days of monitoring is required to reliably estimate habitual physical activity, and 4–7 recording days is required to reliably estimate energy intake using a PDF in adults [11,21]. During both periods of data collection, the monitoring period was 4 days; the participants recorded their entire food intake for one weekend day and three consecutive weekdays and wore the SWA during the same period. Trained researchers telephoned all participants on the second day of the recording period to answer any questions and correct misunderstandings. Participants also received contact information, in order to ask questions to be answered at any time by the trained researchers.

Food Diary and photographic booklet

The PFD, using household measures and photographs for portion size estimation, was originally developed for use among Norwegian children and adolescents [22]. The PFD method provides a detailed dietary registration as it included questions about consumption of 277 food items grouped together according to the typical Norwegian meal pattern [23]. Each food group was supplemented with open-ended alternatives. The design of the PFD was similar to a cross-table with food listed on the left and time span across the top. Food amounts were presented in predefined household units (e.g. glasses, pieces or tablespoons) or as portions estimated from photographs. Along with the food diary, each participant received a validated photography-booklet that contained thirteen series of coloured photographs, each with four different portion sizes ranging from small to large [24]. The participants were instructed to register food and beverage intake immediately after each meal throughout the day. The diaries were scanned using the Teleform program, version 6.0 (Datascan, Oslo, Norway). Daily intake of energy was computed using the food database and software system (KBS, 2012), developed at the Department of Nutrition, University of Oslo. The food database is mainly based on the official food composition table [25].

SenseWear Pro$_3$ Armband (SWA)

The SWA is a portable device that monitors physiological parameters, including heat flux, skin temperature, galvanic skin response and skin temperature, and movement (bi-axial accelerometer) [20]. The participants were instructed to wear the SWA in order to register each day during the data collection period, starting from midnight at the first day of registration. They were instructed on how to apply the armband and informed that the armband should be worn at all times except when taking a bath or shower. The SWA was worn on the right arm over the triceps branchii muscle at the midpoint between the acromion and olecranon processes [20] and data were computed in 1-minute intervals. The participant's SWA data were acceptable for analysis if overall wear time was ≥19.2 hours/day during the period of data collection. SWA has been validated in adult populations, and the results showed underestimation of total EE with 4.7% and 12.5%, compared to estimates derived from doubly labelled water [19,20] and 9% compared to estimates derived from indirect calorimetry [26].

Weight, height, body mass index and lean mass measurements

Body weight and height were measured by trained project staff at two times during each data collection at baseline and post-test, respectively, and mean weight and height for both times were used for statistical analyses. Weight was measured with subjects in light clothing (shorts and t-shirt), and height was measured to the

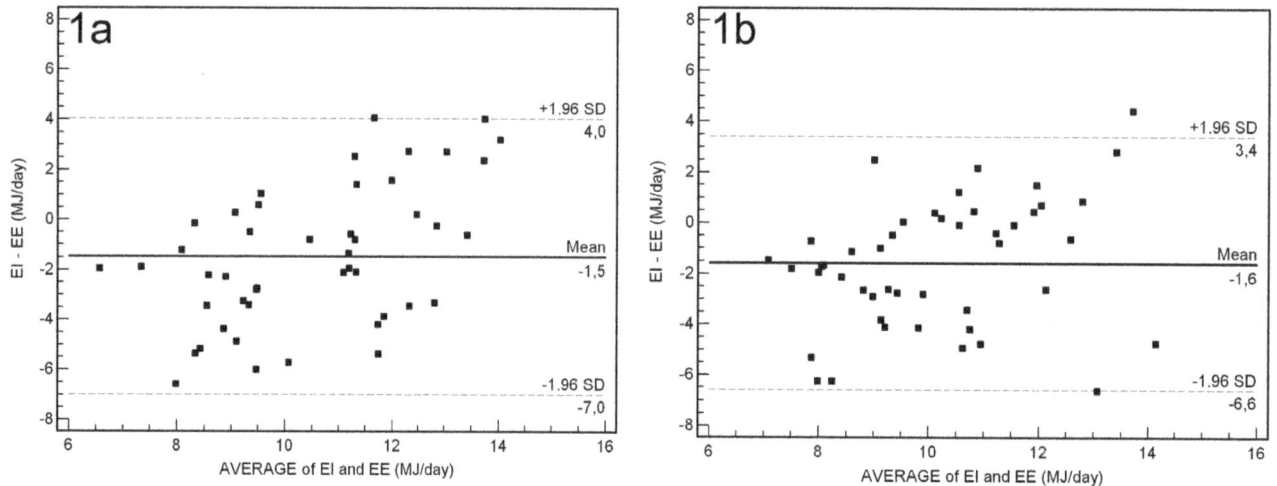

Figure 1. Bland - Altman plots: the baseline difference (Fig.1a) and post-test difference (Fig.1b) between estimated energy expenditure (EE) and estimated energy intake (EI) plotted against the mean of EE and EI. The solid line represents the mean, and the dotted line represents the limits of agreement (plus or minus 1.96 SD).

nearest 0.5 cm, using a measuring tape and body-mass monitor (Seca optima), respectively. Body mass index (BMI) was calculated as weight divided by the square of height (kg/m^2). Criteria for overweight, and obesity used in the present study were consistent with the definitions set forth by the World Health Organization (WHO) where overweigh = BMI 25.0–29.9 kg/m^2 and obesity = BMI ≥30 kg/m^2 [27]. Fat mass measured by one experienced observer was assessed by dual-energy X-ray absorptiometry (DXA; GE-Lunar Prodigy, Madison, WI, USA), which is currently recognized as a well-established reference method for measuring body composition [28], at both baseline and post-test. Participants were scanned from head to toe in supine position.

Statistical methods

The data were normally distributed and parametric statistical analysis was used to detect differences between EE (SWA) and EI (PFD). Table 1 presents physical characteristics of the participants as means and standard deviations. The accuracy of the reported EI was calculated from the ration EI/EE, for which a value of 1 refers to complete agreement between EI and EE. However, energy intake and energy expenditure may vary largely from day to day and exact agreement between EI and EE over several days in one individual is unlikely. Therefore, the accuracy of the reported EI was assessed partly based on the 95% confidence limits of agreement between EI and EE measured by the DLW method as proposed by Black [29]. Under-reporters were defined as EI/EE<0.80, acceptable reporters were defined as having a ration EI/EE in the range 0.80–1.20, while over-reporters were defined as EI/EE>1.20. Visual agreement between the methods was analysed using the procedure proposed by Bland and Altman [30], using a plot of the difference between the two methods against the average of the measurements (Figure 1a and 1b). This type of plot shows the magnitude of disagreement, spot outliers and any trend. A two-way mixed, single measure, parametric intraclass correlation (ICC) was performed for evaluating the extent of agreement between the SWA and the PFD. Difference in self-reported EI and EE among normal weight and overweight/obese participants were analysed using a paired sample t-test (Table 2). Figure 2 shows error bars illustrating mean difference between EI and EE among normal weight and overweight/obese

participants, respectively. A dependent sample t-test was used to analyse whether misreporting of energy intake varied between normal weight and overweight/obese participants. Results were considered statistical significant at p<0.05. Data were analysed using SPSS for Windows release 19.0 (SPSS Inc., Chicago, IL, USA).

Results

Mean age of the participants was 68.4 (SD 6.3) years. Table 1 shows that 29 (61%) and 31 (65%) of the participants were categorized as overweight or obese at baseline and post-test, respectively. Mean body fat was 27% at baseline and 26% at post-test. The mean weight remained stable during both periods of data collection (<1 kg daily variance).

The average EI was 17% lower than the measured EE at baseline and 18% lower at post-test.

Bland-Altman plots, showing the difference between EI estimated from the PFD and EE measured by the SWA plotted against the mean of the two methods, are presented in Figure 1a (baseline) and 1b (post-test). Mean difference from Bland-Altman plot for EI and EE was -1.5 MJ/day at baseline and −1.6 MJ/day at post-test and the width of 95% limits of agreement varied from −7.0 to 4.0 MJ/day at baseline and from −6.6 to 3.4 MJ/day at post-test, respectively. A total of 22 (47%) and 21 (49%) participants were under-reporting and 6 (13%) and 3 (6%) were over-reporting energy intake at baseline and post-test, respectively.

The ICCs were 0.30 (95% confidence interval (CI): 0.02, 0.54) at baseline (p = 0.018) and 0.34 (95% CI: 0.06, 0.57) at post-test (p = 0.009), giving 30 to 34% of the variance explained by differences among individuals.

Measured energy expenditure was significantly higher than self-reported energy intake among overweight/obese participants at both baseline and post-test (p<0.001) (Table 2). This relationship was not shown among normal weight participants. Figure 2 shows that mean difference between EI and EE was −0.2 MJ/day (95% CI: −1.5, 1.1) in normal weight participants and −2.4 MJ/day (−3.4, −1.4) in overweight/obese participants at baseline. Similar results were shown from post-test as mean difference between EI and EE was −0.6 MJ/day (−1.8, 0.52) in normal weight and −2.2 MJ/day (−3.1, −1.2) in overweight/obese participants. Among

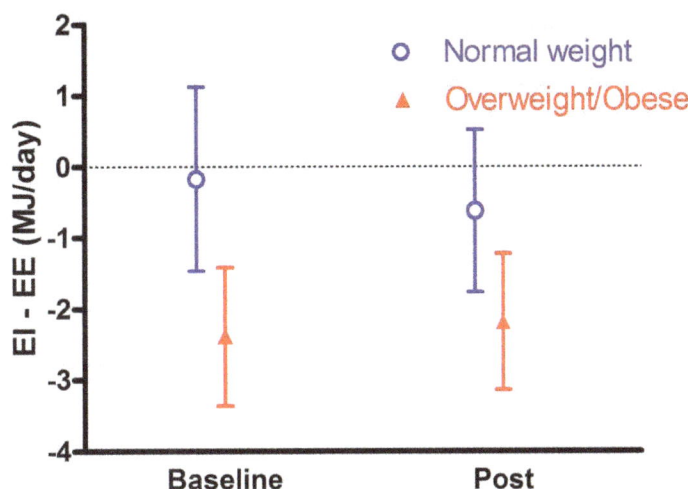

Figure 2. Error bars illustrating mean difference (95% CI) between energy intake (EI) and energy expenditure (EE) in normal weight and overweight/obese participants.

those who underreported EI at baseline, 7 (14.9%) were normal weight and 15 were overweight (31.9%). Among those who underreported EI at post-test, 6 (12.8%) were normal weight and 15 (31.9%) were overweight. Thus, underreporting was significantly more prevalent among overweight/obese participants compared to normal weight participants at both baseline and post-test (p<0.001 for both), respectively.

Discussion

To our knowledge, the PFD used in the present study has never before been used in this age group. The advantage of this method compared with traditional methods like weighed records and dietary history is that it is less time-consuming for the participants and the researchers to conduct. Most of the participants only used approximately 10–15 minutes per day to complete the PFD.

The present study showed that group average of self-reported EI was underreported by 17–18% compared with EE estimated by the SWA. Applying Bland-Altman plots to the energy data showed

a mean difference with a large variance and a scattering of the differences which indicated wide discrepancies between the two methods for individual subjects. Although underreporting was most evident, figure 1a and 1b illustrate the problem with both under- and overreporting of energy intake among the participants. The proportion of participants underreporting EI in the present study was somewhat higher than in other studies (13.6–16.2%) targeting similar age groups [31,32]. Studies among Norwegian children and adolescents that evaluated EI estimated from the same PFD as used in the present study against EE measured with a physical activity monitor (ActiReg), reported corresponding results underreporting ranging from 18% to 34% [12,33].

Different factors may explain the misreporting of energy intake. On the basis of ICC, the results from both baseline and post-test indicated that between 30–34% of the variance in EE and EI was explained by differences among individuals. The present study showed a significant relation between underreporting of energy intake and BMI; the EI seemed to be more valid in normal weight participants compared to overweight/obese participants. Previous

Table 1. Physical characteristics of the participants (n = 47), energy expenditure (EE) measured with SenseWear Pro₃ Armband and energy intake (EI) from the pre-coded food diary.

	Baseline		Post-test	
	Mean	**SD**	**Mean**	**SD**
BMI (kg/m^2)	26.2	3.4	26.5	3.4
Overweight, n (%)	21 (43.8)		22 (45.8)	
Obese, n (%)	8 (16.7)		9 (18.8)	
Percentage fat (%)	26.5	6.6	25.8	6.2
EE (MJ/day)	11.2	1.7	10.9	1.9
EI (MJ/day)	9.7	2.9	9.3	2.5
EI - EE	−1.5	2.8	−1.6	2.5
EI/EE	0.9	0.2	0.9	0.2
Acceptable reporters, n (%)	19 (40.4)		23 (48.9)	
Under-reporters, n (%)	22 (46.8)		21 (44.7)	
Over-reporters, n (%)	6 (12.8)		3 (6.4)	

Table 2. Self-reported energy intake (EI) and measured energy expenditure (EE) among normal weight and overweight/obese participants.

	n	EI (MJ/day)	EE (MJ/day)	p-value*
Baseline				
Normal weight	18	10.8 (9.3, 12.3)	11.0 (10.0, 11.9)	0.784
Overweight/Obese	29	9.0 (8.0, 10.0)	11.4 (10.8, 11.9)	<0.001
Post-test				
Normal weight	16	9.7 (8.4, 11.1)	10.4 (9.3, 11.4)	0.526
Overweight/Obese	31	9.1 (8.2, 10.0)	11.3 (10.6, 11.9)	<0.001

*Dependent sample t-test.

studies which have focused on identifying predictors of misreporting energy intake, confirm a positive relationship between overweight/obesity and underreporting of energy intake among elderly [16,31,34]. A study among 217 elderly women from Perth, Australia, showed higher odds of underreporting in overweight (OR = 2.98, 95% CI: 1.46, 6.09) and obese participants (OR = 5.84, 95% CI: 2.41, 14.14) compared to the rest of the study sample [34]. Furthermore, a study including 2083 elderly Belgian men and women concluded that BMI seemed to be one of the most important factors explaining misreporting [31]. A cohort study among 309 middle-aged Danish men investigated the degree of misreporting of EI and the association between underreporting and previous and current body size [14]. They found that among the participants currently not obese at the mean age of 49 years, underreporting was more than twice as prevalent among those who had been obese at the mean ages of 20 (44%) compared to those who were not obese at this age (21%) [14].

Within a longitudinal study on aging population in Germany, results among 238 female and 105 male participants showed that underreporters (7.6% of females and 16.2% of males), had lower educational level, significantly greater BMI and fat mass compared to adequate reporters [32].

The PFD used in the present study has previously been used in a study among 9 year old participants, and in this age group there was no significant differences in BMI between under-reporters and acceptable reporters (p = 0.77) [33]. In one of two studies among 13 year old girls; however, there was a significant negative relationship between BMI and the difference between EE and EI (EE-EI) (p = 0.003) [12], which is in contrast to most observations [10,35,36].

As the volunteers who participated in the present study were a small group of healthy non-smoking men who did not use medication or supplements, they are most properly not representative for the general elderly population. Another limitation is the choice of reference method in the present study. Validation studies

of SWA indicate that it underestimates EE compared to doubly labelled water (4.7–12.5%) [19,20]. Due to this underestimation, even larger underreporting from the recorded EI than observed may have occurred. However, SWA is a less expensive and complicated method compared with the other objective methods, as doubly labeled water and indirect calorimetry. Moreover, studies have concluded that SWA perform similar to or more accurate than other commonly used portable physical activity monitors [33,37].

It is possible that the participants did change their eating- and physical activity pattern due to increased awareness during the period of diet registration and use of SWA. However, the participants were instructed to maintain their usual daily routines of activity and eating pattern. Finally, the conclusions that have been drawn from the present study are strengthened as similar results were shown at baseline and post-test, respectively.

Conclusion

In summary, the results indicate that the PFD could be a useful tool for estimating energy intake in normal weight elderly men. As overweight/obese participants underestimated energy intake substantially, the PFD seemed to be less suitable for estimating energy intake in this subgroup of elderly men.

Acknowledgments

We would like to thank our dedicated participants, for their efforts throughout the study period.

Author Contributions

Conceived and designed the experiments: THS LFA GP KJH HLS SÅ TB SS SB. Performed the experiments: THS LFA GP KJH HLS SÅ TB SS SB. Analyzed the data: THS SB. Wrote the paper: THS.

References

1. World Health Organization (2013) The European Health Report 2012: charting the way to well-being. Copenhagen: World Health Organization Regional Office for Europe.
2. Australian Government (2010) The 2010 intergenerational report. Australia to 2050: future challenges.
3. Administration on Aging Administration for Community Living U.S. Department of Health and Human Services (2013) A Profile of Older Americans: 2013.
4. Ford DW, Jensen GL, Hartman TJ, Wray L, Smiciklas-Wright H (2013) Association between dietary quality and mortality in older adults: a review of the epidemiological evidence. J Nutr Gerontol Geriatr 32: 85–105.
5. Granic A, Andel R, Dahl AK, Gatz M, Pedersen NL (2013) Midlife dietary patterns and mortality in the population-based study of Swedish twins. J Epidemiol Community Health 67: 578–586.
6. Hsiao PY, Mitchell DC, Coffman DL, Craig Wood G, Hartman TJ, et al. (2013) Dietary patterns and relationship to obesity-related health outcomes and mortality in adults 75 years of age or greater. J Nutr Health Aging 17: 566–572.
7. Huijbregts P, Feskens E, Räsänen L, Fidanza F, Nissinen A, et al. (1997) Dietary pattern and 20 year mortality in elderly men in Finland, Italy, and The Netherlands: longitudinal cohort study. BMJ 315: 13–17.
8. Boeing H (2013) Nutritional epidemiology: New perspectives for understanding the diet-disease relationship? Eur J Clin Nutr 67: 424–429.
9. Long JD, Littlefield LA, Estep G, Martin H, Rogers TJ, et al. (2010) Evidence review of technology and dietary assessment. Worldviews Evid Based Nurs 7: 191–204.
10. Livingstone MBE, Black AE (2003) Markers of the validity of reported energy intake. J Nutr 133: S895–S920.

11. Forrestal SG (2011) Energy intake misreporting among children and adolescents: a literature review. Matern Child Nutr 7: 112–127.

12. Andersen LF, Pollestad ML, Jacobs DR Jr, Løvø A, Hustvedt BE (2005) Validation of a pre-coded food diary used among 13-year-olds: comparison of energy intake with energy expenditure. Public Health Nutr 8: 1315–1321.

13. Biltoft-Jensen A, Matthiessen J, Rasmussen LB, Fagt S, Groth MV, et al. (2009) Validation of the Danish 7-day pre-coded food diary among adults: energy intake v. energy expenditure and recording length. Br J Nutr 102: 1838–1846.

14. Nielsen BM, Nielsen MM, Toubro S, Pedersen O, Astrup A, et al. (2009) Past and current body size affect validity of reported energy intake among middle-aged Danish men. J Nutr 139: 2337–2343.

15. Shahar DR, Yu B, Houston DK, Kritchevsky SB, Newman AB, et al. (2010) Health, Aging, and Body Composition Study: Misreporting of energy intake in the elderly using doubly labeled water to measure total energy expenditure and weight change. J Am Coll Nutr 29: 14–24.

16. Rothenberg EM (2009) Experience of dietary assessment and validation from three Swedish studies in the elderly. Eur J Clin Nutr 63: 64–68.

17. Andersen LF, Pollestad ML, Jacobs DR Jr, Løvø A, Hustvedt BE (2003) Validation of energy intake estimated from a food frequency questionnaire: a doubly labeled water study. Eur J Clin Nutr 57: 279–284.

18. Pinheiro Volp AC, Esteves de Oliveira FC, Duarte Moreira Alves R, Esteves EA, Bressan J (2011) Energy expenditure: components and evaluation methods. Nutr Hosp 26: 430–440.

19. Johannsen DL, Calabro MA, Stewart J, Franke W, Rood JC, et al. (2010) Accuracy of armband monitors for measuring daily energy expenditure in healthy adults. Med Sci Sports Exerc 42: 2134–2140.

20. St-Onge M, Mignault D, Allison DB, Rabasa-Lhoret R (2007) Evaluation of a portable device to measure daily energy expenditure in free-living adults. Am J Clin Nutr 85: 742–749.

21. Trost SG, McIver KL, Pate RR (2005) Conducting accelerometer-based activity assessments in field-based research. Med Sci Sports Exerc 37: S531–S543.

22. Øverby N, Andersen LF (2002) Ungkost 2000: A national representative dietary survey among Norwegian children and adolescents (In Norwegian). Oslo: Directorate for Health and Social Affairs.

23. Øverby NC, Lillegaard ITL, Johanson L, Andersen LF (2004) High intake of added sugar among Norwegian children and adolescents. Public Health Nutr 7: 285–293.

24. Lillegaard ITL, Øverby NC, Andersen LF (2005) Can children and adolescents use photographs of food to estimate portion sizes? Eur J Clin Nutr 59: 611–617.

25. The Norwegian Food Safety Authority, The Norwegian Directorate of Health, The University of Oslo (2013) The Norwegian Food Composition Table. Available: http://www.matvaretabellen.no/?language = en.

26. Berntsen S, Hageberg R, Aandstad A, Mowinckel P, Anderssen SA, et al. (2008) Validity of physical activity monitors in adults participating in free-living activities. Br J Sports Med 44: 657–664.

27. World Health Organization (2004) Global database on body mass index. Available: http://apps.who.int/bmi/index.jsp?introPage = intro_3.html.

28. Kyle UG, Genton L, Pichard C (2002) Body composition: what's new? Curr Opin Clin Nutr Metab Care 5: 427–433.

29. Black AE (2000) The sensitivity and specificity of the Goldberg cut-off for EI:BMR for identifying diet reports of poor validity. Eur Journal Clin Nutr 54: 395–404.

30. Bland JM, Altman DG (1986) Statistical methods for assessing agreement between two methods of clinical measurement. Lancet 1: 307–310.

31. Bazelmans C, Matthys C, De Henauw S, Dramaix M, Kornitzer M, et al. (2007) Predictors of misreporting in an elderly population: the 'Quality of life after 65' study. Public Health Nutr 10: 185–191.

32. Lührmann PM, Herbert BM, Neuhäuser-Berthold M (2001) Underreporting of energy intake in an elderly German population. Nutrition 17: 912–916.

33. Lillegaard ITL, Andersen LF (2005) Validation of a pre-coded food diary with energy expenditure, comparison of under-reporters v. acceptable reporters. Br J Nutr 94: 998–1003.

34. Meng X, Kerr DA, Zhu K, Devine A, Solah VA, et al. (2013) Under-reporting of energy intake in elderly Australian women is associated with a higher body mass index. J Nutr Health Aging 17: 112–118.

35. Johanson G, Wikman A, Ahrén AM, Hallmans G, Johansson I (2001) Underreporting of energy intake in repeated 24-hour recalls related to gender, age, weight status, day of interview, educational level, reported food intake, smoking habits and area of living. Public Health Nutr 4: 919–927.

36. Kretsch MJ, Fong AK, Green MW (1999) Behavioral and body size correlates of energy intake underreporting by obese and normal-weight women. J Am Diet Assoc 99: 300–306.

37. Jakicic JM, Marcus M, Gallagher KI, Randall C, Thomas E, et al. (2004) Evaluation of the SenseWear Pro Armband to assess energy expenditure during exercise. Med Sci Sports Exerc 36: 897–904.

## 8

Estimated Cases of Blindness and Visual Impairment from Neovascular Age-Related Macular Degeneration Avoided in Australia by Ranibizumab Treatment

Paul Mitchell[1]*, Neil Bressler[2], Quan V. Doan[3], Chantal Dolan[4], Alberto Ferreira[5], Aaron Osborne[¤5], Elena Rochtchina[1], Mark Danese[3], Shoshana Colman[6], Tien Y. Wong[7,8]

1 Department of Ophthalmology and Westmead Millennium Institute, University of Sydney, Westmead, New South Wales, Australia, 2 Wilmer Eye Institute, Johns Hopkins University, Baltimore, Maryland, United States of America, 3 Outcomes Insights, Inc., Westlake Village, California, United States of America, 4 CMD Consulting, Inc., Sandy, Utah, United States of America, 5 Novartis, Basel, Switzerland, 6 Genentech, Inc., South San Francisco, California, United States of America, 7 Singapore Eye Research Institute, National University of Singapore, Singapore, Singapore, 8 Centre for Eye Research Australia, University of Melbourne, Parkville, Victoria, Australia

Abstract

Intravitreal injections of anti-vascular endothelial growth factor agents, such as ranibizumab, have significantly improved the management of neovascular age-related macular degeneration. This study used patient-level simulation modelling to estimate the number of individuals in Australia who would have been likely to avoid legal blindness or visual impairment due to neovascular age-related macular degeneration over a 2-year period as a result of intravitreal ranibizumab injections. The modelling approach used existing data for the incidence of neovascular age-related macular degeneration in Australia and outcomes from ranibizumab trials. Blindness and visual impairment were defined as visual acuity in the better-seeing eye of worse than 6/60 or 6/12, respectively. In 2010, 14 634 individuals in Australia were estimated to develop neovascular age-related macular degeneration who would be eligible for ranibizumab therapy. Without treatment, 2246 individuals would become legally blind over 2 years. Monthly 0.5 mg intravitreal ranibizumab would reduce incident blindness by 72% (95% simulation interval, 70–74%). Ranibizumab given as needed would reduce incident blindness by 68% (64–71%). Without treatment, 4846 individuals would become visually impaired over 2 years; this proportion would be reduced by 37% (34–39%) with monthly intravitreal ranibizumab, and by 28% (23–33%) with ranibizumab given as needed. These data suggest that intravitreal injections of ranibizumab, given either monthly or as needed, can substantially lower the number of cases of blindness and visual impairment over 2 years after the diagnosis of neovascular age-related macular degeneration.

Editor: Keisuke Mori, Saitama Medical University, Japan

Funding: This study was funded by Novartis AG and Genentech, Inc. Novartis AG and Genentech, Inc. participated in the design and conduct of the study, in the distribution of the raw data to Outcomes Insights, in the analysis and interpretation of the data and in the preparation of the manuscript. Novartis AG and Genentech, Inc. reviewed the manuscript before submission. Third-party medical writing assistance, but not editorial content sufficient to meet International Committee of Medical Journal Editors (ICMJE) authorship criteria, was funded by Novartis AG.

Competing Interests: The authors have read the journal's policy and have the following conflicts: Dr. Bressler's employer, the Johns Hopkins University (JHU), but not Dr. Bressler himself, receives funding from Bayer, Genentech, Inc., Roche, Novartis and Regeneron, and Steba Pharmaceuticals for sponsored projects by the Department of Ophthalmology for the efforts of Dr. Bressler. Dr. Bressler receives salary support for these sponsored projects; the terms of these projects are negotiated and administered by JHU's Office of Research Administration. Under JHU's policy, support for the costs of research, administered by the institution, does not constitute a conflict of interest. Paul Mitchell has received consultancy fees, lecture fees and travel support from Novartis Pharma AG, Pfizer, Solvay (Abbott), Bayer, Alcon and Allergan. Novartis Pharma AG also funds a retina fellowship at Westmead Hospital, Sydney, which he supervises. Alberto Ferreira is an employee of Novartis Pharma AG. Aaron Osborne is currently with Alcon Research Ltd and is a former employee of Novartis Pharma AG. Shoshana Colman is an employee of Genentech, both Novartis Pharma AG and Genentech sponsored this study. Quan Doan and Mark Danese are employees of Outcomes Insights, Inc., and Chantal Dolan is an employee of CMD Consulting, Inc.; these companies were paid for analysis work. Genentech and Novartis market ranibizumab. No financial benefit is anticipated as a result of this study.

* Email: paul.mitchell@sydney.edu.au

¤ Current address: Alcon Research Ltd., Fort Worth, Texas, United States of America

Introduction

Neovascular age-related macular degeneration (AMD) is the leading cause of blindness in many developed countries, including Australia [1,2]. Over the past 7 years, landmark clinical trials have shown that suppression of vascular endothelial growth factor (VEGF) with monthly or less frequent as-needed intravitreal injections of anti-VEGF agents prevented at least moderate visual acuity (VA) loss in nearly 95% of patients with neovascular AMD

after 1 year and nearly 90% after 2 years, and at least moderate VA improvement has been noted in up to 40% of patients [3-5].

However, despite the clinical efficacy of this treatment and its widespread use in many countries, few studies have investigated the population-wide impact of anti-VEGF therapy on the incidence of blindness and visual impairment [6]. A Danish study recently showed that legal blindness attributable to AMD has halved since the introduction of anti-VEGF therapies and an Israeli study showed a reduction in overall blindness over time after anti-VEGF therapy [7,8].

In the USA, a recent model estimated that the number of cases of legal blindness caused by neovascular AMD would reduce dramatically if monthly ranibizumab (Lucentis, Genentech, Inc., South San Francisco, CA, USA/Novartis AG, Basel, Switzerland) was used when indicated compared with no treatment [9]. Treatment was expected to reduce cases of legal blindness (defined in the USA as best-corrected visual acuity [BCVA] of 20/200 or worse in the better-seeing eye) by approximately 72% (95% confidence interval [CI], 70–74%) and visual impairment (defined as BCVA worse than 20/40 in both eyes) by approximately 37% (95% CI, 35–39%). These data suggested that the impact of neovascular AMD on legal blindness and visual impairment is reduced dramatically when monthly ranibizumab is available.

Additionally, a retrospective US study confirmed that the prevalence of legal blindness and visual impairment 2 years after the diagnosis of neovascular AMD has decreased substantially since the introduction of anti-VEGF therapy [10]. Some patients in this retrospective study received dosing as needed instead of monthly.

In Australia, AMD is the leading cause of blindness and visual impairment in individuals aged 65 years or older and has been estimated to cost the country over $5 billion per year (2010 figures) [11,12]. The impact of ranibizumab therapy on the number of cases of legal blindness and visual impairment caused by neovascular AMD in Australia is unknown. Estimates from the recent model for the USA [9] are unlikely to be directly applicable to Australia due to potential differences in patient characteristics, incidence of neovascular AMD and treatment behaviours. In particular, the US model only considered patients receiving monthly ranibizumab treatment, which is only relevant to a subset of patients with neovascular AMD worldwide. In most other countries, including Australia, patients treated with ranibizumab for visual impairment due to neovascular AMD typically receive therapy on an as-needed basis. Thus, the aim of the present study was to estimate the proportion of cases of legal blindness and visual impairment due to neovascular AMD in Australia that were avoided by treatment with ranibizumab given monthly or as needed over 2 years. A model was constructed assuming that all eligible patients would receive treatment.

Materials and Methods

Subjects

The analysis was based on all Australians aged 60 years or over in 2010 (Table 1). Incident cases of neovascular AMD were derived from the estimated 10-year cumulative incidence of AMD in the Blue Mountains Eye Study (BMES) [13], extrapolated to the Australian population in 2010, and assuming that events occurred evenly over the observation period. Among individuals with neovascular AMD, it was assumed that 33% had existing neovascular AMD in the fellow eye at baseline using information from the Age-Related Eye Disease Study (AREDS), and ANCHOR and MARINA phase 3 ranibizumab trials [3,5,14]. Base-case distribution of lesion types was based on the population used in the recent US model [9]; 5% were predominantly haemorrhagic, 5% extrafoveal, 10% minimally classic, 20% predominantly classic and 60% occult. Patients were classified according to lesion type into three cohorts, which determined their eligibility for treatment (Figure 1). The 'PC lesion' cohort had predominantly classic lesions on fluorescein angiography; the 'OC/MC lesion' cohort had occult with no classic or minimally classic lesions; the 'treatment-ineligible' cohort had lesions that were considered, by the authors, as unlikely to receive ranibizumab treatment and this cohort was not included in the model.

Model structure

The 2-year rates of blindness and visual impairment were estimated using a patient-level simulation developed in TreeAge Pro 2009 Suite (TreeAge Software, Inc., Williamstown, MA, USA) that included three primary health states: 'active treatment', 'no treatment' and 'death' (Figure 1). Each patient began the model on a specific treatment and remained on active treatment until discontinuation or death. The model accounted for VA changes in each eye, treatment discontinuation, risk of AMD in the fellow eye and mortality risk over each monthly interval for 2 years. Separate simulations were run for the PC lesion cohort and the OC/MC lesion cohort to estimate the 2-year rates of outcomes. These rates were then applied to the size of each cohort to determine the magnitude of the outcomes at the population level using @Risk for Excel (version 5.5.1; Palisade Corporation, Ithaca, NY, USA). Change over 2 years in patients with incident neovascular AMD in year 1 was simulated in the model. Model parameters are specified in Table 2.

Treatments

The treatment alternatives were ranibizumab 0.5 mg, given monthly (specified as every 30 ± 7 days) [3,5], ranibizumab dosed as needed (i.e. according to signs of AMD as detected on 4-weekly optical coherence tomography [OCT], as used in the Comparison of AMD Treatment Trials [CATT] study) [4], and photodynamic therapy (PDT) with verteporfin (vPDT) or no treatment if vPDT was not indicated. Across these scenarios, all eligible patients in the model received only the specified treatment. The PC lesion cohort received treatment similar to patients in the ANCHOR trial (ranibizumab, vPDT or no treatment) and the OC/MC lesion cohort received treatment as received by patients in the MARINA trial (ranibizumab or no treatment).

Baseline visual acuity and visual acuity change

The baseline VA for the PC lesion and OC/MC lesion cohorts was based on BCVA distributions in the treated and fellow eyes for patients in ANCHOR and MARINA, respectively [3,5]. Because the results from a subgroup analysis of ANCHOR suggested that the extent of VA change is conditional on baseline VA, the Early Treatment Diabetic Retinopathy Study [ETDRS] chart letter score change over 2 years was sampled from the same patients selected at baseline to preserve the relationship between baseline VA and VA change [15]. For monthly ranibizumab treatment, the VA change from each study and each treatment was applied to the corresponding neovascular AMD lesion subtype and treatment group in the model. For ranibizumab dosed as needed, it was assumed that the gain in VA letter score achieved at 24 months was 2.1 (95% CI, −1.0–5.2) less than that achieved with monthly dosing, based on 2-year data from the CATT study [4]. This adjustment was applied to the patient-level ANCHOR and MARINA data. The model also accounted for the risk of treatment discontinuation each month using discontinuation rates from the ANCHOR and MARINA trials. While the patient was not receiving treatment, VA change was assumed to decline by 1.6% per month based on the 2-year sham-treatment results in MARINA (a loss of 14.9 letters over 24 months) [5]. Patients could not return to active treatment after discontinuation. The VA letter scores in each eye were tracked for each month up to month 24 or the time of death, whichever occurred first. A monthly risk of death was applied using Australian age- and gender-specific mortality data [16,17].

Lesion characteristics

2010 Australia population age ≥ 60 years, N = 4 219 852

Total cases of neovascular AMD, n = 20 184 (95% SI, 11 602–33 477)

Extrafoveal; laser then treatment after recurrence (2.5%)

Predominantly classic (20.0%)

Minimally classic and recent disease progression (10.0%)

Occult with no classic under fovea and recent disease progression at presentation (20.0%) or during year (20.0%)

Predominantly haemorrhagic (5%)

Extrafoveal; laser and no further treatment (2.5%)

Occult with no classic under fovea with no disease progression over 1 year (20.0%)

Treatment options

Treatment-eligible cohort
n = 14 634 (95% SI, 8412–24 271)

Treatment-ineligible cohort
n = 5551 (95% SI, 3191–9206)

Predominantly classic lesion
Ranibizumab, vPDT or
no treatment as in ANCHOR

Occult with no classic and minimally classic lesion
Ranibizumab or no treatment as in MARINA

No treatment
No treatment or laser with no recurrence

Cohort not considered further

Patient-level simulation

No treatment

Treatment discontinuation

Monthly VA change

Active treatment

Death

Outcomes

Blindness: VA of eye worse than 6/60
Visual impairment: VA of eye worse than 6/12

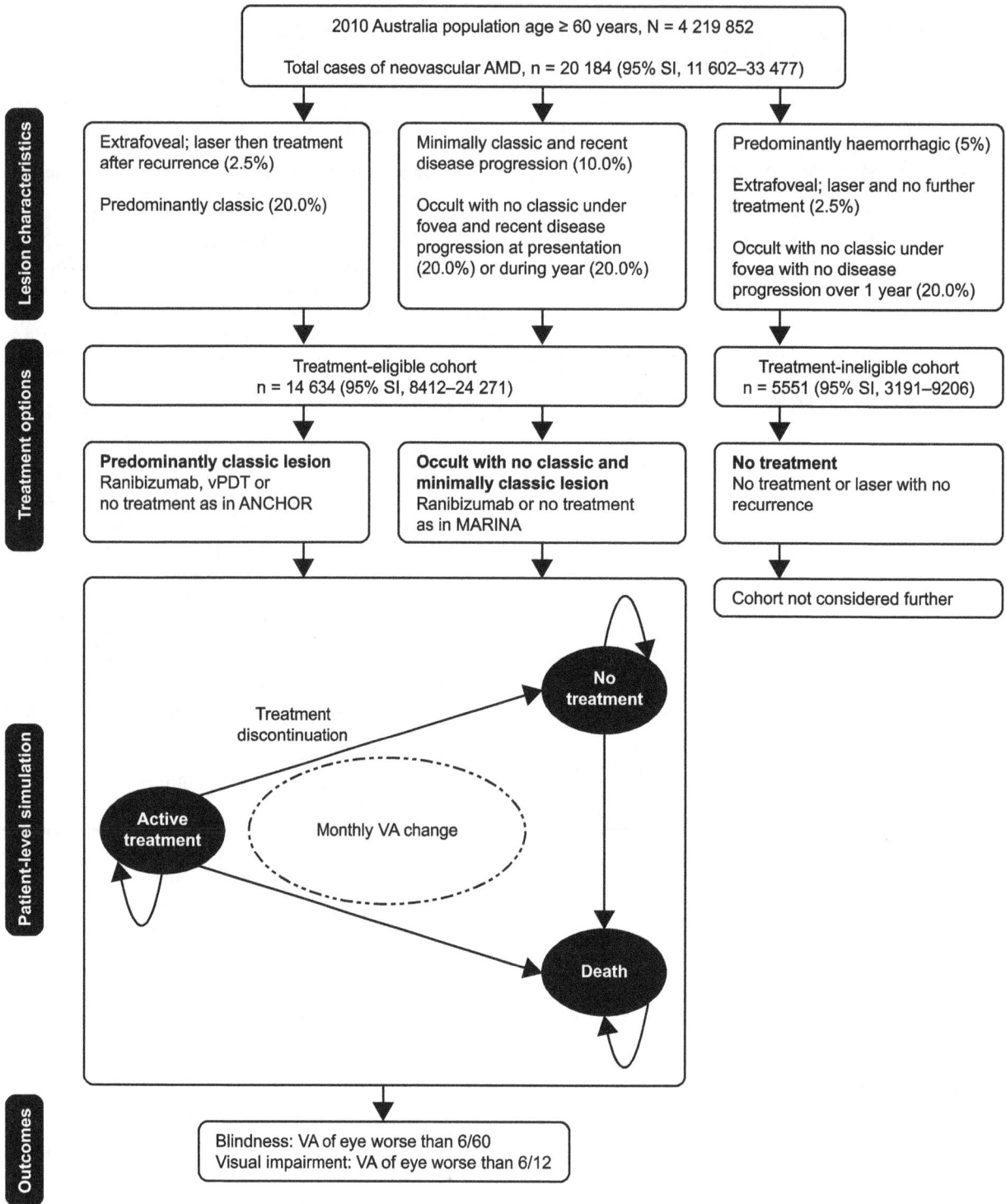

Figure 1. Model schematic. Incident cases of neovascular age-related macular degeneration (AMD) were derived by multiplying the number of individuals in each age group and gender by the respective incidences in the Blue Mountains Eye Study. Incident cases of neovascular AMD from 1 year were in the model for 2 years. Among individuals with AMD in one eye, 33% were estimated to have AMD in the fellow eye at baseline [3,5,14]. SI: simulation interval; VA: visual acuity; vPDT: photodynamic therapy with verteporfin.

Model outcomes

The key outputs from the model were the number of cases of legal blindness, defined as a VA score worse than 6/60 (approximated as a letter score of 38) in the better-seeing eye, and the number of cases of vision impairment, defined as a VA score of worse than 6/12 (approximated as a letter score of 68) in the better-seeing eye, over 2 years, including those patients already classified as having legal blindness [18]. For these outcomes,

Table 1. The Australian population aged 60 years or over in June 2010; distribution by age and gender.

Australian total population	60–69 years	70–79 years	≥ 80 years	Total
Male	1 053 685	599 729	326 947	1 980 361
Female	1 067 032	662 006	510 453	2 239 491
Total	2 120 717	1 261 735	837 400	4 219 852

Australian Bureau of Statistics (2011) 3101.0- Australian Demographic Statistics, Dec 2010. (Accessed September 2013 from http://www.abs.gov.au/AUSSTATS/abs@.nsf/mediareleasesbyCatalogue/251ECE081EC4B2EECA2579190013DCED).

ranibizumab was compared against no treatment, because PDT is now rarely used in Australia.

Sensitivity analyses

One-way sensitivity analyses were conducted on the proportions of neovascular AMD lesion types to assess the impact of these on blindness and visual impairment. Probabilistic sensitivity analysis was undertaken to account for various sources of patient variability and parameter uncertainty. Whenever possible, the distribution of patient-level characteristics was informed by the patient-level variability from trial data (e.g. baseline VA of each eye, VA change at 24 months in each eye). Parameter uncertainty was characterized as either a normal or gamma distribution. Patient-level variability was sampled in the first level, while parameter uncertainty was sampled in the second level, of a two-dimensional Monte Carlo simulation. To achieve stable rates, 300 averages of 10 000 iterations were sampled. Most of the key inputs into the model (Table 2) were evaluated. The confidence in the results is reported as an interval around the expected mean that captured 95% of all possible simulated values (95% simulation interval [SI]) for each outcome.

Results

Incidence of neovascular AMD

The model predicted that 20 184 (95% SI, 11 602–33 477) people would have developed neovascular AMD in Australia in 2010. Of these, 33% (6728) would have had pre-existing neovascular AMD in the fellow eye at the start of 2010.

Patients ineligible to receive ranibizumab

As shown in Figure 1, approximately 27.5% of incident cases of neovascular AMD (n = 5551) would have lesion types that would not be considered eligible for ranibizumab treatment. Assuming that all of the predominantly haemorrhagic cases progressed to a VA of worse than 6/60, and 33% of the extrafoveal and occult with no classic cases for which treatment was not judged to be indicated developed similar disease in the fellow eye, 2553 individuals would become legally blind over the following 2 years.

Patients eligible to receive ranibizumab

If none of the patients eligible to receive ranibizumab who were included in the model received treatment (n = 14 634; 95% SI, 8412–24 271), 2246 (95% SI, 1300–3695) patients would become legally blind over 2 years (Table 3). If they all received ranibizumab on a monthly basis, this number would drop to 624 patients (95% SI, 357–1031), a decrease of 72% (95% SI, 70–74%). If ranibizumab was dosed as needed, 724 patients (95% SI, 414–1211) would become blind, a decrease of 68% (95% SI, 64–71%). Treatment with PDT in those eligible to receive it would

result in a 12% (95% SI, 10–15%) reduction in cases of blindness (n = 1968; 95% SI, 1141–3220) compared with no treatment.

As summarized in Table 3, substantial reductions in the risk of bilateral visual impairment (BCVA worse than 6/60 in the incident eye) were predicted for ranibizumab dosed monthly or as needed. Bilateral visual impairment was predicted to develop over the 2-year period in 4846 patients with no treatment (95% SI, 2782–8027). Risk reductions of 37% and 28%, compared with no treatment, would be achieved with monthly ranibizumab and ranibizumab dosed as needed, respectively (Table 3). The corresponding reduction with PDT would be 1%. A BCVA worse than 6/60 in the incident eye would occur in 7865 patients (95% SI, 4534–13 120) with no treatment over the 2-year period; treatment with monthly or as-needed ranibizumab would achieve risk reductions of 68% and 65%, respectively, compared with no treatment, and the risk reduction for PDT would be 3%. A BCVA worse than 6/12 in the incident eye would occur in 8676 (95% SI, 4987–14 456) patients with no treatment, with risk reductions of 35%, 29% and 1% achieved with monthly ranibizumab, ranibizumab dosed as needed and PDT, respectively.

Sensitivity analyses

In the one-way sensitivity analyses, the proportions of patients with each neovascular AMD lesion type had the greatest impact on the cases of blindness and visual impairment avoided (Figure 2 and Figure 3, respectively). The SIs derived from the probabilistic sensitivity analyses showed moderate uncertainty around the estimates of legal blindness and visual impairment (Table 3).

Discussion

This study estimated the number of cases of blindness and visual impairment caused by neovascular AMD that can be avoided in Australia through the use of intravitreal ranibizumab injections. This model builds and expands on previous work by Bressler et al. [9] by accounting for characteristics specific to the Australian population, including Australian incidence data for neovascular AMD, Australian definitions for legal blindness and visual impairment, and Australian AMD incidence characteristics from population-level data. We modelled VA outcomes using 2-year, phase 3 ranibizumab trial data, which allowed us to use patient-level profiles following monthly treatment [3,5]. Results from the CATT study were used to estimate cases of blindness avoided with as-needed treatment [4]. The inclusion of as-needed therapy is a further important expansion of the previous model [9] because in many countries, including Australia, patients treated with ranibizumab for visual impairment due to neovascular AMD typically receive therapy on an as-needed basis. Furthermore, the inclusion of both monthly and as-needed regimens for the same population permits a comparison of predicted outcomes.

The model predicted that 20 184 people would develop AMD in Australia in 2010. Of these, about 5500 patients would not be

Table 2. Specification of the model parameters.

Model parameter		Value	Data source
Mortality		Overall death rate: 5.63/1000; age- and gender-specific rates used	Australian Bureau of Statistics[16,17]
Patients with health insurance/access problems		All residents of Australia are covered under Medicare plan and ranibizumab is fully covered for subfoveal neovascular AMD	Australian Health Service[a]
1-year incidence (SE) of neovascular AMD, women by age, years	< 60	0	BMES[13]
	60–69	0.0027 (0.0008)	
	70–79	0.0064 (0.0016)	
	≥ 80	0.0155 (0.0093)	
1-year incidence (SE) of neovascular AMD, men by age, years	< 60	0	BMES[13]
	60–69	0.0011 (0.0006)	
	70–79	0.0023 (0.0010)	
	≥ 80	0.0083 (0.0080)	
Patients with neovascular AMD in the fellow eye at baseline, %		33	Bressler et al. 2003[14]
Probability of developing neovascular AMD in the fellow eye, per month		0.0071	AREDS report number 8[b]
Baseline BCVA, LogMAR letter score, mean (SD) for the PC lesion cohort	Treated eye	46.5 (13.1)	ANCHOR trial data [3]; sampled from empirical trial data distribution
	Fellow eye without neovascular AMD at baseline	77.4 (13.7)	
	Fellow eye with neovascular AMD at baseline	34.5 (26.1)	
Baseline BCVA, LogMAR letter score, mean (SD) for the OC/MC lesion cohort	Treated eye	53.5 (13.2)	MARINA trial data;[5] sampled from empirical trial data distribution
	Fellow eye without neovascular AMD at baseline	76.1 (14.7)	
	Fellow eye with neovascular AMD at baseline	38.6 (26.2)	
Distribution of lesion subtypes, %	No treatment	27.5	Assumptions established in Bressler et al. 2011[9]
	PC lesion cohort	22.5	
	OC/MC lesion cohort	50.0	
Change in BCVA at 24 months		From empirical distributions	ANCHOR[3] and MARINA[5] trial data
Difference between monthly versus as-needed ranibizumab dosing in BCVA change at 24 months, letters (95% CI)		−2.1 (−5.2–1.0)	CATT study data[4]
Treatment discontinuation, monthly probability	Ranibizumab (PC lesions)	0.00178	ANCHOR (unpublished data, 2009)[9]
	Ranibizumab (OC/MC lesions)	0.00173	MARINA (unpublished data, 2006)[9]
	Photodynamic therapy	0.00407	ANCHOR (unpublished data, 2009)[9]
Patients, by BCVA letter score, after 2 years without treatment in PC lesion cohort, % (SD)	≤ 38 (worse than 6/60) in incident eye	67 (5.16)	TAP report number 3[c] (predominantly classic CNV)[d], SD reported in Bressler et al. 2011[9]
	≤ 38 (worse than 6/60) in better-seeing eye	22.3 (0.05)	TAP report number 3[d] and ANCHOR[3]
	≤ 68 (worse than 6/12) in incident eye	97.0 (1.86)	Assumption from Bressler et al. 2011[9]
	≤ 68 (worse than 6/12) in both eyes	52.6 (0.10)	Estimated based on TAP report number 3[c,d]
BCVA change per month after discontinuation from active treatment, %		1.6	Based on 2-year sham-treatment results in MARINA (−14.9 letters in 24 months)[5]

[a]Pharmaceutical Benefits Scheme. Ranibizumab. (Accessed September 2013 from www.pbs.gov.au). 2011.
[b]A randomized, placebo-controlled, clinical trial of high-dose supplementation with vitamins C and E, beta carotene, and zinc for age-related macular degeneration and vision loss: AREDS report no. 8. *Arch Ophthalmol* 2001; 119: 1417–1436.
[c]The mean baseline visual acuity of patients in TAP report number 3 is a 50-letter score.
[d]Bressler NM, Arnold J, Benchaboune M, Blumenkranz MS, Fish GE, Gragoudas ES *et al.* (2002) Verteporfin therapy of subfoveal choroidal neovascularization in patients with age-related macular degeneration: additional information regarding baseline lesion composition's impact on vision outcomes-TAP report No. 3. *Arch Ophthalmol*

120: 1443–1454.
AMD: age-related macular degeneration; BCVA: best-corrected visual acuity; CI: confidence interval; CNV: choroidal neovascularization; OC/MC lesion: occult with no classic lesions or minimally classic lesions; PC lesion: predominantly classic lesions; SD: standard deviation; SE: standard error.

eligible for ranibizumab treatment. Without treatment, 2246 of the remaining patients would become legally blind over a 2-year period. The results suggest that monthly ranibizumab would reduce the risk of legal blindness by 72% compared with no treatment, while the risk of visual impairment would be reduced by 37%. Dosing ranibizumab as needed with monthly monitoring provides a comparable reduction in the risk of blindness and visual impairment: 68% and 28%, respectively. Given the comparable VA outcomes between monthly and as-needed dosing regimens observed in the CATT study over 2 years [4], it is not surprising that there were only slightly fewer cases of blindness avoided with as-needed treatment than with monthly treatment, despite less frequent dosing. The extent to which these benefits can be extended beyond the 2-year period considered in this study is currently unknown.

The results of this modelling exercise confirm findings from a real-world database study in Denmark [7]. In that study, cases of blindness due to neovascular AMD were halved during the latter half of a 10-year period during which ranibizumab was introduced with a similar availability as in Australia. Since that study assessed registered blindness and might not have used high-contrast charts to evaluate vision, it is difficult to compare the results with those of our study; however, the Danish study suggests that benefits can be extended beyond the 2-year window that we considered. Although comparison with real-world data was not the aim of this study, future validation of our findings with real-world data on the impact of anti-VEGF therapy in the Australian population is warranted. To date, no studies have been conducted to evaluate real-world reductions in blindness or visual impairment due to neovascular AMD in Australia following the introduction of anti-VEGF therapies. However, several ongoing studies may provide suitable real-world data for future validation in the Australian population [19,20] or for comparison with the UK [21].

Particularly in older populations, blindness and visual impairment have been shown to have substantial clinical, humanistic and economic impacts including increased risk of falls and fractures, reduced mobility and independence, earlier need for supportive care (e.g. entry into a nursing home), and increased risk of mortality [22-30]. Thus, our findings may be of value to healthcare policy experts, recognizing that our results are

Table 3. Blindness and visual impairment outcomes in patients with neovascular age-related macular degeneration with and without monthly treatment with ranibizumab.

Scenario	Number of patients (% of total cohort of 14 634)	95% SI, n (%)	Relative risk reduction compared with no treatment, % (95% SI)
Legal blindness (BCVA worse than 6/60 in better-seeing eye[a])			
No treatment	2246 (15)	1300–3695 (9–25)	–
Monthly ranibizumab	624 (4)	357–1031 (2–7)	72 (70–74)
Ranibizumab dosed as needed	724 (5)	414–1211 (3–8)	68 (64–71)
PDT scenario: PDT indicated and accessible; ranibizumab not accessible	1968 (13)	1141–3220 (8–22)	12 (10–15)
Visual impairment (BCVA worse than 6/12 in better-seeing eye[b])			
No treatment	4846 (33)	2782–8027 (19–55)	–
Monthly ranibizumab	3072 (21)	1763–5114 (12–35)	37 (34–39)
Ranibizumab dosed as needed	3504 (24)	1990–5833 (14–40)	28 (23–33)
PDT scenario: PDT indicated and accessible; ranibizumab not accessible	4773 (33)	2750–7884 (19–54)	1 (−1–4)
BCVA worse than 6/60 in the incident eye			
No treatment	7865 (54)	4534–13 120 (31–90)	–
Monthly ranibizumab	2538 (17)	1463–4197 (10–29)	68 (66–70)
Ranibizumab dosed as needed	2791 (19)	1604–4625 (11–32)	65 (61–68)
PDT scenario: PDT indicated and accessible; ranibizumab not accessible	7635 (52)	4433–12 616 (30–86)	3 (−3–8)
BCVA worse than 6/12 in the incident eye			
No treatment	8676 (59)	4987–14 456 (34–99)	–
Monthly ranibizumab	5632 (38)	3237–9336 (22–64)	35 (33–36)
Ranibizumab dosed as needed	6125 (42)	3513–10 166 (24–69)	29 (26–33)
PDT scenario: PDT indicated and accessible; ranibizumab not accessible	8606 (59)	4943–14 271 (34–98)	1 (−2–2)

[a]Legal blindness was defined as a BCVA letter score worse than 6/60 (approximate ETDRS letter score ≤ 38) in the better-seeing eye.
[b]Visual impairment was defined as a BCVA letter score worse than 6/12 (approximate ETDRS letter score ≤ 68) in the better-seeing eye.
BCVA: best-corrected visual acuity; ETDRS: Early Treatment Diabetic Retinopathy Study; PDT: photodynamic therapy; SI: simulation interval.

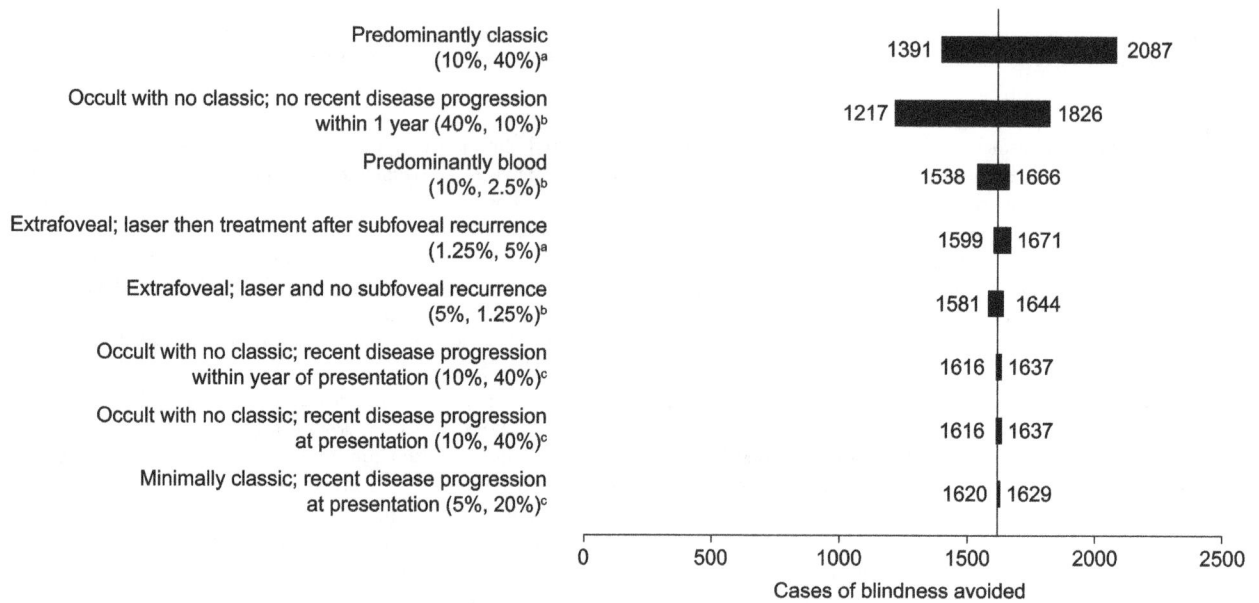

Figure 2. Sensitivity analyses. The impact of neovascular age-related macular degeneration lesion type on the cases of blindness (best-corrected visual acuity in better-seeing eye worse than 6/60) avoided using a monthly ranibizumab scenario compared with a no-treatment scenario. In the base analysis, 1622 cases of legal blindness were avoided with monthly ranibizumab, as indicated by the vertical line. [a]Eligible for PDT and ranibizumab. [b]Ineligible for any treatment. [c]Eligible for ranibizumab, but not for PDT. PDT: photodynamic therapy.

theoretical in nature and need to be considered in context along with factors such as patient preferences for therapy, treatment costs and healthcare resources. The information provided in this study may also be of value to health economists for incorporation in future cost-effectiveness models.

This study has some limitations that need to be considered. First, the incidence rates of neovascular AMD were based on the BMES and there was no allowance for national variability; however, this study is considered representative of the portion of the Australian population that is affected by neovascular AMD (i.e. the Caucasian population), and applies to the older population of Australia in this study [31]. Secondly, there is a lack of patient-level data to estimate results for as-needed dosing. Nevertheless, since the VA profile found in the CATT study after treatment was

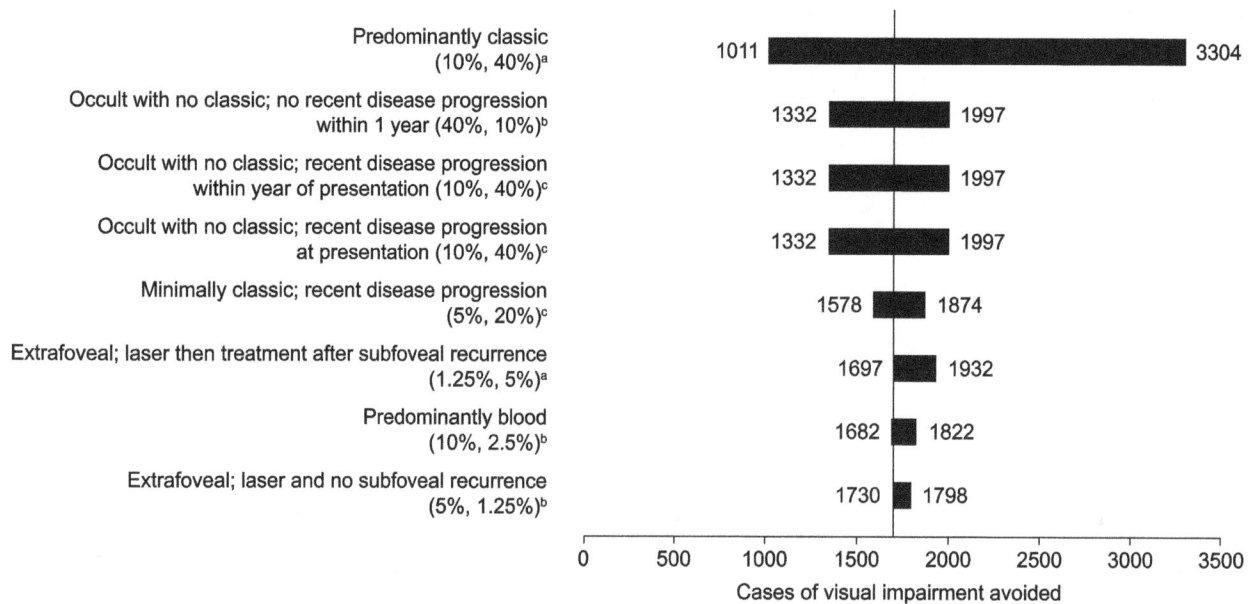

Figure 3. Sensitivity analyses. The impact of neovascular age-related macular degeneration lesion type on the cases of visual impairment (best-corrected visual acuity in better-seeing eye worse than 6/12) avoided using a monthly ranibizumab scenario compared with a no-treatment scenario. In the base analysis, 1774 cases of visual impairment were avoided with monthly ranibizumab, as indicated by the vertical line. [a]Eligible for PDT and ranibizumab. [b]Ineligible for any treatment. [c]Eligible for ranibizumab, but not for PDT. PDT: photodynamic therapy.

consistent across both groups (monthly and as-needed ranibizu-mab) [4], it was considered appropriate to also use the MARINA[5] and ANCHOR[3] profiles for as-needed dosing. Thirdly, there is limited evidence for the distribution of lesion types in patients in Australia. Since lesion type has an impact on avoidable blindness, according to the sensitivity analysis, it is important to know which types of lesions occur in the real world and how they respond to ranibizumab. Fourthly, the results might not be generalizable when the frequency of treatment is reduced below that used in the CATT study, or when monitoring of disease activity is limited to less than the monthly monitoring used in the CATT study. Also, further work is needed to understand the impact of 'treat-and-extend' regimens, as used in some countries, on the prevention of blindness.

To conclude, the results of this study suggest that, in Australia, ranibizumab given for neovascular AMD would reduce the number of cases of legal blindness over a 2-year period by 68% and 72%, and the number of cases of visual impairment by 28% and 37%, with as-needed and monthly treatment, respectively. These results are consistent with the known clinical benefits of anti-VEGF therapy for neovascular AMD, and extend the positive impacts of this treatment to the Australian population. In the future, neovascular AMD may no longer be the leading cause of blindness in older adults in Australia.

Acknowledgments

The authors would like to thank Jennifer Duryea of Outcomes Insights, Inc. for her work on the simulation model and technical report. In addition, Rowena Hughes and Polly Field from Oxford PharmaGenesis Ltd, Oxford, UK, provided editorial assistance in collating and addressing author comments.

Author Contributions

Conceived and designed the experiments: PM NB QVD CD AF AO ER MD SC TYW. Performed the experiments: PM NB QVD CD AF AO ER MD SC TYW. Analyzed the data: PM NB QVD CD AF AO ER MD SC TYW. Contributed reagents/materials/analysis tools: PM NB QVD CD AF AO ER MD SC TYW. Wrote the paper: PM NB QVD CD AF AO ER MD SC TYW.

References

1. Lim LS, Mitchell P, Seddon JM, Holz FG, Wong TY (2012) Age-related macular degeneration. Lancet 379: 1728–1738.

2. Resnikoff S, Pascolini D, Etya'ale D, Kocur I, Pararajasegaram R, et al. (2004) Global data on visual impairment in the year 2002. Bull World Health Organ 82: 844–851.

3. Brown DM, Michels M, Kaiser PK, Heier JS, Sy JP, et al. (2009) Ranibizumab versus verteporfin photodynamic therapy for neovascular age-related macular degeneration: two-year results of the ANCHOR study. Ophthalmology 116: 57–65.

4. Martin DF, Maguire MG, Fine SL, Ying GS, Jaffe GJ, et al. (2012) Ranibizumab and bevacizumab for treatment of neovascular age-related macular degeneration: two-year results. Ophthalmology 119: 1388–1398.

5. Rosenfeld PJ, Brown DM, Heier JS, Boyer DS, Kaiser PK, et al. (2006) Ranibizumab for neovascular age-related macular degeneration. N Eng J Med 355: 1419–1431.

6. Cheung N, Wong TY (2012) Changing trends of blindness: the initial harvest from translational public health and clinical research in ophthalmology. Am J Ophthalmol 153: 193–195.

7. Bloch SB, Larsen M, Munch IC (2012) Incidence of legal blindness from age-related macular degeneration in Denmark: year 2000 to 2010. Am J Ophthalmol 153: 209–213 e202.

8. Skaat A, Chetrit A, Belkin M, Kinori M, Kalter-Leibovici O (2012) Time trends in the incidence and causes of blindness in Israel. Am J Ophthalmol 153: 214–221 e211.

9. Bressler NM, Doan QV, Varma R, Lee PP, Suner IJ, et al. (2011) Estimated cases of legal blindness and visual impairment avoided using ranibizumab for choroidal neovascularization: non-Hispanic white population in the United States with age-related macular degeneration. Arch Ophthalmol 129: 709–717.

10. Campbell JP, Bressler SB, Bressler NM (2012) Impact of availability of anti-vascular endothelial growth factor therapy on visual impairment and blindness due to neovascular age-related macular degeneration. Arch Ophthalmol 130: 794–795.

11. Australian Institute of Health and Welfare (2005) Vision problems among older Australians. Bulletin no. 27. AIHW cat. No. AUS 60. Canberra. 2005. Accessed September 2013. Available: http://www.aihw.gov.au/WorkArea/DownloadAsset.aspx?id = 6442453394.

12. Macular Degeneration Foundation (2011) Eyes on the future. Accessed September 2013. Available: http://www.mdfoundation.com.au/LatestNews/Deloitte_Eyes_on_the_Future_Report_Exec_Summary%20web.pdf.

13. Wang JJ, Rochtchina E, Lee AJ, Chia EM, Smith W, et al. (2007) Ten-year incidence and progression of age-related maculopathy: the Blue Mountains Eye Study. Ophthalmology 114: 92–98.

14. Bressler NM, Bressler SB, Congdon NG, Ferris FL, 3rd, Friedman DS, et al. (2003) Potential public health impact of Age-Related Eye Disease Study results: AREDS report no. 11. Arch Ophthalmol 121: 1621–1624.

15. Kaiser PK, Brown DM, Zhang K, Hudson HL, Holz FG, et al. (2007) Ranibizumab for predominantly classic neovascular age-related macular degeneration: subgroup analysis of first-year ANCHOR results. Am J Ophthalmol 144: 850–857.

16. Australian Bureau of Statistics (2010) 3201.0 Population by Age and Sex, Australian States and Territories. Accessed September 2013. Available: http://www.abs.gov.au/ausstats/abs@.nsf/mf/3201.0/.

17. Australian Bureau of Statistics (2010) 3302.0 - Deaths, Australia, 2009; Table 2: Death rates, Summary, States and territories - 1999 to 2009. 2010. Accessed September 2013. Available: http://www.abs.gov.au/ausstats/abs@.nsf/detailspage/3302.02009.

18. Commonwealth of Australia (2011) Guide to Social Security Law. 7 Jan 2011. Accessed September 2013. Available: http://www.facsia.gov.au/guides_acts/ssg/ssguide-1/ssguide-1.1/ssguide-1.1.p/ssguide-1.1.p.210.html.

19. Abedi F, Wickremasinghe S, Islam AF, Inglis KM, Guymer RH (2014) Anti-VEGF treatment in neovascular age-related macular degeneration: a treat-and-extend protocol over 2 years. Retina Epub ahead of print.

20. Gillies MC, Walton RJ, Arnold JJ, McAllister IL, Simpson JM, et al. (2014) Comparison of outcomes from a phase 3 study of age-related macular degeneration with a matched, observational cohort. Ophthalmology 121: 676-681.

21. Writing Committee for the UK Age-Related Macular Degeneration EMR Users Group (2014) The Neovascular Age-Related Macular Degeneration Database: multicenter study of 92 976 ranibizumab injections: report 1: visual acuity. Ophthalmology 121: 1092–1101.

22. Cruess A, Zlateva G, Xu X, Rochon S (2007) Burden of illness of neovascular age-related macular degeneration in Canada. Can J Ophthalmol 42: 836–843.

23. Hochberg C, Maul E, Chan ES, Van Landingham S, Ferrucci L, et al. (2012) Association of vision loss in glaucoma and age-related macular degeneration with IADL disability. Invest Ophthalmol Vis Sci 53: 3201–3206.

24. Ivers RQ, Cumming RG, Mitchell P, Attebo K (1998) Visual impairment and falls in older adults: the Blue Mountains Eye Study. J Am Geriatr Soc 46: 58–64.

25. Klein BE, Moss SE, Klein R, Lee KE, Cruickshanks KJ (2003) Associations of visual function with physical outcomes and limitations 5 years later in an older population: the Beaver Dam eye study. Ophthalmology 110: 644–650.

26. Lotery A, Xu X, Zlateva G, Loftus J (2007) Burden of illness, visual impairment and health resource utilisation of patients with neovascular age-related macular degeneration: results from the UK cohort of a five-country cross-sectional study. Br J Ophthalmol 91: 1303–1307.

27. Popescu ML, Boisjoly H, Schmaltz H, Kergoat MJ, Rousseau J, et al. (2011) Age-related eye disease and mobility limitations in older adults. Invest Ophthalmol Vis Sci 52: 7168–7174.

28. Soubrane G, Cruess A, Lotery A, Pauleikhoff D, Mones J, et al. (2007) Burden and health care resource utilization in neovascular age-related macular degeneration: Findings of a multicountry study. Arch Ophthalmol 125: 1249–1254.

29. Szabo SM, Janssen PA, Khan K, Lord SR, Potter MJ (2010) Neovascular AMD: an overlooked risk factor for injurious falls. Osteoporos Int 21: 855–862.

30. Wood JM, Lacherez P, Black AA, Cole MH, Boon MY, et al. (2011) Risk of falls, injurious falls, and other injuries resulting from visual impairment among older adults with age-related macular degeneration. Invest Ophthalmol Vis Sci 52: 5088–5092.

31. Mitchell P, Wang JJ, Foran S, Smith W (2002) Five-year incidence of age-related maculopathy lesions: the Blue Mountains Eye Study. Ophthalmology 109: 1092–1097.

## 9

Erectile Dysfunction and Risk of End Stage Renal Disease Requiring Dialysis: A Nationwide Population-Based Study

Yuan-Chi Shen[1,2], Shih-Feng Weng[3,4], Jhi-Joung Wang[3], Kai-Jen Tien[5,6]*

1 Department of Urology, Kaohsiung Chang Gung Memorial Hospital, Kaohsiung, Taiwan, **2** Cheng Shiu University, Kaohsiung, Taiwan, **3** Department of Medical Research, Chi Mei Medical Center, Tainan, Taiwan, **4** Department of Hospital and Health Care Administration, Chia Nan University of Pharmacy and Science, Tainan, Taiwan, **5** Division of Endocrinology and Metabolism, Department of Internal Medicine, Chi Mei Medical Center, Tainan, Taiwan, **6** The Center of General Education, Chia Nan University of Pharmacy and Science, Tainan, Taiwan

Abstract

Background: Previous studies have suggested that erectile dysfunction (ED) is an independent risk factor for macrovascular disease. Very few studies have evaluated the relationship between ED and risk of end stage renal disease (ESRD) requiring dialysis.

Methods: A random sample of 1,000,000 individuals from Taiwan's National Health Insurance database was collected. We selected the control group by matching the subjects and controls by age, diabetes, hypertension, coronary heart disease, hyperlipidemia, area of residence, monthly income and index date. We identified 3985 patients with newly-diagnosed ED between 2000 and 2008 and compared them with a matched cohort of 23910 patients without ED. All patients were tracked from the index date to identify which patients subsequently developed a need for dialysis.

Results: The incidence rates of dialysis in the ED cohort and comparison groups were 10.85 and 9.06 per 10000 person-years, respectively. Stratified by age, the incidence rate ratio for dialysis was greater in ED patients aged <50 years (3.16, 95% CI: 1.62–6.19, p = 0.0008) but not in aged 50–64 (0.94, 95% CI: 0.52–1.69, p = 0.8397) and those aged ≥65 (0.69, 95% CI: 0.32–1.52, p = 0.3594). After adjustment for patient characteristics and medial comorbidities, the adjusted HR for dialysis remained greater in ED patients aged <50 years (adjusted HR: 2.08, 95% CI: 1.05–4.11, p<0.05). The log-rank test revealed that ED patients <50-years-old had significantly higher cumulative incidence rates of dialysis than those without (p = 0.0004).

Conclusion: Patients with ED, especially younger patients, are at an increased risk for ESRD requiring dialysis later in life.

Editor: Chih-Pin Chuu, National Health Research Institutes, Taiwan

Funding: The authors have no support or funding to report.

Competing Interests: The authors have declared that no competing interests exist.

* Email: cmmctkj@gmail.com

Introduction

Erectile dysfunction (ED) is defined as the inability to achieve or maintain an erection sufficient for sexual performance [1]. ED is an important worldwide issue, affecting 152 million men in 1995 and 322 million men in 2025 and negatively impacts life quality, self-esteem, and intimacy [2,3]. One telephone survey of ED prevalence in Taiwan reported that nearly thirty percent of men over 30 years had ED [4]. This medical problem has been associated with endothelial dysfunction and low-grade vascular inflammation and often clusters with hypertension, diabetes mellitus, hyperlipidemia, obesity, and metabolic syndrome [5,6,7]. In addition, it has been reported ED as an independent risk factor for macrovascular diseases such as coronary heart disease, cerebrovascular disease (CVD), and peripheral artery disease [8,9,10,11,12,13].

ED has been extensively studied in relation to metabolic disease and CVD but rarely in relation to microvascular diseases such as end stage renal disease (ESRD). Although ED is commonly found in patients in a late stage of chronic kidney disease (CKD) [14], little attention has been paid to whether it is related to the progression of kidney disease. Several studies have found that there is strong association between CVD and ESRD and that the interaction between the two diseases is bidirectional and complex [5,15,16,17]. Because CVD and ESRD may share a common pathophysiological pathway, it is possible that ED might also be associated with the development of ESRD. One cross-sectional study by Hermans et al., investigating the relationship between ED and microangipathy in diabetes, found ED to be associated with retinopathy but not with level of estimated glomerular filtration rate (eGFR) [18], though another cross-sectional investigation by

Table 1. Demographic characteristics and comorbid medical disorders for patients with and without erectile dysfunction (ED) in Taiwan.

Category	Subcategory	Patients with ED (N = 3985)	Patients without ED (N = 23910)	P-value
Age	0–49	1654(41.51%)	10063(42.09%)	0.7350
	50–64	1475(37.01%)	8818(36.88%)	
	≥65	856(21.48%)	5029(21.03%)	
Diabetes	Yes	541(13.58%)	3058(12.79%)	0.1704
	No	3444(86.42%)	20852(87.21%)	
Hypertension	Yes	905(22.71%)	5422(22.68%)	0.9628
	No	3080(77.29%)	18488(77.32%)	
Coronary heart disease	Yes	327(8.21%)	1935(8.09%)	0.8090
	No	3658(91.79%)	21975(91.91%)	
Hyperlipidemia	Yes	370(9.28%)	2079(8.70%)	0.2233
	No	3615(90.72%)	21831(91.30%)	
Area	North	2143(53.78%)	13387(55.99%)	0.0640
	Central	740(18.57%)	4267(17.85%)	
	South	1003(25.17%)	5729(23.96%)	
	East	99(2.48%)	527(2.20%)	
Income	NT<15840	1801(45.19%)	10646(44.53%)	0.4754
	NT 15841~25000	988(24.79%)	5858(24.50%)	
	NT>25001	1196(30.01%)	7406(30.97%)	

Chuang et al. reported it to be associated with both albuminuria and eGFR [19]. In a meta-analysis by Navaneethan et al., the prevalence of ED in chronic kidney disease was 70%, though one of the limitations with that review was that the studies reviewed were of small sample sizes and had cross-sectional designs [20].

In this longitudinal follow-up study, we used a population-based national insurance dataset in Taiwan to examine the relationship between ED and the risk of ESRD requiring dialysis.

Methods

Data sources

Taiwan launched a single-payer National Health Insurance (NHI) program on March 1, 1995. The NHI database covers nearly all of Taiwan's population, and is one of the largest and most complete population-based datasets in the world. The data used in this study came from the Longitudinal Health Insurance Database 2000 (LHID2000), which is a sub-set of NHI database that contains all claims data (from 1996 to 2011) of one million beneficiaries. This sample was systemic-randomly selected in 2000. There are no significant differences in age, gender and health care costs between the sample group and all enrollees in the NHI program. The LHID2000 provides encrypted patient identification numbers, gender, date of birth, dates of admission and discharge, the ICD-9-CM (International Classification of Diseases, Ninth Revision, Clinical Modification) codes of diagnoses and procedures, details of prescriptions, registry of Catastrophic Illness Patient Database, as well as costs covered and paid for by NHI. The institutional review board of Chi Mei Medical Center approved the protocol of this study. Informed consent was not required because the datasets were devoid of identifiable personal information.

Study sample

A retrospective cohort study was conducted with two study groups: a newly onset ED (erectile dysfunction) group and a matched non-ED control group during the recruitment period of 2000–2008. ED was defined in a patient if he had (1) at least two outpatient service claims with the codes of ED (ICD-9-CM code 60784) at any hospital or local medical clinic or (2) any one single hospitalization with ED listed among the five claims diagnosis codes. Patients diagnosed as having ED before 2000 were excluded. CKD is a well-known strong predictor for ESRD requiring dialysis. To evaluate the true association between ED and ESRD requiring dialysis, any patient with a diagnosis of renal function impairment (ICD9CM code: 582, 583, 585, 586, 588) was excluded. Because the outcome of interest was the occurrence of ESRD requiring dialysis, we also excluded patients identified in the registry of Catastrophic Illness Patient Database as being diagnosed as having chronic kidney disease (ICD-9-CM code 585), which would indicate that they were receiving dialysis for ESRD before their diagnosis of ED.

For each ED patient, six patients not diagnosed with ED were randomly selected from the dataset as a control group match. ED patients were matched with members of the control group by age, diabetes, hypertension, coronary heart disease, hyperlipidemia, area of residence, monthly income and index date. The index date for the ED subjects was the date of their first registration. The year of that index date was used to create the index date for each comparison subject. Demographic data such as gender, age, geographic area of Taiwan, and monthly income (record as NT$) were collected. Baseline co-morbidities of these patients were also recorded. These included diabetes mellitus (ICD9CM code:250), hypertension (ICD9CM code:401–405), coronary heart disease (ICD9CM code:410–414), and hyperlipidemia (ICD9CM code:272), because these co-morbidities are known to affect the risk of ESRD. We counted any of these comorbid conditions if the

Table 2. Risk for end stage renal disease (ESRD) requiring dialysis in patients with and without erectile dysfunction (ED).

		Patients with ED				Patients without ED				IRR (95% CI)	P value
		N	ESRD requiring dialysis	PY#	Rate*	N	ESRD requiring dialysis	PY#	Rate*		
All		3985	33	30412.37	10.85	23910	162	177837.16	9.06	1.20(0.82–1.74)	0.3445
Age	<50	1654	13	12530.70	10.37	10063	25	76264.65	3.28	3.16(1.62–6.19)	0.0008
	50–64	1475	13	11206.17	11.60	8818	80	64914.22	12.32	0.94(0.52–1.69)	0.8397
	≥65	856	7	6675.50	10.49	5029	57	37658.29	15.14	0.69(0.32–1.52)	0.3594
Follow up years	0–2	3985	1	7942.73	1.26	23910	14	47482.70	2.95	0.43(0.06–3.25)	0.4110
	2–4	3955	7	7694.23	9.10	23566	39	45660.37	8.54	1.07(0.48–2.38)	0.8778
	≥4	3575	25	14775.41	16.92	21114	109	85694.09	12.72	1.33(0.86–2.05)	0.1982

#PY, person-years.
*Rate: per 10000 person-years.

condition was diagnosed in an inpatient setting or in three or more ambulatory care claims coded one year before the index medical care date. Follow-up time in person-years (PY) was calculated for each person until diagnosis of ESRD requiring dialysis, death, or the end of 2011.

Statistical Analyses

All statistical operations were performed using the SAS 9.3.1 statistical package (SAS Institute, Inc., Cary, North Carolina, USA). Pearson's $\chi 2$ tests was used to compare differences in the baseline characteristics, co-morbid medical disorders and socio-demographic status between the study and control cohort. The incidence rate was calculated as the number of ESRD requiring dialysis cases during the follow-up, divided by the total person-years for each group by age and duration. The risk of being diagnosed as having ESRD requiring dialysis was compared between the ED group and the control group by estimating the incidence rate ratio using Poisson regression. Moreover, stratified Cox proportional hazard regression (stratified by age group <50 and ≥50) analysis was used to compute the adjusted hazard ratio for developing ESRD requiring dialysis between patients with and without ED after adjusting for possible confounding factors (diabetes, hypertension, coronary heart disease, hyperlipidemia, geographic area and monthly income). Kaplan-Meier analysis was also used to calculate the cumulative incidence rates of ESRD requiring dialysis between two cohorts, and the log-rank test was used to analyze the differences between the survival curves. A two sided P value <0.05 was considered significant.

Results

As can been seen in Table 1, a summary of the baseline characteristics and comorbid conditions of the two groups, 3985 male ED patients and 23910 non-ED patients were enrolled in the study. Because we selected the control group by matching with patients' characteristics and comorbidities, there were no significant differences in diabetes, hypertension, coronary heart disease, hyperlipidemia, geographic area and income.

Table 2 shows the risk for ESRD requiring dialysis in all patients stratified by age and number at risk of follow-up years. During the follow-up period, the incidence rates for ESRD requiring dialysis for the ED and non-ED cohorts were 10.85 and 9.06 per 10000 person-years, respectively. Stratified by age, the younger group <50 years has the most pronounced (IRR = 3.16, 95% CI = 1.62–6.19, p = 0.0008). We found no group differences in risk for ESRD requiring dialysis in the age groups 50–64 years and ≥65 years (IRR = 0.94, 95% CI = 0.52–1.69, p = 0.8397 and IRR = 0.69, 95% CI = 0.32–1.52, p = 0.3594, respectively). Analyzing by number at risk of follow up years, we found that the IRR for ESRD requiring dialysis increased progressively but not significantly along with the duration of ED.

We further analyzed the crude and adjusted HR for ESRD requiring dialysis in patients aged <50 years and those aged ≥50 (Table 3). After adjusting for age, gender, DM, HTN, CHD, hyperlipidemia, geographic area and monthly income, we found ED patients aged <50 years to be 2.08 times more likely to develop ESRD requiring dialysis (adjusted HR = 2.08, 95% CI = 1.05–4.11, P<0.05). There were no group differences in crude and adjusted HRs for ESRD requiring dialysis in those aged ≥ 50 years.

The results of Kaplan-Meier analysis revealed that ED patients <50 years old had a higher cumulative incidence rate for ESRD requiring dialysis than the comparison cohort (log-rank test P = 0.0004) (Figure 1).

Table 3. Crude and adjusted hazard ratios (HR) for the development of end stage renal disease (ESRD) requiring dialysis among the sample patients stratified by age.

		Age <50		Age ≥ 50	
		Crude HR (95% CI)	Adjusted HR (95% CI)	Crude HR (95% CI)	Adjusted HR (95% CI)
Erectile dysfunction	Yes	3.17*(1.62–6.19)	2.08*(1.05–4.11)	0.83(0.52–1.33)	0.85(0.53–1.37)
	No	1.00	1.00	1.00	1.00

*P-value <0.05.
Adjusted for diabetes, hypertension, coronary heart disease, hyperlipidemia, geographic area and monthly income.

Discussion

Many studies have reported ED to be associated with macrovascluar disease, but few have investigated the impact of ED on the progression of a microvascular disease such as kidney disease. This study represents the first nationwide population-based study to investigate the relationship between ED and risk for ESRD requiring dialysis in an Asian population. We found the incidence rate for ESRD requiring dialysis to be 10.85 per 10000 person-years in patients with ED. The risk was especially greater in younger ED patients of age <50 years. After adjusting for patient characteristics and medical comorbidities, we did not find an association between ED and increased risk in patients of age ≥50. The crude and adjusted HR for ESRD dialysis was 3.17-times and 2.08-times higher risk in ED patients of age <50 years than it was in the comparison cohort, respectively. Although the HR decreased after adjustment, ED patients remained at significantly higher risk.

Several studies have investigated the association between ED and microvascular disorders. One cross-sectional study by Siu et al., investigating the prevalence and risk factors of ED in diabetic patients [21], found a significant association between ED and microangiopathy and reported the odd ratios for retinopathy, microalbuminuria, clinical proteinuria and sensory neuropathy to be 2.27, 1.68, 2.27, and 2.05, respectively. Another small cross-sectional study involving 82 male diabetics in Japan reported an association between ED and proteinuria [22], though that study did not address the relationship between ED and eGFR. One study of 221 male diabetes reported an association between ED prevalence of elevated albuminuria [18], but found no difference in eGFR level between patients with ED and those without. Chuang et al., conducting a cross-sectional study to evaluate the association between ED and severity of albuminuria [19], reported that not only was ED associated presence of albuminuria and low eGFR level, but it had a stronger association on the presence of macroalbuminuria than microalbuminuria (odd ratios 4.49 and 2.28, respectively). ED is a common feature of CKD and ESRD. Two studies have closely correlated ED to the stage of CKD [14,20]. Although their results differed somewhat, both studies reported an association between ED and microangiopathy and suggested that it might have an impact on the disease progression.

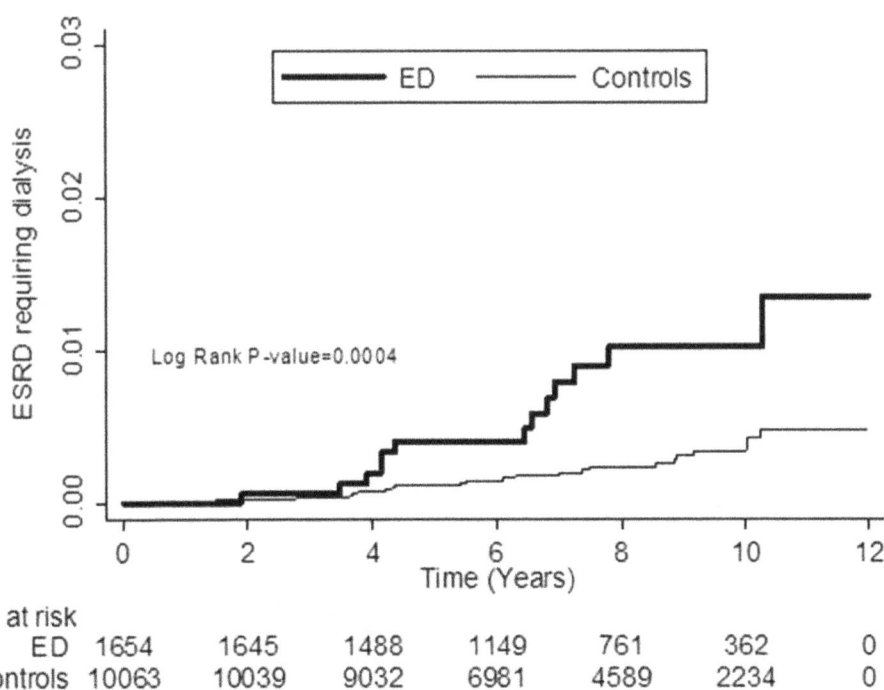

Figure 1. The cumulative incidence rate for end stage renal disease (ESRD) requiring dialysis for patients <50 years of age with erectile dysfunction (ED) and without ED (log-rank P value = 0.0004).

ED is generally thought to be secondarily increased in subjects with CKD and ESRD. However, a cross-sectional study design cannot be used to infer directionality. One important step to clarify the direction of the putative ED-ESRD association is the performance of a longitudinal study of individuals initially free of ESRD at baseline. Because CKD is an extremely strong predictor for ESRD requiring dialysis, we also excluded patients diagnosed as having any form kidney disease. Our study used ESRD requiring regular dialysis as the end point to evaluate the influence of ED on the progression of kidney disease.

Although the underlying mechanism contributing to the association between ED and risk of ESRD requiring dialysis is likely complex, there are some possible explanations that can be considered. First, metabolic comorbidities and cardiovascular disease are highly prevalent in ED patients. One national database in United States reported the crude prevalence rates to be 41.6% for hypertension, 42.4% for hyperlipidemia and 20.2% for diabetes in ED patients [5]. These metabolic comorbidities are the traditional risk factors that can deteriorate renal function. Since metabolic comorbidities were matched and adjusted for in the present study, the relationship between ED and ESRD requiring dialysis survived. The association between ED and ESRD may be in part due to these metabolic comorbidities, but they cannot explain the entire relationship between ED and ESRD. Second, ED is considered as a surrogate marker of endothelial damage, which is an important pathologic change in ED [23]. The hallmark of endothelial dysfunction is reduced synthesis of nitric oxide (NO), increased vasoconstrictor peptide endothelin-1 (ET-1), and increased production of the asymmetric dimethylarginine (ADMA) and inflammatory cytokines, including interleukin-6 (IL-6), C-reactive protein (CRP) and tumor necrosis factor-a (TNF-a) [24]. NO reduction was found to result in increased glomerular capillary pressure, vascular resistance and decreased capillary ultrafiltration in one animal study [25], suggesting that long term endothelial dysfunction might result in irreversible kidney damage. One study by Ravani and colleagues suggested that ADMA is inversely related to GFR and represents a strong and independent marker for progression to ESRD [26]. A population-based cohort study of up to 4926 patients with 15 years of follow-up reported that elevations of most inflammation markers, including TNF-a receptor 2 and IL-6 level, could predict risk of CKD [27]. Therefore, ED might be considered as an early marker and factor predisposing an individual to ESRD and not just diseases secondary to ESRD only.

In the current study, individuals who were diagnosed with ED later in life were at much less risk for ESRD requiring dialysis. The reason for this difference is not known. We speculate this lack of association in an elderly population may be due to several reasons. Compared with ED, the traditional risk factors for ESRD, which include hypertension, hyperlipidemia and diabetes, may have more impact on the disease progression. Marumo et al. evaluated the age-related prevalence of ED and the comorbidities to be common in ED patients in a cross-sectional study [28], and found the prevalence of hypertension, hyperlipidemia and diabetes to be dramatically increased after the age of 50 years. In the present study, the lack of association between ED and ESRD in elderly population may be due to by our adjustment for confounders in our model or may be due to the fact that elderly people with ESRD in Taiwan often refuse chronic dialysis therapy. In addition, the incidence of ESRD requiring dialysis may be underestimated in the elderly population.

This study has some limitations. First, the diagnosis of ED was based on diagnostic codes recorded by the physician in the NHI claims forms; therefore, some registration bias might be involved. The identification of ED and ESRD requiring dialysis diagnoses were based on diagnoses listed in an administrative database and therefore may be less accurate than diagnoses undertaken individually following standard procedures. In Taiwan, the self-administered International Index of Erectile Dysfunction (IIEF-5) questionnaire is usually used to assess and quantify the patients' subjective symptoms of ED. The diagnosis as well as the severity of ED can be evaluated based on the results of self-administered IIEF-5 questionnaire. Because the patients' raw questionnaire scores were not available in the administrative database, we defined ED by ICD-9-CM codes. To ensure the accuracy of these diagnostic codes, only the ED patients diagnosed by two patient claims records citing ED a primary diagnosis were recorded. ESRD requiring dialysis is definitely registered in Catastrophic Illness Patient Database in Taiwan. Patients identified in the registry of Catastrophic Illness Patient Database as having diagnosis of chronic kidney disease (ICD-9-CM code 585), which would indicate that they were receiving dialysis for ESRD. Therefore, registration bias was minimized as much as possible in this study. Another limitation may be related to lack of willingness to discuss possible ED problems in Taiwan. It is possible that some of the controls may have ED but not yet diagnosed. If this were the case, our results would have been biased toward the null leading to a more conservative estimate of association. Another limitation is that disease severity could not be assessed from our dataset. Still another limitation was claims records do not include smoking, Chinese herbal medicine, occupation, and family histories. Nor are environmental data recorded. Despite these limitations, the study is strong because it has a longitudinal, large population-based design and covers nearly all of Taiwan's residents. As such, both referral and selection biases are minimized.

In conclusion, patients with ED, which is conventionally considered as a risk factor of cardiovascular disease, are at increased risk for ESRD, especially in younger adults. Patients with early diagnosed ED are at an increased risk for ESRD with dialysis later in life. Further studies are needed to evaluate the possible underlying mechanisms between these two conditions.

Acknowledgments

This study is based in part on data from the National Health Insurance Research Database provided by the Bureau of National Health Insurance, Department of Health and managed by the National Health Research Institutes (Registered number 100057). The interpretation and conclusions contained herein do not represent those of the Bureau of National Health Insurance, Department of Health, or the National Health Research Institutes. We thank James F. Steed (Di Jian-shi) for editing the English language and reviewing the manuscript.

Author Contributions

Conceived and designed the experiments: YCS KJT. Performed the experiments: YCS SFW JJW KJT. Analyzed the data: SFW KJT. Contributed reagents/materials/analysis tools: YCS SFW JJW KJT. Contributed to the writing of the manuscript: YCS KJT.

References

1. Lewis RW, Fugl-Meyer KS, Corona G, Hayes RD, Laumann EO, et al. (2010) Definitions/Epidemiology/Risk Factors for Sexual Dysfunction. Journal of Sexual Medicine 7: 1598–1607.

2. O'Leary MP, Althof SE, Cappelleri JC, Crowley A, Sherman N, et al. (2006) Self-esteem, confidence and relationship satisfaction of men with erectile dysfunction treated with sildenafil citrate: a multicenter, randomized, parallel

group, double-blind, placebo controlled study in the United States. The Journal of urology 175: 1058–1062.

3. McKinlay JB (2000) The worldwide prevalence and epidemiology of erectile dysfunction. Int J Impot Res 12 Suppl 4: S6–S11.

4. Hwang TI, Tsai TF, Lin YC, Chiang HS, Chang LS (2010) A survey of erectile dysfunction in Taiwan: Use of the erection hardness score and quality of erection questionnaire. The journal of sexual medicine 7: 2817–2824.

5. Seftel AD, Sun P, Swindle R (2004) The prevalence of hypertension, hyperlipidemia, diabetes mellitus and depression in men with erectile dysfunction. The Journal of urology 171: 2341–2345.

6. Viigimaa M, Doumas M, Vlachopoulos C, Anyfanti P, Wolf J, et al. (2011) Hypertension and sexual dysfunction: time to act. Journal of hypertension 29: 403–407.

7. Weinberg AE, Eisenberg M, Patel CJ, Chertow GM, Leppert JT (2013) Diabetes severity, metabolic syndrome, and the risk of erectile dysfunction. The journal of sexual medicine 10: 3102–3109.

8. Blumentals W, Gomez-Caminero A, Joo S, Vannappagari V (2003) Is erectile dysfunction predictive of peripheral vascular disease? The Aging Male 6: 217–221.

9. Chew KK, Finn J, Stuckey B, Gibson N, Sanfilippo F, et al. (2010) Erectile Dysfunction as a Predictor for Subsequent Atherosclerotic Cardiovascular Events: Findings from a Linked-Data Study. The journal of sexual medicine 7: 192–202.

10. Ma RC-W, So W-Y, Yang X, Yu LW-L, Kong AP-S, et al. (2008) Erectile Dysfunction Predicts Coronary Heart Disease in Type 2 Diabetes. Journal of the American College of Cardiology 51: 2045–2050.

11. Ponholzer A, Temml C, Obermayr R, Wehrberger C, Madersbacher S (2005) Is erectile dysfunction an indicator for increased risk of coronary heart disease and stroke? European urology 48: 512–518.

12. Salem S, Abdi S, Mehrsai A, Saboury B, Saraji A, et al. (2009) ORIGINAL RESEARCH—ERECTILE DYSFUNCTION: Erectile Dysfunction Severity as a Risk Predictor for Coronary Artery Disease. The journal of sexual medicine 6: 3425–3432.

13. Thompson IM, Tangen CM, Goodman PJ, Probstfield JL, Moinpour CM, et al. (2005) Erectile dysfunction and subsequent cardiovascular disease. Jama 294: 2996–3002.

14. Bellinghieri G, Santoro D, Mallamace A, Savica V (2008) Sexual dysfunction in chronic renal failure. J Nephrol 21 Suppl 13: S113–117.

15. Stenvinkel P (2010) Chronic kidney disease: a public health priority and harbinger of premature cardiovascular disease. Journal of internal medicine 268: 456–467.

16. Uhlig K, Levey AS, Sarnak MJ (2002) Traditional cardiac risk factors in individuals with chronic kidney disease. pp. 118–127.

17. Zoccali C, Goldsmith D, Agarwal R, Blankestijn PJ, Fliser D, et al. (2011) The complexity of the cardio–renal link: taxonomy, syndromes, and diseases. Kidney International Supplements 1: 2–5.

18. Hermans MP, Ahn SA, Rousseau MF (2009) Erectile dysfunction, microangiopathy and UKPDS risk in type 2 diabetes. Diabetes & metabolism 35: 484–489.

19. Chuang YC, Chung MS, Wang PW, Lee WC, Chen CD, et al. (2012) Albuminuria is an independent risk factor of erectile dysfunction in men with type 2 diabetes. J Sex Med 9: 1055–1064.

20. Navaneethan SD, Vecchio M, Johnson DW, Saglimbene V, Graziano G, et al. (2010) Prevalence and Correlates of Self-Reported Sexual Dysfunction in CKD: A Meta-analysis of Observational Studies. American Journal of Kidney Diseases 56: 670–685.

21. Siu S, Lo SK, Wong K, Ip K, Wong Y (2001) Prevalence of and risk factors for erectile dysfunction in Hong Kong diabetic patients. Diabetic medicine 18: 732–738.

22. Yamasaki H, Ogawa K, Sasaki H, Nakao T, Wakasaki H, et al. (2004) Prevalence and risk factors of erectile dysfunction in Japanese men with type 2 diabetes. Diabetes Research and Clinical Practice 66: S173–S177.

23. Shamloul R, Ghanem H (2013) Erectile dysfunction. The Lancet 381: 153–165.

24. Aversa A, Bruzziches R, Francomano D, Natali M, Gareri P, et al. (2010) Endothelial dysfunction and erectile dysfunction in the aging man. International Journal of Urology 17: 38–47.

25. Reckelhoff J, Manning R (1993) Role of endothelium-derived nitric oxide in control of renal microvasculature in aging male rats. American Journal of Physiology-Regulatory, Integrative and Comparative Physiology 265: R1126–R1131.

26. Ravani P (2005) Asymmetrical Dimethylarginine Predicts Progression to Dialysis and Death in Patients with Chronic Kidney Disease: A Competing Risks Modeling Approach. Journal of the American Society of Nephrology 16: 2449–2455.

27. Shankar A, Sun L, Klein BEK, Lee KE, Muntner P, et al. (2011) Markers of inflammation predict the long-term risk of developing chronic kidney disease: a population-based cohort study. Kidney International 80: 1231–1238.

28. Marumo K, Nakashima J, Murai M (2001) Age-related prevalence of erectile dysfunction in Japan: Assessment by the International Index of Erectile Function. International Journal of Urology 8: 53–59.

## 10

Role of Omega-3 Fatty Acids in the Treatment of Depressive Disorders: A Comprehensive Meta-Analysis of Randomized Clinical Trials

Giuseppe Grosso[1]*, Andrzej Pajak[2], Stefano Marventano[3], Sabrina Castellano[1], Fabio Galvano[1], Claudio Bucolo[1], Filippo Drago[1], Filippo Caraci[4,5]

1 Department of Clinical and Molecular Biomedicine, Section of Pharmacology and Biochemistry, University of Catania, Catania, Italy, 2 Department of Epidemiology and Population Studies, Jagiellonian University Medical College, Krakow, Poland, 3 Department "G.F. Ingrassia", Section of Hygiene and Public Health, University of Catania, Catania, Italy, 4 Department of Educational Sciences, University of Catania, Catania, Italy, 5 IRCCS Associazione Oasi Maria S.S. – Institute for Research on Mental Retardation and Brain Aging, Troina, Enna, Italy

Abstract

Background: Despite omega-3 polyunsaturated fatty acids (PUFA) supplementation in depressed patients have been suggested to improve depressive symptomatology, previous findings are not univocal.

Objectives: To conduct an updated meta-analysis of randomized controlled trials (RCTs) of omega-3 PUFA treatment of depressive disorders, taking into account the clinical differences among patients included in the studies.

Methods: A search on MEDLINE, EMBASE, PsycInfo, and the Cochrane Database of RCTs using omega-3 PUFA on patients with depressive symptoms published up to August 2013 was performed. Standardized mean difference in clinical measure of depression severity was primary outcome. Type of omega-3 used (particularly eicosapentaenoic acid [EPA] and docosahexaenoic acid [DHA]) and omega-3 as mono- or adjuvant therapy was also examined. Meta-regression analyses assessed the effects of study size, baseline depression severity, trial duration, dose of omega-3, and age of patients.

Results: Meta-analysis of 11 and 8 trials conducted respectively on patients with a DSM-defined diagnosis of major depressive disorder (MDD) and patients with depressive symptomatology but no diagnosis of MDD demonstrated significant clinical benefit of omega-3 PUFA treatment compared to placebo (standardized difference in random-effects model 0.56 SD [95% CI: 0.20, 0.92] and 0.22 SD [95% CI: 0.01, 0.43], respectively; pooled analysis was 0.38 SD [95% CI: 0.18, 0.59]). Use of mainly EPA within the preparation, rather than DHA, influenced final clinical efficacy. Significant clinical efficacy had the use of omega-3 PUFA as adjuvant rather than mono-therapy. No relation between efficacy and study size, baseline depression severity, trial duration, age of patients, and study quality was found. Omega-3 PUFA resulted effective in RCTs on patients with bipolar disorder, whereas no evidence was found for those exploring their efficacy on depressive symptoms in young populations, perinatal depression, primary disease other than depression and healthy subjects.

Conclusions: The use of omega-3 PUFA is effective in patients with diagnosis of MDD and on depressive patients without diagnosis of MDD.

Editor: German Malaga, Universidad Peruana Cayetano Heredia, Peru

Funding: Giuseppe Grosso and Sabrina Castellano were supported by the International Ph.D. Program in Neuropharmacology, University of Catania, Catania, Italy. The contributors had no role in the study design, data collection and analysis, decision to publish, or preparation of the manuscript.

Competing Interests: The authors have declared that no competing interests exist.

* E-mail: giuseppe.grosso@studium.unict.it

Introduction

Omega-3 polyunsaturated fatty acids (PUFA) eicosapentaenoic acid (EPA) and docosahexaenoic acid (DHA) have been demonstrated to be effective in cardiovascular disease (CVD) prevention due to their anti-inflammatory and cardio-protective effects [1]. Recently, new therapeutic indications for omega-3 PUFA have been proposed, such as treatment for certain forms of mental illness, including depressive disorders [2]. Indeed, some psychiatric diseases as depression may share certain pathophysiological mechanisms with CVD, namely increased production of pro-inflammatory cytokines, endothelial dysfunction, and elevations in plasma homocysteine levels [3–5]. The positive effects of omega-3 PUFA on depression may depend on their physiological abundant content in the human nervous system and their involvement in neurogenesis and neuroplasticity [6]. Moreover, their anti-inflammatory capacity may counteract inflammatory processes occurring in depression [7,8]. Several ecological, cross-sectional, and prospective studies supported such hypotheses by reporting an inverse association between omega-3 intake and prevalence of depression [2]. Further clinical studies demonstrated lower concentration of omega-3 PUFA in plasma or red blood cell membranes of depressed subjects [9–13]. All together, these observations suggest a correlation between omega-3 PUFA and depressive disorders, justifing the rationale of a number of randomized controlled trials (RCTs) of omega-3 PUFA supplementation for the treatment of depressive disorders. The overall analysis of these studies from previous meta-analyses suggested a general benefit of omega-3 PUFA on depressive symptoms, despite certain variability in results weakened the possible validity of the findings. Indeed, results of such studies are not univocal, jeopardizing the evidence of therapeutic implications of omega-3 PUFA in depressed patients. It has been suggested that the heterogeneity between studies may depend on clinical and methodological issues, such as severity of baseline depression and methods of assessment and diagnosis of depression. Some important issues regarding therapeutic regimen have been explored in more recent meta-analysis, reporting that the positive effects of omega-3 PUFA on depressive symptoms appeared to depend more on EPA administration rather than DHA, severity of depression, and study quality [14]. However, some concerns regarding these findings still persist [15,16]. The analyses previously conducted focused on the effects of omega-3 PUFA supplementation on depressive symptoms, but features associated with the pathophysiological nature of the depression occurring in the patients and their comorbidity status were often lacking. It is reasonable to believe that the biological effects of omega-3 PUFA may result effective in certain subtypes of depressive disorders rather than in others due to the different type of depression or clinical phenotype of the patient. Despite a full understanding of the processes leading to the depressive status is lacking, primary psychiatric disorders, such as major depression disorder (MDD) and bipolar disorders, are specific psychiatric conditions as recognized in the American Psychiatric Association's revised fourth edition of the Diagnostic and Statistical Manual of Mental Disorders (DSM-IV) [17], marking out specific depressive symptoms that should be present as inclusion criteria to determine MDD diagnosis. The mental health examination may include the use of rating scales, such as the Hamilton Rating Scale for Depression [18], the Beck Depression Inventory [19], or the MARDS [20] for MDD, and the bipolar spectrum diagnostic scale [21] for bipolar disorders. These psychiatric diseases have indeed specific biological causes and are often known to be treated with and respond to different pharmacological interventions [22]. Another specific pathological condition is perinatal depression, which indicates the occurrence of depressive and other mood-associated symptoms during pregnancy and lactation, with a range of 5–25% of women developing post-partum depression [23]. Pregnancy and lactation are challenging periods due to a higher demand of omega-3 PUFA from the fetus and the newborn, respectively, and a low DHA status may induce depressive symptoms [24]. Despite the fact that it is not clear if the depressive status is caused by or simply precipitated by pregnancy and lactation conditions, it is however likely associated with these conditions rather than with the aforementioned causes of MDD. Similarly, psychiatric disorders occurring in young populations need special attentions because major differences between adult and juvenile depression have been well-documented, despite the reasons for such dissimilarities are not clear [25]. Actually, there is very limited evidence upon which to base conclusions about the relative effectiveness of psychological interventions or antidepressant medication, but effectiveness of these interventions cannot be fully established [26]. Finally, the occurrence of depression secondary to a different primary disease, for instance schizophrenia, Alzheimer's disease (AD), Parkinson's disease, and CVD, may raise doubts on the pathophysiological mechanisms that cause the depressive symptomatology. In addition, despite it is of interested to examine the role of omega-3 PUFA on potential mood depression in healthy subjects, it is important to underline that preventive and therapeutic pathways may differ each other. Thus, altogether, the choice in previous meta-analyses to pool together studies with such different baseline conditions, in which depression occurred, may have affected the quality of the studies as well as utilizability of the results [27,28]. Moreover, the last meta-analysis included studies up to 2010 [29]. Thus, the aim of this study was to update the current knowledge about the overall clinical efficacy of omega-3 fatty acids (particularly EPA and DHA) in previous and more recent RCTs published in the last years, minimizing, from a clinical point of view, the differences among the populations of patients included in the studies, finally focusing on patients with a DSM-defined diagnosis of MDD.

Methods

A comprehensive search on MEDLINE, EMBASE, PsycInfo, and the Cochrane Database systematic Reviews of all RCTs using omega-3 PUFA on patients with depressive symptoms published up to August 2013 was performed. Articles of potential interest were identified by using the following search terms: "omega-3", "polyunsaturated fatty acids", "PUFA", "trial", "EPA", "DHA", combined with the following terms: "depression", "depressive disorder", "depressed mood", "bipolar", combined with "perinatal", "post-partum", "CVD", "schizophrenia", "Parkinson", "Alzheimer", "diabetes", "angina". Among the 192 articles retrieved, RCTs were identified and screened by reading the abstract and, when necessary, the full text, in order to select those articles relevant for the analysis. The reference list of the relevant reports was also inspected to identify any additional trials not previously identified. The process of identification and inclusion of trials is summarized in Figure 1. Inclusion criteria were the following: (i) studies conducted on humans; (ii) randomized design; (iii) placebo controlled; (iv) use of omega-3 PUFA supplement which relative amount could be quantified; (v) exploring changes in depressive symptoms as primary or secondary outcome. Exclusion criteria were the following: (i) studies reporting insufficient statistics or results; (ii) adopted a dietary intervention design. Study quality was measured in a 13-point scale including the Jadad criteria [30] and specific information regarding (i) registration of RCT before conducting the study, (ii) adequate blinding of the researchers, (iii) the use of an intention-to-treat analysis, (iv) control for patients' diet (i.e., number of servings of fish), (v) assessment of compliance through measurement of plasma fatty acids, (vi) significant differences at baseline, (vii) adequate sample calculation, whether (viii) depression was the primary outcome, and (ix) number and reasons of withdrawal were mentioned. Data were abstracted independently from each identified trial by GG and SM using a standard data abstraction form. This process was independently performed by two researchers and discordances were discussed and risolved.

Out of 59 originally selected studies, one [31] was excluded because of having a non-randomize non-placebo controlled design; two [32,33], because there was used a dietary intervention design; five [34–38], because the depressive status was reported as a categorical variable rather than a rating scale; two [39,40], because an inadequate or poorly comparable rating score of depression was used; two [41,42], because poorly comparable omega-3 PUFA or placebo preparations. This selection strategy resulted in a final selection of 47 studies eligible to be included in the present systematic review.

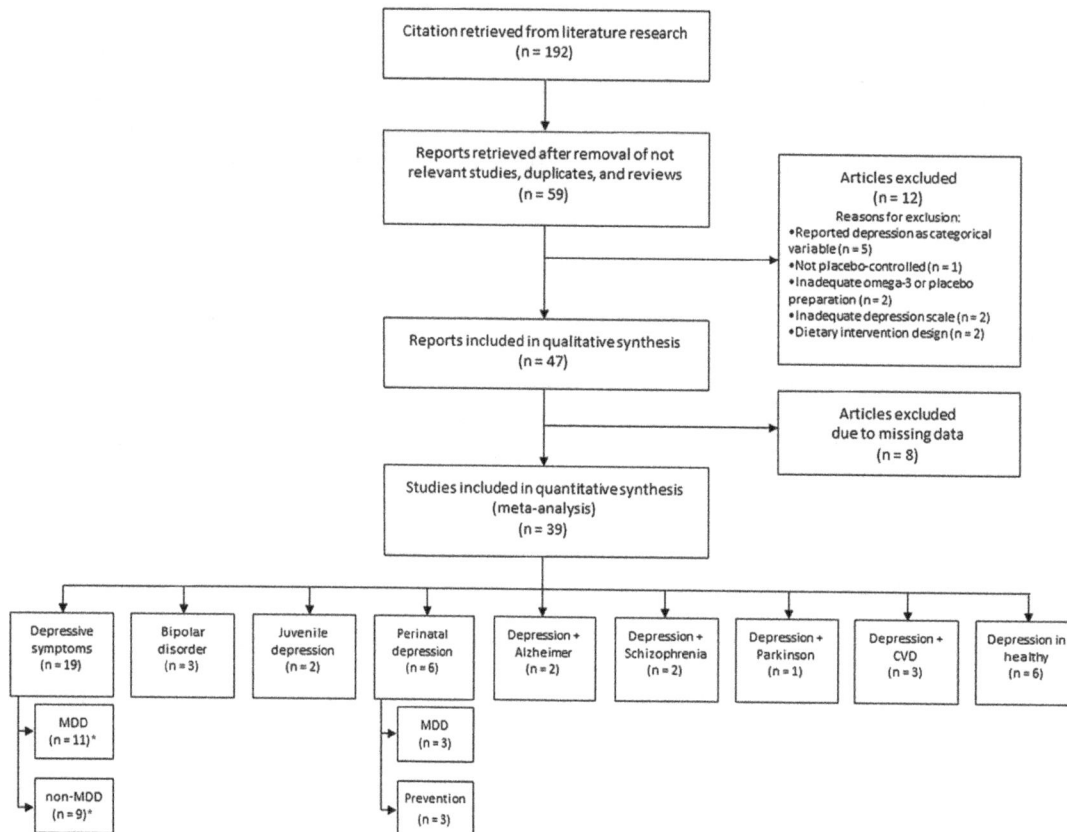

Figure 1. Process of inclusion of trials for systematic review and meta-analysis of studies on omega-3 fatty acids and depressive symptoms.

The clinical outcome of interest was the standardized mean difference in the change from baseline to endpoint scores on a depression rating scale, in patients taking omega-3 PUFA supplements *vs.* patients taking placebo. Preferred rating scales for measuring depression severity were the Hamilton Depression Rating Scale (HDRS), either the 9-item short form, 17-item, 21-item or 25-items scales, and the Montgomery Asberg Depression Rating Scale (MADRS) [20,43,44]. When available, HDRS scores from each study were used. If the HDRS was not available we used the MADRS. If neither HDRS nor MADRS data were available, we used the clinician rated measure of depression that the investigators identified as their primary outcome.

Among selected RCTs lacking in data, such as means and/or standard deviations (SDs), the data of one study [45] were provided by authors; SDs and 95% confidence intervals (CIs) of five studies [46–50] were retrieved from graphs; data of one study [51] were medians; and data of three studies [52–54] were imputed from data from all other trials using the same measure for depression as described elsewhere [55]. Eight studies [56–63] were finally excluded from the meta-analysis due to lacking data, resulting in a total number of 39 studies to be included in the analysis.

Effects due to participant diagnosis were investigated by grouping studies according to the most relevant clinical characteristics of the population on which they were conducted, as follows: (i) Depressed patients (including DSM-defined diagnosis of MDD and general assessment of depression without clinical visit);

(ii) Bipolar disorder patients (including bipolar disorder during pregnancy); (iii) Children or adolescents with depression or bipolar disorder; (iv) Women with perinatal depression (including DSM-defined diagnosis of MDD and prevention of post-partum depression); (v) Mild-cognitive impairment or AD patients; (vi) Schizophrenic patients; (vii) Parkinson's disease patients; (viii) Patients with concomitant CVDs; and (ix) Healthy subjects.

Data regarding type of diagnosis, number of subjects enrolled in the trial, on-going therapy, (TRATT.) type of supplement used in the intervention, type of placebo, daily dose, duration of the intervention, outcome measures, and information to retrieve the study quality were collected. Those RCTs reporting more than one dose of omega-3 PUFA [54,64–68] or more than one formulation (i.e., EPA or DHA separately) [48,51,69], were considered as separate studies in the pooled analyses. One study [70] enrolled different populations (MDD and non-MDD patients), thus each population was also included in the meta-analysis as a separate study.

Statistical Analysis

Continuous data were reported as mean and SDs and listed in descriptive tables. All depression scales' means and SDs at baseline and end of follow-up period of both intervention and control groups were combined [71] and the standardized mean effect for all trials was calculated by using Hedges adjusted g in order to correct for small sample bias [72]. Both random- and fixed-effects models were used to estimate the overall effect size. Heterogeneity

Table 1. Randomized controlled trials investigating effects of omega-3 polyunsaturated fatty acids (PUFAs) on depressed mood listed in chronological order by type of depressive disorder.

Author	Year	Participating Group	Subjects, n (I/C)	Type of treatment	Intervention	Placebo	Daily dose	Duration (weeks)	Outcome measure	Study quality
MDD										
Nemets [76]	2002	Pz with MDD	20 (10/10)	All but 1 used antidepressant	E-EPA	NR	2 g	4	HDRS	8
Marangell [77]	2003	Pz with MDD	36 (18/18)	None	DHA	NR	2 g	6	MADRS HDRS	7
Su [78]	2003	Pz with MDD	28 (14/14)	Mixed antidepressants	EPA+DHA	Olive oil ethyl esters	4.4 g EPA+2.2 g DHA	8	HDRS	8
Grenyer [46]	2007	Pz with MDD	83 (40/43)	Mixed antidepressants	EPA+DHA	Olive oil	0.6 g EPA+2.2 g DHA	16	BDI, HDRS	9
Jazayeri [48]	2008	Pz with MDD	60 (20/20/20)	Fluoxetine	E-EPA, E-EPA+ fluoxetine	Rapeseed oil	1.0 g E-EPA	8	HDRS	10
Mischoulon [83]	2009	Pz with MDD	57 (28/29)	Psychotherapy	EPA (+0.2% dl-alpha-tocopherol)	Paraffin oil and 0.2% dl-alpha-tocopherol	1 g EPA	8	HDRS −17	11
Rondanelli [95]	2010	Pz with MDD (only women >66)	46 (22/24)	None	EPA+DHA	Paraffin oil	1.67 g EPA+0.83 DHA	8	GDS, SF-36	10
Rondanelli [53]	2011	Pz with MDD (only women >66)	46 (22/24)	None	EPA+DHA	Paraffin oil	1.67 g EPA+0.83 DHA	8	GDS, SF-36	10
Gertsik [84]	2012	Pz with MDD	42 (21/21)	Citalopram	EPA+DHA	Olive oil	0.9 g EPA+0.2 g DHA	8	HDRS, BDI, MADRS, CGI	7
Rizzo [96]	2012	Pz with MDD (only women >66)	46 (22/24)	NR	EPA+DHA	Paraffin oil,	2.5 g of n-3 PUFA with EPA/DHA 2:1	8	GDS	8
Non-MDD										
Behan [39]	1990	Pz with post viral fatigue	63 (39/24)	NR	EPA+DHA	Liquid paraffin+ 0.4 g LA	0.14 g EPA+0.09 g DHA	13	4-point Linkert scale	8
Warren [56]	1999	Pz with chronic fatigue syndrome	50 (24/26)	None	EPA+DHA	Sunflower oil	0.14 g EPA+0.9 g DHA	13	BDI	8
Peet [54]	2002	Pz treated for depression	70 (17/18/17/18)	Mixed antidepressants	E-EPA	Liquid paraffin	1 g; 2 g; 4 g	12	HDRS, MADRS, BDI	7

Table 1. Cont.

Author	Year	Partecipating Group	Subjects, n (I/C)	Type of treatment	Intervention	Placebo	Daily dose	Duration (weeks)	Outcome measure	Study quality
Zanarini [91]	2003	Pz with borderline personality disorder	30 (20/10)	Heterogeneous	E-EPA	Mineral oil	1 g	8	MADRS	6
Fux [57]	2004	Pz with obsessive compulsive disorder	11 (11/11) (within-subjects crossover design)	Heterogeneous	E-EPA	Liquid paraffin	2 g	6	HDRS	6
Silvers [79]	2005	Pz treated for depression	77 (40/37)	Mixed antidepressants	EPA+DHA	Olive oil	0.6 g EPA+2.4 g DHA	12	HDRS-SF, BDI	10
Hallahan [49]	2007	Pz with recurrent self-harm	49 (22/27)	Mixed antidepressants	EPA+DHA	Corn oil+1% n23 PUFAs	1.2 g EPA+0.9 DHA	12	BDI, HDRS	9
Rogers [86]	2008	Untreated pz with mild-to-moderate depression	218 (109/109)	None	EPA+DHA	Olive oil	0.63 EPA 0.85 DHA	12	DASS, BDI, GHQ, Mood Diary	12
Lucas [70]	2009	Pz with psychological distress	120 (59/61)	None	EPA +DHA (ethyl esters)	Sunflower oil	1.05 g EPA. 0.15 g DHA	8	PGWB, HDRS, CGI, HSCL-D-20	12
Tajalizadek-hoob [97]	2011	Pz with mild-to-moderate depression (>66 yrs)	66 (33/33)	55 mixed antidepressants, 11 none	EPA+DHA	Coconut oil	0.180 g EPA+0.120 g DHA	24	GDS-15	10
Antypa [89]	2012	Pz with a history of at least one major depressive episode	71 (36/35)	7 mixed antidepressants, 6 heterogeneous, 58 none	EPA+DHA	Olive oil	1.74 g EPA+0.25 g DHA	4	BDI-II	9
Mozaffari-Khosravi [69]	2013	Pz with mild-to-moderate depression	81 (27/27/27)	Mixed antidepressants	EPA or DHA	Coconut oil	1 g EPA or 1 g DHA	12	HDRS-17	12
Sohrabi [40]	2013	Pz with pre-mestrual syndrome	139 (70/69)	113 sedative, 26 none	EPA+DHA	NR	0.24 EPA +0.36 DHA	12	VAS	8
Bipolar disorder										
Stoll [75]	1999	Pz with bipolar disorder	30 (14/16)	Heterogeneous	EPA+DHA	Olive oil	6.2 g EPA+3.4 g DHA	16	HDRS	8
Hirashima [58]	2004	Pz with bipolar disorder	21 (12/9)	Heterogeneous	EPA+DHA	NR	5–5.2 g EPA+3–3.4 g DHA or 1.3 g EPA+0.7 g DHA	4	HDRS	4

Table 1. Cont.

Author	Year	Participating Group	Subjects, n (I/C)	Type of treatment	Intervention	Placebo	Daily dose	Duration (weeks)	Outcome measure	Study quality
Chiu [63]	2005	Pz with bipolar disorder	15 (NR)	Lorazepam, valproate	EPA+DHA	Olive oil	0.44 g EPA+0.24 g DHA	4	HDRS	5
Frangou [65]	2006	Pz with bipolar disorder	75 (24/25/26)	Heterogeneous	E-EPA	Paraffin oil	1 g; 2 g	12	HDRS	9
Keck [59]	2006	Pz with bipolar disorder	116 (59/57)	Mood stabilizing	E-EPA	Liquid paraffin	6 g	17	IDS-C	9
Frangou [80]	2007	Pz with bipolar disorder	14 (7/7)	Lithium	E-EPA	Liquid paraffin	2 g E-EPA	12	HDRS	8
Depression or bipolar disorder in children and adolescents										
Nemets [98]	2006	Children with MDD	28 (13/15)	5 Methylphenidate	EPA+DHA	Olive oil or safflower oil	0.38–0.40 g EPA. 0.18–0.20 g DHA	16	CDRS, CDI, CGI	7
Gracious [61]	2010	Children and adolescents with bipolar disorder	51 (NR)	lithium, atypical antipsychotic	α-LNA	Olive oil	0.55–6.6 α-LNA	16	CDRS-R, CPRS, CGI-BP	11
Amminger [92]	2010	Adolescents at risk of psycosis	81 (41/40)	Heterogeneous	EPA+DHA	Coconut oil	0.70 g EPA+0.48 g DHA	48	MADRS, SCID	11
Peritanal MDD										
Freeman [99]	2008	Pz with MDD during pregnancy	59 (31/28)	Psychotherapy	EPA+DHA	Corn oil+1% fish oil	1.1 g EPA+0.8 g DHA	8	EPDS, HDRS, CGI	8
Su [82]	2008	Pz with MDD during pregnancy	36 (18/18)	None	EPA+DHA	Olive oil ethyl esters	2.2 g EPA 1.2 g DHA	8	HDRS, EPDS, BDI-21	10
Rees [93]	2008	Pz with MDD during pregnancy	26 (13/13)	None	EPA+DHA	Sunola oil	0.42 g EPA. 1.64 g DHA	6	EPDS, HDRS, MADRS	11
Prevention of post-partum depression										
Llorente [85]	2003	Healthy pregnant women	99 (44/45)	None	DHA	NR	0.2 g	16	BDI	10
Doornbos [51]	2009	Healthy pregnant women	119 (42/41/36)	Unclear	DHA DHA+AA	Soybean oil	0.22 g DHA. 0.22 g DHA. 0.22 g AA	28	EPDS (Dutch), PPBQ	5
Mozurkewich [68]	2013	Healthy pregnant women	126	Unclear	EPA+DHA	soy oil	1.06 g EPA+0.27 DHA or 0.9 DHA+0.18 EPA		BDI	12
Depressive symptoms in pz with Alzheimer disease or mild cognitive impairment										
Chiu [81]	2008	Pz with Alzheimer disease or mild cognitive impairment	46 (24/22)	Unclear	EPA+DHA	Olive oil ethyl esters	1.08 g EPA+0.72 g DHA	24	MMSE, HDRS	9
Freund-Levi [50]	2008	Pz with Alzheimer disease	204 (103/101)	Various	EPA+DHA	Corn oil+0.6 g LA	0.6 g EPA. 1.72 g DHA	26	MADRS, NPI	8

Table 1. Cont.

Author	Year	Partecipating Group	Subjects, n (I/C)	Type of treatment	Intervention	Placebo	Daily dose	Duration (weeks)	Outcome measure	Study quality
Sinn [60]	2012	Pz with mild cognitive impairment (>65)	50 (17/18/15)	Unclear	EPA+DHA	LA 2,2 g	1.67 g EPA+0.16 g DHA or 1.55 g DHA+0.40 g EPA	24	GDS	9
Depressive symptoms in pz with schizophrenia										
Fenton [90]	2001	Pz with schizophrenia	87 (43/44)	All but 1 used neuroleptic	E-EPA	Mineral oil	3 g	16	MADRS	10
Peet [64]	2002	Pz with schizophrenia	115 (29/28/27/31)	31 clozapine, 48 atypical antipsychotics, 36 typical psychotic	E-EPA	Liquid paraffin	1 g; 2 g; 4 g	12	MADRS	9
MDD in pz with Parkinson's disease										
Da Silva [47]	2008	Pz with Parkinson's disease and MDD	29 [NAD: 13 (6/7) AD: 16 (8/8)]	26 levodopa, 19 pramipexol, 5 amantadine, 4 COMT inhibitors, 6 SSRI, 4 tricyclics, 2 trazodone	EPA+DHA	Mineral oil	0.72 g EPA. 0.48 g DHA	12	MADRS, BDI, CGI	10
Depressive symptoms in pz with CVD										
Carney [87]	2009	Pz with coronary heart disease and MDD	122 (62/60)	sertraline 50 mg/day	EPA+DHA	Corn oil	0.93 g EPA; 0.75 g DHA	10	BDI-II, HDRS-17	10
Bot [94]	2010	Pz with diabetes mellitus and MDD	25 (13/12)	antidepressant medication	EPA	Rapeseed oil and medium chain triglycerides	1 g	12	MADRS	12
Giltay [100]	2011	Pz post myocardial infarction	4116	antidepressant medication	EPA+DHA		0.4 EPA-DHA/d. 2 ALA/d. 0.4 EPA-DHA+2 ALA	160	GDS, LOT-R	10
Bot [62]	2011	Pz with diabetes mellitus and MDD	25 (13/12)	antidepressant medication	EPA	Rapeseed oil and medium chain triglycerides	1 g	12	MADRS	10
Andreeva [37]	2012	Pz CVD survivors	2501 (620/633/ 622/626)	Antidepressant used by 130 (63/67)	B vitamins and n3B vitamins fatty acids (EPA+DHA), n3 fatty acids, B vitamins		600 mg EPA and DHA in a 2:1 ratio	52	GDS	9
Depressive symptoms in healthy subjects										
Fontani [52]	2005	Healthy subjects	33 (cross-over design)	None	EPA+DHA	Olive oil	1-60 g EPA+0-80 g DHA+0-40 g other omega-3 fatty acids	5	POMS	7

Table 1. Cont.

Author	Year	Partecipating Group	Subjects, n (I/C)	Type of treatment	Intervention	Placebo	Daily dose	Duration (weeks)	Outcome measure	Study quality
Van de Rest [68]	2008	Healthy subjects	302 (96/100/106)	Unclear	EPA+DHA	Sunflower oil	High: 1.093 g EPA. 0.847 g DHA; Low: 0.226 g EPA. 0.176 g DHA	26	CES-D, MADRS, GDS-15	12
Antypa [88]	2009	Healthy subjects	(56;>27/>27)	None	EPA+DHA	Olive oil	1.74 g EPA, 0.25 g DHA	4	MINI, BDI-II, POMS, LEIDS-R	9
Kiecolt-Glaser [102]	2011	Healthy subjects	68 (34/34)	None	EPA+DHA	Palm, olive, soy, canola, and coco butter oils	2.085 g EPA 0.348 g DHA	12	CES-D	11
DeFina [101]	2011	Healthy subjects (overweight)	128 (64/64)	None	EPA+DHA	Soybean and corn oils	3.0 g EPA and DHA in a 5:1 ratio (5 g EPA 1 g DHA)	24	POMS	8
Kiecolt-Glaser [66]	2012	Healthy subjects (overweight)	138 (46/46/46)	None	EPA+DHA	Palm, olive, soy, canola, and coco butter oils	2.09 g EPA+0.35 g DHA; n3 1.25 g middle group	16	CES-D	13

AD: anti-depression; BDI: Beck Depression Inventory; CES-D: Center for Epidemiological Studies Depression Scale; CDRS: Children Depression Rating Scale; CPRS: Comprehensive Psychopathological Rating Scale; GDS: Geriatric Depression Scale; CGI: Clinical Global Impression; CGI-BP: Clinical Global Impression Bipolar; DHA: docosahexaenoic acid; E-EPA: etyl-eicosapentaenoic acid; EPDS: Edinburgh Postnatal Depression Scale; HDRS: Hamilton Depression Rating Scale; I/C: intervention/control; IDS-C: Inventory of Depressive Symptomatology Clinician; LEIDS-R: Leiden Index of Depression Severity Revised; LOT-R: Revised Life Orientation Test; MADRS: Montgomery Åsberg Depression Rating Scale; MINI: Mini International Neuropsychiatric Interview; MMSE: Mini-Mental State Evaluation; NAD: non anti-depression; NPI: Neuropsychiatric Inventory; POMS: Profile of Mood States; PPBQ: Papolos Pediatric Bipolar Questionnaire; SCID: Structural Clinical Interview for Depression; VAS: Visual Analog Score.

Study or Subgroup	Control Mean	SD	Total	Experimental Mean	SD	Total	Weight	Std. Mean Difference IV, Random, 95% CI	Year
MDD									
Nemets 2002	20	8.8	10	11.6	6.2	10	6.5%	1.06 [0.11, 2.01]	2002
Marangell 2003	22.7	9.2	18	15.4	8.3	18	8.4%	0.81 [0.13, 1.50]	2003
Su 2003	15.7	3.2	14	8.9	3.7	14	6.7%	1.91 [0.99, 2.82]	2003
Grenyer 2007	11	12.5	43	14	12.5	40	10.3%	-0.24 [-0.67, 0.19]	2007
Jazayeri 2008	18	6.5	20	14	5.8	20	8.7%	0.64 [-0.00, 1.27]	2008
Jazayeri 2008	18	6.5	20	17	4.9	20	8.9%	0.17 [-0.45, 0.79]	2008
Mischoulon 2009	16	7.6	13	11.2	7.6	11	7.4%	0.61 [-0.22, 1.43]	2009
Lucas 2009	9.2	5.3	14	13.4	4.9	12	7.5%	-0.79 [-1.60, 0.01]	2009
Rondanelli 2010	15.9	5.4	24	12.6	4.3	22	9.0%	0.66 [0.07, 1.26]	2010
Rondanelli 2011	15.9	4.5	24	12.7	4.5	22	9.0%	0.70 [0.10, 1.30]	2011
Rizzo 2012	16.4	4	24	11.6	4.3	22	8.8%	1.14 [0.51, 1.77]	2012
Gertsik 2012	15	11	22	9.9	10	18	8.8%	0.47 [-0.16, 1.11]	2012
Total (95% CI)			246			229	100.0%	0.56 [0.20, 0.92]	

Heterogeneity: Tau² = 0.28; Chi² = 38.25, df = 11 (P < 0.0001); I² = 71%   Test for overall effect: Z = 3.08 (P = 0.002)

Study or Subgroup	Control Mean	SD	Total	Experimental Mean	SD	Total	Weight	Std. Mean Difference IV, Random, 95% CI	Year
non-MDD									
Peet 2002	14.2	6.8	18	12.3	6.8	17	6.4%	0.27 [-0.39, 0.94]	2002
Peet 2002	14.2	6.8	18	13.8	6.8	18	6.6%	0.06 [-0.60, 0.71]	2002
Peet 2002	14.2	6.9	18	10	6.8	17	6.3%	0.60 [-0.08, 1.28]	2002
Zanarini 2003	8	5.5	10	6.2	4.9	20	5.3%	0.34 [-0.42, 1.11]	2003
Silvers 2005	9.4	10.6	37	11.8	10	40	10.1%	-0.23 [-0.68, 0.22]	2005
Hallahan 2007	17.4	8.6	27	12.2	8.5	22	7.7%	0.60 [0.02, 1.17]	2007
Rogers 2008	9.9	6.5	99	10.6	7.6	98	14.3%	-0.10 [-0.38, 0.18]	2008
Lucas 2009	7.6	5.9	37	5.8	4.4	43	10.3%	0.35 [-0.10, 0.79]	2009
Tajalizadekhoob 2011	6.91	3.98	33	6	2.92	33	9.4%	0.26 [-0.23, 0.74]	2011
Antypa 2012	6.5	6.4	35	6.6	7.3	36	9.8%	-0.01 [-0.48, 0.45]	2012
Mozaffari-Khosravi 2013	13.7	2.7	21	13.7	2.7	20	7.2%	0.00 [-0.61, 0.61]	2013
Mozaffari-Khosravi 2013	13.7	2.7	21	10.3	3.2	21	6.6%	1.13 [0.47, 1.78]	2013
Total (95% CI)			374			385	100.0%	0.22 [0.01, 0.43]	

Heterogeneity: Tau² = 0.06; Chi² = 20.44, df = 11 (P = 0.04); I² = 46%   Test for overall effect: Z = 2.07 (P = 0.04)

Overall MDD + non-MDD

Total (95% CI)			620			614	100.0%	0.38 [0.18, 0.59]	

Heterogeneity: Tau² = 0.15; Chi² = 65.71, df = 23 (P < 0.00001); I² = 65%   Test for overall effect: Z = 3.73 (P = 0.0002)

-2 -1 0 1 2
[control]   [experimental]

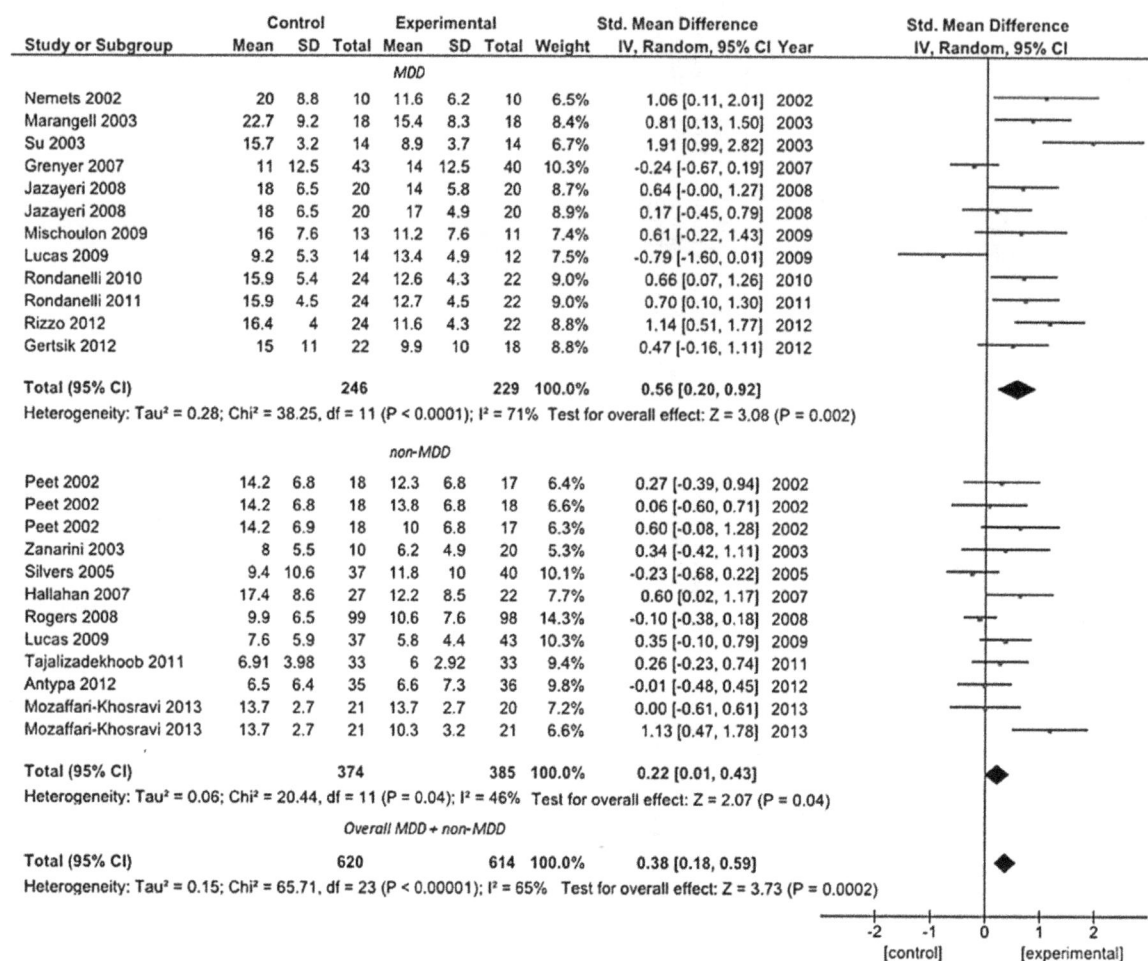

Figure 2. Forest plot showing individual and combined effect size estimates and 95% CIs for 19 trials grouped in those conducted on patients with a DSM-defined diagnosis of major depressive disorder (MDD group, n = 11) and those on patients with an assessment of depression but not rigorously diagnosed according to the DSM criteria (non-MDD group, n = 8). Black squares: indicate the weighting given to the trial in the overall pooled estimate; lines: indicate the 95% CIs; rhombus: indicate the combined effect size.

was investigated by using Higgins' I^2 statistic [73,74]. When heterogeneity between results of the studies exists, the random-effect models were preferred.

Possible publication bias for the analysis regarding RCTs conducted on MDD patients (MDD group, n = 11) and those not diagnosed with DSM-IV criteria (non-MDD group, n = 9) was investigated by drawing a funnel plot to look for funnel plot asymmetry [71] and meta-regression based on study size. Meta-regression was performed using linear regression, with the effect size (SMD) of trials as the dependent variable and the variables of interest as the independent variable. The generic inverse variance method was used to weight trials. Effects due to severity of depressive symptoms, age of patients, and study quality were also investigated by using meta-regression based on standardized baseline depression scores, mean age of the study participants, and our modified Jadad scores of the studies, respectively. The effects of trial duration, EPA and DHA dose in omega-3 preparations, and the use as mono or adjuvant therapy were also examined. Particularly, the qualitative analysis of the type of supplementation used was investigated grouping the studies in those using mainly EPA (EPA >50% of the dose) and mainly DHA (DHA >50% of the dose). A further analysis was computed by splitting the grouping in mainly EPA, pure EPA, mainly DHA,

and pure DHA supplementation. As well, the therapeutic approach was investigated by grouping studies using omega-3 in monotherapy or as adjuvant therapy together with antidepressant drugs. The quantitative analysis of the dose was computed by a meta-regression analysis of the EPA and DHA doses used.

Random- and fixed-effects models, forest and funnel plots, and Higgins' I^2 statistics were performed in Review Manager (RevMan) version 5.2 (Copenhagen: The Nordic Cochrane Centre, The Cochrane Collaboration), meta-regression analyses were performed in SPSS version 17 (SPSS Inc., Chicago, IL, USA).

Results

Overall Studies

The most relevant features of the 47 studies included in this systematic review and meta-analysis are displayed in Table 1. Considerable differences among studies were found for all characteristics examined. The average quality of the studies was about 9 over a maximum score of 13 (range 5–13). The mean length of the trials was about 16 weeks (range 4–160), 36 studies used a mixed intervention with EPA+DHA, 14 pure EPA and 4 pure DHA. The average dose of EPA+DHA was 1.39 g (range 0.63–6.2 of EPA and 0.27–3.4 of DHA), whereas 1.93 g (range

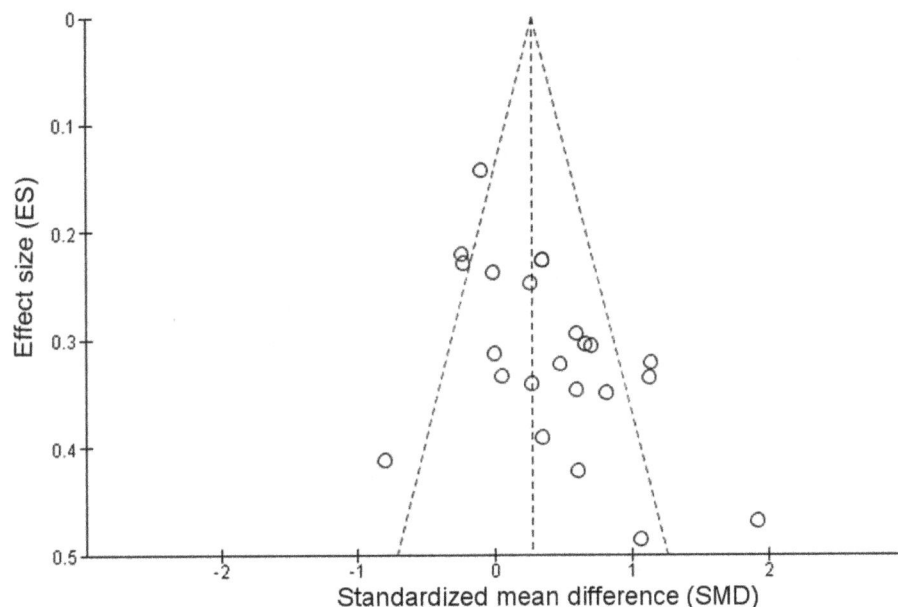

Figure 3. Funnel plot of effect size estimates for individual trials conducted on patients with depressive disorder without secondary comordibities (MDD group and non-MDD group, n = 19).

1–6) and 0.86 g (range 0.22–2) were the average doses of pure EPA and DHA, respectively (Table 1). The most of RCTs used the Hamilton Depression Rating Scale [46,48,49,54,57,58,63,65,69,75–84], 10 studies [46,49,56,68,79,85–89] used the Beck Depression Inventory, and 13 studies [47,50,54,62,64,67,77,84,90–94] the Montgomery-Asberg Depression Scale as the main outcome measure. Among the studies not included in the quantitative analysis,due to lack of data, one was conducted on patients with obsessive-compulsive disorder [57] and one on patients with chronic fatigue syndrome [56], both reporting no relevant effects of omega-3 fatty acids compared with placebo; four studies conducted in bipolar depressed patients [58,59,61,63] reporting that there were no significant differences on any outcome measure between the EPA and placebo groups; one study on diabetes mellitus patients with MDD [62] reporting no effect of omega-3 fatty acids on depression severity; and one on older adults with mild cognitive impairment suggesting that increased intakes of DHA and EPA can reduce depressive symptoms and the risk of progressing to dementia [60].

Depression (MDD and Non-MDD Groups)

A total of 19 studies were included in the first pooled analysis conducted in patients with depressive symptoms (Figure 2). Among them, 11 trials were conducted in patients with a DSM-defined diagnosis of MDD, including 8 studies conducted in adults [46,48,70,76–78,83,84] and 3 studies in elderly patients [53,95,96]. The pooled standardized difference in means using a fixed-effects model for the MDD group was 0.47 SD (95% CI: 0.29, 0.66), which suggests a beneficial effect of omega-3 fatty acids on depressed mood compared with placebo in patients with diagnosis of MDD. The pooled standardized difference in means in a random-effects model was 0.56 SD (95% CI: 0.20, 0.92). The remaining 8 were those conducted on patients with an assessment of depression but not rigorously diagnosed according to the DSM criteria, and included patients with depressive symptoms despite on-going treatment [54,69,79,97], women with borderline personality disorder [91], patients with recurrent self-harm [49],

people with mild to severe depressed mood not taking medications [86], post-menopausal women with psychological distress and depressive symptoms [70], and subjects with a history of at least one major depressive episode [89], whereas two studies were excluded due to lack of data [56,57]. Despite patients pooled in this analysis were not homogeneous in terms of health status, all studies clearly reported to have included subjects with no other psychiatric or neurological illnesses such as AD, Parkinson's disease, as well as no history of any end-stage diseases, CVDs, or any unstable medical conditions, thus to make them comparable each other for our purposes. Similar results were found for this group of patients (standardized mean difference – fixed effects-model: 0.15 SD, 95% CI: 0.01, 0.30; random-effects model: 0.22 SD, 95% CI: 0.01, 0.43). For both MDD and non-MDD groups, there was evidence of heterogeneity (MDD group, $I^2 = 71\%$, $P < 0.001$; non-MDD group, $I^2 = 46\%$, $P = 0.04$).

The overall analysis including both groups was conducted to assess whether results were different considering a mood-improving effect on depressive symptoms in patients with non-organic, metabolic, nor genetic-related neurodegenerative disease. The pooled standardized difference in means using a fixed-effects model was 0.27 SD (95% CI: 0.16, 0.39), and the pooled standardized difference in means using a random-effects model was 0.38 SD (95% CI: 0.18, 0.59). However, there was evidence of heterogeneity ($I^2 = 65\%$, $P < 0.001$). To test this heterogeneity, a funnel plot was drawn and is shown in Figure 3.The funnel plot did not show considerable evidence of asymmetry. Meta-regression of study effect size, based on study size, did not present significant association (regression coefficient = -0.108, 95% CI: -0.224, 0.012; $P = 0.066$) indicating no role of the sample size in determining the results of the analysis.

A meta-regression analysis was performed of standardized mean depression scores on baseline depression scores to test whether the gravity of depression at baseline may play a role in the efficacy of omega-3 fatty supplementation. The analysis showed no relation between baseline depression scores and efficacy for all studies (regression coefficient = 0.019, 95% CI: -0.009, 0.047; $P = 0.167$)

Study or Subgroup	Control Mean	SD	Total	Experimental Mean	SD	Total	Weight	Std. Mean Difference IV, Random, 95% CI	Year
Pure EPA									
Nemets 2002	20	8.8	10	11.6	6.2	10	5.8%	1.06 [0.11, 2.01]	2002
Peet 2002	14.2	6.8	18	13.8	6.8	18	10.4%	0.06 [-0.60, 0.71]	2002
Peet 2002	14.2	6.9	18	10	6.8	17	9.8%	0.60 [-0.08, 1.28]	2002
Peet 2002	14.2	6.8	18	12.3	6.8	17	10.1%	0.27 [-0.39, 0.94]	2002
Zanarini 2003	8	5.5	10	6.2	4.9	20	8.2%	0.34 [-0.42, 1.11]	2003
Jazayeri 2008	18	6.5	20	17	4.9	20	11.2%	0.17 [-0.45, 0.79]	2008
Jazayeri 2008	18	6.5	20	14	5.8	20	10.8%	0.64 [-0.00, 1.27]	2008
Mischoulon 2009	16	7.6	13	11.2	7.6	11	7.3%	0.61 [-0.22, 1.43]	2009
Antypa 2012	6.5	6.4	35	6.6	7.3	36	16.1%	-0.01 [-0.48, 0.45]	2012
Mozaffari-Khosravi 2013	13.7	2.7	21	10.3	3.2	21	10.3%	1.13 [0.47, 1.78]	2013
Total (95% CI)			183			190	100.0%	0.43 [0.18, 0.68]	

Heterogeneity: Tau² = 0.04; Chi² = 12.45, df = 9 (P = 0.19); I² = 28% Test for overall effect: Z = 3.37 (P = 0.0007)

Mainly EPA									
Su 2003	15.7	3.2	14	8.9	3.7	14	5.2%	1.91 [0.99, 2.82]	2003
Lucas 2009	7.6	5.9	37	5.8	4.4	43	22.4%	0.35 [-0.10, 0.79]	2009
Lucas 2009	9.2	5.3	14	13.4	4.9	12	6.8%	-0.79 [-1.60, 0.01]	2009
Rondanelli 2010	15.9	5.4	24	12.6	4.3	22	12.4%	0.66 [0.07, 1.26]	2010
Rondanelli 2011	15.9	4.5	24	12.7	4.5	22	12.3%	0.70 [0.10, 1.30]	2011
Tajalizadekhoob 2011	6.91	3.98	33	6	2.92	33	18.7%	0.26 [-0.23, 0.74]	2011
Rizzo 2012	16.4	4	24	11.6	4.3	22	11.2%	1.14 [0.51, 1.77]	2012
Gertsik 2012	15	11	22	9.9	10	18	11.0%	0.47 [-0.16, 1.11]	2012
Total (95% CI)			192			186	100.0%	0.52 [0.31, 0.73]	

Heterogeneity: Chi² = 25.06, df = 7 (P = 0.0007); I² = 72% Test for overall effect: Z = 4.85 (P < 0.00001)

Pure + mainly EPA									
Total (95% CI)			375			376	100.0%	0.50 [0.27, 0.72]	

Heterogeneity: Tau² = 0.13; Chi² = 38.12, df = 17 (P = 0.002); I² = 55% Test for overall effect: Z = 4.30 (P < 0.0001)

Pure DHA									
Marangell 2003	22.7	9.2	18	15.4	8.3	18	44.6%	0.81 [0.13, 1.50]	2003
Mozaffari-Khosravi 2013	13.7	2.7	21	13.7	2.7	20	55.4%	0.00 [-0.61, 0.61]	2013
Total (95% CI)			39			38	100.0%	0.36 [-0.09, 0.82]	

Heterogeneity: Chi² = 3.03, df = 1 (P = 0.08); I² = 67% Test for overall effect: Z = 1.56 (P = 0.12)

Mainly DHA									
Silvers 2005	9.4	10.6	37	11.8	10	40	19.0%	-0.23 [-0.68, 0.22]	2005
Hallahan 2007	17.4	8.6	27	12.2	8.5	22	11.5%	0.60 [0.02, 1.17]	2007
Grenyer 2007	11	12.5	43	14	12.5	40	20.5%	-0.24 [-0.67, 0.19]	2007
Rogers 2008	9.9	6.5	99	10.6	7.6	98	49.0%	-0.10 [-0.38, 0.18]	2008
Total (95% CI)			206			200	100.0%	-0.07 [-0.27, 0.12]	

Heterogeneity: Chi² = 6.27, df = 3 (P = 0.10); I² = 52% Test for overall effect: Z = 0.72 (P = 0.47)

Pure + mainly DHA									
Total (95% CI)			245			238	100.0%	-0.00 [-0.18, 0.18]	

Heterogeneity: Chi² = 12.26, df = 5 (P = 0.03); I² = 59% Test for overall effect: Z = 0.05 (P = 0.96)

[control] / [experimental]

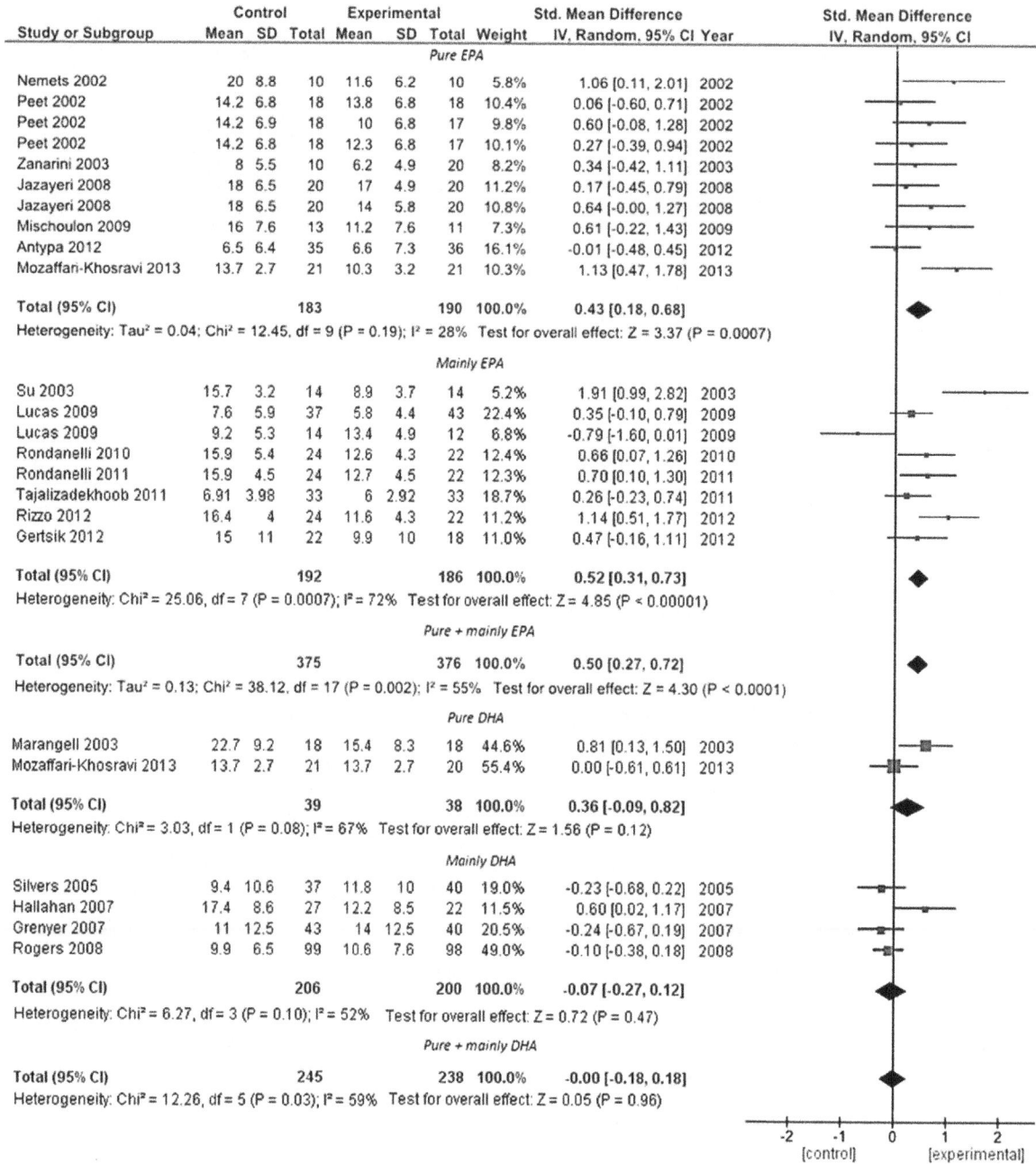

Figure 4. Forest plot examining the effect of the type of omega-3 PUFA supplementation employed on the reduction in depressive symptoms (MDD group and non-MDD group, n = 19).

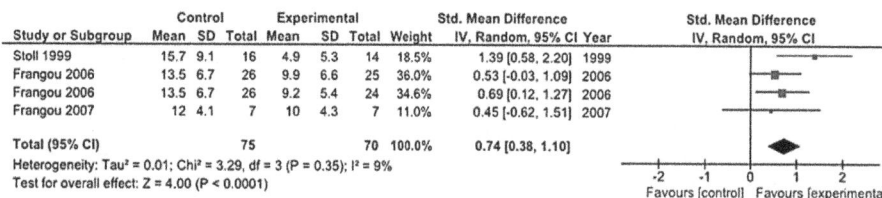

Study or Subgroup	Control Mean	SD	Total	Experimental Mean	SD	Total	Weight	Std. Mean Difference IV, Random, 95% CI	Year
Stoll 1999	15.7	9.1	16	4.9	5.3	14	18.5%	1.39 [0.58, 2.20]	1999
Frangou 2006	13.5	6.7	26	9.9	6.6	25	36.0%	0.53 [-0.03, 1.09]	2006
Frangou 2006	13.5	6.7	26	9.2	5.4	24	34.6%	0.69 [0.12, 1.27]	2006
Frangou 2007	12	4.1	7	10	4.3	7	11.0%	0.45 [-0.62, 1.51]	2007
Total (95% CI)			75			70	100.0%	0.74 [0.38, 1.10]	

Heterogeneity: Tau² = 0.01; Chi² = 3.29, df = 3 (P = 0.35); I² = 9%
Test for overall effect: Z = 4.00 (P < 0.0001)

Favours [control] / Favours [experimental]

Figure 5. Forest plot showing individual and combined effect size estimates and 95% CIs for 3 trials conducted on patients with bipolar depression.

Study or Subgroup	Control Mean	SD	Total	Experimental Mean	SD	Total	Weight	Std. Mean Difference IV, Random, 95% CI	Year
Freeman 2008	9.9	4.7	28	12.8	5.5	31	35.5%	-0.56 [-1.08, -0.04]	2008
Su 2008	14.6	4.8	18	9.9	4.3	18	32.9%	1.01 [0.31, 1.71]	2008
Rees 2008	9.7	5.1	13	7.9	5.1	13	31.6%	0.34 [-0.43, 1.12]	2008
Total (95% CI)			59			62	100.0%	0.24 [-0.73, 1.21]	

Heterogeneity: Tau² = 0.62; Chi² = 12.96, df = 2 (P = 0.002); I² = 85%
Test for overall effect: Z = 0.49 (P = 0.63)

Favours [control]   Favours [experimental]

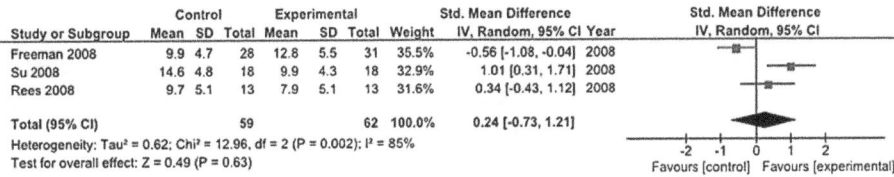

Figure 6. Forest plot showing individual and combined effect size estimates and 95% CIs for 3 trials conducted on pregnant women with major depressive disorder.

as well as for MDD patients (regression coefficient = 0.008, 95% CI: −0.053, 0.068; $P = 0.787$) and non-MDD (regression coefficient = 0.019, 95% CI: −0.017, 0.054; $P = 0.270$) separately. Even taking into account the comparison of studies using the same depression scale (HDRS), no significant relation between baseline depression scores and efficacy was found (data not shown).

Analysis conducted to explore the role of type (namely, the administration of mainly EPA or DHA supplementation) and dose (separately for EPA and DHA) of omega-3 supplement used showed that the use of mainly EPA within the preparation, rather than DHA, appeared to influence final clinical efficacy (standardized mean difference – fixed effects-model: 0.46 SD, 95% CI: 0.31, 0.61; random-effects model: 0.50 SD, 95% CI: 0.27, 0.72) (Figure 4). Despite heterogeneity fallen by 55%, it remained significantly high ($P = 0.002$). When the analysis was split in mainly EPA, pure EPA, mainly DHA, and pure DHA supplementation, both the EPA preparations were significant (for pure EPA, standardized mean difference – fixed effects-model: 0.40 SD, 95% CI: 0.19, 0.61; random-effects model: 0.43 SD, 95% CI: 0.18, 0.68) and the heterogeneity fallen to 28% ($P = 0.19$). This result indicates that despite the overall heterogeneity represented an underlying true difference in effect sizes across studies, it may be strongly affected by type of formulation of omega-3 fatty acids used.

The meta-regression analyses exploring the role of the dose of omega-3 fatty acids revealed that the total dose of DHA were unrelated to efficacy (regression coefficient = −0.066, 95% CI: −0.471, 0.603; $P = 0.801$), whereas the dose of EPA formulation resulted related to efficacy both for all MDD plus non-MDD patients (regression coefficient = 0.477, 95% CI: 0.084, 0.869; $P = 0.02$). However, when the analyses was repeated separately for each group, the association remained significant only for MDD patients (regression coefficient = 0.746, 95% CI: 0.100, 1.392; $P = 0.028$) whereas lost significance for non-MDD patients (regression coefficient = 0.215, 95% CI: −0.288, 0.718; $P = 0.359$).

No relation between study size (regression coefficient = −0.109, 95% CI: −0.231, 0.012; $P = 0.075$, baseline depression severity (regression coefficient = 0.026, 95% CI: −0.007, 0.060; $P = 0.116$), trial duration (regression coefficient = −0.058, 95%

CI: −0.153, 0.038; $P = 0.223$), age of patients (regression coefficient = 0.013, 95% CI: −0.10, 0.036; $P = 0.879$), and study quality (regression coefficient = −0.142, 95% CI: −0.357, 0.072; $P = 0.183$) and omega-3 PUFA efficacy was found, despite study quality almost reached significance when considered only for RCTs conducted on patients with MDD (regression coefficient = −0.403, 95% CI: −0.857, 0.052; $P = 0.077$). On the contrary, fixed- and random-effect models of RCTs grouped by use of omega-3 PUFA as mono- or adjuvant therapy revealed a significant effect when they were used in combination with standard antidepressant therapy (standardized mean difference – fixed effects-model: 0.26 SD, 95% CI: 0.09, 0.44; random-effects model: 0.39 SD, 95% CI: 0.06, 0.71).

Bipolar Disorder

In our systematic review we collected 7 trials conducted on patients with bipolar disorder (both type I and II) [58,59,61,63,65,75,80] (Table 1). The only three studies pooled for the analysis included one study [65] that accounted for more than 70% of the weight of the analysis, that together with others [75,80] resulted in a significant effect of omega-3 fatty acids in ameliorating depressive symptoms in adults with bipolar disorder (standardized mean difference – fixed effects-model: 0.73 SD, 95% CI: 0.39, 1.07; random-effects model: 0.74 SD, 95% CI: 0.38, 1.10; $I^2 = 9\%$, $P = 0.35$) (Figure 5).

Depression or Bipolar Disorder in Children and Adolescents

Among the studies conducted on depression occurring in youth, one study [98] documented a positive effect of omega-3 fatty acids in improving the mood of children diagnosed of MDD and one study conducted on adolescents at high risk of psychosis [92] reported that omega-3 fatty acids significantly reduced positive symptoms, negative symptoms, and improved functioning compared with placebo, but no significant effect was observed on depressive symptoms.

Perinatal Depression

There were six trials aiming to explore the effects of omega-3 PUFA on perinatal depression. We distinguished between those

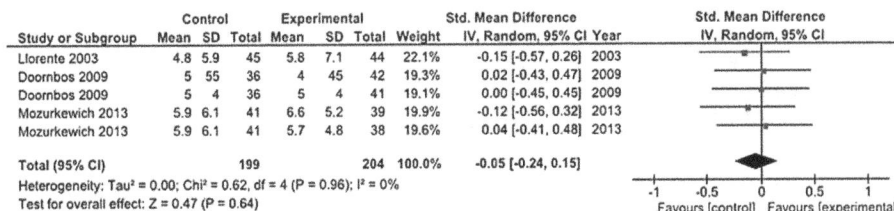

Study or Subgroup	Control Mean	SD	Total	Experimental Mean	SD	Total	Weight	Std. Mean Difference IV, Random, 95% CI	Year
Llorente 2003	4.8	5.9	45	5.8	7.1	44	22.1%	-0.15 [-0.57, 0.26]	2003
Doornbos 2009	5	55	36	4	45	42	19.3%	0.02 [-0.43, 0.47]	2009
Doornbos 2009	5	4	36	5	4	41	19.1%	0.00 [-0.45, 0.45]	2009
Mozurkewich 2013	5.9	6.1	41	6.6	5.2	39	19.9%	-0.12 [-0.56, 0.32]	2013
Mozurkewich 2013	5.9	6.1	41	5.7	4.8	38	19.6%	0.04 [-0.41, 0.48]	2013
Total (95% CI)			199			204	100.0%	-0.05 [-0.24, 0.15]	

Heterogeneity: Tau² = 0.00; Chi² = 0.62, df = 4 (P = 0.96); I² = 0%
Test for overall effect: Z = 0.47 (P = 0.64)

Favours [control]   Favours [experimental]

Figure 7. Forest plot showing individual and combined effect size estimates and 95% CIs for 3 trials conducted on healthy pregnant women for prevention of post-partum depression.

Study or Subgroup	Control			Experimental			Weight	Std. Mean Difference IV, Random, 95% CI	Year	Std. Mean Difference IV, Random, 95% CI
	Mean	SD	Total	Mean	SD	Total				
Freund-Levi 2008	1.6	2.3	101	1.5	2.3	103	87.9%	0.04 [-0.23, 0.32]	2008	
Chiu 2008	3.09	4.59	12	2.71	2.52	17	12.1%	0.11 [-0.63, 0.84]	2008	
Total (95% CI)			113			120	100.0%	0.05 [-0.21, 0.31]		

Heterogeneity: Tau² = 0.00; Chi² = 0.02, df = 1 (P = 0.88); I² = 0%
Test for overall effect: Z = 0.39 (P = 0.70)

Favours [experimental]   Favours [control]

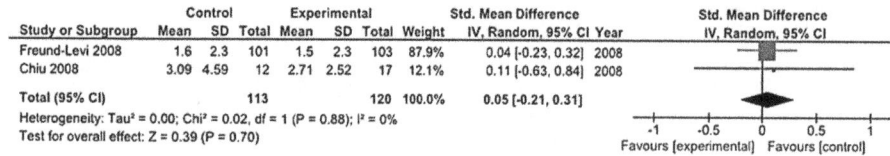

Figure 8. Forest plot showing individual and combined effect size estimates and 95% CIs for 2 trials conducted on patients with Alzheimer or mild cognitive impairment.

studies conducted on pregnant women with MDD [82,93,99] (Figure 6) and those on apparently healthy women (primary prevention) [51,68,85] (Figure 7). However, both analyses led to inconclusive results (MDD in pregnancy, standardized mean difference – fixed effects-model: 0.08 SD, 95% CI: −0.29, 0.45; random-effects model: 0.24 SD, 95% CI: −0.73, 1.21; prevention of post-partum depression, standardized mean difference – fixed effects-model: 0.05 SD, 95% CI: −0.24, 0.15; random-effects model: −0.05 SD, 95% CI: −0.24, 0.15). Only one study [82] concluded that omega-3 fatty acids might have therapeutic benefits in depression during pregnancy. Besides the clinical efficacy of omega-3, in regard to the safety issue, it is important to underline that omega-3 fatty acids supplementation was well tolerated and no adverse effects were reported on the subjects treated and newborns in all studies.

Depression as Secondary Outcome

Among the trials conducted in patients with primary disease other than depression, those conducted on AD or mild cognitive impairment [50,81] (Figure 8), schizophrenia [54,90] (Figure 9), and CVDs [87,94,100] (Figure 10) reported inconclusive results, whereas the only study conducted on Parkinson's disease patients in comorbidity with MDD [47], including those treated with antidepressants and those without, reported improvement in depressive symptoms and indicate that the intake of omega-3 PUFA can be used as adjuvant therapy in Parkinson's disease patients. However, in one study conducted on schizophrenic patients with persistent ongoing symptoms [54], the authors reported a large placebo effect in patients on typical and new atypical antipsychotics and no difference was observed between active treatment and placebo, but in patients on clozapine, there was a clinically important and statistically significant effect of 2 g/day omega-3 PUFA treatment on the PANSS and its sub-scales.

Depressive Symptoms in Healthy Subjects

The trials conducted on healthy subjects aimed to explore potential beneficial effects of omega-3 fatty acids as mood improving medicaments in the general population (Figure 11). Among the tot studies included [52,66,67,88,101,102], the overall analysis showed a nearly null effect of this supplement on depressive symptoms in healthy subjects (standardized mean

difference – fixed and random effects-model: 0.00 SD, 95% CI: −0.13, 0.13).

Discussion

We demonstrated that the use of omega-3 PUFA as therapeutic agents was effective in patients with diagnosis of MDD and on depressive patients without a diagnosis of MDD, whereas inconclusive results were found for patients with other pathological conditions (namely schizophrenia and AD) as well as in healthy subjects and perinatal depression. The analysis of the studies on bipolar disorder showed a positive effect of the omega-3 PUFA, but the evidence is weakened due to the exclusion from the quantitative analysis of three studies that may affect the overall effect of the supplement. When the studies conducted on patients with MDD or those on patients with depressive symptoms but not rigorous evaluation by health professionals were pooled together, a general positive effect of omega-3 PUFA was found.

As previously reported [15], the studies that mostly negatively influenced the pooled results of the non-MDD patients included non-homogenous individuals, since their enrolment was in settings such as general practice surgeries, shopping malls, and university freshman fairs [86], newspaper, radio and television advertising, and flyers posted [70], and through a Community Mental Health Service, general practices, and advertisements in community newspapers [79]. Despite the idea of a widely available low cost supplement that could assist those being treated for a current depressive episode in a community setting is highly desirable, a lack of rigor in patients' selection may lead to the inclusion of subjects with normal emotional states, eventually affecting the results and, thus, challenging the model's credibility. It is noteworthy that negative results came out mostly from studies sharing this methodology [70,79,86]. Moreover, as reported by the authors [79,86], both experimental and control groups improved significantly, usually indicative of a major placebo response which is expected to exert a meaningful clinical effect in the treatment of such "subthreshold" depressed subjects [103]. A recent meta-analysis demonstrated that the relative efficacy of the active drug compared to placebo in clinical trials for MDD is highly heterogeneous across studies, with a worse performance in showing a superiority of the drug *versus* placebo for studies with placebo response rates ≥30% [104]. Thus, the studies quality

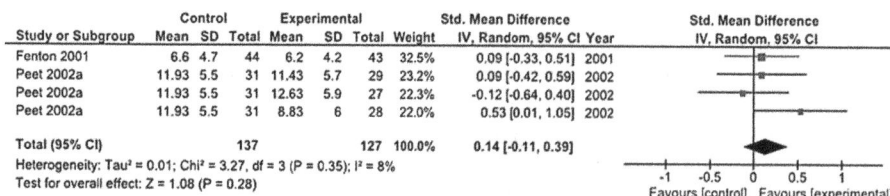

Study or Subgroup	Control			Experimental			Weight	Std. Mean Difference IV, Random, 95% CI	Year	Std. Mean Difference IV, Random, 95% CI
	Mean	SD	Total	Mean	SD	Total				
Fenton 2001	6.6	4.7	44	6.2	4.2	43	32.5%	0.09 [-0.33, 0.51]	2001	
Peet 2002a	11.93	5.5	31	11.43	5.7	29	23.2%	0.09 [-0.42, 0.59]	2002	
Peet 2002a	11.93	5.5	31	12.63	5.9	27	22.3%	-0.12 [-0.64, 0.40]	2002	
Peet 2002a	11.93	5.5	31	8.83	6	28	22.0%	0.53 [0.01, 1.05]	2002	
Total (95% CI)			137			127	100.0%	0.14 [-0.11, 0.39]		

Heterogeneity: Tau² = 0.01; Chi² = 3.27, df = 3 (P = 0.35); I² = 8%
Test for overall effect: Z = 1.08 (P = 0.28)

Favours [control]   Favours [experimental]

Figure 9. Forest plot showing individual and combined effect size estimates and 95% CIs for 2 trials conducted on patients with schizophrenia.

Study or Subgroup	Control Mean	SD	Total	Experimental Mean	SD	Total	Weight	Std. Mean Difference IV, Random, 95% CI	Year
Carney 2009	15	9.7	60	15.9	10.2	62	5.6%	-0.09 [-0.44, 0.27]	2009
Bot 2010	11.6	9.2	12	14	6.9	13	1.1%	-0.29 [-1.08, 0.50]	2010
Giltay 2011	2.1631	2.45905	1030	2.0161	2.32517	1007	93.3%	0.06 [-0.03, 0.15]	2011
Total (95% CI)			1102			1082	100.0%	0.05 [-0.03, 0.13]	

Heterogeneity: Tau² = 0.00; Chi² = 1.36, df = 2 (P = 0.51); I² = 0%
Test for overall effect: Z = 1.14 (P = 0.25)

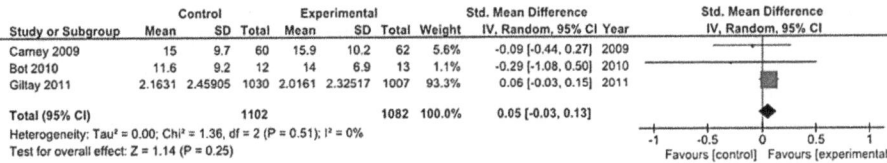

Figure 10. Forest plot showing individual and combined effect size estimates and 95% CIs for 3 trials conducted on patients with cardiovascular disease.

decreased when placebo response rates were not mantained below this critical threshold that may depend on the non-homogenous depressive "phenotypes" of the subjects enrolled. The non-MDD group also included four studies conducted on patients with depressive disorders despite ongoing antidepressant therapy [54,69,79,97]. These results should be considered with caution, because these studies may include those "non-responder" subjects that generally fail to reach remission with the first anti-depressant therapy and have higher relapse rates and poorer outcomes than those who remit [105]. Studies conducted in this subgroup of patients can explain not clearly favorable effects of omega-3 PUFA on depressive symptoms in these studies and puzzling results.

Previous meta-analyses included all RCTs with little distinction among population groups, leading to controversial results, such as overall benefit [106,107] and negligible effects [27,28] of omega-3 PUFA against depressive symptoms, especially due to the high heterogeneity of studies. The following studies improved some methodological issues (i.e., better definition of inclusion criteria, especially in the distinction between the definition of MDD and other depressive disorders) and focused attention on specific aspects of omega-3 administration (i.e., dosage, EPA:DHA ratio) leading to the conclusion that administration of EPA, rather than DHA, is responsible for the beneficial effects of omega-3 PUFA intake as therapeutic agents in patients with depressive disorders [108,109] and supplements containing EPA ≥60%, in dose range from 200 to 2200 mg EPA in excess of DHA, were effective against primary depression. On the contrary, the last meta-analytic study [14] reported small, non-significant benefit of omega-3 PUFA for the treatment of MDD, generally in contrast with the aforementioned previous meta-analyses, but some methodological issues in study selection have arisen [15,16]. Taking into account that pathophysiological processes of depressive symptoms involved in MDD patients are likely to be very different from those in patients with depression occurring in other clinical conditions (i.e., bipolar disorder, pregnancy, primary diseases others than depression) and in non-homogenous patients (i.e., community sample of individuals), we used a different approach to analyze the RCTs using omega-3 PUFA supplementation against depressive symptoms, grouping the studies by type of

diagnosis of depression and taking into account any possible health condition that may influence the onset of the depression as well as the response to therapy. Other meta-analyses reported that the more severe was the depression, the more likely omega-3 PUFA supplementation would reduce depressive symptoms. We failed to demonstrate such a result, and we consider this finding as a surrogate of our observation that, overall, the efficacy of omega-3 PUFA was mostly related to a specific DSM-based diagnosis of MDD. Hence, this latter has been translated in a correlation of efficacy to more severe symptoms whereas, according to our results, we hypothesized that this efficacy may be more related to the specific pathophysiological processes of the MDD rather than to its severity. Compared with previous meta-analyses, the differences of findings may depend on the additional number of RCTs published since the publication of the last study [37,40,53,60,61,66,68,69,84,89,92,94–97,100–102], the increasing number of participants which vary the overall weight of previous studies, the requirement for public registration of trials resulting in an increase of general studies' quality and may be responsible for the decreased evidence of publication bias.

Since the pathophysiological mechanisms and the therapeutic approach for bipolar disorder differ from those of MDD [22,23], when previous analyses included and pooled findings of studies conducted on these groups of different patients, they led to inconclusive results. It has been hypothesized that the efficacy of omega-3 PUFA may be different in the depressive phase rather than the maniacal episode [110], and recent systematic analysis of trials focused on this topic showed positive effects of omega-3 PUFA as an adjunctive treatment for depressive but not mania in bipolar disorder patients [111,112]. Thus, we separately grouped the studies conducted on patients with bipolar disorder and explored efficacy of omega-3 PUFA in ameliorating the depressive symptoms, finding a significant efficacy of the supplement in two [65,75] out of the three trials. Despite the positive results, it is noteworthy to underline that we had to exclude, due to missing of data, four studies [58,59,61,63] conducted on bipolar patients reporting poor effect of the omega-3 PUFA intervention, thus weakening our findings. There is a need of well-designed, high quality studies, which may clarify the potential effects of omega-3

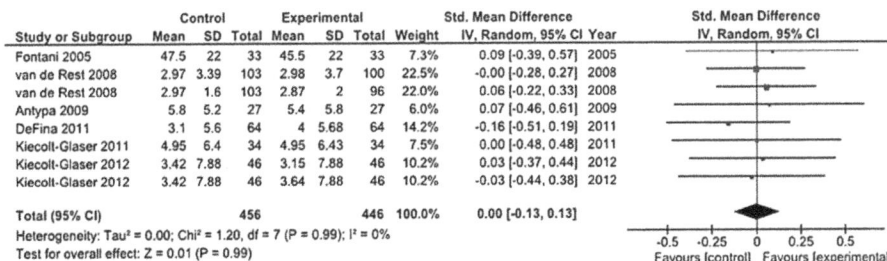

Study or Subgroup	Control Mean	SD	Total	Experimental Mean	SD	Total	Weight	Std. Mean Difference IV, Random, 95% CI	Year
Fontani 2005	47.5	22	33	45.5	22	33	7.3%	0.09 [-0.39, 0.57]	2005
van de Rest 2008	2.97	3.39	103	2.98	3.7	100	22.5%	-0.00 [-0.28, 0.27]	2008
van de Rest 2008	2.97	1.6	103	2.87	2	96	22.0%	0.06 [-0.22, 0.33]	2008
Antypa 2009	5.8	5.2	27	5.4	5.8	27	6.0%	0.07 [-0.46, 0.61]	2009
DeFina 2011	3.1	5.6	64	4	5.68	64	14.2%	-0.16 [-0.51, 0.19]	2011
Kiecolt-Glaser 2011	4.95	6.4	34	4.95	6.43	34	7.5%	0.00 [-0.48, 0.48]	2011
Kiecolt-Glaser 2012	3.42	7.88	46	3.15	7.88	46	10.2%	0.03 [-0.37, 0.44]	2012
Kiecolt-Glaser 2012	3.42	7.88	46	3.64	7.88	46	10.2%	-0.03 [-0.44, 0.38]	2012
Total (95% CI)			456			446	100.0%	0.00 [-0.13, 0.13]	

Heterogeneity: Tau² = 0.00; Chi² = 1.20, df = 7 (P = 0.99); I² = 0%
Test for overall effect: Z = 0.01 (P = 0.99)

Figure 11. Forest plot showing individual and combined effect size estimates and 95% CIs for 6 trials conducted on healthy individuals for prevention of depressive symptoms.

PUFA supplement in patients with rigorously diagnosed bipolar disorder.

Regarding the substantial inefficacy of the omega-3 PUFA in patients with primary diseases other than depression, it may be possible that these studies are more likely to suffer from publication bias, since depression was often a secondary outcome. Despite this methodological issue, the effects of the omega-3 PUFA may have been also affected by factors particularly related to the primary disease. Regarding the studies conducted on patients with CVDs, the analysis included very heterogeneous populations, namely patients with coronary heart disease [87], with diabetes mellitus [94], and post myocardial infarction [100], that may have been responsible for the inconclusive results. Moreover, it has been recently reported that supplementation of EPA in diabetes mellitus patients with comorbid MDD poorly affect biological risk factors for adverse outcome observed in this category of patients [113]. The RCTs conducted on patients with mild cognitive impairment or AD revealed poor efficacy of omega-3 PUFA in ameliorating the depressive symptoms. It has been reported that molecular mechanisms and pathways that underlie the pathogenesis of depression (i.e., impairment in the signaling of some neurotrophins such as Transforming-Growth-Factor-β1 and Brain-derived-neurotrophic-factor) are also involved in the pathogenesis of AD [114,115], thus the omega-3 PUFA supplementation may not be the optimal pharmacological approach for this specific group of patients [116–118]. The two trials (including different dosages) conducted on schizophrenic patients with persistent ongoing symptoms resulted in limited effects of the omega-3 PUFA on patients' affective states. These results may be attributable to some psychotic symptoms (i.e., negative symptoms) that may directly influence (i.e., improve) depression-rating scores. Moreover, these patients were receiving different types of antipsychotics such as first- and second-generation antipsychotics that may differently affect (positively or negatively) the final effects of omega-3 PUFA on depressive symptoms. Equally, we also reported that trials focused on perinatal depression demonstrated scarce efficacy of omega-3 on depressive symptoms. The supplemented omega-3 PUFA may have compensated the increased demand of the developing fetus during pregnancy and neonate during lactation rather than contributing to therapeutic efficacy by reducing depressive symptoms [119]. Finally, depression examined as secondary outcome could suffer by changing of the measurement depending on the improvement (or worsening) of the underlying primary disease.

Regarding the different efficacy of EPA compared with DHA and EPA-DHA combinations, the analysis of RCTs grouped according to type of omega-3 PUFA administered confirmed the findings of previous meta-analysis and substantial stronger pooled results of studies using EPA rather than DHA. However, as previously reported [109], the aforementioned methodological issues may have biased the results in favor of efficacy for EPA-containing preparations suggesting that the reported benefits on depressive symptoms in this group of studies may not therefore be definitively attributed only to the EPA content of the supplementation regimen and also that further studies are needed in this field. Whether EPA, rather than DHA, is effective in ameliorating depression in specific groups of patients, the different effects of these classes of omega-3 PUFA is a challenge to be explained convincingly, since DHA is a major structural component of neuronal membranes, and we can hypothesize that increasing its nutritional availability would have beneficial effects on brain function, rather than EPA, which is present at levels several hundred-fold lower [120]. Possible explanations of the beneficial role of EPA are the following: (i) the anti-inflammatory effects of EPA-derived eicosanoids [121] and its oxidized derivatives [122] (ii) its efficacy at reducing the inflammatory cytokines tumor necrosis factor-alpha (TNF-α), IL-6, and IL-1b [123] through inhibition of the activity of nuclear factor kappa-B (NF-kB) [124]; (iii) *in vivo* evidence of a more effective anti-inflammatory action of dietary EPA compared with DHA [125]. Moreover, DHA has been reported to be poorly incorporated in the human brain [126], and EPA may facilitate an increase in brain DHA levels after its conversion [127]. Finally, EPA supplementation has been associated with N-acetyl-aspartate increase in brain, a marker for neuronal homeostasis, suggesting its role as a neuroprotective agent [80]. Together with the inflammation theory of depression [8], chronic intake of omega-3 fatty acids has been reported to play an important role in neuronal structure and function [128]. However, such hypotheses are not completely exhaustive and further research is needed to better identify the specific molecular mechanisms underlying clinical efficacy of omega-3 PUFA (both EPA and DHA) in preventing or ameliorating depression.

The studies excluded from this systematic review were not comparable in terms of methodology used, and their exclusion was needed in order to reduce differences among RCTs and improve data quality (i.e., reduce selection bias). On the other hand, these trials may still be directly relevant to the topic of the present study, and a specific discussion (e-discussion) may strengthen conclusion retrieved from this meta-analysis. Moreover, we discussed in a specific section of the e-discussion about the studies quality and potential sources of heterogeneity.

The main limitation of this study was the inability to control all the many potential sources of heterogeneity. Despite the fact that a logical grouping of trials was performed, a non-modifiable degree of heterogeneity, due to specific characteristics of all trials included, still weakened the pooled analysis of these studies. However, compared with older studies, the inclusion of the updated RCTs strengthened the conclusions of the effects of omega-3 PUFA intake on depressive disorders.

To sum up, trials conducted in individuals with a diagnosis of MDD provided evidence that omega-3 PUFA supplementation has beneficial clinical effects on depressive status. Evidence of their efficacy was provided also for patients with bipolar disorder, whereas no evidence was found for individuals included in the other diagnostic groups. According to our findings, in RCTs with omega-3 PUFA supplementation in healthy subjects and patients with schizophrenia, AD and CVD seems to result ineffective.

Supporting Information

Checklist S1   PRISMA checklist for meta-analyses studies.

Discussion S1   Additional discussion.

Author Contributions

Conceived and designed the experiments: GG AP FD. Performed the experiments: GG SM FG SC. Analyzed the data: GG SM CB. Wrote the paper: GG FC.

References

1. Kotwal S, Jun M, Sullivan D, Perkovic V, Neal B (2012) Omega 3 Fatty acids and cardiovascular outcomes: systematic review and meta-analysis. Circ Cardiovasc Qual Outcomes 5: 808–818.

2. Grosso G, Galvano F, Marventano S, Malaguarnera M, Bucolo C, et al. (2014) Omega-3 Fatty Acids and Depression: Scientific evidence and Biological Mechanisms. Oxid Med Cell Longev 2014: 313570.

3. Machado-Vieira R, Mallinger AG (2012) Abnormal function of monoamine oxidase-A in comorbid major depressive disorder and cardiovascular disease: pathophysiological and therapeutic implications (review). Mol Med Rep 6: 915–922.

4. Do DP, Dowd JB, Ranjit N, House JS, Kaplan GA (2010) Hopelessness, depression, and early markers of endothelial dysfunction in U.S. adults. Psychosom Med 72: 613–619.

5. Severus WE, Littman AB, Stoll AL (2001) Omega-3 fatty acids, homocysteine, and the increased risk of cardiovascular mortality in major depressive disorder. Harv Rev Psychiatry 9: 280–293.

6. Bourre JM (2004) Roles of unsaturated fatty acids (especially omega-3 fatty acids) in the brain at various ages and during ageing. J Nutr Health Aging 8: 163–174.

7. Hennebelle M, Balasse L, Latour A, Champeil-Potokar G, Denis S, et al. (2012) Influence of omega-3 fatty acid status on the way rats adapt to chronic restraint stress. PLoS One 7: e42142.

8. Maes M, Yirmiya R, Noraberg J, Brene S, Hibbeln J, et al. (2009) The inflammatory & neurodegenerative (I&ND) hypothesis of depression: leads for future research and new drug developments in depression. Metab Brain Dis 24: 27–53.

9. Rees AM, Austin MP, Owen C, Parker G (2009) Omega-3 deficiency associated with perinatal depression: case control study. Psychiatry Res 166: 254–259.

10. Schins A, Crijns HJ, Brummer RJ, Wichers M, Lousberg R, et al. (2007) Altered omega-3 polyunsaturated fatty acid status in depressed post-myocardial infarction patients. Acta Psychiatr Scand 115: 35–40.

11. Frasure-Smith N, Lesperance F, Julien P (2004) Major depression is associated with lower omega-3 fatty acid levels in patients with recent acute coronary syndromes. Biol Psychiatry 55: 891–896.

12. Parker GB, Heruc GA, Hilton TM, Olley A, Brotchie H, et al. (2006) Low levels of docosahexaenoic acid identified in acute coronary syndrome patients with depression. Psychiatry Res 141: 279–286.

13. Assies J, Pouwer F, Lok A, Mocking RJ, Bockting CL, et al. (2010) Plasma and erythrocyte fatty acid patterns in patients with recurrent depression: a matched case-control study. PLoS One 5: e10635.

14. Bloch MH, Hannestad J (2012) Omega-3 fatty acids for the treatment of depression: systematic review and meta-analysis. Mol Psychiatry 17: 1272–1282.

15. Martins JG, Bentsen H, Puri BK (2012) Eicosapentaenoic acid appears to be the key omega-3 fatty acid component associated with efficacy in major depressive disorder: a critique of Bloch and Hannestad and updated meta-analysis. Mol Psychiatry 17: 1144–1149; discussion 1163–1147.

16. Lin PY, Mischoulon D, Freeman MP, Matsuoka Y, Hibbeln J, et al. (2012) Are omega-3 fatty acids antidepressants or just mood-improving agents? The effect depends upon diagnosis, supplement preparation, and severity of depression. Mol Psychiatry 17: 1161–1163; author reply 1163–1167.

17. Association AP (2000) Diagnostic and Statistical Manual of Mental Disorders; 4th, editor. Washington, DC. 317–345 p.

18. Hamilton M (1967) Development of a rating scale for primary depressive illness. Br J Soc Clin Psychol 6: 278–296.

19. Beck AT (1978) Depression Inventory. Center for Cognitive Therapy; Philadelphia.

20. Montgomery SA, Asberg M (1979) A new depression scale designed to be sensitive to change. Br J Psychiatry 134: 382–389.

21. Picardi A (2009) Rating scales in bipolar disorder. Curr Opin Psychiatry 22: 42–49.

22. Geddes JR, Miklowitz DJ (2013) Treatment of bipolar disorder. Lancet 381: 1672–1682.

23. Vesga-Lopez O, Blanco C, Keyes K, Olfson M, Grant BF, et al. (2008) Psychiatric disorders in pregnant and postpartum women in the United States. Arch Gen Psychiatry 65: 805–815.

24. Otto SJ, de Groot RH, Hornstra G (2003) Increased risk of postpartum depressive symptoms is associated with slower normalization after pregnancy of the functional docosahexaenoic acid status. Prostaglandins Leukot Essent Fatty Acids 69: 237–243.

25. Bylund DB, Reed AL (2007) Childhood and adolescent depression: why do children and adults respond differently to antidepressant drugs? Neurochem Int 51: 246–253.

26. Cox GR, Callahan P, Churchill R, Hunot V, Merry SN, et al. (2012) Psychological therapies versus antidepressant medication, alone and in combination for depression in children and adolescents. Cochrane Database Syst Rev 11: CD008324.

27. Appleton KM, Hayward RC, Gunnell D, Peters TJ, Rogers PJ, et al. (2006) Effects of n-3 long-chain polyunsaturated fatty acids on depressed mood: systematic review of published trials. Am J Clin Nutr 84: 1308–1316.

28. Appleton KM, Rogers PJ, Ness AR (2010) Updated systematic review and meta-analysis of the effects of n-3 long-chain polyunsaturated fatty acids on depressed mood. Am J Clin Nutr 91: 757–770.

29. Sublette ME, Ellis SP, Geant AL, Mann JJ (2011) Meta-analysis of the effects of eicosapentaenoic acid (EPA) in clinical trials in depression. J Clin Psychiatry 72: 1577–1584.

30. Jadad AR, Moore RA, Carroll D, Jenkinson C, Reynolds DJ, et al. (1996) Assessing the quality of reports of randomized clinical trials: is blinding necessary? Control Clin Trials 17: 1–12.

31. Clayton EH, Hanstock TL, Hirneth SJ, Kable CJ, Garg ML, et al. (2009) Reduced mania and depression in juvenile bipolar disorder associated with long-chain omega-3 polyunsaturated fatty acid supplementation. Eur J Clin Nutr 63: 1037–1040.

32. Ness AR, Gallacher JE, Bennett PD, Gunnell DJ, Rogers PJ, et al. (2003) Advice to eat fish and mood: a randomised controlled trial in men with angina. Nutr Neurosci 6: 63–65.

33. Beezhold BL, Johnston CS (2012) Restriction of meat, fish, and poultry in omnivores improves mood: a pilot randomized controlled trial. Nutr J 11: 9.

34. Marangell LB, Suppes T, Ketter TA, Dennehy EB, Zboyan H, et al. (2006) Omega-3 fatty acids in bipolar disorder: clinical and research considerations. Prostaglandins Leukot Essent Fatty Acids 75: 315–321.

35. Krauss-Etschmann S, Shadid R, Campoy C, Hoster E, Demmelmair H, et al. (2007) Effects of fish-oil and folate supplementation of pregnant women on maternal and fetal plasma concentrations of docosahexaenoic acid and eicosapentaenoic acid: a European randomized multicenter trial. Am J Clin Nutr 85: 1392–1400.

36. Mattes E, McCarthy S, Gong G, van Eekelen JA, Dunstan J, et al. (2009) Maternal mood scores in mid-pregnancy are related to aspects of neonatal immune function. Brain Behav Immun 23: 380–388.

37. Andreeva VA, Galan P, Torres M, Julia C, Hercberg S, et al. (2012) Supplementation with B vitamins or n-3 fatty acids and depressive symptoms in cardiovascular disease survivors: ancillary findings from the SUpplementation with FOLate, vitamins B-6 and B-12 and/or OMega-3 fatty acids (SU.FOL.OM3) randomized trial. Am J Clin Nutr 96: 208–214.

38. Makrides M, Gibson RA, McPhee AJ, Yelland L, Quinlivan J, et al. (2010) Effect of DHA supplementation during pregnancy on maternal depression and neurodevelopment of young children: a randomized controlled trial. JAMA 304: 1675–1683.

39. Behan PO, Behan WM, Horrobin D (1990) Effect of high doses of essential fatty acids on the postviral fatigue syndrome. Acta Neurol Scand 82: 209–216.

40. Sohrabi N, Kashanian M, Ghafoori SS, Malakouti SK (2013) Evaluation of the effect of omega-3 fatty acids in the treatment of premenstrual syndrome: "a pilot trial". Complement Ther Med 21: 141–146.

41. Sampalis F, Bunea R, Pelland MF, Kowalski O, Duguet N, et al. (2003) Evaluation of the effects of Neptune Krill Oil on the management of premenstrual syndrome and dysmenorrhea. Altern Med Rev 8: 171–179.

42. Puolakka J, Makarainen L, Viinikka L, Ylikorkala O (1985) Biochemical and clinical effects of treating the premenstrual syndrome with prostaglandin synthesis precursors. J Reprod Med 30: 149–153.

43. Beck AT, Ward CH, Mendelson M, Mock J, Erbaugh J (1961) An inventory for measuring depression. Arch Gen Psychiatry 4: 561–571.

44. Hamilton M (1960) A rating scale for depression. J Neurol Neurosurg Psychiatry 23: 56–62.

45. Giltay EJ, Gooren LJ, Toorians AW, Katan MB, Zock PL (2004) Docosahexaenoic acid concentrations are higher in women than in men because of estrogenic effects. Am J Clin Nutr 80: 1167–1174.

46. Grenyer BF, Crowe T, Meyer B, Owen AJ, Grigonis-Deane EM, et al. (2007) Fish oil supplementation in the treatment of major depression: a randomised double-blind placebo-controlled trial. Prog Neuropsychopharmacol Biol Psychiatry 31: 1393–1396.

47. da Silva TM, Munhoz RP, Alvarez C, Naliwaiko K, Kiss A, et al. (2008) Depression in Parkinson's disease: a double-blind, randomized, placebo-controlled pilot study of omega-3 fatty-acid supplementation. J Affect Disord 111: 351–359.

48. Jazayeri S, Tehrani-Doost M, Keshavarz SA, Hosseini M, Djazayery A, et al. (2008) Comparison of therapeutic effects of omega-3 fatty acid eicosapentaenoic acid and fluoxetine, separately and in combination, in major depressive disorder. Aust N Z J Psychiatry 42: 192–198.

49. Hallahan B, Hibbeln JR, Davis JM, Garland MR (2007) Omega-3 fatty acid supplementation in patients with recurrent self-harm. Single-centre double-blind randomised controlled trial. Br J Psychiatry 190: 118–122.

50. Freund-Levi Y, Basun H, Cederholm T, Faxen-Irving G, Garlind A, et al. (2008) Omega-3 supplementation in mild to moderate Alzheimer's disease: effects on neuropsychiatric symptoms. Int J Geriatr Psychiatry 23: 161–169.

51. Doornbos B, van Goor SA, Dijck-Brouwer DA, Schaafsma A, Korf J, et al. (2009) Supplementation of a low dose of DHA or DHA+AA does not prevent peripartum depressive symptoms in a small population based sample. Prog Neuropsychopharmacol Biol Psychiatry 33: 49–52.

52. Fontani G, Corradeschi F, Felici A, Alfatti F, Bugarini R, et al. (2005) Blood profiles, body fat and mood state in healthy subjects on different diets

supplemented with Omega-3 polyunsaturated fatty acids. Eur J Clin Invest 35: 499–507.

53. Rondanelli M, Giacosa A, Opizzi A, Pelucchi C, La Vecchia C, et al. (2011) Long chain omega 3 polyunsaturated fatty acids supplementation in the treatment of elderly depression: effects on depressive symptoms, on phospholipids fatty acids profile and on health-related quality of life. J Nutr Health Aging 15: 37–44.

54. Peet M, Horrobin DF (2002) A dose-ranging study of the effects of ethyl-eicosapentaenoate in patients with ongoing depression despite apparently adequate treatment with standard drugs. Arch Gen Psychiatry 59: 913–919.

55. Furukawa TA, Barbui C, Cipriani A, Brambilla P, Watanabe N (2006) Imputing missing standard deviations in meta-analyses can provide accurate results. J Clin Epidemiol 59: 7–10.

56. Warren G, McKendrick M, Peet M (1999) The role of essential fatty acids in chronic fatigue syndrome. A case-controlled study of red-cell membrane essential fatty acids (EFA) and a placebo-controlled treatment study with high dose of EFA. Acta Neurol Scand 99: 112–116.

57. Fux M, Benjamin J, Nemets B (2004) A placebo-controlled cross-over trial of adjunctive EPA in OCD. J Psychiatr Res 38: 323–325.

58. Hirashima F, Parow AM, Stoll AL, Demopulos CM, Damico KE, et al. (2004) Omega-3 fatty acid treatment and T(2) whole brain relaxation times in bipolar disorder. Am J Psychiatry 161: 1922–1924.

59. Keck PE Jr, Mintz J, McElroy SL, Freeman MP, Suppes T, et al. (2006) Double-blind, randomized, placebo-controlled trials of ethyl-eicosapentanoate in the treatment of bipolar depression and rapid cycling bipolar disorder. Biol Psychiatry 60: 1020–1022.

60. Sinn N, Milte CM, Street SJ, Buckley JD, Coates AM, et al. (2012) Effects of n-3 fatty acids, EPA v. DHA, on depressive symptoms, quality of life, memory and executive function in older adults with mild cognitive impairment: a 6-month randomised controlled trial. Br J Nutr 107: 1682–1693.

61. Gracious BL, Chirieac MC, Costescu S, Finucane TL, Youngstrom EA, et al. (2010) Randomized, placebo-controlled trial of flax oil in pediatric bipolar disorder. Bipolar Disord 12: 142–154.

62. Bot M, Pouwer F, Assies J, Jansen EH, Beekman AT, et al. (2011) Supplementation with eicosapentaenoic omega-3 fatty acid does not influence serum brain-derived neurotrophic factor in diabetes mellitus patients with major depression: a randomized controlled pilot study. Neuropsychobiology 63: 219–223.

63. Chiu CC, Huang SY, Chen CC, Su KP (2005) Omega-3 fatty acids are more beneficial in the depressive phase than in the manic phase in patients with bipolar I disorder. J Clin Psychiatry 66: 1613–1614.

64. Peet M, Horrobin DF (2002) A dose-ranging exploratory study of the effects of ethyl-eicosapentaenoate in patients with persistent schizophrenic symptoms. J Psychiatr Res 36: 7–18.

65. Frangou S, Lewis M, McCrone P (2006) Efficacy of ethyl-eicosapentaenoic acid in bipolar depression: randomised double-blind placebo-controlled study. Br J Psychiatry 188: 46–50.

66. Kiecolt-Glaser JK, Belury MA, Andridge R, Malarkey WB, Hwang BS, et al. (2012) Omega-3 supplementation lowers inflammation in healthy middle-aged and older adults: a randomized controlled trial. Brain Behav Immun 26: 988–995.

67. van de Rest O, Geleijnse JM, Kok FJ, van Staveren WA, Hoefnagels WH, et al. (2008) Effect of fish-oil supplementation on mental well-being in older subjects: a randomized, double-blind, placebo-controlled trial. Am J Clin Nutr 88: 706–713.

68. Mozurkewich EL, Clinton CM, Chilimigras JL, Hamilton SE, Allbaugh LJ, et al. (2013) The Mothers, Omega-3, and Mental Health Study: a double-blind, randomized controlled trial. Am J Obstet Gynecol 208: 313 e311–319.

69. Mozaffari-Khosravi H, Yassini-Ardakani M, Karamati M, Shariati-Bafghi SE (2013) Eicosapentaenoic acid versus docosahexaenoic acid in mild-to-moderate depression: a randomized, double-blind, placebo-controlled trial. Eur Neuropsychopharmacol 23: 636–644.

70. Lucas M, Asselin G, Merette C, Poulin MJ, Dodin S (2009) Ethyl-eicosapentaenoic acid for the treatment of psychological distress and depressive symptoms in middle-aged women: a double-blind, placebo-controlled, randomized clinical trial. Am J Clin Nutr 89: 641–651.

71. Sterne JA, Egger M, Smith GD (2001) Systematic reviews in health care: Investigating and dealing with publication and other biases in meta-analysis. BMJ 323: 101–105.

72. deeks JJ, Altman DG, Bradbrun MJ (2001) Statistical methods for examining heterogeneity and combining results from several studies in metaanalysis. London. 285–312 p.

73. Higgins JP, Thompson SG (2002) Quantifying heterogeneity in a meta-analysis. Stat Med 21: 1539–1558.

74. Higgins JP, Thompson SG, Deeks JJ, Altman DG (2003) Measuring inconsistency in meta-analyses. BMJ 327: 557–560.

75. Stoll AL, Severus WE, Freeman MP, Rueter S, Zboyan HA, et al. (1999) Omega 3 fatty acids in bipolar disorder: a preliminary double-blind, placebo-controlled trial. Arch Gen Psychiatry 56: 407–412.

76. Nemets B, Stahl Z, Belmaker RH (2002) Addition of omega-3 fatty acid to maintenance medication treatment for recurrent unipolar depressive disorder. Am J Psychiatry 159: 477–479.

77. Marangell LB, Martinez JM, Zboyan HA, Kertz B, Kim HF, et al. (2003) A double-blind, placebo-controlled study of the omega-3 fatty acid docosahexaenoic acid in the treatment of major depression. Am J Psychiatry 160: 996–998.

78. Su KP, Huang SY, Chiu CC, Shen WW (2003) Omega-3 fatty acids in major depressive disorder. A preliminary double-blind, placebo-controlled trial. Eur Neuropsychopharmacol 13: 267–271.

79. Silvers KM, Woolley CC, Hamilton FC, Watts PM, Watson RA (2005) Randomised double-blind placebo-controlled trial of fish oil in the treatment of depression. Prostaglandins Leukot Essent Fatty Acids 72: 211–218.

80. Frangou S, Lewis M, Wollard J, Simmons A (2007) Preliminary in vivo evidence of increased N-acetyl-aspartate following eicosapentanoic acid treatment in patients with bipolar disorder. J Psychopharmacol 21: 435–439.

81. Chiu CC, Su KP, Cheng TC, Liu HC, Chang CJ, et al. (2008) The effects of omega-3 fatty acids monotherapy in Alzheimer's disease and mild cognitive impairment: a preliminary randomized double-blind placebo-controlled study. Prog Neuropsychopharmacol Biol Psychiatry 32: 1538–1544.

82. Su KP, Huang SY, Chiu TH, Huang KC, Huang CL, et al. (2008) Omega-3 fatty acids for major depressive disorder during pregnancy: results from a randomized, double-blind, placebo-controlled trial. J Clin Psychiatry 69: 644–651.

83. Mischoulon D, Papakostas GI, Dording CM, Farabaugh AH, Sonawalla SB, et al. (2009) A double-blind, randomized controlled trial of ethyl-eicosapentaenoate for major depressive disorder. J Clin Psychiatry 70: 1636–1644.

84. Gertsik L, Poland RE, Bresee C, Rapaport MH (2012) Omega-3 fatty acid augmentation of citalopram treatment for patients with major depressive disorder. J Clin Psychopharmacol 32: 61–64.

85. Llorente AM, Jensen CL, Voigt RG, Fraley JK, Berretta MC, et al. (2003) Effect of maternal docosahexaenoic acid supplementation on postpartum depression and information processing. Am J Obstet Gynecol 188: 1348–1353.

86. Rogers PJ, Appleton KM, Kessler D, Peters TJ, Gunnell D, et al. (2008) No effect of n-3 long-chain polyunsaturated fatty acid (EPA and DHA) supplementation on depressed mood and cognitive function: a randomised controlled trial. Br J Nutr 99: 421–431.

87. Carney RM, Freedland KE, Rubin EH, Rich MW, Steinmeyer BC, et al. (2009) Omega-3 augmentation of sertraline in treatment of depression in patients with coronary heart disease: a randomized controlled trial. JAMA 302: 1651–1657.

88. Antypa N, Van der Does AJ, Smelt AH, Rogers RD (2009) Omega-3 fatty acids (fish-oil) and depression-related cognition in healthy volunteers. J Psychopharmacol 23: 831–840.

89. Antypa N, Smelt AH, Strengholt A, Van der Does AJ (2012) Effects of omega-3 fatty acid supplementation on mood and emotional information processing in recovered depressed individuals. J Psychopharmacol 26: 738–743.

90. Fenton WS, Dickerson F, Boronow J, Hibbeln JR, Knable M (2001) A placebo-controlled trial of omega-3 fatty acid (ethyl eicosapentaenoic acid) supplementation for residual symptoms and cognitive impairment in schizophrenia. Am J Psychiatry 158: 2071–2074.

91. Zanarini MC, Frankenburg FR (2003) omega-3 Fatty acid treatment of women with borderline personality disorder: a double-blind, placebo-controlled pilot study. Am J Psychiatry 160: 167–169.

92. Amminger GP, Schafer MR, Papageorgiou K, Klier CM, Cotton SM, et al. (2010) Long-chain omega-3 fatty acids for indicated prevention of psychotic disorders: a randomized, placebo-controlled trial. Arch Gen Psychiatry 67: 146–154.

93. Rees AM, Austin MP, Parker GB (2008) Omega-3 fatty acids as a treatment for perinatal depression: randomized double-blind placebo-controlled trial. Aust N Z J Psychiatry 42: 199–205.

94. Bot M, Pouwer F, Assies J, Jansen EH, Diamant M, et al. (2010) Eicosapentaenoic acid as an add-on to antidepressant medication for comorbid major depression in patients with diabetes mellitus: a randomized, double-blind placebo-controlled study. J Affect Disord 126: 282–286.

95. Rondanelli M, Giacosa A, Opizzi A, Pelucchi C, La Vecchia C, et al. (2010) Effect of omega-3 fatty acids supplementation on depressive symptoms and on health-related quality of life in the treatment of elderly women with depression: a double-blind, placebo-controlled, randomized clinical trial. J Am Coll Nutr 29: 55–64.

96. Rizzo AM, Corsetto PA, Montorfano G, Opizzi A, Faliva M, et al. (2012) Comparison between the AA/EPA ratio in depressed and non depressed elderly females: omega-3 fatty acid supplementation correlates with improved symptoms but does not change immunological parameters. Nutr J 11: 82.

97. Tajalizadekhoob Y, Sharifi F, Fakhrzadeh H, Mirarefin M, Ghaderpanahi M, et al. (2011) The effect of low-dose omega 3 fatty acids on the treatment of mild to moderate depression in the elderly: a double-blind, randomized, placebo-controlled study. Eur Arch Psychiatry Clin Neurosci 261: 539–549.

98. Nemets H, Nemets B, Apter A, Bracha Z, Belmaker RH (2006) Omega-3 treatment of childhood depression: a controlled, double-blind pilot study. Am J Psychiatry 163: 1098–1100.

99. Freeman MP, Davis M, Sinha P, Wisner KL, Hibbeln JR, et al. (2008) Omega-3 fatty acids and supportive psychotherapy for perinatal depression: a randomized placebo-controlled study. J Affect Disord 110: 142–148.

100. Giltay EJ, Geleijnse JM, Kromhout D (2011) Effects of n-3 fatty acids on depressive symptoms and dispositional optimism after myocardial infarction. Am J Clin Nutr 94: 1442–1450.

101. DeFina LF, Marcoux LG, Devers SM, Cleaver JP, Willis BL (2011) Effects of omega-3 supplementation in combination with diet and exercise on weight loss and body composition. Am J Clin Nutr 93: 455–462.

102. Kiecolt-Glaser JK, Belury MA, Andridge R, Malarkey WB, Glaser R (2011) Omega-3 supplementation lowers inflammation and anxiety in medical students: a randomized controlled trial. Brain Behav Immun 25: 1725–1734.

103. Barbui C, Cipriani A, Patel V, Ayuso-Mateos JL, van Ommeren M (2011) Efficacy of antidepressants and benzodiazepines in minor depression: systematic review and meta-analysis. Br J Psychiatry 198: 11–16, sup 11.

104. Iovieno N, Papakostas GI (2012) Correlation between different levels of placebo response rate and clinical trial outcome in major depressive disorder: a meta-analysis. J Clin Psychiatry 73: 1300–1306.

105. Souery D, Papakostas GI, Trivedi MH (2006) Treatment-resistant depression. J Clin Psychiatry 67 Suppl 6: 16–22.

106. Freeman MP, Hibbeln JR, Wisner KL, Davis JM, Mischoulon D, et al. (2006) Omega-3 fatty acids: evidence basis for treatment and future research in psychiatry. J Clin Psychiatry 67: 1954–1967.

107. Lin PY, Su KP (2007) A meta-analytic review of double-blind, placebo-controlled trials of antidepressant efficacy of omega-3 fatty acids. J Clin Psychiatry 68: 1056–1061.

108. Ross BM, Seguin J, Sieswerda LE (2007) Omega-3 fatty acids as treatments for mental illness: which disorder and which fatty acid? Lipids Health Dis 6: 21.

109. Martins JG (2009) EPA but not DHA appears to be responsible for the efficacy of omega-3 long chain polyunsaturated fatty acid supplementation in depression: evidence from a meta-analysis of randomized controlled trials. J Am Coll Nutr 28: 525–542.

110. Balanza-Martinez V, Fries GR, Colpo GD, Silveira PP, Portella AK, et al. (2011) Therapeutic use of omega-3 fatty acids in bipolar disorder. Expert Rev Neurother 11: 1029–1047.

111. Montgomery P, Richardson AJ (2008) Omega-3 fatty acids for bipolar disorder. Cochrane Database Syst Rev: CD005169.

112. Sarris J, Mischoulon D, Schweitzer I (2012) Omega-3 for bipolar disorder: meta-analyses of use in mania and bipolar depression. J Clin Psychiatry 73: 81–86.

113. Mocking RJ, Assies J, Bot M, Jansen EH, Schene AH, et al. (2012) Biological effects of add-on eicosapentaenoic acid supplementation in diabetes mellitus and co-morbid depression: a randomized controlled trial. PLoS One 7: e49431.

114. Caraci F, Copani A, Nicoletti F, Drago F (2010) Depression and Alzheimer's disease: neurobiological links and common pharmacological targets. Eur J Pharmacol 626: 64–71.

115. Caraci F, Bosco P, Signorelli M, Spada RS, Cosentino FI, et al. (2012) The CC genotype of transforming growth factor-beta1 increases the risk of late-onset Alzheimer's disease and is associated with AD-related depression. Eur Neuropsychopharmacol 22: 281–289.

116. Salomone S, Caraci F, Leggio GM, Fedotova J, Drago F (2012) New pharmacological strategies for treatment of Alzheimer's disease: focus on disease modifying drugs. Br J Clin Pharmacol 73: 504–517.

117. Caraci F, Spampinato S, Sortino MA, Bosco P, Battaglia G, et al. (2012) Dysfunction of TGF-beta1 signaling in Alzheimer's disease: perspectives for neuroprotection. Cell Tissue Res 347: 291–301.

118. Caraci F, Battaglia G, Bruno V, Bosco P, Carbonaro V, et al. (2011) TGF-beta1 pathway as a new target for neuroprotection in Alzheimer's disease. CNS Neurosci Ther 17: 237–249.

119. Markhus MW, Skotheim S, Graff IE, Froyland L, Braarud HC, et al. (2013) Low omega-3 index in pregnancy is a possible biological risk factor for postpartum depression. PLoS One 8: e67617.

120. Arterburn LM, Hall EB, Oken H (2006) Distribution, interconversion, and dose response of n-3 fatty acids in humans. Am J Clin Nutr 83: 1467S–1476S.

121. Calder PC (2006) n-3 polyunsaturated fatty acids, inflammation, and inflammatory diseases. Am J Clin Nutr 83: 1505S–1519S.

122. Brooks JD, Milne GL, Yin H, Sanchez SC, Porter NA, et al. (2008) Formation of highly reactive cyclopentenone isoprostane compounds (A3/J3-isoprostanes) in vivo from eicosapentaenoic acid. J Biol Chem 283: 12043–12055.

123. Bhattacharya A, Sun D, Rahman M, Fernandes G (2007) Different ratios of eicosapentaenoic and docosahexaenoic omega-3 fatty acids in commercial fish oils differentially alter pro-inflammatory cytokines in peritoneal macrophages from C57BL/6 female mice. J Nutr Biochem 18: 23–30.

124. Zhao Y, Joshi-Barve S, Barve S, Chen LH (2004) Eicosapentaenoic acid prevents LPS-induced TNF-alpha expression by preventing NF-kappaB activation. J Am Coll Nutr 23: 71–78.

125. Sierra S, Lara-Villoslada F, Comalada M, Olivares M, Xaus J (2008) Dietary eicosapentaenoic acid and docosahexaenoic acid equally incorporate as decosahexaenoic acid but differ in inflammatory effects. Nutrition 24: 245–254.

126. Umhau JC, Dauphinais KM, Patel SH, Nahrwold DA, Hibbeln JR, et al. (2006) The relationship between folate and docosahexaenoic acid in men. Eur J Clin Nutr 60: 352–357.

127. Gao F, Kiesewetter D, Chang L, Ma K, Rapoport SI, et al. (2009) Whole-body synthesis secretion of docosahexaenoic acid from circulating eicosapentaenoic acid in unanesthetized rats. J Lipid Res 50: 2463–2470.

128. Chang CY, Ke DS, Chen JY (2009) Essential fatty acids and human brain. Acta Neurol Taiwan 18: 231–241.

## 11

Characterization of Aging-Associated Cardiac Diastolic Dysfunction

Wei-Ting Chang[1,2⦾], Jung-San Chen[3⦾], Yung-Kung Hung[3], Wei-Chuan Tsai[1], Jer-Nan Juang[3]*, Ping-Yen Liu[1,2]*

1 Division of Cardiology, Internal Medicine, National Cheng Kung University Hospital, Tainan, Taiwan, **2** Institute of Clinical Medicine, National Cheng Kung University, Tainan, Taiwan, **3** Department of Engineering Science, National Cheng Kung University, Tainan, Taiwan

Abstract

Aims: Diastolic dysfunction is common in geriatric heart failure. A reliable parameter to predict myocardium stiffness and relaxation under similar end-diastolic pressure is being developed. We propose a material and mathematical model for calculating myocardium stiffness based on the concept of linear correlation between e/e' and wedge pressure.

Methods and Results: We enrolled 919 patients (male: 52.6%[484/919]). Compared with the younger population of controls (mean age: 43.9 ± 11.7 years; $n = 211$; male: 62.1% [131/211]), the elderly (mean age: 76.3 ± 6.2; $n = 708$; male: 52.6% [484/708]) had a greater prevalence of hypertension, diabetes mellitus, and coronary artery disease (all $p < 0.05$). We collected their M-mode and 2-D echocardiographic volumetric parameters, intraventricular filling pressure, and speckle tracking images to establish a mathematical model. The feasibility of this model was validated. The average early diastolic velocity of the mitral annulus assessed using tissue Doppler imaging was significantly attenuated in the elderly (e': 0.09 ± 0.02 vs. 0.08 ± 0.02; $p = 0.02$) and corresponded to the higher estimated wedge (e/e') pressure (7.76 ± 2.44 vs. 8.35 ± 2.64; $p = 0.02$) in that cohort. E (Young's modulus) was calculated to describe the tensile elasticity of the myocardium. With the same intraventricular filling pressure, E was significantly higher in the elderly, especially those with e/e' values >9. Compared with diastolic dysfunction parameters, E also presented sentinel characteristics more sensitive for detecting early myocardial relaxation impairment, which indicates stiffer myocardium in aging hearts.

Conclusion: Our material and geometric mathematical model successfully described the stiffer myocardium in aging hearts with higher intraventricular pressure. Additional studies that compare individual differences, especially in health status, are needed to validate its application for detecting diastolic heart failure.

Editor: Sudhiranjan Gupta, Texas A & M, Division of Cardiology, United States of America

Funding: This research was supported in part by the Headquarters of University Advancement at the National Cheng Kung University, which is sponsored by the Ministry of Education, Taiwan, ROC. The research was also granted from Health Promotion Program: Blood Pressure Control from Health Promotion Administration, Ministry of Health and Welfare, Taiwan, ROC and the grant from NSC101-2314-B-006-075-MY2, sponsored by the Ministry of Science and Technology, Taiwan, ROC. The investigator (PY Liu) was granted by "A Landmark Project to Promote Innovation & Competitiveness of Clinical Trials by the Excellent Clinical Trial and Research Center in National Cheng Kung University Hospital, Ministry of Health and Welfare, Taiwan." The funders had no role in study design, data collection and analysis, decision to publish, or preparation of the manuscript.

Competing Interests: The authors have declared that no competing interests exist.

* E-mail: jjuang@mail.ncku.edu.tw (JNJ); larry@mail.ncku.edu.tw (PYL)

⦾ These authors contributed equally to this work.

Introduction

Heart failure is increasingly prevalent among older adults [1]. Clinically, 40 – 50% of patients with symptomatic heart failure have preserved left heart function, with preserved ventricular ejection fraction ($> 50\%$) [2]. Sometimes this is called "diastolic dysfunction with preserved systolic function" or "diastolic heart failure" [3]. People with diastolic heart failure are generally older and female, and tend to have a greater incidence of systemic hypertension than do those with contractile dysfunction ("systolic heart failure") [4,5]. Physiologically, diastolic heart failure occurs when the ventricle cannot fill properly because it cannot relax or its wall is too rigid [6]. Histological evidence supports the notion that diastolic dysfunction is related to ventricular hypertrophy, increased interstitial collagen deposition into the myocardium [7].

Similarly, aging hearts continuously lose myocytes, which is compensated for by reactive hypertrophy of the remaining cells; thus, these hearts are filled with fibrotic or adipose tissue [8]. Histological samples for measuring the exact tensile elasticity of the myocardium are possible only in animal studies, not human studies. Some mathematical models have been used to describe the dynamics of remodeling in skeletal muscle, arteries, and even the heart [9,10]. However, a mathematical model to study cardiac aging is still lacking. Establishing a model of the aging heart would provide a tool for us to understand underlying mechanisms of cardiac aging and to define the impaired myocardial relaxation process.

It remains uncertain whether current available invasive and noninvasive diagnostic tools can accurately predict myocardium stiffness. The time constant of relaxation (tau, τ), which describes the rate of left ventricular (LV) pressure decay during isovolumic relaxation, is currently the standard parameter for predicting the relaxation function of myocardium [11,12]. However, several confounding factors, when echocardiography is used to measure the deceleration time of mitral inflow, may disturb the equivalence between echocardiographic and catheterized results. Despite the ratio of mitral inflow to annulus tissue, Doppler imaging velocity (e/e') indicates the intraventricular pressure, which is within the borderline range of elevated pressure ($e/e' = 9-14$), the discrimination of diastolic dysfunction remains a dilemma [3]. Therefore, a reliable and noninvasive diagnostic parameter is crucial for facilitating an accurate diagnosis that indicates whether the stiffness is myocardial stiffness.

Studies [13-21] on the elastic properties of the contracting left ventricle have aroused a great deal of interest among scientists and engineers. Many researchers have developed a series of experimental techniques for determining the elastic properties of the left ventricle. A simple and practical approach for in vivo determinations of the properties of the canine left ventricle, proposed in 1972 [13], established the relationship between the effective elastic modulus and the circumferential stress throughout the isovolumetric systolic period. After the concept on the elastic properties of the left ventricle was accepted, some researchers reported that the effective modulus E measured from experiments could also be viewed as an additional indication of the left ventricle having adjusted to the heart disease [14], which showed that normal values of E during the systole directly indicate that the strength of the left ventricle contraction is normal. The nomogram, a clinically usable closed-chest procedure for determining the elastic modulus, was introduced in 1975 [15]. Using a heart-sound-frequency analysis followed by a determination of E, the loss of muscle-medium elasticity can be roughly delineated. In addition to improving data-acquisition techniques, the modeling of the left ventricle is becoming a more important factor for determining myocardial elasticity. These findings showed that the stiffness of the complete ventricle should be considered a function not only of myocardial stiffness but also of the cavity shape, dimensions, and structure of the vessel [16]. A better approximation for ventricular modeling requires assuming that myocardial stiffness is a function of geometry and stress. In other words, the geometry of the left ventricle is essential for simulating it in a model. Thick-walled models are commonly and widely used to study the dynamics of the ventricle. Several studies [17-19] on cardiac muscle mechanics, LV pump function, and LV wall thickening view the left ventricle as a thick-walled cylindrical composite. They report that the thick-walled cylindrical framework seems to be a good and practical approximation sufficient for simulating the left ventricle. One study [20] presented a simple analytical model to describe the relationship between age-related changes in the structure and function of mouse cardiac muscle. It suggested that age-related cardiac sarcopenia likely contributes to depressed LV function in the absence of overt cardiovascular disease. Recently, an alternative mathematical model for investigating cardiac aging characterized by diastolic dysfunction of the left ventricle was introduced [21]. In contrast to the previous study, a spherical thick-walled model and stretch-induced tissue-growth postulate were used to predict LV dimension and wall stiffness changes in aging mice. The Young's modulus of the left ventricle was determined by introducing a smooth monotonic function to fit the experimental data and a simplified version of the linear mixture theory of composite material. It was assumed that the pressure difference and the Young's modulus of the left ventricle are two independent factors that affect end-diastolic dimension/diameter and wall thickness.

The importance of the aging effect on the large vessels and cardiac structure can be also seen from a study [22] on the effect of hypertension on the diameter and elastic modulus of the aortic arch; it showed that the elastic modulus was significantly correlated with age in patients with, but not without, hypertension. In addition, both the aortic arch diameter and the elastic modulus are larger in patients with sustained uncomplicated essential hypertension. Based on the proven linear correlation between mitral e velocity, corrected for the influence of relaxation (e/e' ratio) and intraventricular pressure (similar to wedge pressure; $r = 0.87$; pulmonary capillary wedge pressure (PCWP) $= 1.24$ $[e/e'] + 1.9$) [23], we have created a cardiac mathematical model to simulate the remodeling process under various pressures during the aging process. Unlike other research groups, we hypothesized that the pressure, elastic modulus, and LV dimension are mutually influenced, that the relationship of the elastic modulus to pressure, wall thickness, and age can be established with the mathematical model, and that the aging effect on LV wall thickness can also be determined using the fixed pressure.

Materials and Methods

Patients

We enrolled 919 patients (male: 52.6% [484/919]) and divided them into two cohorts: (1)Echo$^+$: patients given echocardiography on a physical examination at our university hospital between February 2012 and June 2013, and (2) TOP (Echo$^-$): the Tianliao Old People (TOP) study between July 2010 and August 2012 [24,25]. Echocardiographic parameters based on the recommendations of the American Society of Echocardiography [26], medical records, and clinical questionnaires were collected from patients in the cohort. Patients with a poor image window, LV systolic dysfunction, or significant (>moderate severity) valvular heart disease were excluded. This study was approved by the Institutional Review Board of National Cheng Kung University Hospital (IRB no: ER-99-111), and each patient signed an informed consent form before the physical examination.

Echocardiography

Standard echocardiography was done (Vivid I; GE Vingmed Ultrasound AS, Horten, Norway) using a 3.5-MHz multiphase-array probe. The chamber dimensions and LV mass were measured using the two-dimensionally guided M-mode method, and the LV ejection fraction (LVEF) was measured with the two-dimensional M mode (Figure 1A). Intraventricular septal width (IVSd), LV internal dimension (LVIDd), LV posterior wall width (LVPWd), and LV internal dimension (LVIDs) were measured sequentially to calculate geometry and ejection fraction. Transmitral Doppler flow velocity was obtained from an apical four-chamber view, and peak early filling velocity (e), peak atrial velocity (a), and the E/A ratio were recorded. Early diastolic annular velocity (e') and atrial annular velocity (a') were also measured to estimate the LV end-diastolic pressure (e/e'). The average of medial and lateral e/e' was used to represent the estimated intraventricular pressure.

To measure the circumferential strain, 20 patients were randomly selected from the Echo$^+$cohort to receive speckle-tracking echocardiography (STE) (Figure 1B). Short-axis views at the papillary muscle level were recorded in digital loops for a deformation analysis of the left ventricle. The images were acquired at 70-90 frame/sec and stored for three cycles. The images were analyzed offline using computer software (EchoPAC 09; GE-Vingmed Ultrasound AS, Horten, Norway). After tracking the margin of endocardium, the software detected the myocardial

muscle level. C: The model of the cylinder, gross and cross-section.

motion during the entire cardiac cycle. The circumferential strain of six segments was averaged and used in the computation for the condition that $\varepsilon_{\theta\theta} \neq 0$.

Statistical analysis

SPSS 18.0 (SPSS Inc., Chicago, IL) was used for data management and statistical analyses. Data are means ± standard deviation (SD). Continuous variables were compared using Student's t test for normally distributed values. Significant factors in univariate analysis were entered into multivariate analysis. Multivariate logistic regression analysis was used to identify the independent significance of E in patients with diastolic dysfunction. A Pearson's partial correlation coefficient (r) between E and e/e' was calculated. Statistical tests were 2-sided; significance was set at $p < 0.05$.

Mathematical modeling

In this section, a mathematical model for computing the myocardium stiffness of the left ventricle is presented. The left ventricle is assumed to be made of elastic, isotropic, and homogeneous tissue that will completely recover its native form when the forces are removed. To capture LV wall dynamics, a thick-walled cylindrical pressure vessel was used (Figure 1C). The cylinder allows reasonably complex motions of the left ventricle, viz., radial inflation, axial extension, torsion, and transmural shear reflecting a cross-sectional view of the cylinder. The uniform internal (p_i) and external (p_o) pressures are respectively applied to the inner and outer surfaces of the cylinder. The interior radius and exterior radius of the cylinder are denoted by a and b, respectively. The quantity r denotes the radius at an arbitrary position between a and b [27].

For simplification, the strain normal to the cross-sectional plane ($r-\theta$ plane), ε_{zz}, and the shear strains γ_{rz} and $\gamma_{\theta z}$ are assumed to be zero. Hence, the present three-dimensional problem can be reduced to an equivalent two-dimensional one involving approximation. In addition, the cylinder is assumed to be axisymmetric, i.e., the deformation and loading conditions of the cylinder are independent of θ. Then the radial stress σ_{rr} and circumferential stress $\sigma_{\theta\theta}$ can be readily obtained as

$$\sigma_{rr} = \frac{1}{\left(1 - a^2/b^2\right)}\left[\frac{a^2}{b^2}p_i - p_o + \frac{a^2}{r^2}(p_o - p_i)\right] \quad (1)$$

$$\sigma_{\theta\theta} = \frac{1}{\left(1 - a^2/b^2\right)}\left[\frac{a^2}{b^2}p_i - p_o - \frac{a^2}{r^2}(p_o - p_i)\right] \quad (2)$$

The corresponding strains can be acquired from the constitutive relation (stress-strain relation), namely

$$\varepsilon_{rr} = \left(\frac{1+v}{E}\right)[\sigma_{rr} - v(\sigma_{rr} + \sigma_{\theta\theta})] \quad (3)$$

$$\varepsilon_{\theta\theta} = \left(\frac{1+v}{E}\right)[\sigma_{\theta\theta} - v(\sigma_{rr} + \sigma_{\theta\theta})] \quad (4)$$

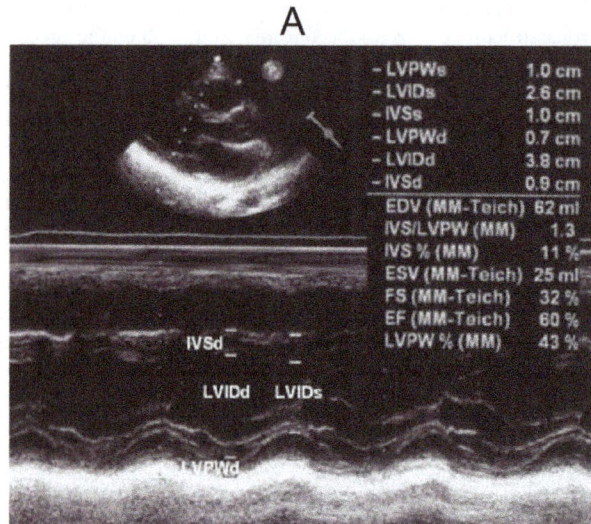

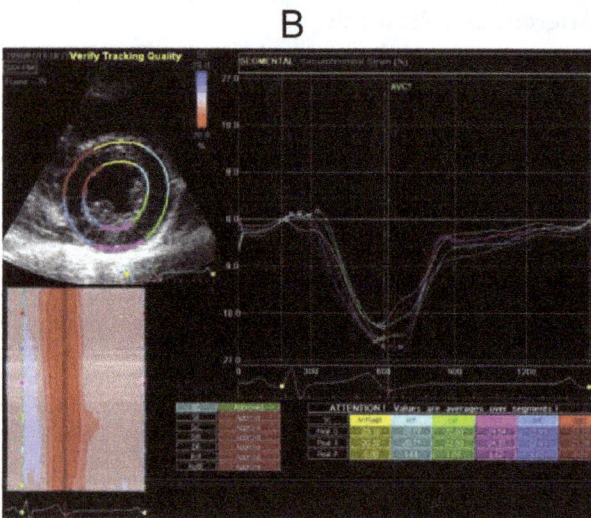

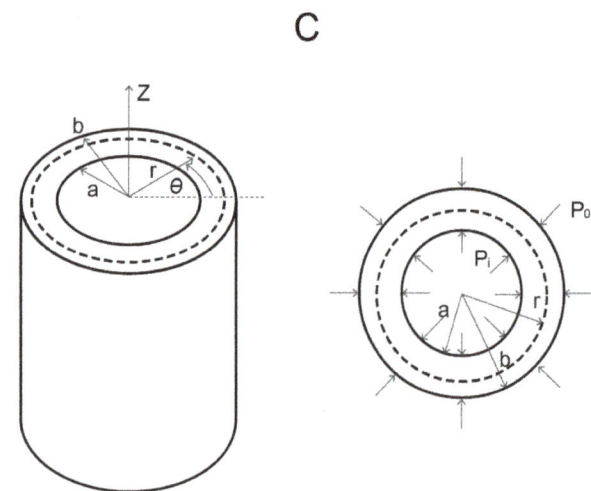

Figure 1. The echocardiographic parameters and the mathematical model for computing the myocardium stiffness of the left ventricle. A: The measured echocardiographic parameters. IVSd: intraventricular septal width in diastole; LVIDd: left ventricular internal dimension in diastole; LVPWd: left ventricular posterior wall width in diastole; and LVIDs: left ventricular internal dimension in systole. B: The measuring circumferential strain in the short-axis, at the papillary

Table 1. The clinical and echocardiographic characteristics of the younger and older cohorts.

Variable	Younger cohort n = 211 (22.9%)	Older cohort n = 708 (77.1%)	p-value
Age (years)	43.88±11.67	76.26±6.2	<0.001
Male	131 (62.08)	484 (68.82)	<0.001
HTN	21 (9.95)	349 (49.22)	<0.001
DM	11 (5.21)	122 (17.2)	<0.001
CAD	6 (2.84)	71 (10.01)	0.02
ECHOCARDIOGRAPHIC PARAMETERS			
IVSd (cm)	0.81±0.2	0.78±0.2	0.14
LVPWd (cm)	0.73±0.1	1.20±6.6	0.31
LVIDd (cm)	4.78±0.5	5.03±0.6	0.01
LVIDs (cm)	2.90±0.4	3.05±0.5	0.01
LVEF (%)	70.02±6.7	68.20±8.4	0.09
e (m/s)	0.74±0.2	0.65±0.3	0.01
e/a	0.80±0.8	0.70±0.3	0.14
e' (m/s)	0.09±0.02	0.08±0.02	0.02
e/e'	7.76±2.44	8.35±2.64	0.02
IVRT	94.44±21.25	107.77±19.1	0.09
DT	210.91±69.52	179.01±94.66	0.67
E (Young's modulus)	28872.72±7710.74	31325.97±10275.77	0.001

Data are n(%) or mean or ± standard error; HTN = hypertension; DM = diabetes mellitus; CAD = coronary artery disease; IVSd = inter-ventricular septal diameter in diastolic phase; LVPWd = left ventricular posterior wall diameter in diastolic phase; LVIDd = left ventricular internal diastolic dimension; LVIDs = left ventricular internal systolic dimension; e = early diastolic mitral inflow velocity; e/a = the ratio of early to late diastolic mitral inflow velocity; e' = the average early diastolic velocity of mitral annulus in tissue Doppler; LVEF = left ventricular ejection fraction.

where ε_{rr} is the radial strain, $\varepsilon_{\theta\theta}$ is the circumferential strain, v is Poisson's ratio, and E is the Young's modulus. Solving Eq. (3) and Eq. (4) yields

$$v = \frac{\sigma_{\theta\theta}\varepsilon_{rr} - \sigma_{rr}\varepsilon_{\theta\theta}}{(\sigma_{rr}+\sigma_{\theta\theta})(\varepsilon_{rr}-\varepsilon_{\theta\theta})} \tag{5}$$

$$E = \left[\frac{(\sigma_{rr}\varepsilon_{rr} - \sigma_{\theta\theta}\varepsilon_{\theta\theta} + 2\sigma_{\theta\theta}\varepsilon_{rr} - 2\sigma_{rr}\varepsilon_{\theta\theta})(\varepsilon_{rr}-\varepsilon_{\theta\theta}-\sigma_{\theta\theta}\varepsilon_{rr}+\sigma_{rr}\varepsilon_{\theta\theta})}{\varepsilon_{rr}(\sigma_{rr}+\sigma_{\theta\theta})(\varepsilon_{rr}-\varepsilon_{\theta\theta})^2}\right] \tag{6}$$

Substituting Eqs. (1) and (2) into Eq. (6) gives

$$E =$$

$$\frac{\frac{a^2}{b^2-a^2}\left\{\left[\frac{a^2}{b^2}p_i - p_o + \frac{a^2}{r^2}(p_o-p_i)\right](\varepsilon_{rr}-2\varepsilon_{\theta\theta}) + \left[\frac{a^2}{b^2}p_i - p_o - \frac{a^2}{r^2}(p_o-p_i)\right](2\varepsilon_{rr}-\varepsilon_{\theta\theta})\right\}}{2\varepsilon_{rr}\left[\frac{a^2}{b^2}p_i - p_o - \frac{a^2}{r^2}(p_o-p_i)\right]}$$

$$\cdot\frac{\left\{\varepsilon_{\theta\theta}\left[\frac{a^2}{b^2}p_i - p_o + \frac{a^2}{r^2}(p_o-p_i)\right] - \varepsilon_{rr}\left[\frac{a^2}{b^2}p_i - p_o - \frac{a^2}{r^2}(p_o-p_i)\right]\right\}}{2\varepsilon_{rr}\left[\frac{a^2}{b^2}p_i - p_o - \frac{a^2}{r^2}(p_o-p_i)\right]} \tag{7}$$

If $\varepsilon_{\theta\theta}$ is not considered, Eqs. (5) and (6) can be reduced to

$$v = \frac{\sigma_{\theta\theta}}{\sigma_{rr}+\sigma_{\theta\theta}} \tag{8}$$

$$E = \left[\frac{(\sigma_{rr}+2\sigma_{\theta\theta})(1-\sigma_{\theta\theta})}{\varepsilon_{rr}(\sigma_{rr}+\sigma_{\theta\theta})}\right] \tag{9}$$

Then the Young's modulus for $\varepsilon_{\theta\theta}=0$ can be readily derived as

$$E = \frac{1}{2\varepsilon_{rr}\left(\frac{a^2}{b^2}p_i - p_o\right)}\left[\frac{3a^2}{b^2}p_i - 3p_o - \frac{a^2}{r^2}(p_o-p_i)\right]$$
$$\cdot\left\{1 - \frac{b^2}{b^2-a^2}\left[\frac{a^2}{b^2}p_i - p_o - \frac{a^2}{r^2}(p_o-p_i)\right]\right\} \tag{10}$$

The parameters a, b, p_i, and p_o can be acquired from experiments and shown as follows:

$$a = \left(\frac{\text{LVIDd}}{2}\right) \tag{11}$$

$$b = \left(\frac{\text{LVIDd}+2\text{LVPWd}}{2}\right) \tag{12}$$

$$p_i = \left(\frac{1.9+1.24e/e'}{0.0075}\right) \tag{13}$$

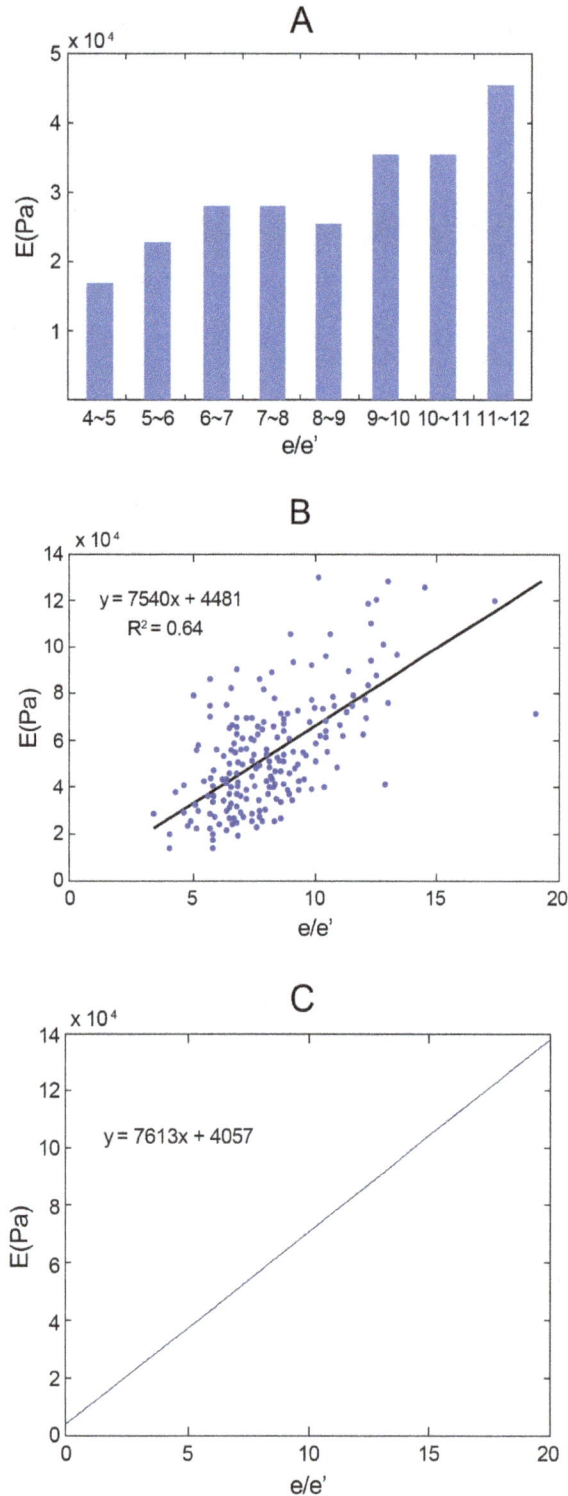

Figure 2. The correlations between e/e' and E both in the clinical statistics and the mathematical models. A and B: The relationship between e/e' and E in clinical statistics, and C: in the mathematical model. e/e' = estimated intraventricular pressure by the ratio of early diastolic mitral inflow velocity and the averaged early diastolic velocity of mitral annulus in tissue Doppler imaging; E = Young's modulus.

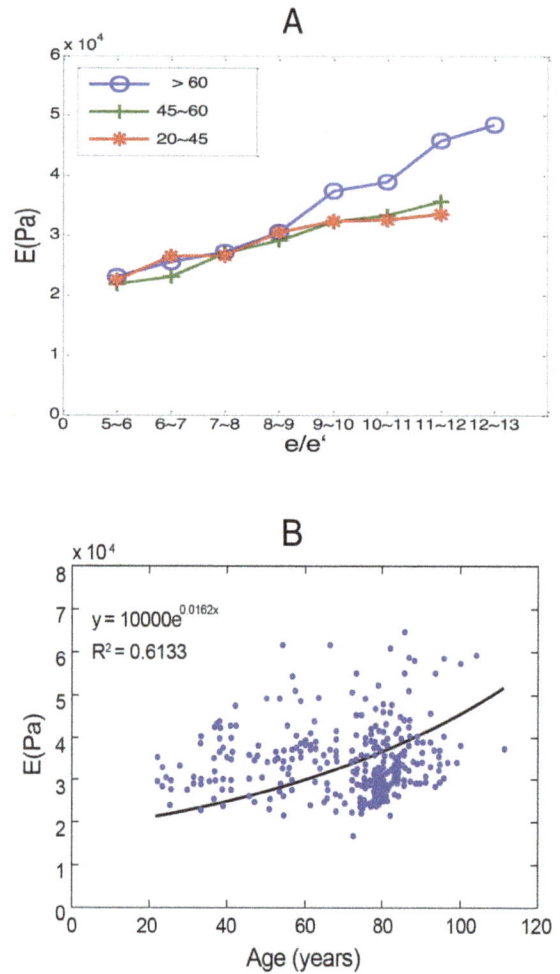

Figure 3. The relationship between E and echocardiographic intraventricular pressure in the younger and older cohorts. A: The relationship between e/e' and E value in various age group. B: The exponential correlation between age and E in the regression analysis.

$$p_o = \left(\frac{1.9 + 1.24 e/e'}{0.0075} \right) \Big/ 10 \qquad (14)$$

Also, ε_{rr} is the ratio of the radial elongation to the diastolic radius, i.e., $\varepsilon_{rr} = (LVIDd - LVIDs)/LVIDd$, and $\varepsilon_{\theta\theta}$ is an average strain for six segments in the circumferential direction. For computation, the parameter r in Eqs. (7) and (10) was chosen as $a + b/2$.

Results

The clinical and echocardiographic characteristics of the younger and older cohorts

The elderly cohort (>65 years old) were significantly older (mean age = 76.26 ± 6.2 vs. 43.88 ± 11.67 years), had a higher prevalence of hypertension (49.2% vs. 10.1%), diabetes mellitus (17.2% vs. 5.2%), and coronary artery disease (9.9% vs. 2.74%; all $p < 0.05$) (Table 1) than did the younger cohort ($n = 211$; male = 62.08%). All of them worked and lived independently. Based on our previous questionnaire in the TOP study [25], most lived an active life (11.8 ± 7.61 h of walking/week).

Table 2. Multivariate regression analyses for the independence of E value in younger patients with diastolic dysfunction.

Variable	Odds Ratio	95% Confidence Interval	p-value
Age	1.33	0.66–2.68	0.41
Diabetes Mellitus	0.46	0.18–1.13	0.09
IVSd	1.02	0.46–2.23	0.96
IVRT	0.99	0.93–1.02	0.11
E (Young's modulus)	1.12	1.03–1.47	0.04

Abbreviations: see Table 1.

To establish a model for predicting the stiffness characteristics of myocardium, we used the M-mode and 2-D echocardiographic volumetric parameters, intraventricular filling pressure, and STE from all clinical patients and the 2 cohorts. The feasibility of this model was validated. Despite a slight but significant ($p=0.01$) difference in intraventricular diameter between the two cohorts ($LVIDd = 5.03 \pm 0.63$ vs. 4.78 ± 0.53), the LV systolic ejection fraction was within the normal range in all patients ($LVEF = 68.20 \pm 8.39$ vs. 70.02 ± 6.72; $p=0.09$). The mean early diastolic velocity of the mitral annulus in tissue Doppler imaging was significantly attenuated in the elderly cohort ($e' = 0.09 \pm 0.02$ vs. 0.08 ± 0.02; $p=0.02$), which corresponds to the higher estimated wedge (e/e') pressure (7.76 ± 2.44 vs. 8.35 ± 2.64; $p=0.02$). E (Young's modulus) was calculated to describe the tensile elasticity of the myocardium, which was also significantly ($p=0.001$) elevated in the elderly cohort ($E = 28{,}872.72 \pm 7710.74$ vs. $31{,}325.97 \pm 10275.77$). Instead of a linear relationship, the regression analysis illustrated a nonlinear association between age and E ($E = 10{,}000e^{0.0162age}$; $r^2 = 0.61$)

After excluding patients with hypertension, diabetes mellitus, and coronary artery disease, the correlation between E and diastolic dysfunction remained significant ($p < 0.05$) in the healthy elderly compared with other echocardiographic parameters (Table S1).

The relationship between E and echocardiographic intraventricular pressure in the younger and older cohorts

There was a positive correlation between e/e' and E ($E = 7699.07e/e' + 2806.7$; $r = 0.87$; $p < 0.001$) both in the clinical statistics (Figure 2A,B) and in the mathematical models (Figure 2C). The slope of the trend line shown in Figure 2B is very close to the one obtained by directly using the mathematical model in Figure 2C. In the group with an $e/e' < 5$, E was estimated as 18,042(Pa), but once the pressure elevated ($e/e' > 11$), E significantly increased (45,030 Pa). Categorizing patients by age groups (20–45y/o, 45–60y/o, >60 y/o) showed that, although under the same intraventricular filling pressure, E was significantly higher in the elderly (>60 y/o), especially with a higher e/e' (>9) ($E = 34{,}633$ in 20–45-year-old group, 33,778 in 45–60-year-old group, and 42,726 in >60-year-old group) (Figure 3A). However, the difference was not significant in younger patients or between genders. Regression analysis showed that an exponential correlation between age and E could be summarized to delineate the soaring E in older patients (Figure 3B). Multivariate analysis, compared with other traditional parameters for diagnosing diastolic dysfunction (deceleration time [DT]; isovolumic relaxation time [IVRT]), E also showed independent elevation for detecting early myocardial relaxation impairment in both younger (odds ratio [OR] = 1.12; 95% confidence interval [CI] = 1.03 − 1.47; $p=0.04$) and older patients ($OR = 1.48$; 95% $CI = 1.22 − 1.94$; $p=0.01$), which indicates stiffer myocardium in aging hearts. (Table 2 and 3; Table S2 and S3)

The corresponding trend in various models

To simulate the human heart, we created a model to obtain the circumferential strain. In addition to the radial strain, the circumferential strain of the actual myocardial contraction was measured using STE Besides a grossly attenuated E, the model reflected a similar trend of geometric and pressure change, regardless of whether the circumferential strain was considered (Figure 4 A,B). Thus, if the major question is the relationship between pressure and the tensile elasticity of the myocardium, rather than the exact values of E, the simpler cylinder model may replace the complex elliptical model to reduce measurement and calculation errors.

The relationship between E and echocardiographic wall thickness in the younger and older cohorts

LV hypertrophy was more prevalent in the elderly than in the younger and middle-aged patients; it led to poor compliance and to difficulty in shape changing; thus, it impaired diastolic function. Although the association between a thicker wall and higher intraventricular pressure has been frequently reported, a suitable model to illustrate it in patients of various ages is lacking. Our mathematical model depicted positive associations between IVSd

Table 3. Multivariate regression analyses for the independence of E value in older patients with diastolic dysfunction.

Variable	Odds Ratio	95% Confidence Interval	p-value
Coronary Artery Disease	1.01	0.97–1.03	0.62
e/a	0.46	0.18–1.13	0.90
E (Young's modulus)	1.48	1.22–1.94	0.01

Abbreviations: see Table 1.

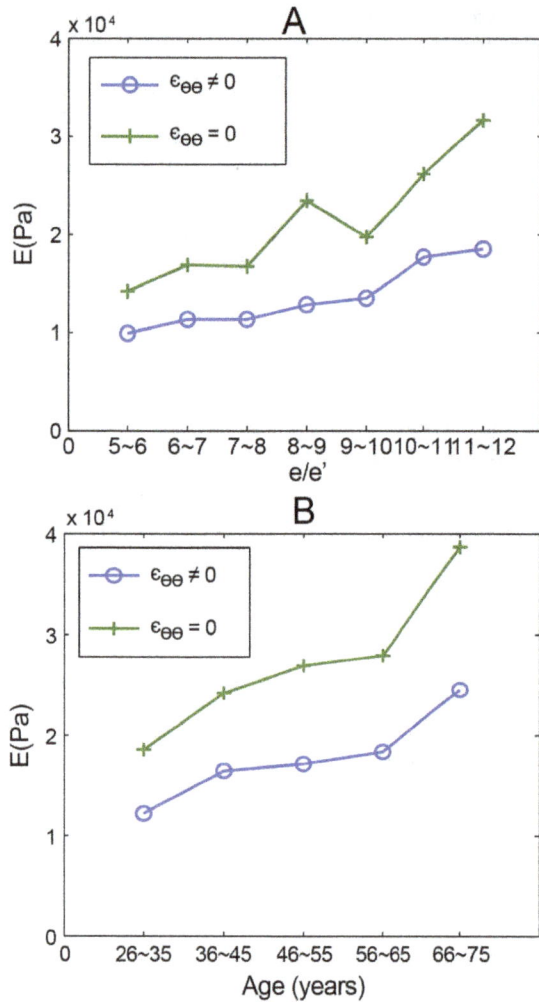

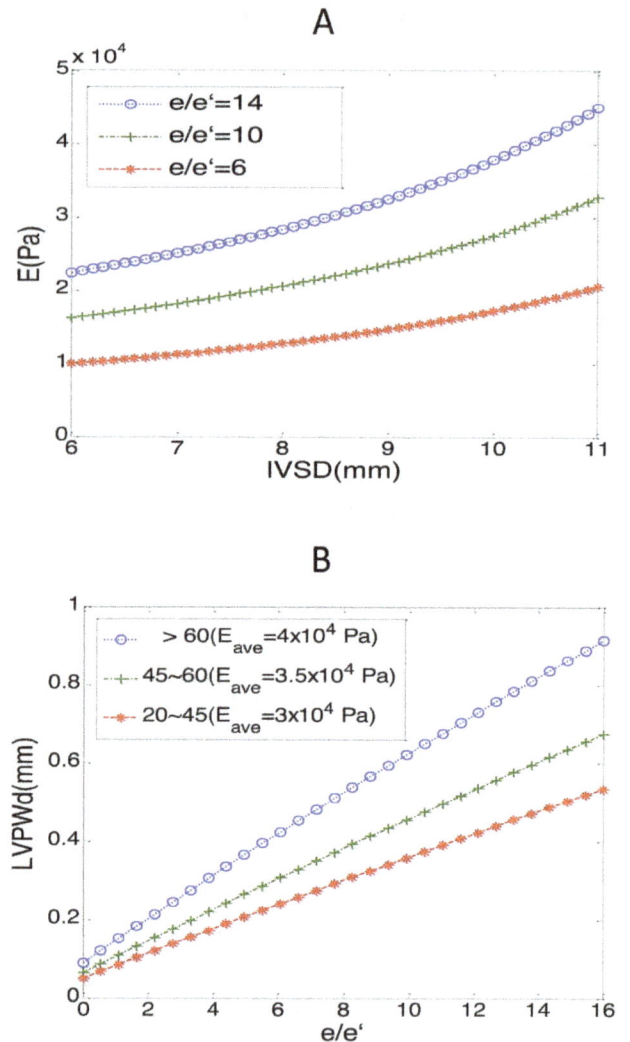

Figure 4. Various models to simulate actual hearts with different conditions. A: The positive association between e/e' and E, and B: between age and E in the mathematical model, whether or not considering circumferential strain. $\varepsilon_{\theta\theta}$ = circumferential strain.

Figure 5. The relationship between E and echocardiographic ventricular wall thickness in the younger and older cohorts. A: In the mathematical model, the positive association between IVSd and E when the value of e/e' is low, moderate, and high. B: The positive correlation between e/e' and IVSd with different average values of E (E_{ave} = 30,000, 35,000, and 40,000 for the 20–45, 45–60, and >60 y/o age groups, respectively). Because circumferential strain = 0, a (internal dimension), pressure, E = f (LVPWd), or E = f (IVSd) was fixed. IVSd = intraventricular septal width in diastole; LVPWd = left ventricular posterior wall width in diastole.

and E, along with the increasing e/e' (Figure 5A). It also indicated that in the same LV wall width, a higher intraventricular pressure correlated to a higher value of E.

In addition, by inputting the representative E (30,000, 35,000, and 40,000 for the 20–45, 45–60, and >60 y/o groups, respectively), we discovered that a higher value of E, along with aging, was associated with a thicker ventricular wall under the same intraventricular pressure (Figure 5B). This may explain the deteriorating myocardial relaxation and higher incidence of signs of heart failure signs in the elderly, who are more vulnerable to the same pressure.

Discussion

This is the first evaluation of the diastolic dysfunction in the aging human heart that uses physiologic and echocardiographic assessments combined with mathematical modeling. Our most important findings are that: (1) E (Young's modulus), the tensile elasticity of the myocardium, can be used clinically to describe myocardial relaxation and to noninvasively detect early diastolic dysfunction; (2) aging myocardium becomes thicker, stiffer, and

less expandable, which agrees with previous clinical findings. Even under the same intraventricular filling pressure, E was significantly higher in elderly patients (>60 y/o), especially with a higher e/e' (>9); (3) our mathematical model similar trends of geometric and pressure changes, regardless of whether circumferential strain was considered.

The criteria for diagnosing diastolic dysfunction and diastolic heart failure remain imprecise [3,11]. Although there are several parameters that indicate myocardial relaxation, none directly describe the tensile property of myocardium. In addition to some measurement errors, the current diagnostic criteria are nsufficient when the borderline value of estimated intraventricular pressure (e/e' = 9 − 14) is considered [12]. Another dilemma is the coexistence of systolic and diastolic dysfunction [27]. Different

Table 4. Comparison of our model and the previous Yang et al. model.

	Yang et al. model [21]	Our model
Geometric assumption	Sphere	Cylinder
Stress-strain relation	Hook's law	Plane elasticity
Material	Composite material	Isotropic material
Factors influencing Young's modulus	Young moduli of collagen	Interior and exterior pressure (measured from experiment)
	Young moduli of muscle	Initial dimension (measured from experiment)
	Volume fraction of collagen (data fitting)	Strains (measured from experiment)

from diastolic dysfunction, which remains preserved in myocardial structure and contractions, systolic dysfunction leads to fatigue and a failure of adequate deformation. Because echocardiographic parameters are too limited to precisely delineate diastolic function in systolic heart failure, using E offers the physician a new opportunity to distinguish it from other types of heart failure based on the change in myocardial stiffness [28].

Researchers have discovered a continuous loss of myocytes surrounded by the adipose and fibrotic tissue deposited in the extracellular matrix (ECM) in the aging process [7]. Therefore, myocardial stiffness is determined by the volume ratio and the combined mechanical properties of the myocytes and ECM. To prove that the age-related increase of collagen content shifts myocardial mechanical properties from a myocyte-based stiffness to a collagen-based stiffness, researchers have created a number of mathematical models [13–21]. To describe myocardial stiffness in various stages, the histological components of myocytes and ECM were transformed to different input numbers in those models. Yang et al. [21] created a mathematical model of LV remodeling in aging mice. Because human myocardial samples are insufficient to support similar models of the aging human heart, we replaced the histological parameters with clinical data. Other studies [22–23] have reported that the e/e' ratios is highly correlated with intraventricular pressure, enabled us to illustrate the geometric and tensile changes under different pressures.

In Yang et al. [21], a spherical thick-walled model and stretch-induced tissue-growth postulate were used to predict left ventricle dimensions and wall stiffness changes in aging mice. A generalized Hook's Law was considered and used for calculating the strain in the radial direction. The Young's modulus of the left ventricle was determined by introducing a smooth monotonic function to fit the experimental data and a simplified version of the linear mixture theory of composite material. It was assumed that the modulus depends only on the volume fraction of collagen and the Young's moduli of collagen and muscle. Also, the pressure difference and the Young's modulus of the left ventricle were assumed to be two independent factors affecting wall thickness and end-diastolic dimension and diameter. The changes in left ventricular mass and pressure with time are important throughout the whole study. It was concluded that senescent mice tend to have a higher modulus and pressure than do young mice.

In our study, the left ventricle considered as a pressurized thick-walled cylinder is assumed to be made of one type of elastic, isotropic, and homogeneous tissue that will be completely restored its native form when the forces are removed. We restricted the equations (stress-strain relations) to the case of plane elasticity. Strains in the radial direction and in the circumferential direction can be taken into account when determining the stiffness of myocardium. The radial and circumferential strains measured

from experiments were directly used to calculate the Young's modulus (E), which is currently regarded as a practical indicator for evaluating cardiac diastolic dysfunction. Also, in our mathematical model, the pressure, elastic modulus, and left ventricle dimensions are mutually influenced. We found that when using the same intraventricular filling pressure to compare the elderly and younger patients, the former had a tendency to have a higher E value. (Table 4) Because data-fitting techniques were not used in our computation, more accurate results could be obtained. In summary, our mathematical model offers an additional practical approach to evaluate cardiac diastolic dysfunction.

STE is an emerging technique, with angle- and load-independent characteristics, for evaluating subtle myocardial dysfunction [29,30]. A close relationship between myocardial strain and long-term outcome in patients with myocardial dysfunction has been reported in a number of studies [31]. In addition, STE recognizes not only the different directions of myocardial strain but also the precise phase of the cardiac cycle [30]. To the best of our knowledge, STE has never been used to develop a mathematical model of the heart; thus, this is the first study that includes circumferential strain in a radial-directed thick-wall model. In contrast to the mathematical model, which does not consider strain, the mechanical model added the lower value of E caused by circumferential strain even while the positive relationship between E and e/e' persisted. If the main purpose is to characterize the aging process of the human heart, the simpler cylinder model is adequate. Otherwise, more delicate factors should be considered (e.g., longitudinal strain).

The present study clearly showed that E was significantly higher in the elderly cohort than in the younger cohort, even under the same intraventricular pressure. E, which has never been used to describe the diastolic function using clinical data, has the potential to detect early diastolic dysfunction with high sensitivity. This will help us understand changes in myocardial stiffness with aging; therefore, we should be able to detect occult diastolic dysfunction in the early stage of systemic chronic diseases like hypertension disorder diabetes mellitus.

This study has several limitations. First, the main hypothesis was based on the linear correlation between the e/e' ratio and intraventricular pressure, but some confounding factors may interfere when measuring e/e' (e.g., tachycardia, frame rate, and different angles when sampling) [23]. Second, lacking sensitive circulating cardiac markers (e.g., troponin and brain natriuretic peptide), validating these formulas might underestimate overestimate asymptomatic heart failure [32,33]. However, most of our patients were relatively healthy, according to the TOP study questionnaires [25]. Moreover, lifestyle-associated information was recorded for patients recruited from the TOP study but not for those given the health examination. Third, in patients without pericardial disease, extracardiac pressure was far lower than intraventricular pressure. One study [34] on 11 dogs with chronic heart failure reported that the pressure in the pericardial space was usually beneath 10 mmHg or 1/3 of the right atrial pressure. Thus, in most LV models, the extra cardiac pressure has been neglected. In our study, E in both models, whether or not extracardiac pressure was considered, showed a trend of changes similar to that of intraventricular pressure or IVSd. Fourth, we assumed the LV to be a hollow axisymmetric cylinder with plane strain, a state of strain in which the strain normal to the $x-y$ plane, ε_z, and the shear strain γ_{xz} and γ_{yz}, are assumed to be zero. The deformation in the axial direction (z direction) is ignored, and the strains in the radial and circumferential directions are independent of θ. In reality, the left ventricle does not have a constant cross-section and does not deform uniformly at different orientations. In addition, the left ventricle was assumed to be made of elastic, isotropic, and homogeneous tissue when we determined the Young's modulus of the myocardium. Nonetheless, the left ventricle usually contains at least two basic raw materials, viz., muscle and collagen.

Although a mathematical model has limitations, it enables us to illustrate the quantitative relationships between structural and functional changes. because diastolic and systolic heart failure share similar poor outcomes [35] detecting diastolic dysfunction early helps to allow early interventions, which may lead to a better prognosis [36]. Furthermore, this model uses echocardiographic parameters instead of histological data, and it is noninvasive, it makes early detection more feasible.

In conclusion, this is the first report to document using a mathematical model to delineate diastolic dysfunction in the aging human heart. The vulnerability of the elderly to higher pressure may contribute to their developing earlier signals for heart failure. E is useful for the early and noninvasive detection of diastolic dysfunction.

Supporting Information

Table S1 After excluding patients with hypertension, diabetes mellitus, and coronary artery disease, the correlation between E and diastolic dysfunction remained significant in the healthy elders.

Table S2 Multivariate analysis on the relationship between E and echocardiographic intraventricular pressure in younger patients.

Table S3 Multivariate analysis on the relationship between E and echocardiographic intraventricular pressure in older patients.

Author Contributions

Conceived and designed the experiments: JNJ PYL. Performed the experiments: WTC JSC YKH WCT. Analyzed the data: WTC JSC YKH. Wrote the paper: WTC JSC JNJ PYL.

References

1. Butler J, Kalogeropoulos A, Georgiopoulou V, Belue R, Rodondi N, et al. (2008) Incident heart failure prediction in the elderly: the health ABC heart failure score. Circ Heart Fail 1: 125–133.
2. Bhatia RS, Tu JV, Lee DS, Austin PC, Fang J, et al. (2006) Outcome of heart failure with preserved ejection fraction in a population-based study. N Engl J Med 355: 260–269.
3. Mor-Avi V, Lang RM, Badano LP, Belohlavek M, Cardim NM, et al. (2011) Current and evolving echocardiographic techniques for the quantitative evaluation of cardiac mechanics: ASE/EAE consensus statement on methodology and indications endorsed by the Japanese Society of Echocardiography. Eur J Echocardiogr 12: 167–120.
4. Tresch DD, McGough MF (1995) Heart failure with normal systolic function: a common disorder in older people. J Am Geriatr Soc 43: 1035–1042.
5. Jaarsma T, Halfens R, Abu-Saad HH, Dracup K, Stappers J, et al. (1999) Quality of life in older patients with systolic and diastolic heart failure. Eur J Heart Fail 1: 151–160.
6. Owan TE, Hodge DO, Herges RM, Jacobsen SJ, Roger VL, et al. (2006) Trends in prevalence and outcome of heart failure with preserved ejection fraction. N Engl J Med 355: 251–259.
7. Anversa P, Hiler B, Ricci R, Guideri G, Olivetti G (1986) Myocyte cell loss and myocyte hypertrophy in the aging rat heart. J Am Coll Cardiol 8: 1441–1448.
8. Khan AS, Sane DC, Wannenburg T, Sonntag WE (2002) Growth hormone, insulin-like growth factor-1 and the aging cardiovascular system. Cardiovasc Res 54: 25–35.
9. Fung Y (1990) Biomechanics: motion, flow, stress, and growth. New York: Springer. 569 p.
10. Taber LA (1998) Biomechanical growth laws for muscle tissue. J Theor Biol 193: 201–213.
11. Nishimura RA, Tajik AJ (1997) Evaluation of diastolic filling of left ventricle in health and disease: Doppler echocardiography is the clinician's Rosetta Stone. J Am Coll Cardiol 30: 8–18.
12. Myreng Y, Smiseth OA (1990) Assessment of left ventricular relaxation by Doppler echocardiography. Comparison of isovolumic relaxation time and transmitral flow velocities with time constant of isovolumic relaxation. Circulation 81: 260–266.
13. Gotteiner NL, Han G, Chandran KB, Vonesh MJ, Bresticker M, et al. (1972) In vivo determination of elastic modulus of canine cardiac muscle. J Basic Eng 94: 912–916.
14. Ghista DN, Sandler H, Vayo WH (1975) Elastic modulus of the human intact left ventricle determination and physiological interpretation. Med Biol Eng 13: 151–161.
15. Ghista DN, Advani SH, Rao BN (1975) In vivo elastic modulus of the left ventricle: its determination by means of a left ventricular vibrational model and its physiological significance and clinical utility. Med Biol Eng 13: 162–170.
16. Yettram AL, Grewal BS, Gibson DG (1992) Modelling the left ventricle for determination of the elasticity of the myocardium. J Eng Med 208: 1–8.
17. Arts T, Renman RS, Veenstra PC (1979) A model of the mechanics of the left ventricle. Ann Biomed Eng 7: 299–318.
18. Dumesnil JG, Shoucri RM, Laurenceau JL, Turcot J (1979) A mathematical model of the dynamic geometry of the intact left ventricle and its application to clinical data. Circulation 59: 1024–1034.
19. Ohayon J, Chadwick RS (1982) Mechanics of the left ventricle. Biophys J 39: 279–288.
20. Lin J, Lopez EF, Jin Y, Van Remmen H, Bauch T, et al. (2008) Age-related cardiac muscle sarcopenia: combining experimental and mathematical modeling to identify mechanisms. Exp Gerontol 43: 296–306.
21. Yang T, Chiao YA, Wang Y, Voorhees A, Han HC, et al. (2012) Mathematical modeling of left ventricular dimensional changes in mice during aging. BMC Syst Biol 6: 1–12.
22. Isnard RN, Pannier BM, Laurent S, London GM, Diebold B, et al. (1989) Pulsatile diameter and elastic modulus of the aortic arch in essential hypertension: a noninvasive study. J Am Coll Cardiol 13: 399–405.
23. Nagueh SF, Middleton KJ, Kopelen HA, Zoghbi WA, Quinones MA (1997) Doppler tissue imaging: a noninvasive technique for evaluation of left ventricular relaxation and estimation of filling pressures. J Am Coll Cardiol 30: 1527–1533.
24. Chang CS, Chang YF, Liu PY, Chen CY, Tsai YS, et al. (2012) Smoking, habitual tea drinking and metabolic syndrome in elderly men living in rural community: the Tianliao old people (TOP) study 02. PLOS One 7: e38874.
25. Chang CL, Lee PT, Chang WT, Chang CS, Chen JH, et al. (2013) The interplay between inflammation, physical activity and metabolic syndrome in a remote male geriatric community in Southern Taiwan: the Tianliao Old People (TOP) study 03. Diabetol Metab Syndr 5: 60.
26. Lang RM, Bierig M, Devereux RB, Flachskampf FA, Foster E, et al. (2005) Recommendations for chamber quantification: a report from the American Society of Echocardiography's Guidelines and Standards Committee and the Chamber Quantification Writing Group, developed in conjunction with the European Association of Echocardiography, a branch of the European Society of Cardiology. J Am Soc Echocardiogr 18: 1440–1463.
27. Reismann H, Pawlik PS (1980) Elasticity theory and applications. New York: John Wiley & Sons.
28. Tei C, Ling LH, Hodge DO, Bailey KR, Oh JK, et al. (1995) New index of combined systolic and diastolic myocardial performance: a simple and reproducible measure of cardiac function–a study in normals and dilated cardiomyopathy. J Cardiol 26: 357–366.
29. Liu YW, Su CT, Lin CC, Chen JH (2009) Evidence of left ventricular systolic dysfunction detected by automated functional imaging in patients with heart failure and preserved left ventricular ejection fraction. J Cardiac Fail 15: 782–789.

30. Perk G, Kronzon I (2009) Non-Doppler two dimensional strain imaging for evaluation of coronary artery disease. Echocardiography 26: 299–306.

31. Bertini M, Ng AC, Antoni ML, Nucifora G, Ewe SH, et al. (2012) Global longitudinal strain predicts long-term survival in patients with chronic ischemic cardiomyopathy. Circ Cardiovasc Imaging 5: 383–391.

32. Lukowicz TV, Fischer M, Hense HW, Döring A, Stritzke J, et al. (2005) BNP as a marker of diastolic dysfunction in the general population: importance of left ventricular hypertrophy. Eur J Heart Fail 4: 525–531.

33. Huang XP, Du JF (2004) Troponin I, cardiac diastolic dysfunction and restrictive cardiomyopathy. Acta Pharmacol Sin 12: 1569–1575.

34. Horne SG, Belenkie I, Tyberg JV, Smith ER (2000) Pericardial pressure in experimental chronic heart failure. Can J Cardiol 5: 607–613.

35. Warren SE, Grossman W (1991) Prognosis in heart failure: is systolic or diastolic dysfunction more important? Herz 16 Spec No 1: 324–329.

36. Galderisi M (2005) Diastolic dysfunction and diastolic heart failure: diagnostic, prognostic and therapeutic aspects. Cardiovasc Ultrasound 3: 9.

## 12

Association between Reproductive Factors and Age-Related Macular Degeneration in Postmenopausal Women: The Korea National Health and Nutrition Examination Survey 2010-2012

Bum-Joo Cho[1,2], Jang Won Heo[1,2]*, Jae Pil Shin[3], Jeeyun Ahn[1,4], Tae Wan Kim[1,4], Hum Chung[1,2]

1 Department of Ophthalmology, Seoul National University College of Medicine, Seoul, Korea, 2 Department of Ophthalmology, Seoul National University Hospital, Seoul, Korea, 3 Department of Ophthalmology, Kyungpook National University School of Medicine, Daegu, Korea, 4 Department of Ophthalmology, Seoul Metropolitan Government Seoul National University Boramae Medical Center, Seoul, Korea

Abstract

Purpose: To examine the association between female reproductive factors and age-related macular degeneration (AMD) in postmenopausal women.

Design: Nationwide population-based cross-sectional study.

Methods: A nationally representative dataset acquired from the 2010–2012 Korea National Health and Nutrition Examination Survey was analyzed. The dataset involved information for 4,377 postmenopausal women aged ≥50 years with a fundus photograph evaluable for AMD in either eye. All participants were interviewed using standardized questionnaires to determine reproductive factors including menstruation, pregnancy, parity, lactation, and hormonal use. The association between reproductive factors and each type of AMD was investigated.

Results: The mean age of the study participants was 63.1 ± 0.2 years. Mean ages at menarche and menopause were 16.1 ± 0.0 and 49.2 ± 0.1 years, respectively. The overall prevalence rates of early and late AMD were 11.2% (95% confidence interval [CI], 10.1–12.5) and 0.8% (95% CI, 0.5–1.2), respectively. When adjusted for age, neither smoking nor alcohol use was associated with the presence of any AMD or late AMD. Multivariate logistic regression analysis revealed age (OR, 1.12 per 1 year), duration of lactation (OR, 0.91 per 6 months), and duration of use of oral contraceptive pills (OCP) (OR, 1.10 per 6 months) as associated factors for late AMD. The other variables did not yield a significant correlation with the risk of any AMD or late AMD.

Conclusion: After controlling for confounders, a longer duration of lactation appeared to protect against the development of late AMD. A longer duration of OCP use was associated with a higher risk of late AMD.

Editor: Demetrios Vavvas, Massachusetts Eye & Ear Infirmary, Harvard Medical School, United States of America

Funding: The authors have no support or funding to report.

Competing Interests: The authors have declared that no competing interests exist.

* Email: jangwonheo@gmail.com

Introduction

The leading cause of blindness and visual impairment in elderly individuals of developed countries is age-related macular degeneration (AMD) [1,2]. With the expanding human lifespan, AMD has garnered increasing interest among researchers. Several risk factors have been identified for this condition, including cigarette smoking, hyperopia, and genetic variation in complement factor H [3–5].

Among those risk factors, female sex has been associated with a higher prevalence of AMD in many population-based studies [6]. Recent researches have suggested gender differences in the pathophysiology of AMD arising from dissimilar hormonal status [5,6]. However, there have not been sufficient data on the association between female own risk factors and AMD. Only a few epidemiological studies were performed, and the results have been inconclusive to date [7–10]. Identification of female risk factors for AMD would help to understand the pathogenesis of the disease and screen the patients at risk. Because most female patients at risk for AMD are post-menopausal, the associated hormonal changes must be examined closely as well.

Therefore, in this study, we investigated the association between female reproductive factors and each type of AMD in postmenopausal women. Various factors related to menstruation, pregnancy, delivery, lactation, and the use of hormonal drugs were explored. To acquire representative data for the general population, we analyzed the nationwide data obtained as part of the Korea National Health and Nutrition Examination Survey (KNHANES) on behalf of the Korean Ophthalmological Society (KOS) [11]. The ethnic homogeneity of Korea might facilitate to reveal the risk factors of AMD by minimizing the bias resulting from interracial differences [12]. To the authors' knowledge, this is the first study to analyze this association in an Asian population.

Materials and Methods

Study population

The data analyzed in this study were obtained from the fifth cycle of the KNHANES which was performed from 2010 through 2012. The KNHANES is an ongoing nationally representative cross-sectional survey to examine the health, physical, and nutritional status of the general Korean population [11,12]. The survey was first administered in 1998 and has been conducted annually since 2007 by the Korea Center for Disease Control and Prevention (KCDC). Ophthalmologic examinations were included since the second half of 2008. Details relating to the KNHANES design and methods have been presented elsewhere [11,12]. To summarize briefly, the study methodology involves stratified multistage cluster-sampling to prevent subject omission or overlap. The rolling-sampling method makes each annual survey results representative for the entire Korean population and mergeable with the past results. During the period from 2010–2012, the KNHANES annually included 3,800 households from 192 enumeration districts. From each household, all family members aged ≥ 1 year were included as eligible subjects [11]. The eligible subjects were asked to take part in health interviews and physical examinations including comprehensive ophthalmologic assessments in mobile centers by trained teams. Non-mydriatic $45°$ color fundus photographs were obtained for each subject aged ≥ 19 years in a dark room using a digital fundus camera (TRC-NW6S; Topcon, Tokyo, Japan). When the non-mydriatic photograph was of insufficient quality for grading due to media opacity or a small pupil, mydriatic fundus photographs were obtained at the point of maximal pupillary dilation, with the patients' consent.

Among the participants, only postmenopausal women were included in this study. As suggested previously, premenopausal women, women aged <50 years, women who experienced menopause before the age of 30, or those who did not report the age of menopause were excluded [10,13]. Subjects without any fundus photograph evaluable for the presence of AMD were also excluded from this study. Ultimately, only postmenopausal women who were aged ≥ 50 years and who had ≥ 1 assessable fundus photograph were included. The study described here adhered to the tenets of the Declaration of Helsinki, and written informed consent was obtained from all participants. The survey protocol was approved by the Institutional Review Board of the KCDC (IRB No: 2010-02CON-21-C, 2011-02CON-06-C, 2012-01EXP-01-2C).

Assessment of Reproductive factors

Female reproductive factors, demographic variables, and health behavioral factors were assessed on the basis of self-reported answers to a standardized questionnaire. The reproductive factors evaluated included the following: age at menarche, age at menopause, type of menopause, number of pregnancies, number of spontaneous and/or artificial abortions, parity (the number of children given birth to), lactation, use of oral contraceptive pills (OCP), and use of postmenopausal female hormone replacement therapy (HRT).

The type of menopause was dichotomized as natural vs. artificial (e.g., hysterectomy or oophorectomy). The duration of lactation, OCP use, or HRT use was recorded as the total number of experienced months. The drug components of HRT and/or OCP were not specified. Length of the reproductive period was calculated as follows: age at menopause – age at menarche. Duration of the postmenopausal period was designated as follows: age – age at menopause. Duration of lactation per child was calculated from the division of duration of lactation by the number of parity.

Assessment of AMD

The presence of each AMD type was determined on the fundus photographs [11]. Each fundus photograph was preliminarily evaluated for the presence of AMD on site by dispatched ophthalmologists who were trained for grading by the National Epidemiologic Survey Committee of the KOS and used the International Age-related Maculopathy Epidemiological Study Group grading system [14]. Detailed grading was later performed by nine retina specialists with experience in grading AMD, who were masked to the patients' characteristics. Any discrepancy between the preliminary and detailed grading was resolved by an independent ophthalmologist (J.P.S.). Drusen were classified on the basis of size, appearance, and edge sharpness [14]. Retinal pigmentary abnormalities were graded as hypo- or hyperpigmentation [14]. Patients were defined as having early AMD if they met any one of the following criteria: (1) the presence of soft indistinct drusen or reticular drusen; (2) the presence of hard or soft distinct drusen with pigmentary abnormalities in the absence of late AMD [14]. Late AMD was defined as either the presence of neovascularization or geographic atrophy [14]. AMD was classified as neovascular if associated with detachment of the retinal pigment epithelium (RPE), serous detachment of the neurosensory retina, subretinal or sub-RPE hemorrhages, or subretinal fibrous scars [14]. Geographic atrophy was defined as a circular area with a sharp edge ≥ 175 μm in diameter showing hypopigmented RPE and apparent choroidal vessels, in the absence of signs for neovascular AMD [14]. When the severity of AMD differed between eyes, the subject was assigned the more advanced grade, and when only one eye could be assessed, the subject was assigned the grade of that eye. The presence of any AMD was defined as having either early AMD or late AMD. The quality of the grading was verified by the KOS. Grading agreement between the preliminary graders and the standard reading specialists ranged from 94.1–96.2%.

Statistical Analysis

Statistical estimations were performed using the sampling weights adjusted for response rate, extraction rate, and the distribution of the general Korean population. Continuous variables were expressed as mean ± standard error or mean with 95% confidence intervals (CIs). Categorization was performed for some of the continuous variables. In order to assess the association with AMD, the odds ratios (ORs) of continuous and categorical variables were calculated.

Prior to main analyses, the confounders for the risk of AMD were investigated among demographic and health behavioral variables by age-adjusted univariate logistic regression analyses. Next, univariate logistic regression analyses were performed to screen the potential reproductive risk factors for any AMD or late AMD after controlling for confounders. Risk factors with $P<0.1$ were selected, and multicollinearity among them was examined by calculating the variance inflation factors (VIFs). Those with a VIF ≥5 were excluded from subsequent analyses. Finally, multivariate logistic regression analyses were performed using a stepwise selection method. Final models for the presence of AMD were constructed using the set of risk factors with P<0.05 in the multivariate analysis. All statistical analyses were performed using SPSS 20.0 for Windows (SPSS Inc., Chicago, IL).

Results

During the period from 2010–2012, among 16,593 eligible women, 13,298 women were interviewed and underwent physical examinations (response rate, 80.1%) (Fig. 1). Participation rates during the period from 2010–2012 ranged from 79.5–80.5%. Of these, 4,922 subjects were postmenopausal and aged ≥50 years old. Among these, 4,377 (88.9%) subjects with a fundus photograph for either eye that could be used to assess the presence of AMD were ultimately included in this study.

Demographics of Study Participants

The mean age of the all study participants was 63.1±0.2 years (range, 50–97 years). Mean ages at menarche and menopause were 16.1±0.0 years (range, 8–28 years) and 49.2±0.1 years (range, 30–72 years), respectively. The age-stratified reproductive characteristics of the study group are presented in Table 1. In younger generations, reproductive years were longer and the numbers of pregnancy and parity were smaller compared to those in older generations (P<0.001 for all). Duration of lactation was shorter in the younger generations than in the older generations (P<0.001), while both the periods of OCP use and HRT use tended to be longer in the younger generations than in the older generations (P<0.001).

The overall prevalence rates of early, late, and any AMD among the study participants were 11.2% (95% CI, 10.1–12.5), 0.8% (95% CI, 0.5–1.2), and 12.0% (95% CI, 10.8–13.2), respectively. The overall prevalence of neovascular AMD and geographic atrophy was 0.6% (95% CI, 0.4–1.0) and 0.1% (95% CI, 0.0–0.5).

Data pertaining to demographic and reproductive characteristics are presented according to the type of AMD in Table 2. Both early AMD subjects and late AMD subjects were significantly older than those without any AMD (P<0.001 and P=0.006, respectively). Postmenopausal period was also significantly longer in early AMD subjects and in late AMD subjects than in those without any AMD (P<0.001 and P=0.010, respectively).

Univariate binary logistic regression analysis showed that age was highly associated with the presence of any AMD and that of late AMD (OR 1.08; 95% CI, 1.07–1.09 and OR 1.07; 95% CI, 1.02–1.14, respectively). When adjusted for age, the presence of any AMD was not associated with a history of ever smoking, current smoking, or current alcohol use (P=0.826, P=0.139, and P=0.701, respectively). The same trend was observed for late AMD (P=0.439, P=0.795, and P=0.798, respectively).

Association between Reproductive Factors and AMD

The association of reproductive factors with any AMD and late AMD is summarized in Table 3. Age-adjusted univariate logistic regression analysis did not reveal any associated factor (P<0.1) for the presence of any AMD. On the other hand, age-adjusted univariate logistic regression analysis showed that the following factors were correlated with the presence of late AMD (P<0.1): number of pregnancy, number of parity, duration of lactation per child, duration of lactation, and duration of OCP use. Among these variables, the VIFs of number of parity, duration of lactation

per child, and duration of lactation were ≥5 (5.618, 5.025, and 10.000, respectively). Duration of lactation per child was excluded from next analyses, because it was obtained from the calculation with number of parity and duration of lactation, and the authors reached a consensus that it would be a less meaningful variable than total duration of lactation in the development of AMD. After the exclusion, the corresponding VIFs of number of pregnancy, number of parity, duration of lactation, and duration of OCP use were all <5 (1.852, 3.300, 2.538, and 1.009, respectively).

In a multivariate logistic regression analysis using these variables, number of pregnancy and number of parity yielded insignificant correlations. Ultimately, the final regression model for late AMD included age (OR, 1.12 per year; 95% CI, 1.06–1.18), duration of lactation (OR per 6 months, 0.91; 95% CI 0.86–0.95), and duration of OCP use (OR, 1.10 per 6 months; 95% CI, 1.02–1.18) as associated factors. Among these, duration of lactation was shown to protect against late AMD, with a 9% risk reduction per 6-month breast-feeding. The other factors were positively correlated with the risk of late AMD (Table 4).

Discussion

The present study examined the association of various reproductive factors with the risk of AMD, in a representative population of postmenopausal Korean women. The investigated factors included menstruation, pregnancy, abortion, parity, lactation, as well as the use of OCP and HRT. After controlling for confounders, the duration of lactation was inversely associated with the risk of late AMD. In contrast, the use of OCP increased the risk of late AMD.

An interesting finding in this study is that breast-feeding has a protective effect against late AMD. More specifically, a 6-month increment in the total duration of lactation was associated with a 9% decrease in the risk of late AMD. This finding was first suggested by Erke et al in a recent research [7]. The authors stated that an increase in the total duration of lactation was significantly associated with a reduced risk of late AMD (OR per 3 months, 0.84) and a 1-month increase in the duration of lactation per child decreased the risk of late AMD by 20% [7]. The current study consisted with this result and identified the protective effect in a period-dependent manner. The amount of protective effect was less than that in the previous study [7]. Thus far, no other prior study has explored the association between lactation and AMD in the literature. Notably, the duration of lactation appeared to be significantly higher in the early AMD group in this study compared to that in the control group. However, this difference was eliminated in the regression analysis after age-adjustment, indicating that the increase in the duration of lactation in the early AMD group may have arisen from the increased age of the group.

The mechanism underlying the association between lactation and AMD is not well understood, but it might be approached in consideration of the protective effect of breast-feeding against several cardiovascular diseases [7,15]. In Women's Health Initiative study that included 139,681 postmenopausal women, those who had breastfed for >12 months were less likely to have hypertension (OR, 0.88), diabetes mellitus (OR, 0.80), hyperlipidemia (OR, 0.81), and cardiovascular disease (OR, 0.91) than those who had never breastfed [15]. In a Norwegian prospective population-based cohort study, lactation for ≥24 months decreased the cardiovascular mortality significantly among parous women aged <65 years (hazard ratio, 0.36) [16]. Additionally, lactation is known to improve the subclinical vascular indices of cardiovascular disease [17], to promote lipid metabolism [18], and to reduce serum concentrations of C-reactive protein [19].

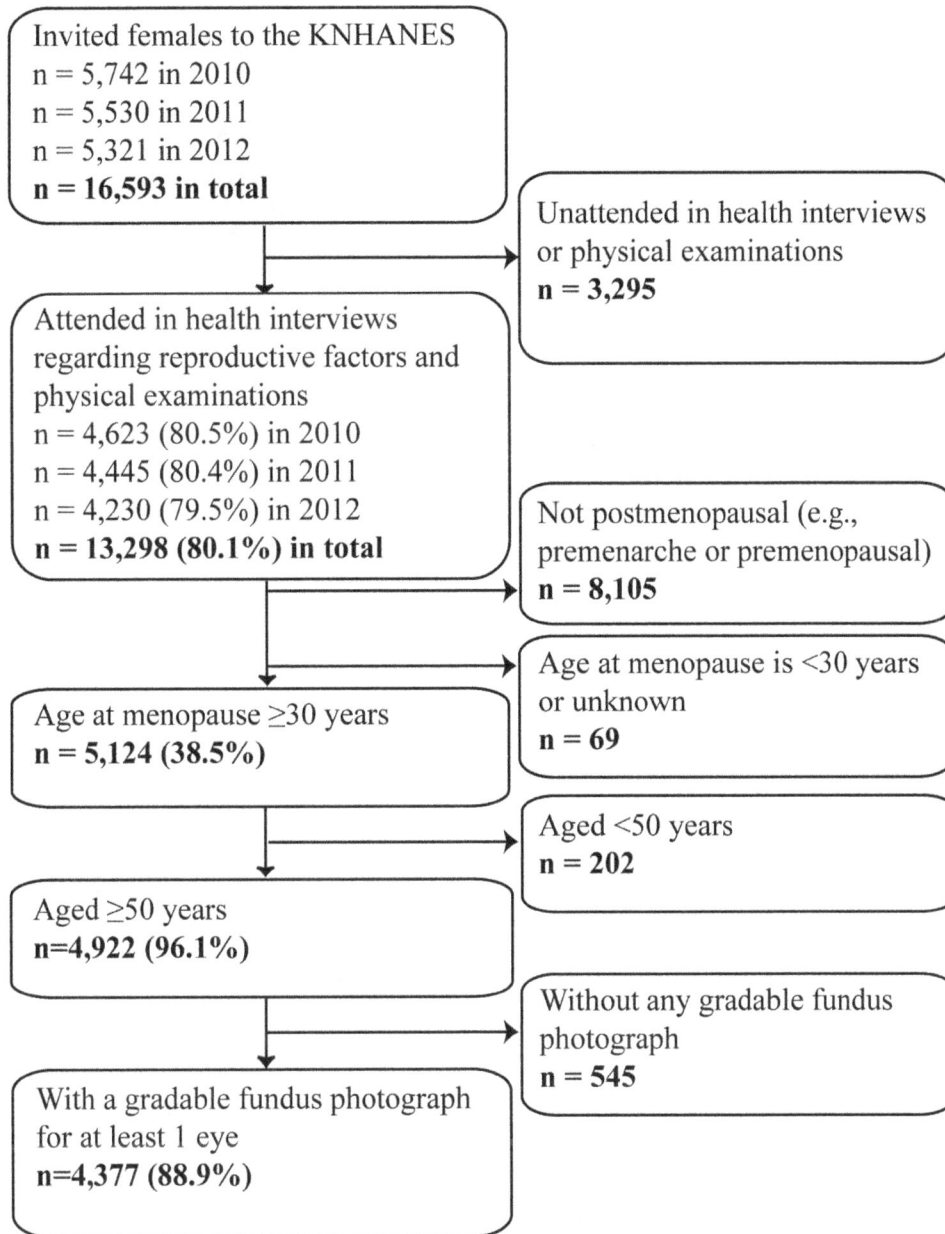

Figure 1. Participation flow-chart for the Korea National Health and Nutrition Examination Survey (KNHANES) during the period from 2010–2012.

Moreover, these effects were found to be long-lasting in a large cohort study [20]. Late AMD has been associated with cardio-vascular diseases in several studies [21,22], thus the protective effect of lactation against cardiovascular diseases might also help to reduce the risk of late AMD. This might be mediated by the effects on the microvasculature of choroid or retina. On the other hand, lactation has an inhibitory effect on the female hormonal axis, including estrogen exposure [15]. Considering that estrogen exposure has shown a protective effect against development of AMD in some previous studies [23], the protective effect of lactation against late AMD described above may override the anti-protective effect mediated by the inhibition of the hormonal axis.

Another novel finding presented here is the positive correlation between the use of OCP and the risk of late AMD. The present

study showed a 10% increase in the risk of late AMD per 6-month increase of OCP use. Thus far, there have been only a few studies on the association between AMD and OCP use [5,7,10,24]. One study reported a reduced risk of neovascular AMD (OR, 0.55) in women who had used OCP at least once [5], and another found a decreased risk of early AMD (OR, 0.5) in those who had used OCP ever [24]. Other researchers have reported that the use of OCP was not associated with the risk of early or late AMD in postmenopausal women [7,10]. On the other hand, since the introduction of OCP, a variety of vascular complications have been reported to be associated with it [25]. The risky diseases associated with OCP include deep-vein thrombosis, pulmonary embolism, stroke, and myocardial infarction (MI) [25]. A recent meta-analysis revealed a three-fold increase in the risk of venous

Table 1. Age-based stratification of postmenopausal women aged ≥50 years in the KNHANES 2010–2012.

	50–59[a] (n = 1586)	60–69[a] (n = 1516)	70–79[a] (n = 1080)	≥80[a] (n = 195)	P Value
Age, y	54.6±0.1	64.3±0.1	74.1±0.1	82.6±0.2	<0.001[b]
Prevalence of early AMD, %	4.8±0.7	11.8±1.0	20.7±1.7	22.2±4.0	<0.001[c]
Prevalence of late AMD, %	0.3±0.2	0.7±0.3	1.1±0.3	3.4±1.6	0.002[c]
Age at menarche, y	15.7±0.1	16.3±0.1	16.7±0.1	16.6±0.2	<0.001[b]
Age at menopause, y	49.4±0.1	49.9±0.2	48.0±0.2	47.7±0.5	<0.001[b]
Reproductive years, y	33.7±0.1	33.6±0.2	31.3±0.2	31.2±0.5	<0.001[b]
Postmenopausal period, y	5.2±0.1	14.4±0.2	26.1±0.2	34.9±0.5	<0.001[b]
Number of pregnancy	3.9±0.1	5.0±0.1	6.2±0.1	6.2±0.2	<0.001[b]
Number of spontaneous abortion	0.3±0.0	0.3±0.0	0.3±0.0	0.3±0.1	0.988[b]
Number of artificial abortion	1.3±0.0	1.5±0.1	1.4±0.1	0.6±0.1	<0.001[b]
Number of parity	2.3±0.0	3.2±0.0	4.5±0.1	5.2±0.2	<0.001[b]
Duration of lactation, m	25.2±0.8	50.0±1.2	90.8±2.1	107.9±5.4	<0.001[b]
Duration of OCP use, m	4.1±0.6	7.6±0.7	6.0±0.7	1.0±0.5	<0.001[b]
Duration of HRT use, m	5.3±0.5	7.4±0.8	1.8±0.5	0.9±0.6	<0.001[b]

AMD = age-related macular degeneration; OCP = oral contraceptive pills; HRT = hormone replacement therapy.
[a]Age in years.
[b]General linear model for complex samples.
[c]Pearson's chi-square test for complex samples.

thromboembolism, a two-fold increase in the risk of ischemic stroke, and an indeterminate effect on the risk of MI [25]. The positive association between OCP use and late AMD in this study is in line with the increased rate of cardiovascular disease observed for OCP users.

The pathophysiology of the association of OCP with cardiovascular diseases or late AMD is not clearly elucidated yet. OCP are typically either a combination of progestin and lower doses of estrogen or progestin only [26]. OCP increase the levels of prothrombin fragments, fibrinogen, plasmin–antiplasmin complex, and protein C activity, and decrease antithrombin activity and the level of tissue-plasminogen activator [27,28]. These hemostatic effects are known to be modulated by the progestin's potency as an androgen [27]. Progestin is also suggested to increase the level of aminopeptidase P and the breakdown of bradykinin, and thereby to increase blood pressure [29]. The hemodynamic and hemostatic effects of OCP might contribute to the risk of cardiovascular disease, and thus affect the development

Table 2. Demographics of postmenopausal women aged ≥50 years by the type of age-related macular degeneration (AMD) in the KNHANES 2010–2012.

	No AMD (n = 3845)	Early AMD (n = 500)	P value[a]	Late AMD (n = 32)	P value[a]
Age, y	62.4±0.2	68.9±0.5	<0.001	69.6±2.7	0.006
Age at menarche, y	16.1±0.0	16.4±0.1	0.005	16.9±0.4	0.084
Age at menopause, y	49.2±0.1	48.9±0.3	0.242	48.8±0.9	0.661
Reproductive years, y	33.1±0.1	32.5±0.3	0.044	32.0±0.8	0.141
Postmenopausal period, y	13.2±0.2	20.0±0.6	<0.001	20.8±3.0	0.010
Number of pregnancy	4.7±0.0	5.5±0.1	<0.001	4.4±0.4	0.369
Number of spontaneous abortion	0.3±0.0	0.3±0.0	0.657	0.2±0.1	0.220
Number of artificial abortion	1.3±0.0	1.3±0.1	0.708	1.0±0.4	0.485
Number of parity	3.1±0.0	3.8±0.1	<0.001	3.1±0.2	0.948
Duration of lactation, m	48.4±1.1	69.7±3.1	<0.001	44.5±6.7	0.565
Duration of OCP use, m	5.2±0.4	5.9±0.9	0.495	27.7±21.5	0.296
Duration of HRT use, m	5.0±0.4	4.5±0.9	0.570	4.1±2.6	0.724

OCP = oral contraceptive pills; HRT = hormone replacement therapy.
[a]Comparison with no AMD group, not adjusted for any covariate.

Table 3. Age-adjusted odds ratios (ORs) of age-related macular degeneration (AMD) for reproductive risk factors in postmenopausal women in the KNHANES 2010–2012.

Reproductive risk factors	Increment	Any AMD			Late AMD		
		OR	95% CI	P Value	OR	95% CI	P Value
Age at menarche	1 year	1.01	0.96–1.06	0.705	1.13	0.90–1.41	0.289
Age at menopause	1 year	1.00	0.98–1.03	0.746	1.00	0.94–1.07	0.911
Reproductive years	1 year	1.00	0.98–1.02	0.878	0.99	0.94–1.04	0.634
Postmenopausal period	1 year	1.00	0.97–1.02	0.744	1.00	0.94–1.06	0.908
Number of pregnancy	1	1.00	0.95–1.04	0.911	0.81	0.67–0.97	0.025
Number of spontaneous abortion	1	0.97	0.82–1.14	0.677	0.79	0.47–1.32	0.364
Number of artificial abortion	1	1.00	0.94–1.06	0.963	0.92	0.64–1.32	0.644
Number of parity	1	1.00	0.92–1.08	0.999	0.74	0.62–0.88	0.001
Duration of lactation per child	1 month	1.00	0.98–1.01	0.415	0.96	0.91–1.00	0.053
Duration of lactation[a]	6 months	1.00	0.98–1.01	0.616	0.91	0.87–0.95	<0.001
Duration of OCP use[a]	6 months	1.03	0.99–1.07	0.149	1.09	1.01–1.18	0.025
Duration of HRT use[a]	6 months	1.01	0.99–1.04	0.436	1.00	0.93–1.09	0.881
Artificial menopause	Yes	0.92	0.62–1.37	0.667	0.87	0.26–2.91	0.818
Bilateral oophorectomy	Yes	1.08	0.61–1.90	0.798	1.66	0.45–6.16	0.449

CI = confidence interval; OCP = oral contraceptive pills; HRT = hormone replacement therapy.
[a]Total years of experience.

Table 4. Multivariate-adjusted odds ratios (ORs) of late age-related macular degeneration (AMD) for reproductive risk factors in postmenopausal women in the KNHANES 2010–2012.

	Risk factors	Increment	OR	95% CI	P Value
Model 1	Age	1 year	1.12	1.06–1.17	<0.001
	Number of pregnancy	1	0.82	0.53–1.28	0.386
	Number of parity	1	1.11	0.61–2.02	0.725
	Duration of lactation[a]	6 months	0.92	0.85–1.00	0.043
	Duration of OCP use[a]	6 months	1.10	1.02–1.19	0.013
Model 2[b]	Age	1 year	1.12	1.06–1.18	<0.001
	Duration of lactation[a]	6 months	0.91	0.86–0.95	<0.001
	Duration of OCP use[a]	6 months	1.10	1.02–1.18	0.019

CI = confidence interval; OCP = oral contraceptive pills.
[a]Total years of experience.
[b]Final multivariate model consisted of risk factors of p value<0.05.

of AMD. However, further studies with larger sample sizes will be necessary in the future to validate the findings of this study.

Estrogen is considered one of the most important reproductive hormones in women. Endogenous exposure to estrogen starts with the release of estrogen from the ovary, and is related to the age at menarche, age at menopause, and the number of pregnancies [23]. The Aravind Comprehensive Eye Survey showed age at menarche ≥14 years, which means the late start of estrogen release, is a risk factor for overall AMD (OR, 2.3) [30], and the Rotterdam Study showed an increased risk of AMD in those who experienced early menopause following oophorectomy (OR, 3.8) [3]. The Blue Mountain Eye Study reported that a long reproductive period was associated with a decreased prevalence of early AMD [31]. These findings provide further support for the notion that a shorter duration of estrogen exposure may increase the risk of AMD. However, no such association was found in this study.

The association between AMD and exogenous exposure to estrogen in the form of HRT has been inconsistent in previous studies [5,9,13,23,32]. A 34% increase in the risk of early AMD was observed among current HRT users in one report as compared to that in individuals who had never used HRT [10]. To the contrary, HRT was associated with a lower risk of neovascular AMD (RR, 0.52) among female nurses aged 30–55 years [10], and reduced the risk of exudative AMD (OR, 0.6) in the Eye Disease Case–Control Study [33]. A postulated explanation for this association is that estrogen deficiency results in a down-regulation of matrix metalloproteinase–2 activity and an up-regulation of YKL-40 protein which may accelerate choroidal neovascularization [24,34]. However, most studies to date have reported no association between estrogen treatment and early or late AMD [3,7,8,24,30,32]. In the current study, we were also unable to find an association between HRT and any AMD or late AMD. This result might stem from our limited sample size.

The present study has several limitations. As it was a cross-sectional survey, the association between risk factors and late AMD does not guarantee causality. The result means only a cross-sectional distribution of AMD in a certain population, and a survivorship bias may intervene. Therefore, a longitudinal cohort study is required to validate the findings presented here and disclose the causality. It will also help to examine the incidence of AMD in the population at risk. In addition, as the information for

several reproductive factors in this survey was based on self-reported answers from the participants, and not on their medical records, there could be an intervening recall bias. To minimize biases, the health interviews in this survey were performed using a standardized questionnaire by trained teams. However, because most participants were old, there may be some recall bias remaining in this study. Moreover, although we tried to control for several potential confounders, the possibility of a confounding effect between the risk factors studied and AMD still remains. The small number of late AMD patients represents another limitation that may have reduced the statistical power of our conclusions. Regarding OCP use, more specific data such as the drug components were not investigated in the current survey. Future studies involving the drug components of OCP are necessary in order to reveal the association of OCP use with AMD more clearly. Lastly, subjects who could not have an evaluable fundus photograph taken due to mature cataract or other media opacity were excluded. Because these patients tended to be older [12] and thus were more likely to have had AMD, the prevalence of AMD may have been underestimated. The strength of this study derives largely from our use of data from a large, nationally representative sample population.

In conclusion, the current study suggests a longer period of lactation might protect against late AMD. We also presented our novel finding that a longer use of OCP increases the risk of late AMD. These findings could elucidate the development of AMD and help the screening of patients at risk as well as the prevention of AMD among postmenopausal women in public health.

Acknowledgments

The authors appreciate the Epidemiologic Survey Committee of the Korean Ophthalmological Society for the dedication to designing and accomplishment of the Korea National Health and Nutrition Examination Survey, acquisition and verification of the data, and opening of the data to the public.

Author Contributions

Conceived and designed the experiments: BJC JWH HC. Performed the experiments: BJC JWH JPS TWK. Analyzed the data: BJC JA TWK. Contributed reagents/materials/analysis tools: BJC JWH JPS. Contributed to the writing of the manuscript: BJC JA.

References

1. Pascolini D, Mariotti SP, Pokharel GP, Pararajasegaram R, Etya'ale D, et al. (2004) 2002 global update of available data on visual impairment: a compilation of population-based prevalence studies. Ophthalmic Epidemiol 11: 67–115.

2. Congdon N, O'Colmain B, Klaver CC, Klein R, Munoz B, et al. (2004) Causes and prevalence of visual impairment among adults in the United States. Arch Ophthalmol 122: 477–485.

3. Tomany SC, Wang JJ, Van Leeuwen R, Klein R, Mitchell P, et al. (2004) Risk factors for incident age-related macular degeneration: pooled findings from 3 continents. Ophthalmology 111: 1280–1287.

4. Gemmy Cheung CM, Li X, Cheng CY, Zheng Y, Mitchell P, et al. (2013) Prevalence and risk factors for age-related macular degeneration in Indians: a comparative study in Singapore and India. Am J Ophthalmol 155: 764–773, 773 e761–763.

5. Edwards DR, Gallins P, Polk M, Ayala-Haedo J, Schwartz SG, et al. (2010) Inverse association of female hormone replacement therapy with age-related macular degeneration and interactions with ARMS2 polymorphisms. Invest Ophthalmol Vis Sci 51: 1873–1879.

6. Rudnicka AR, Jarrar Z, Wormald R, Cook DG, Fletcher A, et al. (2012) Age and gender variations in age-related macular degeneration prevalence in populations of European ancestry: a meta-analysis. Ophthalmology 119: 571–580.

7. Erke MG, Bertelsen G, Peto T, Sjolie AK, Lindekleiv H, et al. (2013) Lactation, female hormones and age-related macular degeneration: the Tromso Study. Br J Ophthalmol 97: 1036–1039.

8. Klein BE, Klein R and Lee KE (2000) Reproductive exposures, incident age-related cataracts, and age-related maculopathy in women: the beaver dam eye study. Am J Ophthalmol 130: 322–326.

9. Haan MN, Klein R, Klein BE, Deng Y, Blythe LK, et al. (2006) Hormone therapy and age-related macular degeneration: the Women's Health Initiative Sight Exam Study. Arch Ophthalmol 124: 988–992.

10. Feskanich D, Cho E, Schaumberg DA, Colditz GA, Hankinson SE (2008) Menopausal and reproductive factors and risk of age-related macular degeneration. Arch Ophthalmol 126: 519–524.

11. Yoon KC, Mun GH, Kim SD, Kim SH, Kim CY, et al. (2011) Prevalence of eye diseases in South Korea: data from the Korea National Health and Nutrition Examination Survey 2008–2009. Korean J Ophthalmol 25: 421–433.

12. Cho BJ, Heo JW, Kim TW, Ahn J, Chung H (2014) Prevalence and risk factors of age-related macular degeneration in Korea: the Korea National Health and Nutrition Examination Survey 2010–2011. Invest Ophthalmol Vis Sci 55: 1101–1108.

13. Snow KK, Cote J, Yang W, Davis NJ, Seddon JM (2002) Association between reproductive and hormonal factors and age-related maculopathy in postmenopausal women. Am J Ophthalmol 134: 842–848.

14. Bird AC, Bressler NM, Bressler SB, Chisholm IH, Coscas G, et al. (1995) An international classification and grading system for age-related maculopathy and age-related macular degeneration. The International ARM Epidemiological Study Group. Surv Ophthalmol 39: 367–374.

15. Schwarz EB, Ray RM, Stuebe AM, Allison MA, Ness RB, et al. (2009) Duration of lactation and risk factors for maternal cardiovascular disease. Obstet Gynecol 113: 974–982.

16. Natland Fagerhaug T, Forsmo S, Jacobsen GW, Midthjell K, Andersen LF, et al. (2013) A prospective population-based cohort study of lactation and cardiovascular disease mortality: the HUNT study. BMC Public Health 13: 1070.

17. McClure CK, Catov JM, Ness RB, Schwarz EB (2012) Lactation and maternal subclinical cardiovascular disease among premenopausal women. Am J Obstet Gynecol 207: 46. e41–48.

18. Kjos SL, Henry O, Lee RM, Buchanan TA, Mishell DR Jr (1993) The effect of lactation on glucose and lipid metabolism in women with recent gestational diabetes. Obstet Gynecol 82: 451–455.

19. Williams MJ, Williams SM, Poulton R (2006) Breast feeding is related to C reactive protein concentration in adult women. J Epidemiol Community Health 60: 146–148.

20. Stuebe AM, Rich-Edwards JW, Willett WC, Manson JE, Michels KB (2005) Duration of lactation and incidence of type 2 diabetes. Jama 294: 2601–2610.

21. Klein R, Klein BE, Tomany SC, Cruickshanks KJ (2003) The association of cardiovascular disease with the long-term incidence of age-related maculopathy: the Beaver Dam eye study. Ophthalmology 110: 636–643.

22. van Leeuwen R, Ikram MK, Vingerling JR, Witteman JC, Hofman A, et al. (2003) Blood pressure, atherosclerosis, and the incidence of age-related maculopathy: the Rotterdam Study. Invest Ophthalmol Vis Sci 44: 3771–3777.

23. Connell PP, Keane PA, O'Neill EC, Altaie RW, Loane E, et al. (2009) Risk factors for age-related maculopathy. J Ophthalmol 2009: 360764.

24. Fraser-Bell S, Wu J, Klein R, Azen SP, Varma R (2006) Smoking, alcohol intake, estrogen use, and age-related macular degeneration in Latinos: the Los Angeles Latino Eye Study. Am J Ophthalmol 141: 79–87.

25. Peragallo Urrutia R, Coeytaux RR, McBroom AJ, Gierisch JM, Havrilesky LJ, et al. (2013) Risk of acute thromboembolic events with oral contraceptive use: a systematic review and meta-analysis. Obstet Gynecol 122: 380–389.

26. Christin-Maitre S (2013) History of oral contraceptive drugs and their use worldwide. Best Pract Res Clin Endocrinol Metab 27: 3–12.

27. Sitruk-Ware R, Nath A (2013) Characteristics and metabolic effects of estrogen and progestins contained in oral contraceptive pills. Best Pract Res Clin Endocrinol Metab 27: 13–24.

28. Wiegratz I, Lee JH, Kutschera E, Winkler UH, Kuhl H (2004) Effect of four oral contraceptives on hemostatic parameters. Contraception 70: 97–106.

29. Cilia La Corte AL, Carter AM, Turner AJ, Grant PJ, Hooper NM (2008) The bradykinin-degrading aminopeptidase P is increased in women taking the oral contraceptive pill. J Renin Angiotensin Aldosterone Syst 9: 221–225.

30. Nirmalan PK, Katz J, Robin AL, Ramakrishnan R, Krishnadas R, et al. (2004) Female reproductive factors and eye disease in a rural South Indian population: the Aravind Comprehensive Eye Survey. Invest Ophthalmol Vis Sci 45: 4273–4276.

31. Smith W, Mitchell P, Wang JJ (1997) Gender, oestrogen, hormone replacement and age-related macular degeneration: results from the Blue Mountains Eye Study. Aust N Z J Ophthalmol 25 Suppl 1: S13–15.

32. Abramov Y, Borik S, Yahalom C, Fatum M, Avgil G, et al. (2004) The effect of hormone therapy on the risk for age-related maculopathy in postmenopausal women. Menopause 11: 62–68.

33. The Eye Disease Case-Control Study Group (1992) Risk factors for neovascular age-related macular degeneration. Arch Ophthalmol 110: 1701–1708.

34. Rakic JM, Lambert V, Deprez M, Foidart JM, Noel A, et al. (2003) Estrogens reduce the expression of YKL-40 in the retina: implications for eye and joint diseases. Invest Ophthalmol Vis Sci 44: 1740–1746.

## 13

Quantified Self and Comprehensive Geriatric Assessment: Older Adults Are Able to Evaluate Their Own Health and Functional Status

Olivier Beauchet[1,2]*, Cyrille P. Launay[1], Christine Merjagnan[1,2], Anastasiia Kabeshova[1], Cédric Annweiler[1,3]

1 Department of Neuroscience, Angers University Hospital, Angers, France, **2** Biomathics, Paris, France, **3** Department of Medical Biophysics, the University of Western Ontario, London, Canada

Abstract

Background: There is an increased interest of individuals in quantifying their own health and functional status. The aim of this study was to examine the concordance of answers to a self-administered questionnaire exploring health and functional status with information collected during a full clinical examination performed by a physician among cognitively healthy adults (CHI) and older patients with mild cognitive impairment (MCI) or mild-to-moderate Alzheimer disease (AD).

Methods: Based on cross-sectional design, a total of 60 older adults (20 CHI, 20 patients with MCI, and 20 patients with mild-to-moderate AD) were recruited in the memory clinic of Angers, France. All participants completed a self-administered questionnaire in paper format composed of 33 items exploring age, gender, nutrition, place of living, social resources, drugs daily taken, memory complaint, mood and general feeling, fatigue, activities of daily living, physical activity and history of falls. Participants then underwent a full clinical examination by a physician exploring the same domains.

Results: High concordance between the self-administered questionnaire and physician's clinical examination was showed. The few divergences were related to cognitive status, answers of AD and MCI patients to the self-administered questionnaire being less reliable than those of CHI.

Conclusion: Older adults are able to evaluate their own health and functional status, regardless of their cognitive status. This result needs to be confirmed and opens new perspectives for the quantified self-trend and could be helpful in daily clinical practice of primary care.

Editor: Sonia Brucki, University Of São Paulo, Brazil

Funding: The authors have no support or funding to report.

Competing Interests: The authors have declared that no competing interests exist.

* Email: olbeauchet@chu-angers.fr

Introduction

Quantified self (QS) is a recent trend in general population based on self-measure of health and functional status using new digital technologies to become healthier or remain healthy [1]. Nowadays, the miniaturization of devices combined with new digital technologies allow the measure of human physiological parameters reflecting health status (e.g., caloric expenditures or blood pressure). The advantage of this "high-tech" QS is to provide objective measures, but its main disadvantage is to consider the individual more as a measurement object, than an actor of his own health, the latter point being yet crucial for health improvement. It has been reported that improvements of health and functional status, as well as reduced adverse consequences on health systems, depend in part on the active participation of individuals [2–4]. For this reason, the World Health Organization (WHO) recommends the use of self-administered questionnaires to rate and monitor individuals' own health [4–6]. This approach is also thought to educate people about wellness and promote

healthy lifestyles [2–6]. Because of the increasing popularity of QS, self-administered questionnaires evaluating health and functional status in complement or not to high-tech QS could be an interesting solution to improve older adults' health and functional status, and thus to limit adverse consequences of age-related disorders on health systems. However, an obstacle to this self-rated health approach could be the decline of cognition encountered in older adults, which may affect their ability to provide answers objectively reflecting their actual situation.

Older adults' health and functional status is heterogeneous because of the various cumulative effects of chronic diseases and physiologic decline, contributing to a vicious cycle of increased frailty [7–9]. Thanks to advances in medicine and hygiene, a growing number of older adults spend more years with a greater range of disorders causing disability but not mortality [10]. Health systems thus need to face this new challenge [10,11]. Quantification of the burden of non-fatal health outcomes is crucial to understand how efficiently health systems may respond to this situation.

In daily practice, adapted care plans for older patients arise from an assessment process called comprehensive geriatric assessment (CGA), which is a multidimensional, interdisciplinary diagnostic process to determine the medical, psychological, and functional capabilities of older adults [12,13]. The implementation of systematic CGA among older community-dwellers with accumulation of chronic diseases and disability remains difficult in daily practice because of a number of issues. First, while the number of older community-dwellers keeps increasing, the number of health care professionals with geriatric skills does not [14,15]. Second, the CGA is a complex and time-consuming process [15,16]. Third, the CGA requires multidisciplinary geriatric teams that cannot support alone the care of all older adults due to their limited number [13–16].

Because of these issues preventing performing a CGA in every older community-dweller with cumulative chronic diseases, and because of the increased interest of individuals in their own health and functional status, we hypothesized that it was possible to perform a self-CGA using a self-administered questionnaire among older adults with and without cognitive decline. The aim of this study was to examine, among cognitively healthy adults (CHI) and older patients with mild cognitive impairment (MCI) or mild-to-moderate Alzheimer disease (AD), the concordance of answers to a self-administered questionnaire with information collected by a physician during a full clinical examination.

Methods

Participants

Between March and May 2013, 60 older adults (i.e., 20 CHI, 20 patients with MCI, and 20 patients with mild-to-moderate AD) were recruited in this cross-sectional study. All participants were sent for a memory complaint by their primary care physician to the memory clinic of Angers University Hospital, France. Eligibility criteria were age 65 years and over, outpatients, able to understand and speak French, and no acute medical illness in the past month. For the present analysis, exclusion criteria were severe AD (i.e., Mini-Mental State Examination score (MMSE) ≤ 9), low near vision, neurological diseases including Parkinson's disease, cerebellar disease, myelopathy, peripheral neuropathy, and major orthopaedic impairments of the upper limbs [17].

Self-administered questionnaire

A self-administered questionnaire in format paper was given to each patient meeting the selection criteria at their arrival in the memory clinic. This questionnaire consisted of 33 items (Table S1). Except age and weight, all items corresponded to a question with a forced choice in closed-ended format (i.e., yes or no, or calling for a specific answer). The French version of questionnaire is presented in Appendix S1.

Neuropsychological assessment

Neuropsychological assessment was performed during a face-to-face examination carried out by a neuropsychologist. The memory complaint was characterized using the same 6 questions exploring memory as for the self-administered questionnaire. All answers were coded as a binary variable (i.e., yes or no). In addition, the following standardized tests were used to probe several aspects of cognition: MMSE, frontal assessment battery (FAB), ADAS-cog, trail making test parts A and B and French version of the free and cued selective reminding test [17–22]. The diagnoses of MCI and AD were made during multidisciplinary meetings involving geriatricians, neurologists and neuropsychologists of Angers University Memory Clinic, and were based on the neuropsycho-

logical tests mentioned above, medical examination findings, blood tests and Magnetic Resonance Imaging (MRI) of the brain. MCI was diagnosed according to Winblad et al. consensus criteria [23]. Participants with all categories of MCI were included in this study, i.e. amnestic and non-amnestic as well as single and multiple affected domains. The diagnosis of AD followed the DSM-IV and NINCDS/ADRDA consensus criteria [24]. Mild and moderate stages of AD were defined as MMSE score ≥ 10. Participants who were neither MCI nor dementia/AD and who had normal neuropsychological and functional performance were considered as CHI, regardless of the presence or not of underlying non-cognitive chronic diseases.

Medical examination

Participants underwent a full clinical examination by a physician. Age, gender, weight (kg), height (m), the number and the type of therapeutic classes of drugs used per day were recorded. The body mass index (BMI, in kg/m^2) was calculated based on anthropometric measurements. A loss of 4 kg and over in past year was also sought. The usual place of life (i.e., home-living versus institution-dwelling defined as living in nursing homes or in senior housing facilities), and the use of formal and/or informal home and social services were also recorded and coded as a binary variable (i.e., yes or no). Activities of daily living scale (ADL) and instrumental activities of daily living scale (IADL) were performed [25,26]. Depression was evaluated by the 4-item short Geriatric Depression Scale (GDS) score [27]. A score ≥1 indicated symptoms of depression. Participants were also questioned on their feeling and fatigue using the same questions as for the self-administered questionnaire. Physical activity was considered if participants practiced at least one recreational physical (walking, gymnastics, cycling, swimming or gardening) activity for at least one hour a week for the past month or more. Participants were also interviewed on their history of falls over the past year. A fall was defined as an event resulting in a person coming to rest unintentionally on the ground or at other lower level, not as the result of a major intrinsic event or an overwhelming hazard, according to the French society of geriatrics and gerontology (SFGG) and the French national agency for health (HAS) [28]. In the case of falls, the severity was recorded using the same items as for the self-administered questionnaire. In addition, education level was evaluated with the number of years of school completed.

Standard Protocol Approvals, Registrations, and Participant Consents

In the present study, a written informed consent was obtained from the patients themselves in the presence of their trusted person, usually a family member, who helped them to make decision. The study was conducted in accordance with the ethical standards set forth in the Helsinki Declaration (1983). The entire study protocol was approved by the Ethical Committee of Angers Hospital University, France (2013/25 – "Auto-évaluation de l'état de santé de la personne âgée").

Statistics

Participants' baseline characteristics were summarized using means and standard deviations or frequencies and percentages, as appropriate. Participants were separated into three groups based on their cognitive status (i.e., CHI, MCI and AD). A second stratification into two groups of all participants based on their education level and using a threshold of the median value (i.e., 11 years spent at school) was also done. Comparisons between groups of participants were performed using Kruskal-Wallis or one-way analysis of variance with Bonferroni corrections, t-test, Mann-Whitney test, and Chi-Square test, as appropriate. Comparison of answers from the self-administered questionnaire and the full clinical examination were performed using paired t-tests, Wilcoxon signed rank test or McNemar test, as appropriate.

Results

Table S2 reports the characteristics of participants obtained with the self-questionnaire according to their cognitive status. AD patients were older than MCI patients and CHI (P = 0.001). There were fewer women in the group of CHI compared to MCI patients (P = 0.025) and AD patients (P = 0.004). CHI were taller than MCI patients (P = 0.043) and AD (P = 0.015). CHI and MCI patients (P = 0.017) lived more frequently at home compared to AD patients. AD patients used more frequently formal and/or informal home help services (P<0.002) compared to CHI and MCI patients. Patients with AD took more drugs than CHI (P = 0.049) and MCI patients (P = 0.047). AD patients felt more frequently discouraged and sad compared to CHI (P = 0.002). In addition, AD (P<0.001) and MCI (P = 0.008) patients had more often a positive 4-item GDS than CHI. AD patients were less independent for toileting than CHI and MCI (P = 0.043). AD patients were less independent for the abilities to use transportation independently (P<0.001) and to handle finances (P<0.002) and for the responsibility for own medications (P<0.004) compared to CHI and MCI. Patients with AD had more mobility problems than MCI (P = 0.035). Furthermore, the IADL score was lower in AD compared to CHI and MCI (P<0.002). In final, AD patients had less often a feeling happy than CHI (P = 0.002), and they practiced less often physical activity than MCI and CHI (P< 0.001). There was no between-group difference for education level (10.8±3.2years for CHI, 11.5±3.2years for MCI patients, and 10.9±3.3years for AD patients, with P = 0.757). Stratification of the participants according to education level showed that there was no significant difference between self-administered questionnaire and full clinical examination among participants with higher education level (i.e., >11 years of school) and those with lower education level, exept for number of drugs daily taken, incontinence and ADLs score (Table S3). Indeed, there was a significant difference for individuals with low level of education (i.e., ≤11 years of school) for the number of drugs daily taken (P< 0.001). In addition, there was also a significant difference, whatever the education level group, for incontinence (P<0.006) and ADLs score (P<0.03).

Comparison between self- and hetero-assessments underscored that only the answers regarding height, number of drugs daily taken, ADLs score and items, and feeling of fatigue were significantly different (Table S4). AD patients declared to be taller than they actually were (P = 0.033). MCI and AD patients reported on self-administered questionnaire taking fewer drugs compared to physician assessment (P = 0.015 and P = 0.001). MCI patients declared to be less independent in ADLs (P = 0.002) and more often incontinent than estimated by the physician (P = 0.008). In contrast, CHI declared to be less often incontinent than estimated by the physician (P = 0.004). Finally, all participants declared to be more tired on self-administered questionnaire compared to physician assessment (P = 0.003), without any significant difference according to cognitive status. The magnitude of difference between results of self-questionnaire and physician examination for quantitative variables was low, regardless of the group of individuals (i.e., total population, CHI, MCI or patients with AD; please see Appendix S2).

Discussion

The present findings show that there were few divergences between a self-administered questionnaire in older adults and a CGA performed by a physician during a full clinical examination, and that these few divergences were mainly related to the cognitive status of participants. Answers of AD and MCI patients to the self-administered questionnaire were less reliable than those of CHI.

To the best of our knowledge, we report here the first evidence that older adults are able to assess accurately their own health and functional status, with a high concordance with physician comprehensive geriatric assessment. Only few divergences were observed. First, AD patients declared to be taller than there actually were. An explanation could rely on the onset of osteoporotic vertebral fractures, which lead to decreased height in older individuals. AD patients were older than CHI and MCI patients in our study. Because of their episodic memory disorders, they were also more likely to forget and underreport this loss of height. A second divergence concerned the drugs daily taken, AD and MCI patients having declared taking fewer drugs than they actually took. This result is consistent with the fact that it may be difficult for an older adult to know precisely what kind of drugs she/he takes, particularly in the case of cognitive decline. Third, another divergence has been found with the ADLs, notably regarding incontinence among CHI and participants with MCI. An explanation could rely on the misunderstanding of the wording by participants. Indeed, incontinence is a medical term that can be unknown or misinterpreted in its definition, and thus this misunderstanding may lead to error in answers. Fourth, the ADLs score, which was calculated based on the addition of 6 items, was also divergent for patients with MCI, who answered to be more frequently dependent than they actually were. It was not the case while analyzing each item separately. Subjective perception rather than objective difficulties could be an explanation for this result. The perception of difficulties to perform activities of daily living for an individual with memory episodic disorders may be important, whilst s/he can perform them correctly, which may lead to a discrepancy between subjective perception and the absence of objective difficulties. One explanation could be related to the higher level of attention required to prepare an action compared to executing it.

Fifth, our results underscored that, regardless of their cognitive status, older patients declared to be more frequently tired on the self-administered questionnaire than they expressed to the physician. To explain this result, it could be suggested that the concept of fatigue was misinterpreted or understood differently by participants while answering to the self-administered questionnaire. It is also possible that participants showed modesty or bravery when facing the doctor, and underestimated their actual fatigue during the medical examination.

Patients' characteristics in the studied sample showed many similarities with previous studies. First, AD patients in our study were older than CHI and MCI, which is in concordance with age as a first risk factor for AD [29–31]. Second, participants with cognitive decline (i.e., MCI and AD) were more frequently women, fact which was also reported in previous studies [30,31]. Third, we observed that AD patients took more drugs per day and used more frequently home services, were more depressed, practiced less physical activity and were less independent in ADLs and iADLs than CHI and MCI patients. All these characteristics are usually associated with AD and are adverse consequences of cognitive decline [30,31]. Despite these similarities, the translation of our findings to the general elderly population should be cautious. Our sample size was relatively small and could not be calculated *a priori*. However, post-hoc power analysis using either the number of drugs for AD patients or the fact to live alone for CHI showed that the number of participants should have been between 9 and 77. Furthermore, recruitment in our study was performed in only one memory clinic. Finally, limitations include the fact that socio-economic conditions not measured could have influenced the participants' answers to the self-administered questionnaire.

The high concordance of a self-administered questionnaire and physician's CGA among older adults suggest a number of perspectives in terms of primary care. The CGA is a complex and time-consuming process that cannot be performed systematically by all general practitioners (GPs) for every geriatric patient during routine office visits [15,16]. An active participation of the patients themselves in CGA is therefore required. We showed that a self-administered questionnaire corresponding to a self-CGA is feasible and accurate in older adults. Because the older patient may answer to the questionnaire in the waiting room, this approach is easy to implement in clinical practice. In addition, the result of this questionnaire could be used by GPs to screen frail older adults, and propose adapted care plans at the right time to the right patient.

Our results open also new perspectives in the field of QS. Nowadays, the miniaturization of devices combined with new digital technologies allow the measure of several physiological parameters reflecting health status. Therefore, QS focuses on different aspects of individuals' daily life in terms of inputs and/or outputs (e.g., food consumed, caloric expenditures, etc.), health status (e.g., blood pressure, blood oxygen levels, heart rythm, etc.), or physical performance (e.g., number of steps per day, etc.). As a result, the development of "high-tech" QS is allowing to acquire full data on older individuals, which only wait to be dissected, analyzed and interpreted. This explains that one current challenge is to transform raw data into structured and relevant material, to normalize it for analysis and to exchange it at the right time and place. As a consequence, feedbacks to individuals are still limited, and the expected beneficial impact on health remains to be demonstrated. A major forgotten step with this "high-tech" approach of QS is that individuals are not active actors of their own health, although improvements of health and functional status require individuals' active participation. Our results suggest that the use of a "low-tech" self-administered questionnaire, which captures a variety of health and functional information, could be an attractive solution for addressing this need. Among the possible perspectives, the development of a digital form accessible by touchpad or smartphone could serve both to gather health and functional information, and also to provide interactive feedback and generic and/or specific advice based on the responses entered by the patients.

In conclusion, our study shows that older adults are able to evaluate their own health and functional status, regardless of their cognitive status (i.e., CHI and patients with MCI or mild-to-moderate AD). Further research is needed to corroborate this finding but now this result opens new perspectives in the approach of geriatric patients, and could be extremely useful in daily clinical practice. A comprehensive geriatric assessment performed by an older adult could provide valuable information to the physicians to guide the medical examination and easily identify older patients requiring additional expertise and particular medical attention.

Supporting Information

Table S1 Items of self-administered questionnaire.

Table S2 Participants' characteristics obtained with the self-administered questionnaire, and comparisons according to their cognitive status (n = 60). CHI = cognitively healthy individuals; MCI = mild cognitive impairment; AD = Alzheimer disease; n: number of participants; BMI = body mass index; SD: Standard deviation; IQR: interquartile range; GDS: Geriatric depression scale; ADL: Activities of daily living; IADL: Instrumental activities of daily living; *: results from the self-administered questionnaire; †: Mild-to-moderate AD; ‡: Comparison between groups of participants based on Kruskal-Wallis with Bonferroni corrections, *t*-test, Mann-Whitney test and Chi-square test, as appropriate; §: >2 answers 'yes' among the 6 questions on memory complaint; #: Answer 'happy' or 'very happy' to the feeling question; ¶: Answer 'yes' to the question on fatigue. **: Considered if participants practiced at least one recreational physical (walking, gymnastics, cycling, swimming or gardening) activity for at least one hour a week for the past month or more; ††: A fall was defined as an event resulting in a person coming to rest unintentionally on the ground or at other lower level, not as the result of a major intrinsic event or an overwhelming hazard; P significant (<0.05) indicated in bold.

Table S3 P-values* of comparisons between self-administered questionnaire and physician examination according to educational level† (n = 60). n: number of participants; BMI = body mass index; SD: Standard deviation; IQR: interquartile range; ADL: Activities of daily living; IADL: Instrumental activities of daily living; ¶: Answer 'happy' or 'very happy' to the feeling question; *: Answer 'yes' to the question on fatigue; †: Considered if participants practiced at least one recreational physical (walking, gymnastics, cycling, swimming or gardening) activity for at least one hour a week for the past month or more; ‡: A fall was defined as an event resulting in a person coming to rest unintentionally on the ground or at other lower level, not as the result of a major intrinsic event or an overwhelming hazard; P significant (<0.05) indicated in bold.

Table S4 Comparisons between answers to the self-administered questionnaire and results of the full medical examination, according to the cognitive status of participants (n = 60). CHI = cognitively healthy individuals; MCI = mild cognitive impairment; AD = Alzheimer disease; n: number of participants; BMI = body mass index; SD: Standard deviation; GDS: Geriatric depression scale; ADL: Activities of daily living; IADL: Instrumental activities of daily living; *: Mild-to-moderate AD; †: >2 answers 'yes' among the 6 questions on memory complaint; ‡: Item of Geriatric Depression Scale; §: Item of Activities of Daily Living scale; #: Item of Instrumental Activities of Daily Living scale; ¶: Answer 'happy' or 'very happy' to the feeling question; **: Answer 'yes' to the question on fatigue; ††: Considered if participants practiced at least one recreational physical (walking, gymnastics, cycling, swimming or gardening) activity for at least one hour a week for the past month or more; ‡‡: A fall was defined as an event resulting in a person coming to rest unintentionally on the ground or at other lower level, not as the result of a major intrinsic event or an overwhelming hazard; All P-value are based on paired *t*-test, Wilcoxon signed rank test or McNemar test, as appropriate.

Appendix S1 Items of self-administered questionnaire in French.

Appendix S2 Mean value, standard deviation, median and interaquartil range of difference between self-questionnaire and physician examination for quantitative variables (n = 60). CHI = -cognitively healthy individuals; MCI = mild cognitive impairment; AD = Alzheimer disease; n: number of participants; BMI = body mass index; ADLs: Activities of daily living; IADLs: Instrumental activities of daily living.
(DOC)

Acknowledgments

The authors would like to thank "l'Agence Régionale de Santé de la région des Pays de la Loire", Denis Granger from PatientsWorld, Kevin Galery and all participants of the study.

Author Contributions

Conceived and designed the experiments: OB CA. Performed the experiments: OB CA CPL. Analyzed the data: OB CPL CM AK CA. Contributed reagents/materials/analysis tools: OB CPL CM AK CA. Wrote the paper: OB CPL CM AK CA.

References

1. den Braber M (2013) Quantified Self: insight in yourself through self-monitoring. Ned Tijdschr Geneeskd 157: A7028.
2. Salomon JA, Nordhagen S, Oza S, Murray CJL (2009) Are Americans feeling less healthy? The Puzzle of Trends in self-rated health. American Journal of Epidemiology 170: 343–351.
3. Kramers PGN (2003) The ECHI project - Health indicators for the European community. Eur J Public Health 13: 101–106.
4. World Health Organization (1996) Health interview surveys: Towards international harmonization of methods and instruments. WHO Regional Publications - European Series, 58.
5. Andrews G, Kemp A, Sunderland M, Von Korff M, Ustun TB (2009) Normative data for the 12 item WHO Disability Assessment Schedule 2.0. PLoS One 4: e8343.
6. Ustün TB, Chatterji S, Kostanjsek N, Rehm J, Kennedy C, et al. (2010) Developing the World Health Organization Disability Assessment Schedule 2.0. Bull World Health Organ 88: 815–823.
7. Sternberg SA, Wershof Schwartz A, Karunananthan S, Bergman H, Mark Clarfield A (2011) The identification of frailty: a systematic literature review. J Am Geriatr Soc 59: 2129–2138.
8. Berrut G, Andrieu S, Araujo de Carvalho I, Baeyens JP, Bergman H, et al. (2013) Promoting access to innovation for frail old persons. IAGG (International Association of Gerontology and Geriatrics), WHO (World Health Organization) and SFGG (Société Française de Gériatrie et de Gérontologie) Workshop—Athens January 20-21, 2012 Tool (GFST). J Nutr Health Aging 17: 688–693.
9. Rockwood K, Bergman H (2012) FRAILTY: A Report from the 3(rd) Joint Workshop of IAGG/WHO/SFGG, Athens, January 2012. Can Geriatr J 15: 31–36.
10. Vos T, Flaxman AD, Naghavi M, Lozano R, Michaud C, et al. (2012) Years lived with disability (YLDs) for 1160 sequelae of 289 diseases and injuries 1990–2010: a systematic analysis for the Global Burden of Disease Study 2010. Lancet 380: 2163–2196.
11. Barnett K, Mercer SW, Norbury M, Watt G, Wyke S, et al. (2012) Epidemiology of multimorbidity and implications for health care, research, and medical education: A cross-sectional study. Lancet 380: 37–43.
12. Li CM, Chen CY, Li CY, Wang WD, Wu SC (2010) The effectiveness of a comprehensive geriatric assessment intervention program for frailty in community-dwelling older people: A randomized, controlled trial. Arch Gerontol Geriatr. 50:S39–42.
13. Van Craen K, Braes T, Wellens N, Denhaerynck K, Flamaing J, et al. (2010) The effectiveness of inpatient geriatric evaluation and management units: a systematic review and meta-analysis. J Am Geriatr Soc 58: 83–92.
14. McCusker J, Verdon J, Tousignant P, de Courval LP, Dendukuri N, et al. (2001) Rapid emergency department intervention for older people reduces risk of functional decline: Results of a multicenter randomized trial. J Am Geriatr Soc 49: 1272–1281.
15. Lang PO, Zekry D, Michel JP, Drame M, Novella JL, et al. (2010) Early markers of prolonged hospital stay in demented inpatients: A multicentre and prospective study. J Nutr Health Aging 14: 141–147

16. Hoogerduijn JG, Schuurmans MJ, Duijnstee MS, de Rooij SE, Grypdonck MF (2007) A systematic review of predictors and screening instruments to identify older hospitalized patients at risk for functional decline. J Clin Nurs 16: 46–57.
17. Folstein MF, Folstein SE, McHugh PR (1975) "Mini-mental state". A practical method for grading the cognitive state of patients for the clinician. J Psychiatr Res12: 189–198.
18. Dubois B, Slachevsky A, Litvan I, Pillon B (2000) The FAB: a Frontal Assessment Battery at bedside. Neurology 55: 1621–1626.
19. Rosen WG, Mohs RC, Davis KL (1984) A new rating scale for Alzheimer's disease. Am J Psychiatry 141: 1356–1364.
20. Brown EC, Casey A, Fisch RI, Neuringer C (1958) Trail making test as a screening device for the detection of brain damage. J Consult Psychol. 22:469–474.
21. Grober E, Buschke H, Crystal H, Bang S, Dresner R (1988) Screening for dementia by memory testing. Neurology 38: 900–903.
22. Van der Linden M, Coyette F, Poitrenaud F, Kalafat M, Calicis F, et al. (2004) L'épreuve de rappel libre/rappel indicé à 16 items (RL/RI-16). In L'évaluation des troubles de la mémoire, (Eds. Solal), Marseille.
23. Winblad B, Palmer K, Kivipelto M, Jelic V, Fratiglioni L, et al. (2004) Mild cognitive impairment—beyond controversies, towards a consensus: Report of the International Working Group on Mild Cognitive Impairment. J Intern Med 256: 240–246.
24. McKhann G, Drachman D, Folstein M, Katzman R, Price D, et al. (1984) Clinical diagnosis of Alzheimer's disease: Report of the NINCDS-ADRDA Work Group under the auspices of Department of Health and Human Services Task Force on Alzheimer's Disease. Neurology 34: 939–944.
25. Katz S, Downs TD, Cash HR, Grotz RC (1970). Progress in development of the index of ADL. Gerontologist 10: 20–30.
26. Pérès K, Chrysostome V, Fabrigoule C, Orgogozo JM, Dartigues JF, et al. (2006) Restriction in complex activities of daily living in MCI: Impact on outcome. Neurology 67: 461–466.
27. Shah A, Herbert R, Lewis S, Mahendran R, Platt J, et al. (1997) Screening for depression among acutely ill geriatric inpatients with a short Geriatric Depression Scale. Age Ageing 26: 217–221.
28. Beauchet O, Dubost V, Revel Delhom C, Berrut G, Belmin J, et al. (2011) How to manage recurrent falls in clinical practice: Guidelines of the French Society of Geriatrics and Gerontology. J Nutr Health Aging 15: 79–84.
29. Popa-Wagner A, Buga AM, Popescu B, Muresanu D (2013). Vascular cognitive impairment, dementia, aging and energy demand. A vicious cycle. J Neural Transm [Epub ahead of print]
30. Matthews FE, Arthur A, Barnes LE, Bond J, Jagger C, et al. (2013) A two-decade comparison of prevalence of dementia in individuals aged 65 years and older from three geographical areas of England: Results of the Cognitive Function and Ageing Study I and II. Lancet. 382: 1405–1412.
31. Prince M, Bryce R, Albanese E, Wimo A, Ribeiro W, et al. (2013). The global prevalence of dementia: A systematic review and metaanalysis. Alzheimers Dement 9: 63–75.

## 14

Does Improved Survival Lead to a More Fragile Population: Time Trends in Second and Third Hospital Admissions among Men and Women above the Age of 60 in Sweden

Korinna Karampampa[1]*, Tomas Andersson[1,2], Sven Drefahl[1,3], Anders Ahlbom[1], Karin Modig[1]

1 Institute of Environmental Medicine, Unit of Epidemiology, Karolinska Institutet, Stockholm, Sweden, 2 Centre for Occupational and Environmental Medicine, Stockholm County Council, Stockholm, Sweden, 3 Department of Sociology, Demography Unit, Stockholm University, Stockholm, Sweden

Abstract

Background: Life expectancy and time to first hospitalization have been prolonged, indicating that people live longer without needing hospital care. Life expectancy increased partially due to improved survival from severe diseases, which, however, could lead to a more fragile population. If so, time to a subsequent hospitalization could decrease. Alternatively, the overall trend of improved health could continue after the first hospitalization, prolonging also the time to subsequent hospitalizations. This study analyzes trends in subsequent hospitalizations among Swedish men and women above the age of 60, relating them to first hospitalization. It also looks at trends in the proportion of never hospitalized.

Methods: Individuals were followed in national registers for hospital admissions and deaths between 1972 and 2010. The proportion of never hospitalized individuals at given ages and time points, and the annual change in the risks of first and subsequent hospitalizations, were calculated.

Findings: An increase in the proportion of never hospitalized was seen over time. The risks of first as well as subsequent hospitalizations were reduced by almost 10% per decade for both men and women. Improvements were observed mainly for individuals below the ages of 90 and up to the year 2000.

Conclusions: The reduction in annual risk of both first *and* subsequent hospitalizations up to 90 years of age speaks in favor of a postponement of the overall morbidity among the elderly and provides no support for the hypothesis that the population becomes more fragile due to increased survival from severe diseases.

Editor: Angelo Scuteri, INRCA, Italy

Funding: Funding was received from the Swedish Research Council for Health, Working Life and Social Research (Forskningsrådet för hälsa, arbetsliv och välfärd, FAS) grant number: 2011-0843), and the Swedish Society of Medicine (Svenska Läkaresällskapet). The funders had no role in study design, data collection and analysis, decision to publish, or preparation of the manuscript.

Competing Interests: The authors have declared that no competing interests exist.

* E-mail: korinna.karampampa@ki.se

Introduction

Due to the increasing life expectancy, the question regarding the health of the elderly has become very important [1,2]. By the year 2020, 33% of the population in developed countries is projected to be older than 60 years [3], a potential challenge for medical and social care [4].

One way to understand the general health status of the population is to examine time trends in incidence and mortality rates of major diseases, such as cardiovascular diseases (CVD). CVD are major causes of morbidity and death in the older population, and a decrease in both incidence and mortality has been observed since the 1960s [5–8]. While such trends provide important insights for specific diseases, they do not necessarily reflect overall health trends. The annual change in hospitalization rates for all diagnoses is an alternative measure that provides information regarding the overall health of the population. The interpretation of such a change, however, is not straightforward since healthcare practices have evolved simultaneously.

In an earlier study we have shown that in parallel with an increase in life expectancy, the mean age at first hospital admission after the age of 60 has been postponed in Sweden by approximately 2 years between 1995 and 2010 [9]. Improved survival from severe diseases explains part of the increased life expectancy and the survivors may constitute a particularly fragile part of the population. This raises the question of whether the time to a subsequent hospitalization decreases. Alternatively, the overall trend of improved health could continue also after the first hospital event in which case one would expect a prolongation also of the time to a subsequent hospitalization.

This study aims to describe trends in subsequent hospitalizations among Swedish men and women above the age of 60, relating them to first hospitalization. It also examines the proportion of individuals never hospitalized in order to provide an overview of the overall health trends in the Swedish population from a novel perspective.

Materials and Methods

Study material

Our study population was created from the Total Population Register in Sweden [10]. Information regarding the date of birth and migration status of individuals was collected. In addition, the Total Population Register was used together with the Longitudinal Integration Database for Health Insurance and Labour Market Studies (LISA) [11], which includes yearly information about individuals' income, pensions and social transfers, in order to identify the individual's place of residence from 1972 onwards.

The Patient Register includes individual data regarding all hospital admissions in Sweden; it was used to obtain information about hospitalizations. This register has nation-wide coverage since 1987; however, Stockholm and Uppsala counties have had full coverage in this register since 1972 [12]. To be able to describe hospitalization trends for the longest period possible, we limited our study cohort to these two counties - combined they represent about 20% of the entire Swedish population above the age of 60.

Information on death was obtained from the Cause of Death Register. It includes deaths occurring within or outside Sweden for individuals who were registered in Sweden at the time of death [13].

Information about inpatient care and death was linked to the study cohort using a unique personal identification number that every person residing in Sweden holds. The linking procedure was done by Statistics Sweden and the researchers received a de-identified dataset.

Setting

All men and women above the age of 60, who were living in the Stockholm and Uppsala counties since 1972, were included in the study population. They were followed from the year 1972 to 2010. The follow-up ended when one of the following events occurred: hospitalization, death, or December 31, 2010. Individuals who moved away from Stockholm and Uppsala counties after 1972 were censored at the time they left.

Statistical analyses

The outcome under study was hospital admission due to any cause, which had a minimum duration of two nights, and took place after individuals turned 60. The first, second, and third hospital admissions were analyzed, regardless of the outcome being fatal or not. The second and the third hospital admissions had to occur at least 91 days apart from the previous admission.

Proportion of non-hospitalized men and women over the period 1972 to 2010. A Kaplan-Meier estimator was used to calculate the proportion of individuals that had never been admitted to the hospital at a given age. Five different birth cohorts, 1912, 1916, 1920, 1924, and 1928 were analyzed and the proportions of non-hospitalized individuals were compared for six ages; 70, 75, 80, 85, 90, and 95 years-old.

Hospitalization risks over the period 1972–2010. Using a discrete time logistic model with a complementary *loglog* link [14], the annual relative change in the age-specific annual risk (RR) of being admitted to the hospital for the first, second, and the third time after the age of 60 was estimated. For example, the relative change in the age-specific annual risk for being admitted to the hospital for the first time in 1999 was compared with that of 1998. The average annual relative change over all ages, stratified first in nine different age groups (60–64, 65–69, 70–74, 75–79, 80–84, 85–89, 90–94, 95–99, and 100+), and additionally in four different time periods (1972–1980, 1981–1990, 1991–2000, and 2001–2010) was calculated. Then, the annual change in the risk was estimated by subtracting the relative change from one (1-RR).

For the relative risk of the first admission to the hospital, age at first hospitalization (treated as a categorical variable) was used as a time-varying predictor of the outcome in a regression model. For the second hospital admission, both the age of individuals (treated as a categorical variable), and the time (in years) since the first admission to the hospital, were considered to have an impact on the regression outcome. Therefore an interaction term "*age×years since first hospitalization*" was included in the regression model to capture the effect of both parameters simultaneously. The model predictor (time varying) was age at second admission to the hospital. A similar analysis was done for the relative risk of the third hospitalization with age (treated as a categorical variable) being the model predictor, and adjusted for the interaction "*age×years since second hospitalization*".

Sensitivity analyses

In order to explore the impact of three of the most important causes of death and hospital admissions of older individuals, analyses were made where hospitalizations related to (1) CVD, (2) neoplasms, and (3) mental, behavioral and neurodevelopmental disorders (including dementia and Alzheimer's disease) where removed one at a time. The International Classification of Diseases (ICD) codes were used to identify and exclude the relevant hospital admissions. CVD were defined as; ICD 8 & 9 codes: 390–460, ICD 10 codes: I00-I99. Neoplasms were defined as; ICD 8 & 9 codes: 140–206, ICD 10 codes: C00-C97 and D00-D99. Mental, behavioral and neurodevelopmental disorders were defined as ICD 8&9 codes: 290–319, and 331, ICD 10 codes: F00-F99, and G30.

Additional sensitivity analyses were conducted by altering the minimum duration of hospital stay from two nights to one and three nights respectively. Since there have been changes in the health care policy in Sweden over time affecting the length of stay in hospitals, going from longer and fewer to shorter and more frequent admissions [15], we also tested the minimum transition time from first to second and from second to third hospital admission by running the analysis with 365 days as a minimum time apart between the events.

Ethical permission

An ethics approval for this study was obtained from the regional ethics committee in Stockholm, Dnr 2011/136-31/5. All databases used in this study were linked using the individuals' personal identification number (*personnumer*). The linkage was conducted by Statistics Sweden and researchers received anonymized data.

Results

Proportion of non-hospitalized men and women over the period 1972 to 2010

Tables 1a and 1b present the proportion of individuals without any admission to the hospital at different ages, across different birth cohorts, for men (Table 1a) and women (Table 1b). An increase in the proportion of never hospitalized was seen over time. Even among the 90-year olds, the proportion has increased although the proportion of never hospitalized 90-year olds was rather small (0.7% among men and 1.8% among women). Overall, the proportion of women never hospitalized was smaller compared to men.

Hospitalization risks over the period 1972–2010

In Tables 2a and 2b the annual decrease in the risk of a first, second, and third admission to the hospital between 1972 and 2010 is presented. Results are shown as an average effect for all ages above 60 as well as stratified in nine age groups, for men (Table 2a) and women (Table 2b). In Tables 3a and 3b, results are presented, stratified in four different time periods, for men (Table 3a) and women (Table 3b).

The risks of being hospitalized both for the first and the second time after the age of 60 decreased on average by about 9% per decade for men as well as for women. This risk reduction for the first admission to the hospital was observed in almost all age groups - it was higher among the youngest and tended to level off at the highest ages. However, for the second hospital admission, the risk reduction was only observed for men and women up to the age of 89.

For the third admission to the hospital, the reduction in the risk was slightly lower compared to the one estimated for the first and second hospital admission; for men, a reduction of 8% per decade was observed and for women 6%. Among the oldest (90+), an increase in the risk of a third admission to the hospital was observed.

When stratifying the results in four different time periods, for both men and women, a rather high reduction in the risk of subsequent admissions was observed between the years 1972 and 1980 (about 3% per year for the second admission and about 4%

per year for the third admission to the hospital). However, results pointed in the opposite direction for the first hospital admission; a 4% increase per year in the risk was observed for men and a 3% increase for women.

Between the years 1980 and 2000, for the first *and* subsequent hospital admissions, an annual risk reduction of 2% was observed for both men and women. During the latest decade, a small annual increase in the risk was observed for the first admission to the hospital for both men and women (0.4% per year), among women with a second hospital admission (0.7% per year), and for both men and women with a third hospital admission (0.7% per year). Among men, no change in the risk of a second admission to the hospital was observed between 2001 and 2010.

Results from the sensitivity analyses

Excluding CVD, neoplasms, and mental, behavioral and neurodevelopmental disorders, or altering the minimum duration of the admission to the hospital to one and three days respectively, had no impact on the observed trends of the proportion of never hospitalized individuals or the annual change in the risk of first, second, and third hospitalization. Similarly, changing the minimum time between a first and a second hospital admission from 91 to 365 days did not have any impact on the trends. The change in the minimum time between a second and a third admission to the hospital resulted in a slightly lower annual risk reduction for men for the third hospital admission (0.7% reduction instead of 0.8%) while no changes were observed for women.

Discussion

This study investigated trends in subsequent hospital admissions above the age of 60. In an earlier study, we concluded that individuals nowadays suffer less from illnesses leading to hospitalization [9]. Such a reduction, however, reflects only an initial improvement. Individuals may be more fragile once they have survived the disease that led to the first hospital stay and, hence, subsequent hospitalizations may occur more rapidly. However, our analyses of the change in the risk of subsequent hospital admissions showed no support for this, at least not for ages up to 90 years.

Table 1. Proportion of men and women at different ages without any admission to hospital.

A - Men						
Birth Cohorts	Age 70	Age 75	Age 80	Age 85	Age 90	Age 95
1912	28.80%	14.30%	5.80%	2.10%	0.60%	0.10%
1916	28.50%	14.90%	6.10%	2.10%	0.50%	
1920	29.90%	15.90%	7.40%	3.00%	0.70%	
1924	31.20%	18.00%	9.00%	3.40%		
1928	33.10%	19.80%	10.30%			
B - Women						
Birth Cohorts	Age 70	Age 75	Age 80	Age 85	Age 90	Age 95
1912	42.10%	25.90%	13.70%	5.40%	1.50%	0.20%
1916	39.40%	25.10%	12.90%	5.40%	1.60%	
1920	40.00%	24.90%	13.60%	6.20%	1.80%	
1924	40.10%	25.10%	14.40%	6.60%		
1928	42.00%	28.20%	15.20%			

Table 2. Annual decrease in the risk of first, second, and third hospital admission after the age of 60, for men and women.

A – Men

	Average across all ages	age 60–64	age 65–69	age 70–74	age 75–79	age 80–84	age 85–89	age 90–94	age 95–99	age 100 +
First hospital admission, risk+ (95% CI)	0.91% (0.88%, 0.94%)	1.20% (1.15%, 1.26%)	0.85% (0.78%, 0.92%)	0.73% (0.65%, 0.81%)	0.71% (0.62%, 0.81%)	0.65% (0.52%, 0.78%)	0.26% (0.02%, 0.5%)	−0.12% (−0.66%, 0.42%)	0.48% (−1.02%, 1.96%)	1.19% (−4.96%, 6.98%)
Second hospital admission, risk+,* (95% CI)	0.86% (0.82%, 0.91%)	0.73% (0.65%, 0.8%)	1.01% (0.92%, 1.11%)	1.08% (0.97%, 1.2%)	0.91% (0.77%, 1.04%)	0.75% (0.57%, 0.93%)	0.35% (−0.01%, 0.72%)	−0.38% (−1.27%, 0.49%)	−1.30% (−4.4%, 1.71%)	n.a. n.a. n.a.
Third hospital admission, risk+,# (95% CI)	0.77% (0.71%, 0.83%)	0.45% (0.33%, 0.58%)	0.74% (0.62%, 0.86%)	1.19% (1.06%, 1.32%)	1.11% (0.97%, 1.26%)	0.66% (0.48%, 0.85%)	0.05% (−0.26%, 0.37%)	−0.32% (−1.05%, 0.41%)	−0.78% (−3.54%, 1.91%)	−1.72% (−29.81%, 20.29%)

B – Women

	Average across all ages	age 60–64	age 65–69	age 70–74	age 75–79	age 80–84	age 85–89	age 90–94	age 95–99	age 100 +
First hospital admission, risk+ (95% CI)	0.67% (0.64%, 0.7%)	0.85% (0.8%, 0.9%)	0.60% (0.53%, 0.66%)	0.59% (0.52%, 0.66%)	0.51% (0.44%, 0.59%)	0.82% (0.73%, 0.91%)	0.47% (0.32%, 0.61%)	−0.21% (−0.51%, 0.09%)	−1.44% (−2.26%, −0.62%)	0.14% (−2.7%, 2.9%)
Second hospital admission, risk+,* (95% CI)	0.73% (0.69%, 0.77%)	0.55% (0.48%, 0.63%)	0.87% (0.78%, 0.96%)	0.98% (0.89%, 1.08%)	0.99% (0.88%, 1.09%)	0.51% (0.38%, 0.63%)	0.05% (−0.16%, 0.26%)	−0.47% (−0.93%, −0.01%)	−1.57% (−3.11%, −0.06%)	0.0179 (−4.48%, 7.69%)
Third hospital admission, risk+,# (95% CI)	0.64% (0.59%, 0.69%)	0.16% (0.04%, 0.29%)	0.76% (0.64%, 0.88%)	0.98% (0.87%, 1.1%)	1.08% (0.97%, 1.2%)	0.53% (0.4%, 0.65%)	−0.02% (−0.2%, 0.17%)	−0.08% (−0.46%, 0.3%)	0.28% (−1.02%, 1.56%)	−2.01% (−7.87%, 3.53%)

+ annual decrease in the risk of hospitalization. A negative percentage indicates an annual increase in the risk.
* adjusted for the interaction between age and the number of years since the first hospital admission.
# adjusted for the interaction between age and the number of years since the second hospital admission.
n.a. measurement not available due to very few observations.

Table 3. Annual decrease in the risk of first, second, and third hospital admission after the age of 60, stratified in four different time periods, for men and women.

A - Men

Period:	1972–1980	1981–1990	1991–2000	2001–2010
First hospital admission, risk+ (95% CI)	−4% (−12.3%, 3.69%)	1.53% (1.25%, 1.81%)	3.38% (3.09%, 3.67%)	−0.45% (−0.78%, −0.11%)
Second hospital admission, risk+,* (95% CI)	2.74% (2.26%, 3.22%)	1.34% (1.02%, 1.66%)	2.14% (1.81%, 2.47%)	0.11% (−0.29%, 0.5%)
Third hospital admission, risk+,*,# (95% CI)	3.56% (2.88%, 4.25%)	1.29% (0.91%, 1.67%)	2.01% (2.01%, 2.01%)	−0.69% (−1.15%, −0.23%)

B - Women

Period:	1972–1980	1981–1990	1991–2000	2001–2010
First hospital admission, risk+ (95% CI)	−2.70% (−2.92%, −2.47%)	2.11% (1.88%, 2.34%)	1.93% (1.69%, 2.17%)	−0.44% (−0.73%, −0.15%)
Second hospital admission, risk+,* (95% CI)	3.04% (2.63%, 3.45%)	1.76% (1.5%, 2.03%)	1.51% (1.24%, 1.78%)	−0.71% (−1.04%, −0.38%)
Third hospital admission, risk+,*,# (95% CI)	3.55% (2.95%, 4.14%)	1.62% (1.3%, 1.93%)	1.60% (1.3%, 1.9%)	−0.66% (−1.03%, −0.29%)

+ annual decrease in the risk of hospitalization. A negative percentage indicates an annual increase in the risk.
* adjusted for the interaction between age and the number of years since the first hospital admission.
# adjusted for interaction between age and the number of years since the second hospital admission.

The annual risk for a second hospitalization decreased by almost 10% per decade for ages up to 90 years, a similar improvement as for the risk of first admission. The risk for a third admission to the hospital also decreased but less than the one for the first and second admission. Above age 90, no clear improvement over time was observed for subsequent hospital admissions, which may be a consequence of a more fragile population. On the other hand no worsening was seen either – the risk remained stable.

Since the analyses of changes in the risk of subsequent hospital admissions are based only on the part of the population that has been hospitalized previously, changes in the risk must be interpreted in conjunction with the change in the proportion of the population that has never been hospitalized. An improvement for subsequent hospital admissions alone does not necessarily an improvement for the whole population as the proportion of the population never hospitalized could have decreased at the same time. However, during our observation period we observed both a decreasing risk for subsequent hospital admissions and a simultaneous increase in the proportion of never hospitalized – in all ages up to 90.

The finding of a lack of improvement regarding the risk of subsequent admissions among the very oldest, above 90, is in line with a previous study of Swedish centenarians where death rates above age 100 appeared to have been stable between 1969 and 2008 [16,17], in contrast to younger ages where a continuous reduction has been observed.

This risk reduction for hospitalization was mainly evident during the 1980s and 1990s, and no improvements were seen for the most recent decade (2000–2010). We have no clear explanation to this. It may be a temporal stagnation that will not affect the overall trend when allowing longer follow up in the next decade, or it may be a sign of a real stagnation of improvements. It could also be the effect of a single (period-) factor such as the increase in elective surgery like hip replacement during the past decade [18]. On the other hand, such procedures still constitute a minor part of all hospital admissions in Sweden and therefore the impact on the general trends should be minor.

Even if our results speak in favor of a postponement of morbidity and an amelioration of the overall health of the population, other explanations must be considered as well. The shift of some treatments from inpatient to outpatient care, the availability of home care services to serve the needs of the elderly or other sensitive groups outside a hospital setting [19], and the cut in the number of hospital beds, are factors that need to be considered. A report from the Swedish National Board of Health and Welfare showed a significant reduction in the inpatient care (in favor of outpatient care) received for diseases of the eye and adnexa, asthma, ulcers and inguinal hernia between 1987 and 2010 [20]. However, this shift is unlikely to fully explain the observed trends since only a minority (depending on the disease) of individuals is receiving inpatient care due to these diseases [9].

Home care programs have been designed to enable the elderly to continue an independent lifestyle as opposed to being admitted to the hospital for very long periods, becoming institutionalized in nursing homes and other care facilities [19]. It is therefore possible that such programs would be the underlying mechanism of a shift in second and third hospitalization to higher ages over time – elderly individuals receiving home care may not be admitted to a hospital for conditions that can be treated/monitored through home care services. However, it is difficult to evaluate how much the effect of such programs would be, given that there are other factors as well contributing to the observed trends for the risk of subsequent hospitalizations.

Regarding the cut in number of hospital beds, it is difficult to separate any effect of this on the risk of hospitalization since it is reasonable to believe that the cut is an effect of a more effective health care and a better control of diseases in primary care making the outcome of diseases less severe. It can be observed in the data that over time inpatient care has shifted from longer to shorter and more frequent hospitalizations.

Finally, interpreting our results of a reduction in the risk of both first *and* subsequent hospital admissions, together with findings from other studies showing declining trends in the incidence and mortality of several important diseases among the elderly such as CVD [8], malignancies [21,22], and dementia [23], lead us to believe that it is conceivable that there has been a postponement of overall severe morbidity in line with the decrease in mortality over the years. Whether these improvements will be extended also to the very oldest, above 90 and 100 years of age, remains to be answered, together with the question of whether less severe morbidity that is treated in primary care has improved as well.

Conclusions

The risk of a subsequent hospitalization has not increased suggesting that the health of the general population is not worsened due to a higher proportion of people with compromised health that could follow from the improved survival in severe diseases. The lack of improvements in the most recent decade suggests the need for further surveillance of the trends.

Author Contributions

Analyzed the data: KK TA. Wrote the paper: KK TA SD AA KM.

References

1. Bronnum-Hansen H, Petersen I, Jeune B, Christensen K (2009) Lifetime according to health status among the oldest olds in Denmark. Age and ageing 38: 47–51.
2. Vaupel JW, Zhang Z, van Raalte AA (2011) Life expectancy and disparity: an international comparison of life table data. BMJ open 1: e000128.
3. Rasmussen LJ, Sander M, Wewer UM, Bohr VA (2011) Aging, longevity and health. Mechanisms of ageing and development 132: 522–532.
4. Larsson K, Thorslund M (2006) Chapter 8: old people's health. Scandinavian journal of public health Supplement 67: 185–198.
5. Cooper R, Cutler J, Desvigne-Nickens P, Fortmann SP, Friedman L, et al. (2000) Trends and disparities in coronary heart disease, stroke, and other cardiovascular diseases in the United States: findings of the national conference on cardiovascular disease prevention. Circulation 102: 3137–3147.
6. Kesteloot H, Sans S, Kromhout D (2006) Dynamics of cardiovascular and all-cause mortality in Western and Eastern Europe between 1970 and 2000. European heart journal 27: 107–113.
7. Levi F, Chatenoud L, Bertuccio P, Lucchini F, Negri E, et al. (2009) Mortality from cardiovascular and cerebrovascular diseases in Europe and other areas of the world: an update. European journal of cardiovascular prevention and rehabilitation: official journal of the European Society of Cardiology, Working Groups on Epidemiology & Prevention and Cardiac Rehabilitation and Exercise Physiology 16: 333–350.
8. Modig K, Andersson T, Drefahl S, Ahlbom A (2013) Age-specific trends in morbidity, mortality and case-fatality from cardiovascular disease, myocardial infarction and stroke in advanced age: evaluation in the Swedish population. PloS one 8: e64928.
9. Karampampa K, Drefahl S, Andersson T, Ahlbom A, Modig K (2013) Trends in age at first hospital admission in relation to trends in life expectancy in Swedish men and women above the age of 60. BMJ open 3: e003447.
10. Statistics Sweden [Statistika Centralbyrån] (2013) Total Population Register [Registret över totalbefolkningen (RTB)]. Available: http://www.scb.se/Pages/List____257499.asp. Accessed: 31 October, 2013.
11. Statistics Sweden [Statistika Centralbyrån] (2013) Longitudinal integration database for health insurance and labour market studies (LISA by Swedish acronym). Available from: http://www.scb.se/Pages/List____257743.aspx. Accessed: 31 October, 2013.
12. National Board of Health and Welfare [Socialstyrelsen] (2013) Patient Register [Patientregistret]. Available: http://www.socialstyrelsen.se/register/halsodataregister/patientregistret. Accessed: 31 October, 2013.
13. National Board of Health and Welfare [Socialstyrelsen] (2013) Cause of Death Register [Dödsorsaksregistret]. Available: http://www.socialstyrelsen.se/register/dodsorsaksregistret. Accessed: 31 October, 2013.
14. Modig K, Drefahl S, Ahlbom A (2013) Limitless longevity: Comment on the Contribution of rectangularization to the secular increase of life expectancy. International journal of epidemiology.
15. Socialstyrelsen [National Board of Health and Welfare] (2012) Patientregistret för 2010 ur ett DRG-perspektiv [National In-patient Care Register in 2010, from a DRG perspective]. Available: http://www.socialstyrelsen.se/publikationer2012/2012-5-25. Accessed: 16 Nov 2012.
16. Drefahl S, Lundstrom H, Modig K, Ahlbom A (2012) The era of centenarians: mortality of the oldest old in Sweden. Journal of internal medicine 272: 100–102.
17. Modig K, Drefahl S, Ahlbom A (2013) Limitless longevity: Comment on the Contribution of rectangularization to the secular increase of life expectancy. International journal of epidemiology 42: 914–916.
18. Garellick G, Kärrholm J, Rogmark C, Rolfson O, Herberts P (2011) Swedish Hip Arthroplasty Register, Annual Report. Swedish Hip Arthroplasty Register.
19. Holosko MJ, Holosko DA, Spencer K (2009) Social services in Sweden: an overview of policy issues, devolution, and collaboration. Social work in public health 24: 210–234.
20. National Board of Health and Welfare [Socialstyrelsen] (2011) Inpatient diseases in Sweden 1987–2010 [Sjukdomar i sluten vård 1987–2010]. Available: http://www.socialstyrelsen.se/Lists/Artikelkatalog/Attachments/18410/2011-9-5.pdf. Accessed: 16 November, 2012.
21. Bosetti C, Bertuccio P, Malvezzi M, Levi F, Chatenoud L, et al. (2013) Cancer mortality in Europe, 2005–2009, and an overview of trends since 1980. Annals of oncology: official journal of the European Society for Medical Oncology/ESMO.
22. Karim-Kos HE, de Vries E, Soerjomataram I, Lemmens V, Siesling S, et al. (2008) Recent trends of cancer in Europe: a combined approach of incidence, survival and mortality for 17 cancer sites since the 1990s. European journal of cancer 44: 1345–1389.
23. Qiu C, von Strauss E, Backman L, Winblad B, Fratiglioni L (2013) Twenty-year changes in dementia occurrence suggest decreasing incidence in central Stockholm, Sweden. Neurology 80: 1888–1894.

## 15

A Self-Reported Screening Tool for Detecting Community-Dwelling Older Persons with Frailty Syndrome in the Absence of Mobility Disability: The FiND Questionnaire

Matteo Cesari[1,2]*, **Laurent Demougeot**[1], **Henri Boccalon**[1], **Sophie Guyonnet**[1], **Gabor Abellan Van Kan**[1,2], **Bruno Vellas**[1,2], **Sandrine Andrieu**[1,2]

1 Institut du Vieillissement, Gérontopôle, Centre Hospitalier Universitaire de Toulouse, Toulouse, France, **2** Inserm UMR1027, Université de Toulouse III Paul Sabatier, Toulouse, France

Abstract

Background: The "frailty syndrome" (a geriatric multidimensional condition characterized by decreased reserve and diminished resistance to stressors) represents a promising target of preventive interventions against disability in elders. Available screening tools for the identification of frailty in the absence of disability present major limitations. In particular, they have to be administered by a trained assessor, require special equipment, and/or do not discriminate between frail and disabled individuals. Aim of this study is to verify the agreement of a novel self-reported questionnaire (the "Frail Non-Disabled" [FiND] instrument) designed for detecting non-mobility disabled frail older persons with results from reference tools.

Methodology/Principal Findings: Data are from 45 community-dwelling individuals aged ≥60 years. Participants were asked to complete the FiND questionnaire separately exploring the frailty and disability domains. Then, a blinded assessor objectively measured the frailty status (using the phenotype proposed by Fried and colleagues) and mobility disability (using the 400-meter walk test). Cohen's kappa coefficients were calculated to determine the agreement between the FiND questionnaire with the reference instruments. Mean age of participants (women 62.2%) was 72.5 (standard deviation 8.2) years. Seven (15.6%) participants presented mobility disability as being unable to complete the 400-meter walk test. According to the frailty phenotype criteria, 25 (55.6%) participants were pre-frail or frail, and 13 (28.9%) were robust. Overall, a substantial agreement of the instrument with the reference tools (kappa = 0.748, quadratic weighted kappa = 0.836, both p values < 0.001) was reported with only 7 (15.6%) participants incorrectly categorized. The agreement between results of the FiND disability domain and the 400-meter walk test was excellent (kappa = 0.920, p < 0.001).

Conclusions/Significance: The FiND questionnaire presents a very good capacity to correctly identify frail older persons without mobility disability living in the community. This screening tool may represent an opportunity for diffusing awareness about frailty and disability and supporting specific preventive campaigns.

Editor: Antony Bayer, Cardiff University, United Kingdom

Funding: The MINDED project is funded as a Chair of Excellence of the Agence Nationale de Recherche assigned to Dr. Cesari. The funders had no role in study design, data collection and analysis, decision to publish, or preparation of the manuscript.

Competing Interests: The authors have declared that no competing interests exist.

* Email: macesari@gmail.com

Introduction

The aging of our societies combined with the high costs of healthcare directed towards older persons (especially if disabled) represent major threats for the sustainability of public health services. In these last years, early actions aimed at implementing strategies against the onset of disabling conditions have been repeatedly advocated [1,2]. Programs of primary prevention aimed at avoiding the beginning of the irreversible disabling process are indeed urgently needed. Obviously, they should target individuals who are not already experiencing the outcome of interest (i.e. disability), but are still exposed to specific risk factors

for it. In this context, the so-called "frailty syndrome" is largely recognized as an interesting and promising pre-disability state to consider [3]. Frailty is described as a multi-systemic disruption of the organism's homeostasis and characterized by an extreme vulnerability to endogenous and exogenous stressors [4]. The detection of frail older individuals living in the community has repeatedly been advocated as the first step for building up effective prevention strategies against its negative health-related consequences (including falls, disability, institutionalizations, and mortality) [5,6].

A wide range of instruments has been developed over the years for identifying frailty in the elderly. Unfortunately, available screening tools for the identification of non-disabled frail older persons still present two major limitations: 1) very few are valid for self-completion, and 2) none enables to differentiate frailty from disability.

As mentioned, although some exceptions exist (e.g., the PRISMA-7 tool [7,8], or the Sherbrooke Postal Questionnaire [9]), most of the available instruments are not designed to be self-administered. This represents a relevant issue if the screening has to target large populations, such as in the case of preventive campaigns against disability requiring the evaluation of community-dwelling older persons. For example, the well-known frailty phenotype [10] is not feasible without the help of an assessor trained at 1) conducting the interview (including a complex questionnaire such as the Minnesota Leisure Time Activity for estimating the kcal/week of energy consumption [11]), and 2) administer the physical function tests (i.e. usual gait speed test and handgrip strength measurement). It is noteworthy that the frailty phenotype also requires the use of a dynamometer, which tends to be rarely available even in the clinical setting (especially in primary care). For facilitating the clinical implementation of the frailty syndrome, Ensrud and colleagues [12] proposed and validated the use of the three defining criteria (i.e. fatigue, involuntary weight loss, and chair stand test) in the Study of Osteoporotic Fractures (SOF). Nevertheless, such simplification did not still completely solve the problem concerning the need of an assessor/supervisor. In fact, there might be safety issues (e.g. risk of falls) at promoting the self-assessment of the chair stand test (i.e. ability to rise from a chair 5 times without using the arms) without supervision, especially if the target population may include frail older persons. The Gérontopôle Frailty Screening Tool (GFST) [13] and the 7-point Clinical Frailty Scale [14] again require the presence of an assessor. In particular, they are largely based on the subjective clinical judgment of a clinician. When searching for the right instrument for screening frailty in community-dwelling older persons, it is also important to keep in mind the dynamic nature of the frailty syndrome. This means that it is easily foreseeable the need of repeatedly screening the target population on a regular basis. Such need poses serious problems in terms of feasibility due to the consequent high demands of resources, budget, and personnel to devote, confirming the implementation of self-reported questionnaires as the most solid solution. Recently, Morley and colleagues proposed the FRAIL questionnaire which has the characteristics for being easily be self-assessed by the older person [15]. Nevertheless, this tool has not the capacity to well differentiate a frail person from one with disability. Such limitation (common to all the existing frailty screening tools) makes this as well as the other instruments inadequate for identifying possible candidates to preventive interventions against disability.

In order to foster the identification of non-disabled older persons at risk of negative health-related outcomes living in the community, we designed the "Frail non-Disabled" (FiND) questionnaire. The novel instrument follows the main multidimensional construct of the widely adopted frailty phenotype [10]. At the same time, it also includes a specific section for excluding the presence of mobility disability (an early stage of the disabling process) [16–18]. In the present study, we formally test the agreement of results obtained from the FiND questionnaire with those coming from reference instruments measuring the frailty syndrome and disability in a sample of community-dwelling older persons.

Methods

Study sample

A total of 144 individuals randomly drawn from the electoral lists of the general population living in the area of Labastide-Murat (Lot department, France) were invited at undergoing a clinical visit at the Centre Médicale "La Roseraie" (Montfaucon, France). Data are from the 45 subjects accepting to participate (see the "sample size calculation" section).

At the study center, a study physician assessed whether the subject met the eligibility criteria of the study. The inclusion criteria were 1) age of 60 years and older, 2) Mini Mental State Exam (MMSE) [19] score $\geq 18/30$, and 3) absence of any acute disease or injury. Exclusion criteria were 1) failure to provide informed consent, 2) living in nursing home, and 3) systolic blood pressure ≥ 170 mmHg and/or diastolic blood pressure ≥ 110 mmHg. In order to not include individuals with acute or subacute conditions preventing the safe conduction of the 400-meter test [20], recent (previous 6 months) overnight hospitalizations for the following conditions (not considered absolute non-inclusion criteria) were investigated: heart attack, stroke, cancer, arthritis, diabetes mellitus, and hip fracture.

Participants were asked to autonomously complete the FiND questionnaire. Then, a blinded assessor objectively measured the frailty and mobility disability status of each participant.

All participants signed an informed consent for participating in the study. The study protocol was approved by the local Institutional Review Board (Comité de Protection des Personnes Sud-Ouest et Outre-Mer, Toulouse).

The FiND questionnaire

The FiND questionnaire (Table 1) consists of five different questions. Two questions (A and B) are specifically aimed at identifying individuals with mobility disability (an early stage of the disabling process [16,21]). For the present analyses, the presence of mobility disability was defined as "a lot of difficulties" or "inability" at performing at least one of these two tasks.

Three additional questions (items C–E) were aimed at assessing signs, symptoms, or conditions commonly considered as components of the frailty syndrome [10]: weight loss (item C), exhaustion (item D), and sedentary behavior (item E). In the present analyses, participants presenting one or more frailty criteria in the absence of mobility disability (items A and B) were considered as "frail". It is noteworthy that the weight loss and exhaustion criteria included in the FiND questionnaire are exactly the same of those originally proposed in the frailty phenotype.

Participants reporting no mobility disability as well as no frailty criterion were considered as robust at the FiND questionnaire.

Mobility disability

Mobility disability was defined as the incapacity to complete a 400-meter walk test [20]. The dichotomous result of the 400-meter walk test (i.e. ability versus inability to successfully complete the test) has been used in major clinical trials on mobility disability as primary outcome [16,21]. As mentioned above, mobility disability represents an early stage of the disabling cascade and a proxy for community ambulation. In fact, the 400-meter distance mirrors the minimum distance an older person should be able to cover in order to maintain his/her full independence [16–18].

The 400-meter walk test was conducted over a track marked using two cones placed 20 meters apart. Participants were asked to start from a still standing position, walk down the corridor at their usual pace, turn around the cones in a continuous loop, and repeat the course 10 times in order to complete a 400-meter walk. During

Table 1. The FiND questionnaire.

Domain	Questions	Answers	Score
Disability	**A.** Have you any difficulties at walking 400 meters?	a. No or some difficulties	0
		b. A lot of difficulties or unable	1
	B. Have you any difficulties at climbing up a flight of stairs?	a. No or some difficulties	0
		b. A lot of difficulties or unable	1
Frailty	**C.** During the last year, have you involuntarily lost more than 4.5 kg?	a. No	0
		b. Yes	1
	D. How often in the last week did you feel than everything you did was an effort or that you could not get going?	a. Rarely or sometimes (twice or less/week)	0
		b. Often or almost always (3 or more times per week)	1
	E. Which is your level of physical activity?	a. Regular physical activity (at least 2–4 hours per week)	0
		b. None or mainly sedentary	1

If A+B≥1, the individual is considered as "disabled".
If A+B=0 and C+D+E≥1, the individual is considered as "frail".
If A+B+C+D+E=0, the individual is considered as "robust".

the test, participants could not use any assistive device. If participants felt the need to stop and rest, they were allowed to do it provided that 1) resumed the walking within 60 seconds, and 2) did not sit down. There were no limits to the number of allowable stops to rest as long as the participant could complete the walk within 15 minutes.

Participants unable to complete the 400-meter walk, taking more than 15 minutes to complete it, and/or sitting during a rest stop were considered to be mobility disabled [22].

Frailty

The frailty phenotype proposed by Fried and colleagues [10] was used in the present study as reference measure of frailty. The frailty phenotype has shown to be predictive of major health-related negative outcomes in older persons [6]. It was assessed using the five items originally validated in the Cardiovascular Health Study [10], as follows:

- Slow gait speed. Usual gait speed was measured over a 4.57-meter (15-feet) track starting from a standing still position. The slow gait speed criterion was defined as present if the measured gait speed was below the gender- and height-specific cut-points proposed in the original description of the frailty phenotype [10].
- Poor muscle strength. Muscle strength was assessed by using a hand-held dynamometer (model Jamar, Sammons Preston, United Kingdom). Participants were asked to perform the test twice with each hand. The best result was used for the present analyses. The presence of the poor muscle strength criterion was considered as present if below the originally defined thresholds adjusted for gender and body mass index [10].
- Exhaustion. This criterion was considered as present if the participant answered "often" or "most of the time" to either of the two following questions part of the Center for Epidemiological Studies-Depression (CES-D) scale [23]: a) How often in the last week you felt that everything you did was an effort?, and b) How often in the last week you felt that you could not get going?

- Involuntary weight loss. It was defined as unintentional loss of more than 4.5 kg in the past year.
- Sedentary behavior. Participants' physical activity level was measured by means of the Leisure Time Physical Activity questionnaire [24], the modified version of the Minnesota Leisure Time Activity Questionnaire originally used in the Cardiovascular Health study [11,25]. The criterion was considered as present if the physical activity level fell below the gender-specific thresholds (i.e. <383 kcal/week in men, < 270 kcal/week in women) originally proposed by Fried and colleagues [10].

After exclusion of those failing the 400-meter walk test (identified as mobility disabled), the frail, the remaining participants were defined as frail, pre-frail, and robust according to the presence of ≥3, 1-2, and no frailty criteria, respectively [10].

Statistical analysis

Sample size calculation. In a test for agreement between two assessments using the Kappa statistics, a sample of 45 subjects was identifying as achieving 90.4% power (at significance level of 0.05) to detect a true Kappa value of 0.7 in a test of H0: Kappa = 0.30 vs. H1: Kappa <>0.30 [26]. Sample size analyses were conducted considering 3-level categorical variables with frequencies equal to 16% (disabled), 59% (pre-frail and frail), and 25% (robust) as described in literature for the French population [27].

Data analysis. Data are presented as percentages, or means ± standard deviations (SD). Cohen's kappa coefficients were calculated to determine the agreement between the FiND questionnaire (and its components) with the reference instruments (i.e. frailty phenotype and mobility disability). For 3×3 tables, quadratic weights (i.e. 1, 0.75, 0) were also applied in the calculation of agreements and kappa coefficients. Sensitivity and specificity of the FiND questionnaire for the identification of non-disabled frail participants were also calculated. SPSS (version 20.0 for Mac, SPSS Inc., Chicago, IL) and Stata (version 12.0SE, StataCorp, College Station, TX) were used for the present analyses.

Table 2. Characteristics of the study sample (n = 45).

	Mean ± SD, or n (percentage)
Age (years)	72.5±8.2
Gender (women)	28 (62.2)
Body Mass Index (kg/m²)	26.5±3.8
Mini Mental State Examination	28.2±2.6
Arthritis	21 (46.7)
Cardiovascular disease	7 (15.6)
Diabetes	7 (15.6)
Depression	5 (11.1)
History of cancer	7 (15.6)
Hypertension	14 (31.1)
Osteoporosis	5 (11.1)
Respiratory disease	8 (17.8)
Systolic blood pressure (mmHg)	132.4±17.6
Diastolic blood pressure (mmHg)	73.7±12.4

SD: standard deviation.

Results

Main characteristics of the study sample (n = 45) are presented in Table 2. Mean age of participants was 72.5 (SD 8.2) years, and women were slightly more prevalent than men (62.2% versus 37.8%).

Seven (15.6%) participants presented mobility disability as being unable to complete the 400-meter walk test. Participants with mobility disability had a slower gait speed at the 4.57-meter (0.71 [SD 0.49] m/sec as well as the 400-meter walk (0.25 [SD 0.24] m/sec, taking into account the exact distance they covered, i.e. 154.3 [SD 176.1] m) tests compare to those who were not mobility disabled (1.13 [SD 0.34] m/sec and 1.19 [SD 0.23] m/sec, respectively; all p values <0.01).

According to the criteria proposed by Fried and colleagues [10], 25 (55.6%) participants were defined as pre-frail or frail, and 13 (28.9%) were robust. The prevalence of the frailty criteria (after exclusion of participants with mobility disability) was (in descending order): sedentary behavior (57.9%), exhaustion (13.2%), poor muscle strength (10.5%), slow gait speed (2.6%), and involuntary weight loss (2.6%).

Table 3 presents the comparison of results from the FiND questionnaire and the reference instruments. Overall, it was reported a substantial agreement between the two assessments (84.4%; kappa = 0.748, p<0.001), which also increased when quadratic weights (i.e. 1, 0.75, 0) were applied in the 3×3 table (96.1%, weighted kappa = 0.836, p<0.001). Only 7 (15.6%) participants were incorrectly categorized.

The agreement between results of the FiND disability domain and the 400-meter walk test (dichotomous variable) was excellent (97.8%; kappa = 0.920, p<0.001). For what concerns the FiND frailty domain, the agreements with the reference items of the frailty phenotype were (in descending order): involuntary weight loss (100%; kappa = 1.000, p<0.001), exhaustion (86.7%; kappa = 0.615, p<0.001), and sedentary behavior (77.8%; kappa = 0.537, p<0.001).

Results from analyses aimed at evaluating the capacity of the FiND questionnaire to correctly identify non-disabled frail older persons (that is differentiating the pre-frail and frail subjects from the robust and disabled ones) are presented in Table 4. Again, a substantial agreement of the questionnaire with the reference instruments was found (84.4%; kappa = 0.693, p<0.001). The FiND questionnaire presented a 95% specificity (95%CI 75.1–99.2%) and 76% (95%CI 54.9–90.6%) in the identification of non-disabled frail participants.

Discussion

In this study, we formally tested the agreement between a novel self-reported screening tool aimed at identifying non-disabled frail older persons with reference instruments. Aim of the FiND questionnaire is to support the identification of community-dwelling older persons presenting an increased risk profile (i.e. frailty syndrome) in the absence of mobility disability. Main characteristic of the instrument is design allowing the individual's self-assessment. Overall, our study shows a substantial agreement between results of the FiND questionnaire with those obtained from reference assessment tools.

Non-disabled frail older persons are frequently indicated in literature as the ideal target population for preventive interventions against disability in the elderly [1–3,6]. The identification of such individuals (particularly prevalent in our societies) represents a crucial preliminary step in the development of effective prevention against disability and age-related conditions. As occurring for every primary prevention campaign, the screening of a risk factor or early sign of the disease should not be only delegated to general practitioners, but go through a cultural modification in the society. This means that the single individual should be made aware of the modifiable risk condition, its consequences, and the possible available counteractions to take. An increased knowledge about the frailty syndrome and the disabling process in the general population may promote the adoption of healthier lifestyles. Moreover, shifting the screening phase from the general practitioner to the individual him/herself will likely 1) anticipate the identification of possible health problems (thus potentially facilitating the reversion of the risk condition), and 2) reduce the tasks already overcharging the general practitioners' activities.

Table 3. Comparison of results from the FiND questionnaire with those obtained from the frailty phenotype and 400-meter walk test.

| | | Frailty phenotype + 400-meter walk test | | |
		Robust	Pre-frail or frail	Mobility disabled
FiND	Robust	12 (26.7)	5 (11.1)	0 (-)
	Frail	1 (2.2)	19 (42.2)	0 (-)
	Disabled	0 (-)	1 (2.2)	7 (15.6)

Results are presented as number of participants (percentage of the overall sample).
Unweighted agreement: 84.4%; unweighted Cohen's kappa coefficient: k = 0.748, p<0.001
Quadratic weighted agreement: 96.1%; Quadratic weighted Cohen's kappa coefficient: k = 0.836, p<0.001.

To our knowledge, the FiND questionnaire is the only assessment tool designed for differentiating frailty from disability. In fact, current frailty instruments provide estimates of the individual's risk profile, but do not inform whether disability is already present. This means that the identification of the non-disabled frail elder could not be conducted without an additional assessment tool specifically measuring the disability status. Such second evaluation is obviously time-consuming and limits the feasibility of the screening, especially when to be applied on a large population. Indeed, the FiND questionnaire fills this gap in the field. In fact, it supports the identification of elders who are experiencing an increased risk of negative events without yet showing signs of mobility disability.

It might be argued that our operationalization might have limited the relevance of gait speed in the definition of frailty, as potentially suggested by the low prevalence of "slow gait speed" after mobility disabled individuals were excluded. It is noteworthy that the choice of focusing the disability assessment only considering the mobility domain is motivated by the hypothesized use of the FiND questionnaire in the framework of preventive actions against disability. By using mobility disability to censor the frailty status, we have confined frailty between robustness and an early stage of the disabling process when the individual is starting to lose his/her capacity to adequately interact with the surrounding environment [16–18]. The fact that non-disabled frail older persons present a low prevalence of slow gait speed may be explained by the strong relationship between this parameter and the disability condition. In fact, it is possible that below a certain threshold of gait speed (here operationalized according to the cut-points proposed by Fried and colleagues [10]), it might be particularly unlikely to find non-disabled individuals (especially if the disability definition is centered on the mobility domain as in our study).

The provision of a self-assessment screening tool as the FiND questionnaire may thus support preventive campaigns against disability by indicating to the general population that specific symptoms and signs should not be underestimated and worth to be verified by a clinician. In fact, in a hypothetical scenario, the positive results of the FiND questionnaire should drive the individual at looking for medical advice and verified by the general practitioner (remaining the primary responsible for the individual's health). If the presence of the frailty syndrome will be confirmed, the general practitioner will then consider the need of further diagnostic procedures (e.g. comprehensive geriatric assessment) in order to understand the nature and causes of the frailty syndrome. In particular, the identification of frailty in the absence of mobility disability may support the extension of the comprehensive geriatric assessment technology from its current use (mostly in already disabled individuals) to the novel scenario of disability prevention. Given the large size of the target population (i.e. elders living in the community), it would be otherwise unfeasible delegating to the general practitioner such screening procedures. Furthermore, such hypothetical clinical pathway is common to what already in place for many other preventable diseases. For example, women have been informed about the importance of breast cancer screening and instructed about how to conduct a regular self-assessment. In case of abnormal findings at the self-palpation, the woman seeks for medical advice to plan the eventual diagnostic process.

To date, although the theoretical foundations of the frailty syndrome are quite well described and agreed, no operational definition has been able to attire general consensus. In the present study, we adopted the frailty phenotype [10] as the most commonly used operational definition. Moreover, given its design rendering frailty as a syndrome, this instrument seems particularly suitable for designing preventive strategies against a multidimensional condition as disability. Nevertheless, it should always be considered the difference between the assessment instrument and the measured condition. As the frailty phenotype is not the frailty syndrome *per se* (but its reflection through an *ad hoc* designed

Table 4. Comparison of results aimed at isolating frail non-disabled participants (thus potential candidates to preventive interventions against disability) with the FiND questionnaire versus the combination frailty phenotype and 400-meter walk test.

| | | Frailty phenotype + 400-meter walk test | |
		Robust or mobility disabled	Pre-frail or frail
FiND	Robust or disabled	19 (42.2)	6 (13.3)
	Frail	1 (2.2)	19 (42.2)

Results are presented as number of participants (percentage of the overall sample).
Agreement: 84.4%; Cohen's kappa coefficient: k = 0.693, p<0.001.

instrument), the FiND questionnaire was not designed to propose a "novel" operational definition for the condition of interest. As most of the other existing instruments, it remains a screening tool for a complex and heterogeneous risk condition (i.e. frailty). Therefore, as mentioned above, its positive results should necessarily be followed by a specific diagnostic pathway (i.e. comprehensive geriatric assessment) to understand the underlying biological, clinical, and social foundation of the risk condition.

The present study has several limitations worth to be mentioned. The study population was recruited in a rural area in France. The living environment might modify the frailty profile [28], thus potentially affecting our results. Nevertheless, since the FiND questionnaire was designed for mirroring as much as possible the reference instrument, we would not expect major differences in the agreement when testing other populations. Moreover, it should be considered that the FiND questionnaire is indeed very similar to the original frailty phenotype, having 2 of the 5 original criteria (i.e. involuntary weight loss and exhaustion) exactly replicated. Different results might have been obtained if the FiND questionnaire was tested versus other frailty (e.g. Frailty Index [14]) or disability (e.g. Activities of Daily Living [29]) reference tools. However, the choice of using the frailty phenotype and the 400-meter walk test was motivated by their widespread use and capacity to detect early phases of the disabling process, respectively. Furthermore, the adoption as reference of a frailty instrument rather than another may have secondary importance at this time when a largely agreed operational definition is still lacking. Finally, although based on *ad hoc* sample size analyses, the relatively small number of participants in our study might have affected some of findings. In particular, the evaluation of specific sub-populations in which the agreement of the FiND question-

naire may differ (e.g. subjects with low cognitive function) was not possible. In this context, further studies are needed to confirm and expand our findings.

In conclusion, the proposed screening tool (i.e. FiND questionnaire) may represent an opportunity for diffusing awareness about frailty and disability among community-dwelling older persons and supporting specific preventive campaigns. Moreover, allowing older persons to self-evaluate their health status profile will 1) avoid to delegate the screening of such burdening and highly prevalent conditions to healthcare professionals, and 2) potentially anticipate possible preventive interventions against the disabling process (under the coordination of the general practitioner).

Acknowledgments

The present study was possible thanks to the enthusiastic support received by the populations, local authorities (majors, Communauté de Communes du Causse de Labastide-Murat, Agence Regionale de Santé) and public health professionals (general practitioners, nurses, physical therapists, pharmacist, social assistants, home care personnel) of the following participating towns: Beaumat, Blars, Caniac du Causse, Fontanes du Causse, Frayssinet, Ginouillac, Labastide-Murat, Lunegarde, Montfaucon, Saint Sauveur La Vallée, Senaillac Lauzes, Seniergues, Soulomes, Vaillac. Special thanks also go to Mrs. Virginie Bruyere for her crucial help in the practical organization and conduction of the study.

Author Contributions

Conceived and designed the experiments: MC SG GAVK BV SA. Performed the experiments: MC LD HB SG. Analyzed the data: MC LD. Contributed reagents/materials/analysis tools: MC LD. Wrote the paper: MC LD HB SG GAVK BV SA. Critical revision of the manuscript: MC LD HB SG GAVK BV SA.

References

1. Morley JE, Vellas B, Abellan van Kan G, Anker SD, Bauer JM, et al. (2013) Frailty consensus: a call to action. J Am Med Dir Assoc 14: 392–397.
2. Vellas B, Cestac P, Morley JE (2012) Implementing frailty into clinical practice: we cannot wait. J Nutr Health Aging 16: 599–600.
3. Subra J, Gillette-Guyonnet S, Cesari M, Oustric S, Vellas B (2012) The integration of frailty into clinical practice: preliminary results from the gérontopôle. J Nutr Health Aging 16: 714–720.
4. Rodríguez-Mañas L, Féart C, Mann G, Viña J, Chatterji S, et al. (2012) Searching for an Operational Definition of Frailty: A Delphi Method Based Consensus Statement. The Frailty Operative Definition-Consensus Conference Project. J Gerontol A Biol Sci Med Sci 68: 62–67.
5. Ferrucci L, Guralnik JM, Studenski S, Fried LP, Cutler GB, et al. (2004) Designing randomized, controlled trials aimed at preventing or delaying functional decline and disability in frail, older persons: a consensus report. J Am Geriatr Soc 52: 625–634.
6. Clegg A, Young J, Iliffe S, Rikkert MO, Rockwood K (2013) Frailty in elderly people. Lancet 381: 752–762.
7. Hebert R, Raiche M, Dubois MF, Gueye NR, Dubuc N, et al. (2010) Impact of PRISMA, a coordination-type integrated service delivery system for frail older people in Quebec (Canada): A quasi-experimental study. J Gerontol B Psychol Sci Soc Sci 65B: 107–118.
8. Hoogendijk EO, van der Horst HE, Deeg DJ, Frijters DH, Prins BA, et al. (2013) The identification of frail older adults in primary care: comparing the accuracy of five simple instruments. Age Ageing 42: 262–265.
9. Hebert R, Bravo G, Korner-Bitensky N, Voyer L (1996) Predictive validity of a postal questionnaire for screening community-dwelling elderly individuals at risk of functional decline. Age Ageing 25: 159–167.
10. Fried LP, Tangen CM, Walston J, Newman AB, Hirsch C, et al. (2001) Frailty in older adults: evidence for a phenotype. J Gerontol A Biol Sci Med Sci 56: M146–M156.
11. Taylor HL, Jacobs DRJ, Schucker B, Knudsen J, Leon AS, et al. (1978) A questionnaire for the assessment of leisure time physical activities. J Chronic Dis 31: 741–755.
12. Ensrud K, Ewing SK, Taylor BC, Fink HA, Cawthon P, et al. (2008) Comparison of 2 frailty indexes for prediction of falls, disability, fractures, and death in older women. Arch Intern Med 168: 382–389.
13. Vellas B, Balardy L, Gillette-Guyonnet S, Abellan Van Kan G, Ghisolfi-Marque A, et al. (2013) Looking for Frailty in Community-Dwelling Older Persons: The Gerontopole Frailty Screening Tool (GFST). J Nutr Health Aging 17: 629–631.
14. Rockwood K, Song X, MacKnight C, Bergman H, Hogan DB, et al. (2005) A global clinical measure of fitness and frailty in elderly people. CMAJ 173: 489–495.
15. Morley JE, Malmstrom TK, Miller DK (2012) A Simple Frailty Questionnaire (FRAIL) Predicts Outcomes in Middle Aged African Americans. J Nutr Health Aging 16: 601–608.
16. Fielding RA, Rejeski WJ, Blair S, Church T, Espeland MA, et al. (2011) The Lifestyle Interventions and Independence for Elders Study: Design and Methods. J Gerontol A Biol Sci Med Sci 66: 1226–1237.
17. Hirvensalo M, Rantanen T, Heikkinen E (2000) Mobility difficulties and physical activity as predictors of mortality and loss of independence in the community-living older population. J Am Geriatr Soc 48: 493–498.
18. Hardy SE, Kang Y, Studenski S, Degenholtz HB (2011) Ability to walk 1/4 mile predicts subsequent disability, mortality, and health care costs. J Gen Intern Med 26: 130–135.
19. Folstein MF, Folstein SE, McHugh PR (1975) "Mini-mental state". A practical method for grading the cognitive state of patients for the clinician. J Psychiatr Res 12: 189–198.
20. Newman AB, Simonsick EM, Naydeck BL, Boudreau R, Kritchevsky SB, et al. (2006) Association of long-distance corridor walk performance with mortality, cardiovascular disease, mobility limitation, and disability. JAMA 295: 2018–2026.
21. Pahor M, Blair SN, Espeland M, Fielding R, Gill TM, et al. (2006) Effects of a physical activity intervention on measures of physical performance: Results of the lifestyle interventions and independence for Elders Pilot (LIFE-P) study. J Gerontol A Biol Sci Med Sci 61: 1157–1165.
22. Rolland YM, Cesari M, Miller ME, Penninx BW, Atkinson HH, et al. (2004) Reliability of the 400-m usual-pace walk test as an assessment of mobility limitation in older adults. J Am Geriatr Soc 52: 972–976.
23. Orme JG, Reis J, Herz EJ (1986) Factorial and discriminant validity of the Center for Epidemiological Studies Depression (CES-D) scale. J Clin Psychol 42: 28–33.
24. Martin MY, Powell MP, Peel C, Zhu S, Allman R (2006) Leisure-time physical activity and health-care utilization in older adults. J Aging Phys Act 14: 392–410.
25. Siscovick DS, Fried L, Mittelmark M, Rutan G, Bild D, et al. (1997) Exercise intensity and subclinical cardiovascular disease in the elderly. The Cardiovascular Health Study. Am J Epidemiol 145: 977–986.
26. Flack VF, Afifi AA, Lachenbruch PA, Schouten HJA (1988) Sample size determinations for the two rater Kappa statistic. Psychometrika 53: 321–325.

27. Santos-Eggimann B, Cuénoud P, Spagnoli J, Junod J (2009) Prevalence of frailty in middle-aged and older community-dwelling Europeans living in 10 countries. J Gerontol A Biol Sci Med Sci 64: 675–681.

28. Raphael D, Cava M, Brown I, Renwick R, Heathcote K, et al. (1995) Frailty: a public health perspective. Can J Public Health 86: 224–227.

29. Katz S, Downs TD, Cash HR, Grotz RC (1970) Progress in development of the index of ADL. Gerontologist 10: 20-30.

## 16

The Adherence to Initial Processes of Care in Elderly Patients with Acute Venous Thromboembolism

Anna K. Stuck[1]*, Marie Méan[1], Andreas Limacher[2], Marc Righini[3], Kurt Jaeger[4], Hans-Jürg Beer[5], Joseph Osterwalder[6], Beat Frauchiger[7], Christian M. Matter[8,13], Nils Kucher[9], Michael Egloff[10], Markus Aschwanden[4], Marc Husmann[11], Anne Angelillo-Scherrer[12], Nicolas Rodondi[1], Drahomir Aujesky[1]

1 Division of General Internal Medicine, Bern University Hospital, Bern, Switzerland, 2 CTU Bern, Department of Clinical Research, and Institute of Social and Preventive Medicine, University of Bern, Bern, Switzerland, 3 Division of Angiology and Hemostasis, Geneva University Hospital, Geneva, Switzerland, 4 Division of Angiology, Basel University Hospital, Basel, Switzerland, 5 Cantonal Hospital of Baden, Baden, Switzerland, 6 Emergency Department, Cantonal Hospital of St. Gallen, St. Gallen, Switzerland, 7 Department of Internal Medicine, Cantonal Hospital of Frauenfeld, Frauenfeld, Switzerland, 8 Cardiovascular Research, Institute of Physiology, Zurich Center for Integrative Human Physiology, University of Zurich, Zurich, Switzerland, 9 Division of Angiology, Bern University Hospital, Bern, Switzerland, 10 Division of Diabetology, Geneva University Hospital, Geneva, Switzerland, 11 Clinic of Angiology, Zurich University Hospital, Zurich, Switzerland, 12 University Clinic of Hematology and Hematology Central Laboratory, Bern University Hospital, Bern, Switzerland, 13 Division of Cardiology, Zurich University Hospital, Zurich, Switzerland

Abstract

Background: We aimed to assess whether elderly patients with acute venous thromboembolism (VTE) receive recommended initial processes of care and to identify predictors of process adherence.

Methods: We prospectively studied in- and outpatients aged ≥65 years with acute symptomatic VTE in a multicenter cohort study from nine Swiss university- and non-university hospitals between September 2009 and March 2011. We systematically assessed whether initial processes of care, which are recommended by the 2008 American College of Chest Physicians guidelines, were performed in each patient. We used multivariable logistic models to identify patient factors independently associated with process adherence.

Results: Our cohort comprised 950 patients (mean age 76 years). Of these, 86% (645/750) received parenteral anticoagulation for ≥5 days, 54% (405/750) had oral anticoagulation started on the first treatment day, and 37% (274/750) had an international normalized ratio (INR) ≥2 for ≥24 hours before parenteral anticoagulation was discontinued. Overall, 35% (53/153) of patients with cancer received low-molecular-weight heparin monotherapy and 72% (304/423) of patients with symptomatic deep vein thrombosis were prescribed compression stockings. In multivariate analyses, symptomatic pulmonary embolism, hospital-acquired VTE, and concomitant antiplatelet therapy were associated with a significantly lower anticoagulation-related process adherence.

Conclusions: Adherence to several recommended processes of care was suboptimal in elderly patients with VTE. Quality of care interventions should particularly focus on processes with low adherence, such as the prescription of continued low-molecular-weight heparin therapy in patients with cancer and the achievement of an INR ≥2 for ≥24 hours before parenteral anticoagulants are stopped.

Editor: Hugo ten Cate, Maastricht University Medical Center, Netherlands

Funding: The study was funded by a grant from the Swiss National Science Foundation (33CSCO-122659/139470). The funders had no role in study design, data collection and analysis, decision to publish, or preparation of the manuscript.

Competing Interests: The authors have declared that no competing interests exist.

* Email: anna.stuck@insel.ch

Introduction

The incidence of acute venous thromboembolism (VTE), defined as acute deep vein thrombosis (DVT) or pulmonary embolism (PE), rises exponentially with age [1,2]. In the geriatric population, VTE not only carries a higher mortality but also a higher rate of VTE recurrence and major bleeding than in younger patients [3].

The American College of Chest Physicians (ACCP) Evidence-based Clinical Practice Guidelines recommend specific processes of care for the management of patients with acute VTE [4,5]. Several of these processes have the potential to improve patient outcomes and to reduce the length of hospital stay and health care costs [6–12]. These recommended processes include the administration of parenteral anticoagulation for at least five days, initiation of oral anticoagulation on the first treatment day, maintenance of an International Normalized Ratio (INR) ≥2 for at least 24 hours before parenteral anticoagulation is discontinued, continued therapy with low-molecular-weight heparin (LMWH) in patients with cancer, and the use of compression stockings in

Table 1. Patient Baseline Characteristics

Characteristic	n (%)[a]
Age>80 years	261 (28)
Female sex	443 (47)
BMI>30 kg/m^2	226 (24)
Nursing home care	24 (3)
Higher level of educational[b]	427 (45)
Symptomatic PE[c]	654 (69)
Hospital-acquired VTE[d]	175 (18)
History of major bleeding	92 (10)
Active cancer[e]	153 (16)
Cardiovascular comorbidity[f]	231 (24)
Diabetes mellitus	147 (15)
Renal impairment[g]	197 (21)
Anemia[h]	374 (39)
Low platelet count (<150×10^9/L)	131 (14)
Concomitant antiplatelet medication[i]	315 (33)
Polypharmacy[k]	489 (51)

Abbreviations: BMI = body mass index; PE = pulmonary embolism; VTE = venous thromboembolism.
[a]Overall, missing values were 0.5% for BMI, 0.1% for nursing home care, 0.2% for higher level of education, 0.1% for history of major bleeding, 6.6% for hemoglobin level, and 6.6% for platelet count.
[b]High school or post high school attendance.
[c]Symptomatic PE with or without a deep vein thrombosis.
[d]VTE event occurring during a hospital stay.
[e]Requiring chemotherapy, radiotherapy, surgery, or palliative care during the last three months.
[f]Acute heart failure or history of heart failure or coronary heart disease.
[g]Glomerular filtration rate <30 ml/min or a history of chronic renal failure.
[h]Hemoglobin level <13 g/dL for men or <12 g/dL for women.
[i]Use of aspirin, clopidogrel, prasugrel, and/or dipyridamol.
[k]Concomitant use of more than four drugs.
(n = 950).

patients with symptomatic DVT [4,5]. Prior studies demonstrated wide practice variation and suboptimal adherence to these processes of care [13–15].

Despite the higher VTE incidence and complication rates in elderly patients, to our knowledge, only two retrospective studies have examined the adherence to VTE-related processes of care in patients aged ≥65 years [16,17]. In a large multicenter prospective cohort study, we therefore assessed whether elderly patients aged 65 years or over with VTE received recommended processes of care in the early phase of VTE and to identify predictors of process adherence.

Methods

Ethics statement

We asked eligible patients to provide written informed consent. The study was approved by the Institutional Review Board of each participating site (Commission cantonale (VD) d'éthique de la recherche sur l'être humain, Commission cantonale d'éthique de la recherche, Kantonale Ethikkommission Bern, Kantonale Ethikkommission Zürich, Kantonale Ethikkommission Kanton Aargau, Ethikkommission des Kanton St. Gallen, Ethikkommission des Kantons Thurgau, Ethikkommission Luzern, Ethikkommission Basel). The committees approved the consent procedure of participants.

Cohort sample

The study was conducted between September 1, 2009 and March 31, 2011 as part of a prospective, multicenter cohort study to assess medical outcomes of patients aged ≥65 years with acute, symptomatic VTE from all five Swiss university and four high-volume non-university hospitals [18]. Potential participants were consecutively identified in the inpatient and outpatient services of all participating study sites. We defined DVT as the acute onset of leg pain or swelling plus incomplete compressibility of a venous segment on ultrasonography or an intraluminal filling defect on contrast venography) [19]. Because the iliac vein and the inferior vena cava may be technically difficult to compress, iliac/caval DVT was defined as abnormal duplex flown patterns compatible with thrombosis or an intraluminal filling defect on contrast computed tomography or magnetic resonance imaging venography [20]. Given that ultrasonography has a reduced sensitivity and specificity for distal DVT [21] patients with distal DVT were included only if the incompressible distal vein transverse diameter was at least 5 mm. We defined PE as the acute onset of dyspnea, chest pain, or syncope coupled with a new high-probability ventilation/perfusion lung scan; a new contrast filling defect on spiral computed tomography or pulmonary angiography; or the new documentation of a proximal DVT either by venous ultrasound or contrast venography [22,23]. Radiographic studies used to diagnose VTE were interpreted by on-site vascular specialists or radiologists.

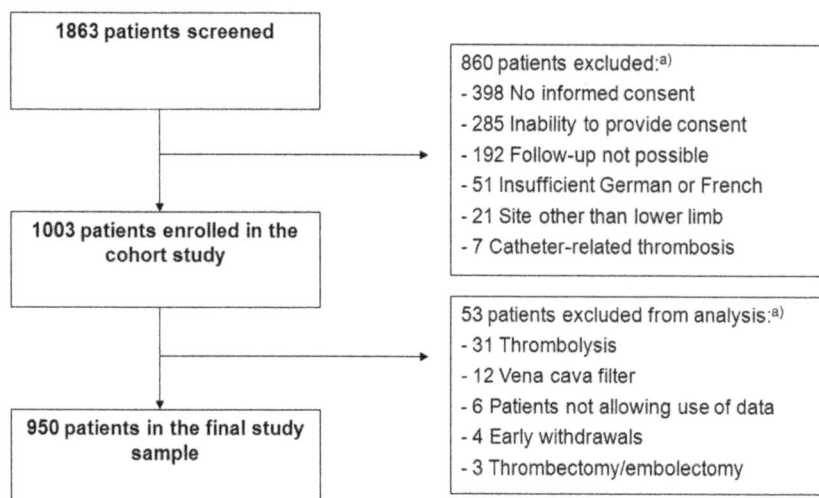

Figure 1. Flow chart. Abbreviations: DVT = deep vein thrombosis. A) Multiple reasons for exclusion may apply.

Exclusion criteria were inability to provide informed consent (i.e., severe dementia), conditions incompatible with follow-up (i.e., terminal illness or place of living too far away from the study center), insufficient German or French speaking ability, thrombosis at a different site than lower limb, catheter-related thrombosis, or previous enrollment in the cohort. We also excluded patients who received thrombolytic therapy, surgical treatment (i.e., thrombo-/embolectomy), or a vena cava filter.

Treatment of VTE, e.g., the type of anticoagulant used (i.e., parenteral anticoagulant followed by vitamin K antagonists or parenteral anticoagulation alone) and the prescription of compression stockings, was entirely left to the discretion of the managing physicians.

Baseline data collection

For all enrolled patients, baseline demographic information (age, gender, weight, height, level of education and place of living), type (PE, DVT, or both) and occurrence of VTE (hospital-acquired vs. home-acquired), comorbid conditions (history of major bleeding, cardiovascular comorbidity, diabetes mellitus, renal impairment), laboratory findings (anemia, low platelet count), concomitant use of platelet inhibitors, and the number of concomitant drug treatments were prospectively collected by medical record review by trained research nurses and recorded on

standard data collection forms. Information was also gathered on pharmacological (type, timing, and duration of anticoagulant treatment) and non-pharmacological treatments (prescription of compression stockings).

Processes of care

We assessed whether the following five processes of care, which were recommended in the 2008 ACCP guidelines [4], were performed in each patient: (1) administration of parenteral anticoagulants for ≥5 days; (2) start of oral anticoagulation on the first treatment day (defined as the administration of the first dose of vitamin K antagonists within 24 hours after VTE diagnosis); (3) continuation of parenteral anticoagulants until an international normalized ratio [INR] ≥2 for at least 24 hours; (4) continued use of LMWH without switching to vitamin K antagonists in patients with an active cancer (defined as active solid or hematologic cancers requiring chemotherapy, radiotherapy, or surgery within the previous three months); and (5) prescription of compression stockings in patients with symptomatic DVT. For our analysis of processes of care 1–3, we considered only patients who were switched from parental anticoagulants to vitamin K antagonists within 21 days. We collected data up to 90 days following the index VTE.

Table 2. Adherence to Recommended Processes of Care.

Processes of care	n/N (%)[a]
1) Duration of parenteral anticoagulation ≥5 days	645/750 (86)
2) Start of oral anticoagulation on the first treatment day	405/750 (54)
3) Parenteral anticoagulation until an INR ≥2 for at least 24 hours	274/750 (37)
4) Continued treatment with LMWH for active cancer	53/153 (35)
5) Prescription of compression stockings for symptomatic DVT	304/423 (72)

Abbreviations: INR = international normalized ratio; LMWH = low-molecular-weight heparin; DVT = deep vein thrombosis.
[a]Denominators change because of different subgroup analyses.
For instance, for processes of care 1–3, we analyzed the 750 patients who were switched from LMWH to oral anticoagulants. For processes of care 4 and 5, we analyzed the 153 with cancer and the 423 patients with symptomatic DVT, respectively.

Table 3. Stratified Analyses by Type of Venous Thromboembolism.

	Overt PE[a] n/N (%)	DVT only n/N (%)	P-value
Parenteneral anticoagulation for ≥5 days	465/546 (85)	180/204 (88)	0.281
Initiation of oral anticoagulation on the first treatment day	283/546(52)	122/204 (60)	0.051
INR ≥2 during at least 24 hours before discontinuation of parenteral anticoagulation	219/546 (40)	55/204 (27)	<0.001
Continued treatment with LMWH for cancer	26/101 (26)	27/52 (52)	0.001
Prescription of compression stockings for symptomatic DVT	88/127 (69)	216/296 (73)	0.440

Abbreviations: PE = pulmonary embolism; DVT = deep vein thrombosis; INR = international normalized ratio; LMWH = low-molecular-weight heparin.
[a]With or without concomitant DVT.

Statistical analyses

Baseline characteristics are shown as numbers and percentages. Analyzed and non-analyzed patients were compared using the chi-squared test or the Wilcoxon rank-sum test as appropriate. For each of the five processes of care, as well as for the combination of the three anticoagulation-related processes of care, the number and proportion of guideline adherence was calculated.

We used logistic regression to explore associations between baseline patient characteristics shown in Table 1 and the adherence to three processes of care: (1) duration of parenteral anticoagulation ≥5 days, (2) start of oral anticoagulation on the first treatment day, and (3) continuation of parenteral anticoagulation until the INR is ≥2 for 24 hours. The sample sizes of the subpopulations with cancer and symptomatic DVT were not large enough to conduct robust multivariable analyses. For missing values, we performed multiple imputation by chained equations [24], assuming missing data to be missing at random. A total of twenty imputed datasets were generated based on all baseline variables, the three outcome variables and study site. Adjusted odds ratios (OR) and corresponding 95% confidence intervals (CI) and P-values were calculated applying Rubin's rules [25]. Adjustment was done for all baseline variables as fixed effects and study site as a random effect in a mixed-effects logistic model. In a sensitivity analysis, a complete case analysis was performed, excluding any cases with missing values. All analyses were performed using STATA statistical software, Version 12.0.

Results

Patient identification and baseline characteristics

Of 1863 patients screened during the study period, 1003 were originally enrolled in the cohort study (Figure 1). Of these, 53 were excluded, leaving a study sample of 950 analyzed patients. Non-analyzed patients were statistically significantly older (mean age 77 vs. 76 years; P<0.001) and more likely to be women (59% vs. 47%; P<0.001) than analyzed patients.

Overall, 28% of patients were aged >80 years, 47% (443/950) were women, and 3% (24/950) were nursing home residents (Table 1). Eighteen percent (175/950) had hospital-acquired VTE. Of the 775 patients who developed VTE in an outpatient setting (community-acquired VTE), 589 (76%) were admitted to the hospital.

Adherence to recommended processes of care

Overall, 750 patients were switched from parental anticoagulants to vitamin K antagonists. Of these, 86% (645/750) received parenteral anticoagulation for ≥5 days, 54% (405/750) had oral anticoagulation started on the first treatment day, and 37% (274/750) had an INR ≥2 for ≥24 hours before parenteral anticoagulation was discontinued (Table 2). Only 18% (138/750) of patients received all three anticoagulation-related processes of care.

Among the 153 patients with active cancer, only 35% (53/153) received continued LMWH, 25% (39/153) received unfractionated heparin or fondaparinux followed by oral anticoagulation, 23% (35/153) unfractionated heparin or fondaparinux alone, 14% (21/153) LMWH followed by oral anticoagulation, 2% (3/153) oral anticoagulation alone, and 1% (2/153) no anticoagulation at all. Of 423 patients who had symptomatic DVT, 72% (304/423) were prescribed compression stockings.

There was some variation by type of VTE. As shown in Table 3, patients with PE were more likely to have an INR ≥2 for ≥ 24 hours before parenteral anticoagulation was stopped than patients with DVT only (40% vs. 27%; P<0.001). On the other hand, patients with cancer who had DVT only were more likely to receive continued treatment with LMWH than patients with PE (52% vs. 26%; P = 0.001).

There was a substantial variation across study sites: adherence varied from 79% to 94% for parenteral anticoagulation for ≥5 days, from 47% to 62% for the start of oral anticoagulation on the first treatment day, from 13% to 50% for an INR ≥2 for ≥ 24 hours before parenteral anticoagulation was discontinued, from 0% to 64% for continued LMWH in patients with cancer, and from 61% to 90% for the prescription of compression stockings in patients with symptomatic DVT.

Predictors of process adherence

In multivariable analyses, patients with hospital-acquired VTE (OR, 2.60; 95% CI, 1.10–6.14) were statistically significantly more likely to receive parenteral anticoagulation for ≥5 days (Figure 2A). Patients with hospital-acquired VTE (OR, 0.37; 95% CI, 0.23–0.60) and overt PE (OR, 0.70; 95% CI, 0.50–0.99) were less likely to receive oral anticoagulation on the first treatment day (Figure 2B). Finally, patients with overt PE (OR, 1.50; 95% CI, 1.02–2.20) and cardiovascular comorbidity (OR, 1.52; 95% CI, 1.01–2.28) were more likely to continue parenteral anticoagulation until the INR was ≥2 for 24 hours, whereas patients with concomitant antiplatelet medication were less likely to have two INR values ≥2 for 24 hours before parenteral anticoagulation was stopped (OR, 0.61; 95% CI, 0.41–0.92) (Figure 2C). Age >80 years was not a significant predictor of process adherence. When patients with missing values were excluded from analyses, results remained similar.

A.

Characteristics		Adjusted[a] OR (95% CI)
Age >80 years		0.72 (0.44 to 1.17)
Female sex		0.88 (0.56 to 1.37)
BMI >30kg/m^2		1.74 (0.99 to 3.08)
Overt PE		0.73 (0.44 to 1.23)
Hospital-acquired VTE		2.60 (1.10 to 6.14)
History of major bleeding		2.41 (0.83 to 6.99)
Cardiovascular comorbidity		1.30 (0.72 to 2.36)
Antiplatelet medication		1.15 (0.66 to 1.98)
Polypharmacy		1.11 (0.67 to 1.84)

B.

Characteristics		Adjusted[a] OR (95% CI)
Age >80 years		1.33 (0.93 to 1.90)
Female sex		0.93 (0.68 to 1.27)
BMI >30kg/m^2		0.72 (0.50 to 1.03)
Overt PE		0.70 (0.50 to 0.99)
Hospital-acquired VTE		0.37 (0.23 to 0.60)
History of major bleeding		0.60 (0.34 to 1.05)
Cardiovascular comorbidity		1.05 (0.71 to 1.56)
Antiplatelet medication		0.81 (0.56 to 1.17)
Polypharmacy		0.85 (0.60 to 1.21)

C.

Characteristics		Adjusted[a] OR (95% CI)
Age >80 years		1.09 (0.75 to 1.57)
Female sex		1.16 (0.84 to 1.61)
BMI >30kg/m^2		1.14 (0.79 to 1.65)
Overt PE		1.50 (1.02 to 2.20)
Hospital-acquired VTE		0.69 (0.42 to 1.14)
History of major bleeding		0.95 (0.54 to 1.68)
Cardiovascular comorbidity		1.52 (1.01 to 2.28)
Antiplatelet medication		0.61 (0.41 to 0.92)
Polypharmacy		1.42 (0.98 to 2.05)

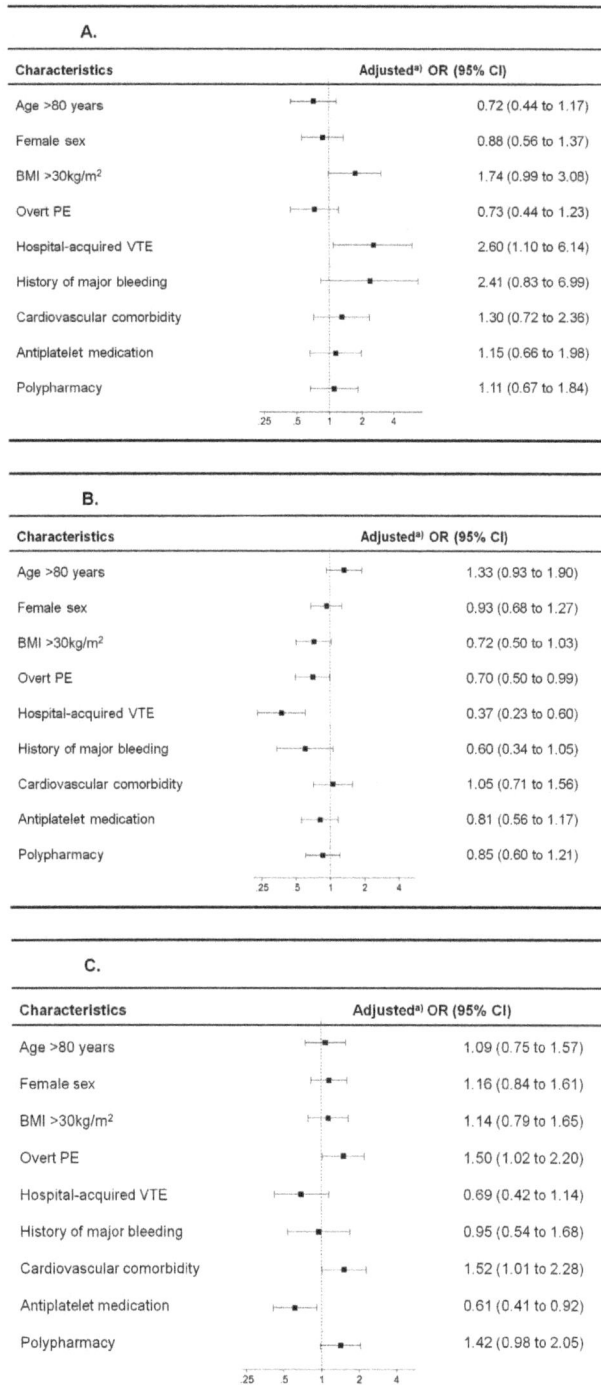

Figure 2. A. Predictors for using parenteral anticoagulation for ≥5 days (n = 750). Abbreviations: OR = odds ratio; CI = confidence interval; BMI = body mass index; VTE = venous thromboembolism; PE = pulmonary embolism. A. a) Adjusted for all baseline characteristics shown in Table 1 as a fixed effect and for study site as a random effect. A selection of variables is displayed in the figures to improve legibility i.e. age, sex and all variables with statistical significant numbers. **B. Predictors for starting oral anticoagulation on the first treatment day (n = 750). C. Predictors for continuing parenteral anticoagulation until an international normalized ratio of ≥2 for 24 hours (n = 750).**

Discussion

In this prospective multicenter cohort study of 950 elderly patients with acute symptomatic VTE, we found that adherence to five recommended processes of care was variable and partially suboptimal. The adherence rate varied from 86% for treatment with parenteral anticoagulants for at least five days to a mere 35% for continued treatment with LMWH in patients with active cancer. Overall, our findings are consistent with prior studies demonstrating that the use of recommended processes of care and the achievement of treatment goals for patients with VTE leaves room for improvement [6,13–17,26].

If anything, adherence rates were even lower in our elderly population (mean age 76 years) for several processes of care than in previous studies enrolling younger patients with VTE (mean age 56–66 years) [6,13–15]. Compared to a retrospective study of U.S. veterans in which oral anticoagulation was initiated on the first treatment day in 64% of cases [6], we found a substantially lower rate in our study sample (54%). In a prospective study of Canadian outpatients with VTE [15], 60% of patients with cancer-related VTE received LMWH monotherapy compared to 35% in our study. While the proportion of patients who had parenteral anticoagulation continued until an INR value ≥2.0 for 24 hours was 37% only in our sample, this target was achieved in about 50% of patients in younger patients [13,14].

Our results demonstrating a low adherence rate to anticoagulation-related processes of care in elderly patients are consistent with prior evidence showing that the rate of anticoagulation is low in hospitalized elderly patients with atrial fibrillation [27]. Elderly, multimorbid medical inpatients have also a low rate of venous thromboprophylaxis [28]. It remains unclear whether the low adherence rate is due to lack of physicians' knowledge, physicians' fear to induce bleeding, the presence of comorbid conditions that are not compatible with guideline adherence, or patient preferences [29]. For instance, elderly patients with cancer who develop VTE are more likely to have severe renal failure and therefore, may not be candidates for extended LMWH treatment. Similarly, although LMWHs seem to be acceptable to patients with cancer [30], many elderly patients may prefer to receive oral anticoagulants rather than daily injections with LMWH. One study found that 30% of physicians did not believe it is necessary to have a therapeutic INR for ≥2 days before discontinuing heparin [14].

Prior evidence about the effect of age on VTE-related anticoagulation practices is limited. While age did not influence the duration of anticoagulant therapy in one study [16], older patients were more likely to have continuation of parenteral anticoagulation until INR was ≥2 for 24 hours in another study [6]. In an Italian registry, compression stockings were 1.6 times more likely to be prescribed in patients aged 40–60 years than in patients aged >80 years [31].

To our knowledge, there are no studies examining the effectiveness of interventions to improve anticoagulation-related processes of care for established VTE. Although evidence from studies on VTE prophylaxis suggests that active, multifaceted strategies, including provider education, electronic alerts, and regular audit and feedback to medical staff, appear to be the most promising interventions [29,32–34], whether such interventions have the potential to improve therapeutic anticoagulation-related care and outcomes of VTE must be further examined.

We could not identify a clear pattern of consistent predictors of suboptimal process adherence that may become potential targets for quality improvement interventions. While hospital-acquired VTE was associated with delayed initiation of oral anticoagulation, patients with the same condition were more likely to get parenteral anticoagulation for ≥5 days. Given that hospitalized patients often undergo diagnostic or therapeutic procedures, parenteral anticoagulation is easier to control and thus possibly preferred. Similarly, patients with PE, who are hospitalized in most instances, were less likely to get oral anticoagulants on the first treatment day but were more likely to have two INR values ≥ 2.0 before parental anticoagulation was stopped. Our finding that patients with concomitant antiplatelet therapy were less likely to have two INR values before stopping parenteral anticoagulation may reflect physicians' underlying fear of bleeding in such patients [29].

Our study has potential limitations. First, our sample may not reflect the full spectrum of elderly patients with VTE because analyzed patients were younger and more likely to be men than non-analyzed patients. Moreover, given that patients were enrolled from hospital inpatient and outpatient services, patients with DVT who were diagnosed and entirely managed in the primary care or nursing home setting may be underrepresented in our sample. This could explain the relatively high proportion of patients who had symptomatic PE (69%) in our cohort. Because we excluded patients with severe dementia who may have a lower process adherence, our study may overestimate the true process adherence rates [35]. However, given that our multicenter cohort study enrolled a broad population of in- and outpatients aged ≥65 years from university- and non-university hospitals, our study sample should be fairly representative for elderly patients with VTE. Second, as treating physicians were aware that patients were included in a cohort study, they may have altered their behavior and better followed recommended processes of care. Thus, we cannot exclude that the adherence rates in our study may overestimate the true process adherence rates. Third, because data on physician characteristics (e.g., type and duration of training) were not available in our database, we could not examine whether these factors were associated with adherence to VTE-related

processes of care. Similarly, we could not explore potential physician barriers to antithrombotic guideline adherence in elderly patients with VTE, which must be done in a further study. Fourth, because patient enrollment in our study started in 2009, we used the 2008 version of the ACCP guidelines as a benchmark for VTE-related quality of care and not the latest 2012 version [4,5]. However, the recommendations with respect to the processes of care examined in our study are basically the same in both versions. Finally, our goal was to examine adherence rates to initial processes of care in elderly patients with VTE and to identify predictors of process adherence. Thus, we did not examine the impact of process adherence on patient outcomes, which must be done in another study.

In conclusion, adherence to recommended processes of care was variable and partially suboptimal in elderly patients with VTE. Additional efforts are needed to increase process adherence and quality of care in such patients. Quality of care interventions should particularly focus on recommended processes with low adherence rates, such as the prescription of continued LMWH in patients in cancer and the achievement of an INR ≥2 for ≥ 24 hours before parenteral anticoagulants are stopped.

Acknowledgments

The authors would like to thank all collaborators of the SWITCO65+ study.

Author Contributions

Conceived and designed the experiments: AKS MM DA. Performed the experiments: MR KJ HJB BF JO NK AAS NR CMM ME MA MH. Analyzed the data: AL. Wrote the paper: AKS DA MM AL. Obtained funding from the Swiss National Foundation: DA MR KJ HJB BF JO NK AAS NR.

References

1. White RH (2003) The epidemiology of venous thromboembolism. Circulation 107: I4–8.
2. Deitelzweig SB, Johnson BH, Lin J, Schulman KL (2011) Prevalence of clinical venous thromboembolism in the USA: current trends and future projections. Am J Hematol 86: 217–220.
3. Spencer FA, Gore JM, Lessard D, Emery C, Pacifico L, et al. (2008) Venous thromboembolism in the elderly. A community-based perspective. Thromb Haemost 100: 780–788.
4. Kearon C, Kahn SR, Agnelli G, Goldhaber S, Raskob GE, et al. (2008) Antithrombotic therapy for venous thromboembolic disease: American College of Chest Physicians Evidence-Based Clinical Practice Guidelines (8th Edition). Chest 133: 454S–545S.
5. Kearon C, Akl EA, Comerota AJ, Prandoni P, Bounameaux H, et al. (2012) Antithrombotic therapy for VTE disease: Antithrombotic Therapy and Prevention of Thrombosis, 9th ed: American College of Chest Physicians Evidence-Based Clinical Practice Guidelines. Chest 141: e419S–494S.
6. Aujesky D, Long JA, Fine MJ, Ibrahim SA (2007) African American race was associated with an increased risk of complications following venous thromboembolism. J Clin Epidemiol 60: 410–416.
7. Smith SB, Geske JB, Maguire JM, Zane NA, Carter RE, et al. (2010) Early anticoagulation is associated with reduced mortality for acute pulmonary embolism. Chest 137: 1382–1390.
8. Mohiuddin SM, Hilleman DE, Destache CJ, Stoysich AM, Gannon JM, et al. (1992) Efficacy and safety of early versus late initiation of warfarin during heparin therapy in acute thromboembolism. Am Heart J 123: 729–732.
9. Gallus A, Jackaman J, Tillett J, Mills W, Wycherley A (1986) Safety and efficacy of warfarin started early after submassive venous thrombosis or pulmonary embolism. Lancet 2: 1293–1296.
10. Kakkos SK, Daskalopoulou SS, Daskalopoulos ME, Nicolaides AN, Geroulakos G (2006) Review on the value of graduated elastic compression stockings after deep vein thrombosis. Thromb Haemost 96: 441–445.
11. Leroyer C, Bressollette L, Oger E, Mansourati J, Cheze-Le Rest C, et al. (1998) Early versus delayed introduction of oral vitamin K antagonists in combination with low-molecular-weight heparin in the treatment of deep vein thrombosis. a randomized clinical trial. The ANTENOX Study Group. Haemostasis 28: 70–77.
12. Akl EA, Vasireddi SR, Gunukula S, Barba M, Sperati F, et al. (2011) Anticoagulation for the initial treatment of venous thromboembolism in patients with cancer. Cochrane Database Syst Rev: CD006649.
13. Tapson VF, Hyers TM, Waldo AL, Ballard DJ, Becker RC, et al. (2005) Antithrombotic therapy practices in US hospitals in an era of practice guidelines. Arch Intern Med 165: 1458–1464.
14. Caprini JA, Tapson VF, Hyers TM, Waldo AL, Wittkowsky AK, et al. (2005) Treatment of venous thromboembolism: adherence to guidelines and impact of physician knowledge, attitudes, and beliefs. J Vasc Surg 42: 726–733.
15. Kahn SR, Springmann V, Schulman S, Martineau J, Stewart JA, et al. (2012) Patterns of management and adherence to venous thromboembolism (VTE) treatment guidelines in a national prospective cohort study of VTE management in the Canadian outpatient setting: The Recovery Study. Thromb Haemost 108: 493–8.
16. Ganz DA, Glynn RJ, Mogun H, Knight EL, Bohn RL, et al. (2000) Adherence to guidelines for oral anticoagulation after venous thrombosis and pulmonary embolism. J Gen Intern Med 15: 776–781.
17. Whittle J, Johnson P, Localio AR (1998) Anticoagulation therapy in patients with venous thromboembolic disease. J Gen Intern Med 13: 373–378.
18. Mean M, Righini M, Jaeger K, Beer HJ, Frauchiger B, et al. (2013) The Swiss cohort of elderly patients with venous thromboembolism (SWITCO65+): rationale and methodology. J Thromb Thrombolysis 36: 475–483.
19. Dauzat M, Laroche JP, Deklunder G, Ayoub J, Quere I, et al. (1997) Diagnosis of acute lower limb deep venous thrombosis with ultrasound: trends and controversies. J Clin Ultrasound 25: 343–358.
20. Fraser DG, Moody AR, Morgan PS, Martel AL, Davidson I (2002) Diagnosis of lower-limb deep venous thrombosis: a prospective blinded study of magnetic resonance direct thrombus imaging. Ann Intern Med 136: 89–98.
21. Kearon C, Ginsberg JS, Hirsh J (1998) The role of venous ultrasonography in the diagnosis of suspected deep venous thrombosis and pulmonary embolism. Ann Intern Med 129: 1044–1049.
22. Buller HR, Davidson BL, Decousus H, Gallus A, Gent M, et al. (2003) Subcutaneous fondaparinux versus intravenous unfractionated heparin in the initial treatment of pulmonary embolism. N Engl J Med 349: 1695–1702.
23. Le Gal G, Righini M, Sanchez O, Roy PM, Baba-Ahmed M, et al. (2006) A positive compression ultrasonography of the lower limb veins is highly predictive

of pulmonary embolism on computed tomography in suspected patients. Thromb Haemost 95: 963–966.

24. Royston P (2004) Multiple imputation of missing values. The Stata Journal 4: 227–241.

25. Rubin DB (1987) Multiple Imputation for Nonresponse in Surveys. New York: J Wiley & Sons.

26. Spirk D, Husmann M, Willenberg T, Banyai M, Frank U, et al. (2011) Inconsistencies in the planning of the duration of anticoagulation among outpatients with acute deep-vein thrombosis. Results from the OTIS-DVT Registry. Thromb Haemost 105: 239–244.

27. Marcucci M, Iorio A, Nobili A, Tettamanti M, Pasina L, et al. (2010) Factors affecting adherence to guidelines for antithrombotic therapy in elderly patients with atrial fibrillation admitted to internal medicine wards. Eur J Intern Med 21: 516–523.

28. Marcucci M, Iorio A, Nobili A, Tettamanti M, Pasina L, et al. (2013) Prophylaxis of venous thromboembolism in elderly patients with multimorbidity. Intern Emerg Med 8: 509–520.

29. Caprini JA, Hyers TM (2006) Compliance with antithrombotic guidelines. Manag Care 15: 49–50, 53–60, 66.

30. Noble SI, Nelson A, Turner C, Finlay IG (2006) Acceptability of low molecular weight heparin thromboprophylaxis for inpatients receiving palliative care: qualitative study. BMJ 332: 577–580.

31. Arpaia G, Carpenedo M, Pistelli R, Mastrogiacomo O, Cimminiello C, et al. (2009) Attitudes to prescribing compression stockings for patients with acute DVT: the MASTER registry. J Thromb Thrombolysis 28: 389–393.

32. Mahan CE, Spyropoulos AC (2010) Venous thromboembolism prevention: a systematic review of methods to improve prophylaxis and decrease events in the hospitalized patient. Hosp Pract (Minneap) 38: 97–108.

33. Merli G (2010) Improving venous thromboembolism performance: a comprehensive guide for physicians and hospitalists. Hosp Pract (Minneap) 38: 7–16.

34. Kahn SR, Morrison DR, Cohen JM, Emed J, Tagalakis V, et al. (2013) Interventions for implementation of thromboprophylaxis in hospitalized medical and surgical patients at risk for venous thromboembolism. Cochrane Database Syst Rev 7: CD008201.

35. Rose AJ, Miller DR, Ozonoff A, Berlowitz DR, Ash AS, et al. (2013) Gaps in monitoring during oral anticoagulation: insights into care transitions, monitoring barriers, and medication nonadherence. Chest 143: 751–757.

## 17

Combining Neuroprotectants in a Model of Retinal Degeneration: No Additive Benefit

Fabiana Di Marco[1]*, **Mattia Di Paolo**[1], **Stefania Romeo**[1], **Linda Colecchi**[1], **Lavinia Fiorani**[1], **Sharon Spana**[2], **Jonathan Stone**[2,3], **Silvia Bisti**[1,3]

1 Department of Biotechnology and Applied Clinical Science, University of L'Aquila, L'Aquila, Italy, **2** Discipline of Physiology and Bosch Institute, University of Sydney, Sydney, New South Wales, Australia, **3** ARC Centre of Excellence in Vision Science, The Australian National University, Canberra, Australia

Abstract

The central nervous system undergoing degeneration can be stabilized, and in some models can be restored to function, by neuroprotective treatments. Photobiomodulation (PBM) and dietary saffron are distinctive as neuroprotectants in that they upregulate protective mechanisms, without causing measurable tissue damage. This study reports a first attempt to combine the actions of PBM and saffron. Our working hypothesis was that the actions of PBM and saffron in protecting retinal photoreceptors, in a rat light damage model, would be additive. Results confirmed the neuroprotective potential of each used separately, but gave no evidence that their effects are additive. Detailed analysis suggests that there is actually a negative interaction between PBM and saffron when given simultaneously, with a consequent reduction of the neuroprotection. Specific testing will be required to understand the mechanisms involved and to establish whether there is clinical potential in combining neuroprotectants, to improve the quality of life of people affected by retinal pathology, such as age-related macular degeneration, the major cause of blindness and visual impairment in older adults.

Editor: Steven Barnes, Dalhousie University, Canada

Funding: This work was supported by the Australian Research Council Centre of Excellence in Vision Science, by the Sir Zelman Cowen Universities Fund and the Lord Mayor's Charitable Foundation, by Australian Travel Awards for L'Aquila Researchers (ARIA) to FDM and SR and by a Ministero dell'Istruzione, dell'Università e della Ricerca dedicato ai PRIN, Progetti di Ricerca di Interesse Nazionale (MIUR-PRIN) (2010-2011) research grant to SB. The funders had no role in study design, data collection and analysis, decision to publish, or preparation of the manuscript.

Competing Interests: SB holds a non-remunerative relation with HN P/L, (hortusnovus.it) which supports research. JS is a director of CSCM Pty Ltd.

* Email: dm.fabiana@hotmail.it

Introduction

The central nervous system in mammals has only a limited ability to repair its neuronal circuitry. Its functional stability is achieved by ensuring the stability of individual neurons and by redundancy that enables normal function despite substantial loss of neurons. Age-related loss of retinal stability results in diseases such as age related macular degeneration (AMD).

Inflammation is an important feature of the aged retina and in many retinal diseases, including AMD. Recent studies have demonstrated that exposure to 670 nm light reduces inflammation in the retina undergoing degeneration [1,2,3], mitigates the light-induced upregulation of Müller cell- specific markers, for example glial fibrillary acid protein (GFAP) [5] and vimentin [1,3], and reduces lipid peroxidation and complement activation in degenerating retina [2,3].

Saffron has been used for a long time in traditional medicine. Its effectiveness as a neuroprotectant was pioneered by Maccarone and colleagues [4], who showed that dietary saffron maintains photoreceptor morphology and function after exposure to damaging light in rat retina, and reduces the overexpression of fibroblast growth factor 2 (FGF-2). This neuroprotective action of saffron has been confirmed in models of photoreceptor degener-

ation [5] and Parkinson's disease [6] and in clinical trials with AMD [7,8].

Microarray analysis [9] showed that both PBM and saffron treatment were able to change the gene expression induced by light damage, but their effects were not identical. Preconditioning by both PBM and saffron mitigated a damage-induced reduction in *GPX3*, which codes for a glutathione peroxidase; and reduced the expression of *CCL2*, which codes for a cytokine which recruits monocytes, memory T-cells and dendritic cells to sites of inflammation; and both reduced the expression of many ncRNAs. Saffron preconditioning, but not PBM, on the other hand, regulated *EDN2*, which codes for a vasoconstrictive peptide, and the ncRNAs regulated by saffron and PBM differed significantly (Tables 4 and 5 in [9]), These differences suggested that the simultaneous application of the two neuroprotectants might have an additive and more powerful protective activity.

Our previous study has described the time course of protection for dietary saffron and photobiomodulation (PBM), in an animal model of light damage [5]. Both treatments are effective in reducing retinal degeneration, and present low toxicity. This paper describes a first attempt to define their protective efficacy when simultaneously applied.

Methods

Light damage model

All experiments conducted were in accordance with the policies of the Association for Research in Vision and Ophthalmology (ARVO) and with the approval of the Animal Ethics Committee at the University of Sydney (Approval number: K22/5-2009/2/5003). Animals were raised and experiments conducted in cyclic 5 lux light (12 hrs: 12 hrs). Adult Sprague Dawley (SD) albino rats were born and raised in dim cyclic light conditions (12 h at 5 lux, 12 h dark)

Light damage (LD) was generated by exposing the animals to 1000 lux light for 24 h. The light was generated by fluorescent tubes located above the cage. For the exposure period, the animals were provided with food and water from containers on the floor of the cage, to ensure consistent exposure to the light. After LD the animals were returned to dim cyclic illumination for a post-exposure period of one week (1 w). The animals were euthanized (Lethobarb 60 mg/kg intraperitoneal) and retinal tissues were obtained for analysis.

Five groups of animals were used:

- Control: These animals (n = 4) were raised in 5 lux cyclic light, as above.
- Light damaged (LD) control: These animals (n = 10) were raised in dim cyclic light, then exposed to bright light for 24 h, and returned to dim cyclic light for 1 w.
- Saffron-conditioned LD: These animals (n = 10) were raised in dim cyclic light and, prior to exposure to bright light, were preconditioned for 10 days with saffron at 1 mg/kg/day. Saffron (stigmata of *Crocus sativus*, "L'Aquila Saffron", Italy) was soaked in water (at 2 mg of spice/ml H_2O) and 12 h was allowed for the major antioxidants, which are water soluble [10], to dissolve. The solute was then fed to the rats by injecting a small volume into a piece of the vegetable matrix, which the animal readily ingested. The volume for each daily feed was calculated to provide the solutes from 1 mg of saffron/kg body weight.
- Photobiomodulation (PBM) conditioned LD: These animals (n = 10) were raised in dim cyclic light, exposed to bright light and kept for a further week, as above. For 7d prior to exposure to the bright light, each animal was exposed to 670 nm red light from a WARP 75 source (Quantum Devices Inc, Barneveld, WI, USA). Animals were gently restrained under a plexiglass platform with the eyes ~2.5 cm below the platform. The WARP 75 device was placed on top of the platform and turned on for 3 min. This arrangement provided a fluence of 4.0–4.5 J/cm^2 at the eye, calculated from an estimate of power at 2.5 cm from the LED array, made using a calibrated sensor provided by Quantum Devices (Barneveld, Wisconsin). The animals did not hide from or appear agitated by the red light.
- Combined conditioned: These animals (n = 10) were raised in dim cyclic light, exposed to bright light and kept for a further week, as above. For 10d prior to the exposure to bright light, each was exposed simultaneously to both the saffron and the PBM conditioning described above.

Preparation of retinal material

The superior aspect of the eye was marked with an indelible marker by a stitch in the conjunctiva, after anaesthesia and prior to euthanasia. After euthenasia, the eyes were dissected free and fixed by immersion in 4% paraformaldehyde fixative buffer at 4°C

for 1 h. After three rinses in 0.1 M phosphate-buffered saline (PBS), eyes were left overnight in a 15% sucrose solution to provide cryoprotection. Eyes were embedded in mounting medium (Tissue Tek OCT compound; Sakura Finetek, Torrance, CA) by snap freezing in liquid nitrogen. Cryosections were cut at 20 μm (CM1850 Cryostat; Leica, Wetzlar, Germany) with the eyes oriented so that the sections extended from superior to inferior edge. Sections were mounted on gelatin and poly-L-lysine-coated slides and were then dried overnight in 50°C oven and stored at −20°C until processed.

Detection of cell death (TUNEL)

Sections were labelled for apoptotic cell death using the terminal deoxynucleotidyl transferase dUTP nick end labelling (TUNEL) technique [11] following protocols published previously [12]. To demonstrate cellular layers, sections were also labelled with the DNA-specific dye bisbenzimide (Calbiochem, La Jolla, CA), by incubating them for 2 min in a 1:10.000 solution in 0.1 M PBS. Sections cut adjacent to or through the optic nerve head were chosen, to minimise variations in retinal length and position. Counts of TUNEL+ profiles (apoptotic cells) were made using a calibrated 20 x objective and an eyepiece graticule. Each section was scanned from the superior to inferior edge, and the number of TUNEL+ profiles was recorded for each 400 μm length of the section. Counts were averaged from at least four sections per animal and were recorded separately for the outer nuclear layer (ONL) and inner nuclear layer (INL).

Immunohistochemistry: GFAP staining

Retinal sections were washed with 0.1 M PBS (10 min twice) and incubated in 10% normal goat serum in 0.1 M PBS for 1 hour at room temperature, to block non-specific binding. Sections were then incubated overnight at 4°C in rabbit polyclonal anti GFAP (1:700; DakoCytomation, Campbellfield, Australia). After 3 rinses in PBS for 10 minutes each, sections were incubated with an appropriate secondary antibody (1:1.000 ALEXA Fluor 594; Molecular Probes, Invitrogen Carlsbad, CA), for 1 h at room tempertaure

Outcome measures

Three measures of neuroprotection were used, the surviving population of photoreceptors, the rate of photoreceptor death, and the expression of the stress-inducible protein GFAP in Müller cells. All were assessed 1 w after exposure to damaging light.

Photoreceptor survival. We estimated photoreceptor survival by measuring the thickness of the outer nuclear layer (ONL). Specifically, we recorded the ratio of the thickness of the ONL to the thickness of the retina (from the inner to the outer limiting membrane), measured at 0.40 mm intervals, from the superior to the inferior edge of the retina. The ratio of ONL to retinal thickness was used as a measure of ONL thickness, rather than the absolute thickness of the ONL (μm), to compensate for oblique sectioning.

Extent of GFAP labelling. We measured the length of Müller cells along which GFAP expression was evident (μm), as a proportion of retinal thickness (from the inner to the outer limiting membrane), This was recorded at 0.4 mm steps along retinal sections, from the superior to the inferior edge. Measurements were made in at least 2 sections from one eye of each animal studied.

Electroretinographic Recording

Electroretinograms (ERGs) were recorded in control and treated animals 1 day before and 1 week after high intensity light exposure (light damage LD). Albino rats were previously dark adapted overnight. Ketamine : xylazine anaesthesia was used with intra peritoneal injection of 100 mg/kg ketamine, 12 mg/kg xylazine (Ketavet 100 mg/ml, Intervet production srl; Xylazine 1 g, Sigma Co.). Corneas were anesthetized with a drop of novocaine, and pupils were dilated with 1% atropine sulfate (Allergan, Westport, IR). Body temperature was maintained at $37 \pm 0.5°C$ with a heating pad controlled by a rectal temperature probe. Recordings were made from the left eyes, with a gold electrode loop (2 mm in diameter) placed on the cornea while the right eye was fully covered with a bandage. The reference electrode was placed on the right cornea under the bandage, and the ground electrode was inserted in the anterior scalp, between the eyes. The rat's head was positioned just inside the opening of the Ganzfeld dome (Biomedica Mangoni, Pisa, Italy). This electronic flash unit generated flashes of a range of intensities from $0.001–100$ cd/m^2. Responses were recorded over 300 ms plus 25 ms of pre-trial baseline, amplified differentially, bandpass filtered at 0.3 to 300 Hz, digitized at 0.25- to 0.3-ms intervals by a personal computer interface (LabVIEW 8.2; National Instruments, Milan, Italy), and stored on a disc for processing. Responses from several trials were averaged ($n = 5$), with an interstimulus interval ranging from 60 seconds for dim lights to 5 minutes for the brightest flashes. The amplitude of the b-wave was measured from the most negative point of the average trace to the highest positive point, without subtracting oscillatory potentials. The distributions of ERG response, across several experimental groups at different light intensities, were described by means and standard deviations. The between-group differences were compared using one-way ANOVA for repeated measurement data to account for potential correlations among readings from the same rats.

Statistical tests

The significance of differences in ONL thickness and GFAP labelling associated with conditioning were assessed using ANOVA, followed by a Tukey test. The Tukey test was used for all pairwise comparisons of the mean values. Results are expressed as the mean $\pm$ SE. $p < 0.05$ was considered significant.

Results

Single and combined conditioning: rate of photoreceptor death

In control retina (dim-reared, not exposed to bright light, unconditioned by saffron or PBM) the rate of photoreceptor death, assessed by the frequency of TUNEL+ cells in the ONL (Figure 1, blue bar) was low (Figure 1). Exposure to damaging light (white bar) increased the count of TUNEL+ cells, most prominently in superior retina [13] (for reasons discussed in Section 3.2.2). When the retina was preconditioned with 7 d PBM, 10 d saffron or with both saffron and PBM, the TUNEL count in superior retina was reduced (orange, red, green bars). Because, in the current experiments, retinas were examined 1 w after the bright light exposure that induced cell death, the numbers of TUNEL+ profiles were lower than in earlier studies [4], in which the retina was examined immediately after damaging light exposure. For all three treatments a reduction in cell death from the unconditioned light damage level was evident and significant, but greater reduction was not achieved with PBM and saffron given simultaneously.

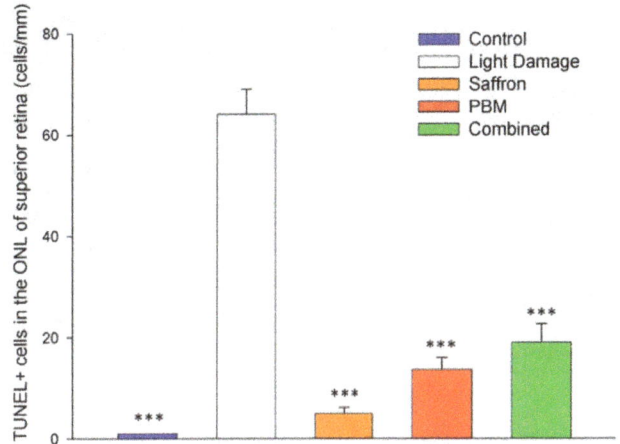

Figure 1. Impact of single and combined neuroprotectants on TUNEL-positive cells in the ONL of superior retina one week after light exposure. We tested whether the number of TUNEL+ cells were significantly different among 5 experimental groups. In all three treated groups, the number of TUNEL+ profiles was significantly smaller than in the light damage (LD) group. The histogram bars show mean numbers of TUNEL+ cells/mm ONL, for each experimental group; the error bars show standard error of the means. Statistical significance indicator: [***] $p < 0.001$.

Single and combined conditioning: photoreceptor survival

Figure 2 shows representative images of superior mid-peripheral retina, in a control retina (A), and in retinas from the four experimental groups (B-E). The ONL is 50-80 μm thick in the control retina (A), and is sharply reduced in thickness by exposure to bright light for 24 h (B). Preconditioning with PBM (C) or saffron (D) was protective, limiting the thinning on the ONL; this confirms prior reports [1,4,5,14]. Conditioning with both PBM and saffron (E) was also protective, but did not improve survival, compared to saffron or PBM conditioning separately.

The result is shown quantitatively in Figures 2F, G, which show ONL thickness as a function of distance between the superior and inferior edges of the retina. ONL thinning induced by LD is most marked in the superior retina (as reported in [15,16]); the thinning is reduced by conditioning. Figure 2G shows the mean ONL thickness averaged across superior retina, in the five experimental groups. Comparisons were made using the four measures of ONL thickness available between 2.2 mm and 3.4 mm from the superior edge, thus excluding all inferior retina, and the more peripheral regions of superior retina. The difference between the unconditioned and PBM conditioned light damage groups was highly significant ($p < 0.0001$), as were the differences between the saffron-conditioned and unconditioned groups ($p < 0.0001$), and between the combined-conditioned and unconditioned groups ($p < 0.0004$). The thinning of the ONL in the combined conditioned group, relative to the single conditioned groups, was significant for both saffron ($p < 0.0001$) and PBM ($p < 0.001$). The difference in thickness between PBM-and saffron-conditioned groups was not significant in these data ($p = 0.0626$; Figure 2G). In conclusion, combining saffron and PBM was not additive; indeed the thinning of the ONL was greater in the combined group than in the PBM or saffron groups.

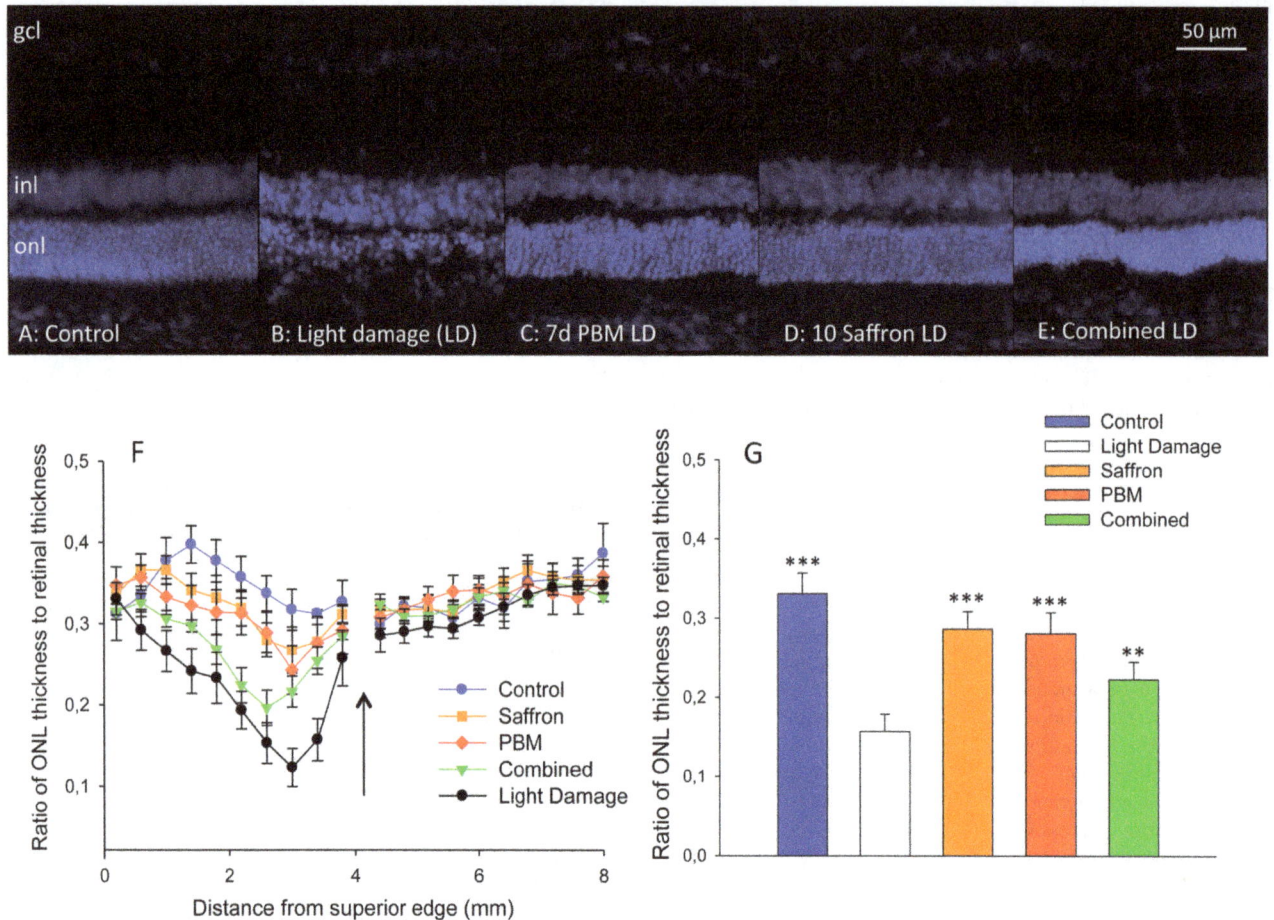

Figure 2. Impact of single and combined neuroprotectants on the thickness of the ONL in superior retina. A–E: Representative bisbenzimide labelling in control (A), light damage (B), 7 days PBM (C), 10 days saffron (D) and combined treatment (E) groups, 1 w after light damage. Images are taken one millimeter dorsal from optic disc. F: The ratio of ONL thickness to retinal thickness from the superior to the inferior edge. The arrow shows the position of the optic disc. Different symbols represent different experimental groups. For each group, each point shows the mean of the group; the error bars show standard errors of the mean. G: The ratio of ONL thickness to retinal thickness, in the hot spot area (the area of greatest light-induced damage), 1 mm superior to the optic disc. For each group, each point shows the mean of the group; the error bars show standard errors of the mean. Statistical significance indicators: (***) p<0.001; (**) p<0.01, for the difference of each group from the light damage group value.

Single and combined conditioning: impact on GFAP expression

Figure 3 shows GFAP expression in the retina, in the five experimental groups. Without light damage or conditioning, GFAP expression is confined to the astrocytes at the inner surface of the retina (Figure 3A). Light damage induced the upregulation of GFAP in the radially oriented Müller cells; the protein was visible along the full length of the Müller cell (Figure 3B). The length of the Müller cell that expressed GFAP was shortened by 7d conditioning with PBM and by 10d conditioning with saffron, confirming previous study [5] (Figures 3C, D). The length of Müller cells labelled by combined conditioning is shown in Figure 3E.

The result is shown quantitatively in Figures 3F, G. The length of Müller cells labelled was consistent along sections of the retina, extending from the superior to the inferior edge. The difference in the length of Müller cell that was GFAP+ was highly significant between unconditioned and PBM conditioned light damaged groups (p<0.0001), between unconditioned and saffron conditioned groups (p<0.0001) and between the unconditioned and

combined conditioned groups (p<0.0001; Figure 3G). That is, the unpregulation in GFAP expression caused in Müller cells by light damage was reduced by saffron, by PBM and by combined conditioning. As with the ONL, combined conditioning did not provide greater reduction in GFAP labelling than saffron single conditioning or PBM single conditioning. The biggest difference between the ONL and GFAP measures was that combined conditioning reduced GFAP upregulation less than saffron conditioning, but not less than PBM conditioning; saffron-conditioning reduced GFAP labelling significantly more than did PBM-conditioning (p<0.0001; Figure 3G).

Single and combined conditioning: retinal function

Figure 4 shows the impact of PBM, saffron and combined conditioning on the preservation of retinal function. We recorded ERG responses as a function of increasing flash intensity (Figure 4A), from threshold to saturation. Figure 4C shows representative ERG traces obtained at a fixed luminance (10 cd/m^2), less than saturation. Quantitative results for different treatments are summarized in Figure 4B as a percentage of

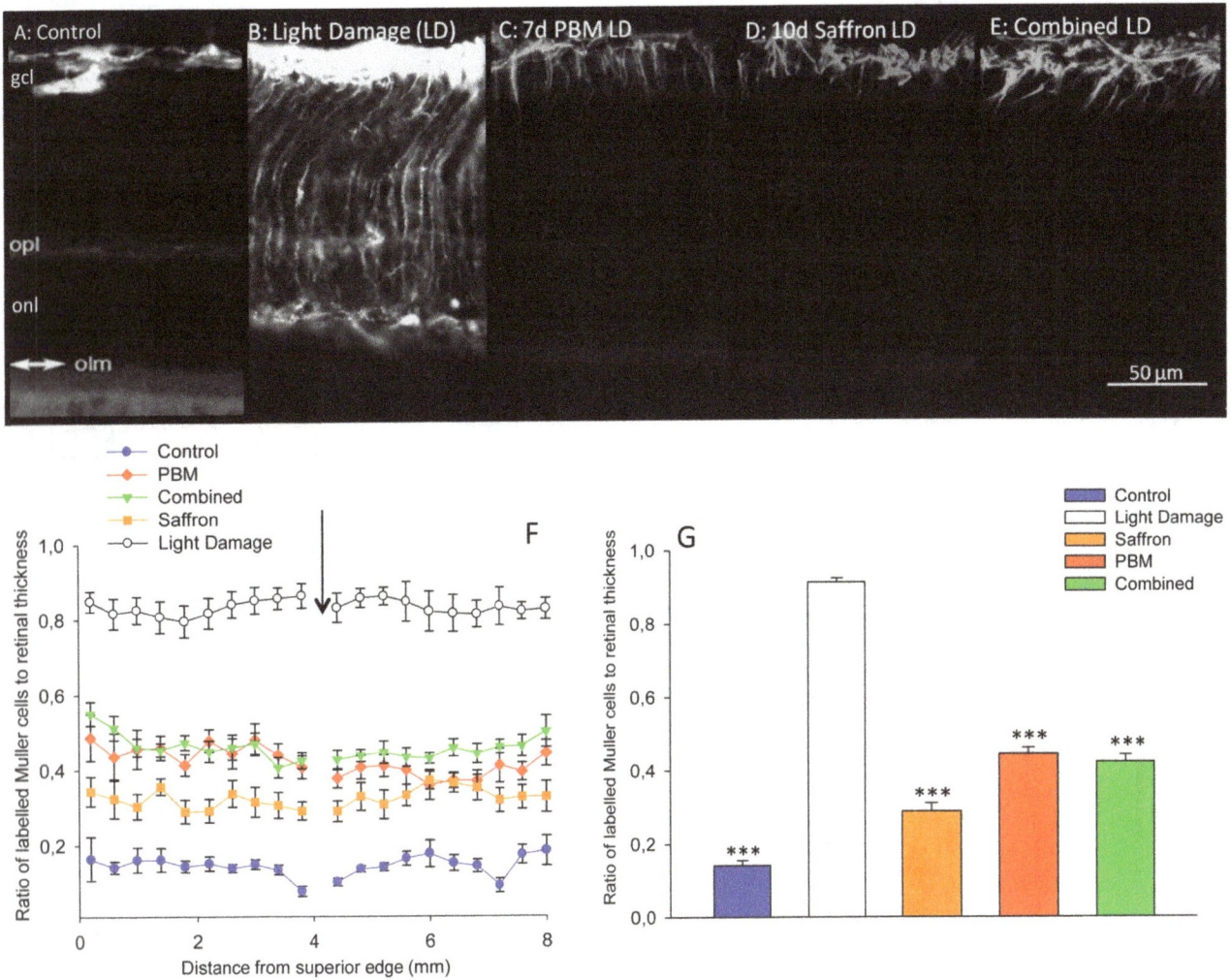

Figure 3. Impact of single and combined neuroprotectants on GFAP labelling of Müller cells. A–E: Representative GFAP labelling in control (A), light damage (B), 7 d PBM (C), 10 d saffron (D) and combined treatment (E) groups, 1 w after light damage. Light damage induced the up-regulation of GFAP in the radially oriented Müller cells; the protein is visible along the full length of the Müller cells, from the ILM to the OLM. F: Length of the Müller processes expressing GFAP as a function of distance from superior edge in the five experimental groups. The arrow shows the position of the optic disc. Each point shows the mean labelled length; error bars show standard deviations of the mean. G: Mean length of Müller processes expressing GFAP, averaged across superior retina, in: Control (A), Light Damage (B), 7 days PBM (C), 10 days saffron (D) and combined (E) groups. In all treated groups, the length of Müller cells expressing GFAP was less than in the light damage group. The error bars show standard errors of the mean. Statistical significance indicator: [***] $p < 0.001$.

control amplitude of the b-wave. The amplitude was strongly reduced after light damage (70% reduction). Pre-conditioning with 7 d PBM and 10 d saffron mitigated the reduction, to 40% and 50% respectively. Preconditioning with both PBM and saffron, given simultaneously did not increase the mitigation. We recorded responses as a function of increasing luminance from threshold to saturation. Comparison were made from data obtained at a fixed value of luminance (10 cd/m^2), which was non-saturating.

The difference in the amplitude of the b-wave is significant between unconditioned and PBM conditioned light damaged group ($p < 0.05$) and between unconditioned and saffron conditioned light damaged group ($p < 0.01$; Figure 4B). The difference between unconditioned and combined conditioning is not significant ($p = 0.244$; Figure 4B). In agreement with morphologic data, these data demonstrate that both treatments are effective in preserving retinal function when separately applied but their protective efficacy is lower, and in this case not significant, when simultaneously applied.

Discussion

The present observation, that neuroprotective effects of saffron and PBM are not additive, does not support our working hypothesis, formulated on the basis of results obtained in a microarray study [9], where we observed a limited overlap of gene regulation patterns during saffron- and PBM-induced neuroprotection. We hypothesized from that data that saffron and PBM would activate separate but complementary, and therefore potentially additive, protective pathways. The lack of any additive effect suggests that saffron and PBM compete to activate the same neuroprotective pathway or pathways. The dose-effect data in a previous study [5] suggest that the mechanism involved is

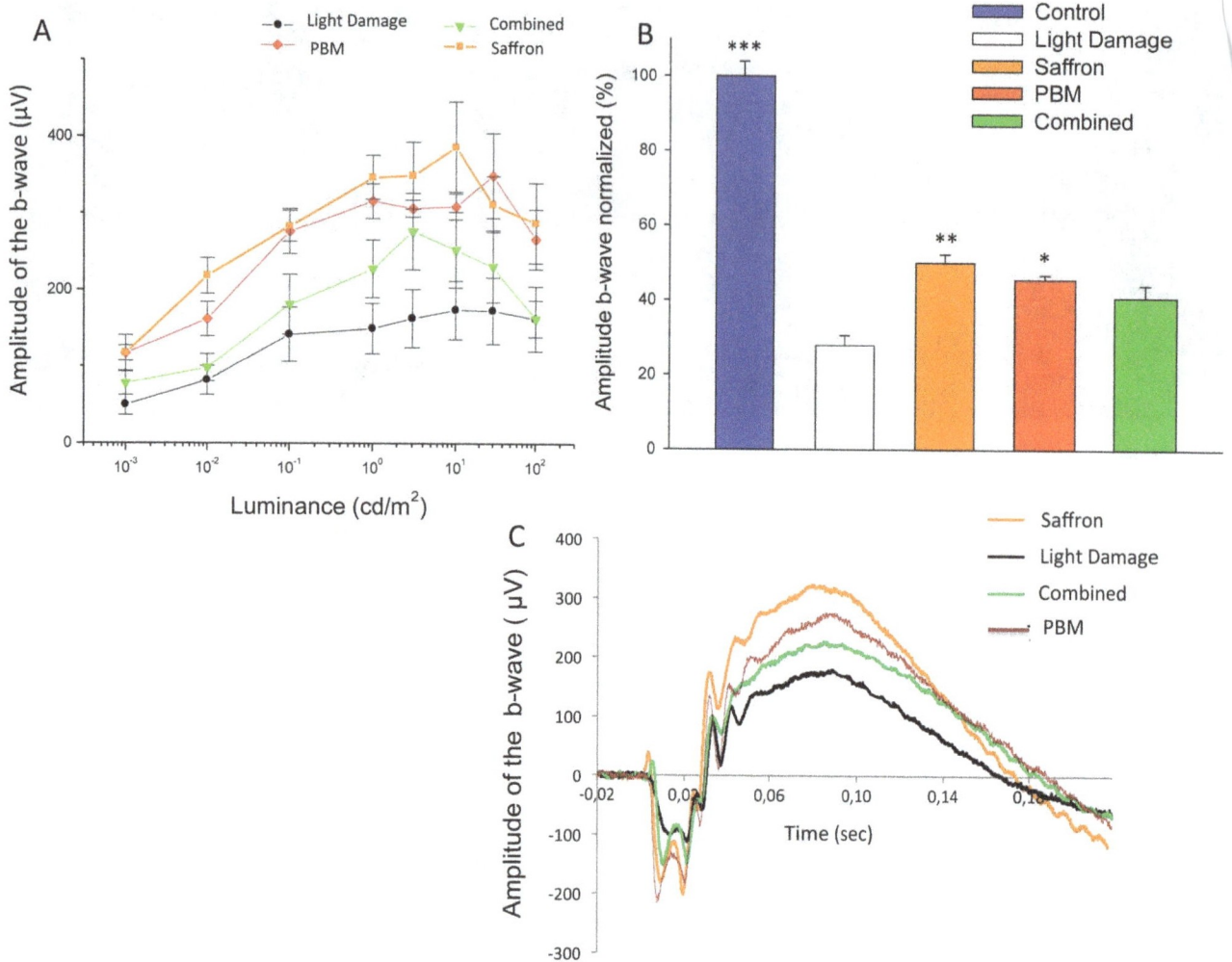

Figure 4. Impact of single and combined neuroprotectants on the ERG. A: ERG b-wave amplitude (µV) as a function of flash brightness (cd/m²) in four experimental groups. As for other data, each point represents the group mean and error bars show standard deviations of the mean. B: The amplitude of the b-wave normalized to control values in the 5 experimental groups. Histogram bars show means for each experimental group; error bars show standard deviations of the mean. The comparisons were made from data obtained at a fixed value of luminance (10 cd/m²) before saturation. Single treatment with saffron and PBM mitigated the b-wave reduction induced by light damage, and the differences between treated and untreated groups were significant. Combined treatment also mitigated the reduction of the b-wave, but the difference was not statistically significant. C: Representative traces for each group to a stimulus flash of 10 cd/m² of luminance. The error bars show standard errors of the mean. Statistical significance indicators: (***) p<0.001; (**) p<0.01, (*) p<0.05.

activated progressively, over 5–10d, but further work is required for it to be identified.

The experimental stress we used (bright continuous light exposure) induces oxidative stress, to which neurons are vulnerable. Oxidative stress can also contribute to tissue damage indirectly, by activating pathways that induce the expression of stress sensitive genes, and by glia-mediated inflammation that causes secondary neuronal damage [17]. The neuroprotective activity of saffron probably is not limited to the trapping of free radicals, as an antioxidant, but likely involves regulation of genes which control the release of pro-inflammatory cytokines by glial cells. While acting as neuroprotectants, both saffron and PBM downregulate chemokine gene expression [9].

Do PBM and saffron interfere with each other's actions?

In both the ONL and GFAP data, combined treatment gave a poorer outcome than in single saffron conditioning; the differences

were statistically significant. This suggests a limited degree of interference between the two forms of conditioning. Confirmation of this interference and more knowledge of the underlying mechanisms seem necessary for progress towards the successful combination of neuroprotectants. The suggestion of interference gives weight to the main outcome of this study, that the protective effects of PBM and saffron are not additive; greater protection is not gained when both forms of conditioning are applied.

More positively, our results show that combination of saffron and PBM preconditioning does not introduce major side effects or induce a major reduction in neuroprotection. The general idea of combining different treatments to reach a better results remains valid, but needs further investigation to form a basis in animal models for human trials of combinations of protectants.

different studies for clinical reference. In this study, we aimed to provide pooled rates of non-union, re-operation, infection, and approach related complications after surgical treatment of unstable odontoid fractures using AOSF. Furthermore, we tried to explore potential factors that affected these outcomes.

Materials and Methods

Search strategy and inclusion criteria

A computerized systematic search was conducted up to August 2013 using MEDLINE database. We screened all fields by the term "odontoid fracture" or "odontoid screw" or "odontoid fixation". Articles were limited to those published in English. We also searched the reference lists and relevant journals by hand. This meta-analysis was performed in accordance with the preferred reporting items for systematic reviews and meta-analyses (PRISMA) guidelines (when appropriate) (Checklist S1).

We included studies which were carried out on humans. The studies that discussed fusion results, and/or re-operations, and/or infections, and/or approach related complications after odontoid screw fixation for type II or type III odontoid fractures were selected. We also required a minimum sample size of five to ensure quality and comparability of data. Biomechanical studies, cadaveric studies, animal studies, case report, duplications, and review articles were excluded. Clinical studies with inadequate information or incomplete data were also excluded. We carefully reviewed the department/institute of each potential eligible study to screen whether there were any papers from the same surgical team. For papers that had overlapping patients determined through the overlapping research time, we only included the paper with the largest sample size for analysis.

Data extraction

Two investigators reviewed all identified articles to determine if an individual study was eligible for inclusion. Data from each study was extracted using a standardized form. Disagreements on eligibility and data between reviewers were resolved by consensus with the third reviewer. Studies were categorized into levels of evidence according to those published in the Journal of Bone and Joint Surgery (American) [78].

Data extracted consisted of study year, country, level of evidence, patients' mean age, sex proportion, mean follow-up duration, classification of the odontoid fracture, number of patients, number of non-unions, number of re-operations, number of infections, and number of approach related complications. Fusion status should be assessed according to radiological (static or dynamic) and/or computed tomography (CT) examinations. Because the fusion criteria might be different among the included studies, we used a universal definition of fusion for data extraction. Criteria for fusion success included formation of trabecular and cortex bony bridges through the fracture site, absence of sclerotic borders adjacent to the fracture site, and absence of movement of the fracture site confirmed on radiographs and/or CT scan. Radiolucent cleft, clear fracture line, fibrous union, or any movement at the fracture site were considered as non-union. Re-operation represented secondary surgical intervention for any reason after odontoid screw fixation. Infections indicated only those located at the surgical site including both superficial and deep ones. We extracted data on five types of approach related complications including postoperative dysphagia, postoperative hoarseness, esophageal /retropharyngeal injury, wound hematomas, and spinal cord injury. In this meta-analysis, data regarding the study characteristics and the outcomes of interest were extracted based on the average value of each study. For studies

with overlapping patients, only the one with the largest sample size was entered into meta-analysis.

Statistical analysis

Meta-analyses were performed to pool the rates of non-union, re-operation, infection, and approach related complications. A Freeman-Tukey Double arcsine transformation was implemented to calculate the overall proportion. A test of heterogeneity was carried out, and cut-off p value of 0.1 was established as a threshold of homogeneity. Pooled estimates and 95% confidence intervals (CIs) were summarized by forest plots. Fixed-effect models were applied unless statistical heterogeneity was significant, in which case random-effect models were used. We further investigated potential sources of heterogeneity by arranging groups of studies according to relevant characteristics (year of publication, level of evidence, patients' mean age, sex, follow-up duration, fracture type, and study sample size) and by meta-regression analysis. Factors were examined both individually and in multiple-variable models. To avoid model instability, only factors that showed significant effects individually were enrolled into a multiple regression model. Publication bias was assessed using Egger test. All analyses were done in the statistical software R 3.0.1.

Results

In the initial screening, 972 potential studies were selected according to the search strategy. Hand-searching resulted in 12 additional papers. After reviewing titles and abstracts, 814 papers were found to be unrelated to the current topic. Of the remaining 170 papers, the full texts were read and 104 publications which did not meet eligibility criteria were excluded. Further three papers [71,73,76] were excluded due to potential overlapping patients. Consequently, sixty three papers met all inclusion criteria and were selected (Figure 1) [12–70,72,74,75,77]. Based on the level of evidence, there were 1 level II, 17 level III, and 45 level IV studies. The mean age ranged from 35 to 85.4 years. We divided the studies into five age subgroups (age ≤40, age 40 to <50, age 50 to <60, age 60 to <70, and age ≥70). The male to female ratio was 1.74. The follow-up duration ranged from 1.5 months to 9 years. 88.9% of the injuries were type II dens fractures according to Anderson and D'Alonzo's classification [8]. The characteristics of selected studies were summarized in Table S1 and Table S2.

54 studies [12–20,22–29,31–51,53–60,62,63,65–70] that reported fusion results were pooled. Six studies [21,52,61,72,74,75] were excluded from data synthesizing because of potential patients overlapping. Imaging methods used for fusion assessment included radiograph (static and/or dynamic) and CT scan. Radiograph was used in fifty two studies. CT scan was used in twenty six papers. Twenty five studies used both methods. In selected studies, a total of 1425 patients were evaluated. The non-union rates ranged from 0% to 62%. The pooled estimate for all studies was 10% (95% CI: 7%–13%). However, the estimate was associated with substantial heterogeneity (p<0.001) (Figure 2). We observed that the pooled non-union rate based on CT scan (12%, 95% CI: 7%–17%) was higher than that based on only X-rays (8%, 95% CI: 4%–13%). Nevertheless, the difference was statistically insignificant (p = 0.234) after univariate meta-regression analysis. Therefore, we combine both image modalities into one database. Univariate meta-regression analysis showed that old age (p = 0.002), less than one year follow-up (p = 0.017), and publication after 2000 (p = 0.012) were significantly predictive of non-union. The non-union rate increased with age, as estimates in the five age groups were 7%, 6%, 11%, 15%, and 25%, respectively (Figure 3). Subgroup comparisons showed that the non-union rate in age ≥

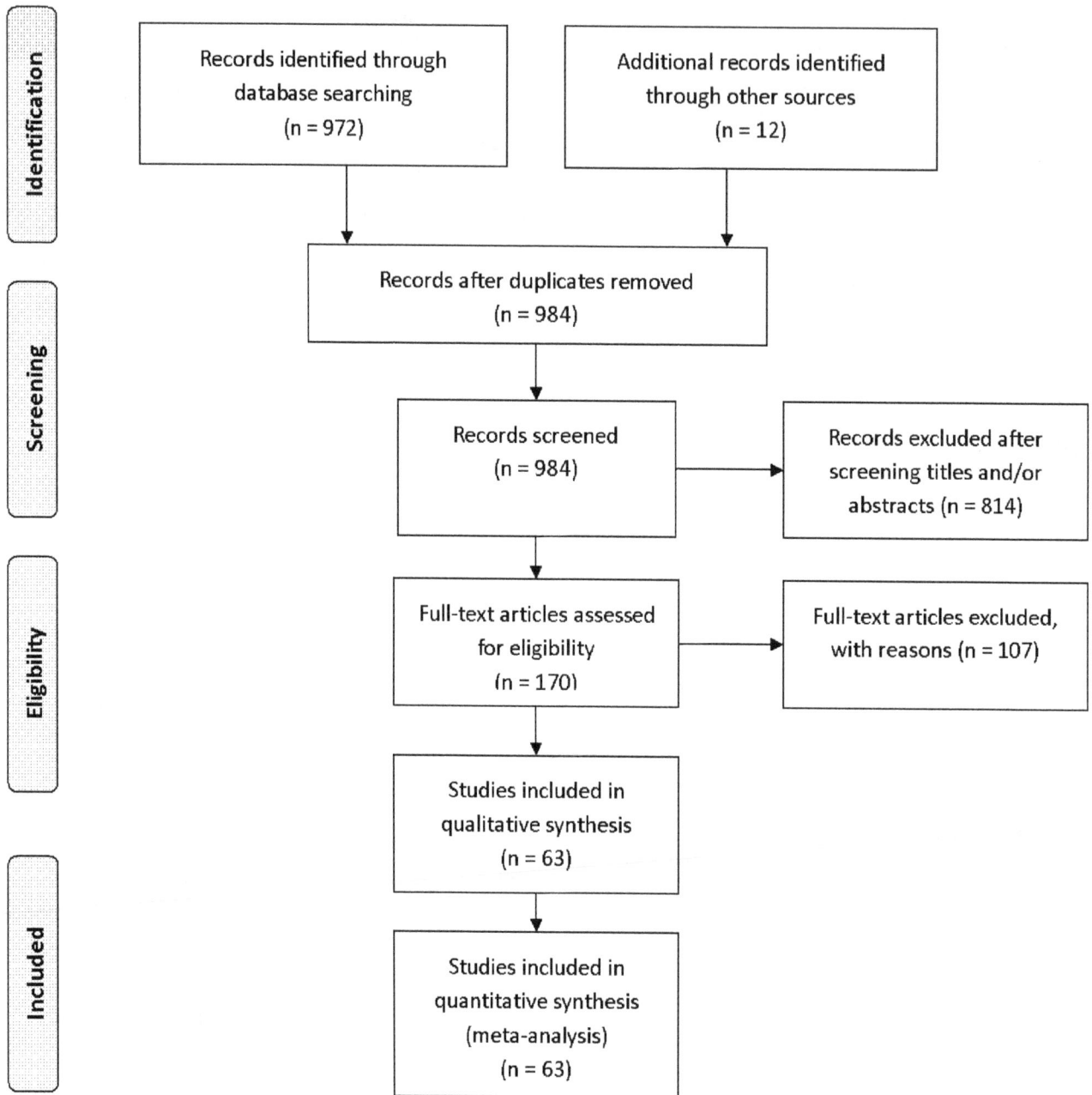

Figure 1. Selection of relevant publications, reasons for exclusion.

70 was significant higher than that in age ≤40 (p = 0.015) and in age 40 to <50 (p = 0.015). After multivariate meta-regression analysis, only age (p = 0.016) remained significant. No significant publication bias was detected (p = 0.699).

48 citations [12,14,15,17–20,22–24,26–31,33–35,38–56,58–60,62–67,69] provided re-operation information following odontoid screw fixation. Reasons for re-operation included screw loosening/pullout/cut-out/mal-position, fracture re-dislocation, unstable non-union, hematoma, and so on. The re-operation rates ranged from 0% to 24%. The random-effect pooled proportion was 5% (95% CI: 3%–7%) with pronounced heterogeneity (p = 0.029) (Figure 4). Meta-regression analysis revealed that none of the examined variables (year of publication, age, gender, follow-up duration, fracture type, or sample size)

significantly influenced the re-operation rate. Egger test for publication bias showed no significant evidence for bias (p = 0.343).

Surgical site infection was assessed in 20 studies [15,19,21,22,24,31,33,34,41,45,47,49,50,60–62,66,67,69,70] with 563 surgeries. The reported infection rate was low, with estimates varied from 0% to 6%. The overall infection rate of all included studies was 0.2% (95% CI: 0%–1.2%) (Figure 5). As there was no substantial significant heterogeneity, further meta-regression analysis was not carried out. There was no significant publication bias (p = 0.549).

The main approach related complication was postoperative dysphagia. The pooled rate was 10% (95% CI: 4%–17%) with statistically significant heterogeneity (Figure 6). Meta-regression

Study	Events	Total	Proportion	95%-CI	W(random)
Bohler 1982	0	15	0.00	[0.00; 0.22]	1.7%
Lesoin 1987	0	5	0.00	[0.00; 0.52]	0.9%
Borne 1988	0	7	0.00	[0.00; 0.41]	1.1%
Geisler 1989	0	7	0.00	[0.00; 0.41]	1.1%
Esses 1991	0	9	0.00	[0.00; 0.34]	1.3%
Jeanneret 1991	0	13	0.00	[0.00; 0.25]	1.6%
Etter 1991	2	22	0.09	[0.01; 0.29]	2.0%
Montesano 1991	2	13	0.15	[0.02; 0.45]	1.6%
Knoringer 1992	3	63	0.05	[0.01; 0.13]	2.6%
Pointillart 1994	2	43	0.05	[0.01; 0.16]	2.4%
Verheggen 1994	1	17	0.06	[0.00; 0.29]	1.8%
Chang 1994	0	12	0.00	[0.00; 0.26]	1.5%
Dickman 1995	0	14	0.00	[0.00; 0.23]	1.6%
Rainov 1996	2	34	0.06	[0.01; 0.20]	2.3%
Chiba 1996	3	45	0.07	[0.01; 0.18]	2.4%
Jenkins 1998	12	36	0.33	[0.19; 0.51]	2.3%
Henry 1999	5	61	0.08	[0.03; 0.18]	2.6%
Subach 1999	1	26	0.04	[0.00; 0.20]	2.1%
Ziai 2000	0	5	0.00	[0.00; 0.52]	0.9%
ElSaghir 2000	0	28	0.00	[0.00; 0.12]	2.2%
Andersson 2000	2	8	0.25	[0.03; 0.65]	1.2%
Harrop 2000	1	9	0.11	[0.00; 0.48]	1.3%
Apfelbaum 2000	28	133	0.21	[0.14; 0.29]	2.9%
Alfieri 2001	0	9	0.00	[0.00; 0.34]	1.3%
Borm 2003	7	27	0.26	[0.11; 0.46]	2.1%
Lee 2004	2	48	0.04	[0.01; 0.14]	2.5%
Chibbaro 2005	0	10	0.00	[0.00; 0.31]	1.4%
Fountas 2005	4	42	0.10	[0.03; 0.23]	2.4%
Bhanot 2006	1	17	0.06	[0.00; 0.29]	1.8%
Moon 2006	0	32	0.00	[0.00; 0.11]	2.2%
Platzer 2007	8	110	0.07	[0.03; 0.14]	2.8%
Chi 2007	1	10	0.10	[0.00; 0.45]	1.4%
Song 2007	1	16	0.06	[0.00; 0.30]	1.7%
Ahmed 2007	11	30	0.37	[0.20; 0.56]	2.2%
Srinivasan 2008	2	11	0.18	[0.02; 0.52]	1.5%
Agrillo 2008	2	9	0.22	[0.03; 0.60]	1.3%
Sucu 2008	1	5	0.20	[0.01; 0.72]	0.9%
Collins 2008	4	15	0.27	[0.08; 0.55]	1.7%
Omeis 2009	10	16	0.62	[0.35; 0.85]	1.7%
Eap 2010	1	36	0.03	[0.00; 0.15]	2.3%
Mayer 2011	9	18	0.50	[0.26; 0.74]	1.8%
Osti 2011	5	33	0.15	[0.05; 0.32]	2.3%
Yang 2011	1	29	0.03	[0.00; 0.18]	2.2%
Wang 2011	2	42	0.05	[0.01; 0.16]	2.4%
Hou 2011	6	42	0.14	[0.05; 0.29]	2.4%
Kim 2011	1	6	0.17	[0.00; 0.64]	1.0%
Henaux 2012	5	9	0.56	[0.21; 0.86]	1.3%
Konieczny 2012	3	13	0.23	[0.05; 0.54]	1.6%
Mashhadinezhad 2012	2	15	0.13	[0.02; 0.40]	1.7%
Cho 2012	8	41	0.20	[0.09; 0.35]	2.4%
Rizvi 2012	7	20	0.35	[0.15; 0.59]	1.9%
Steltzlen 2013	1	14	0.07	[0.00; 0.34]	1.6%
Fan 2013	4	24	0.17	[0.05; 0.37]	2.0%
Martirosyan 2013	4	51	0.08	[0.02; 0.19]	2.5%
Random effects model		**1425**	**0.10**	**[0.07; 0.13]**	**100%**

Heterogeneity: I-squared=65.9%, tau-squared=0.0729, p<0.0001

0   0.2   0.4   0.6   0.8

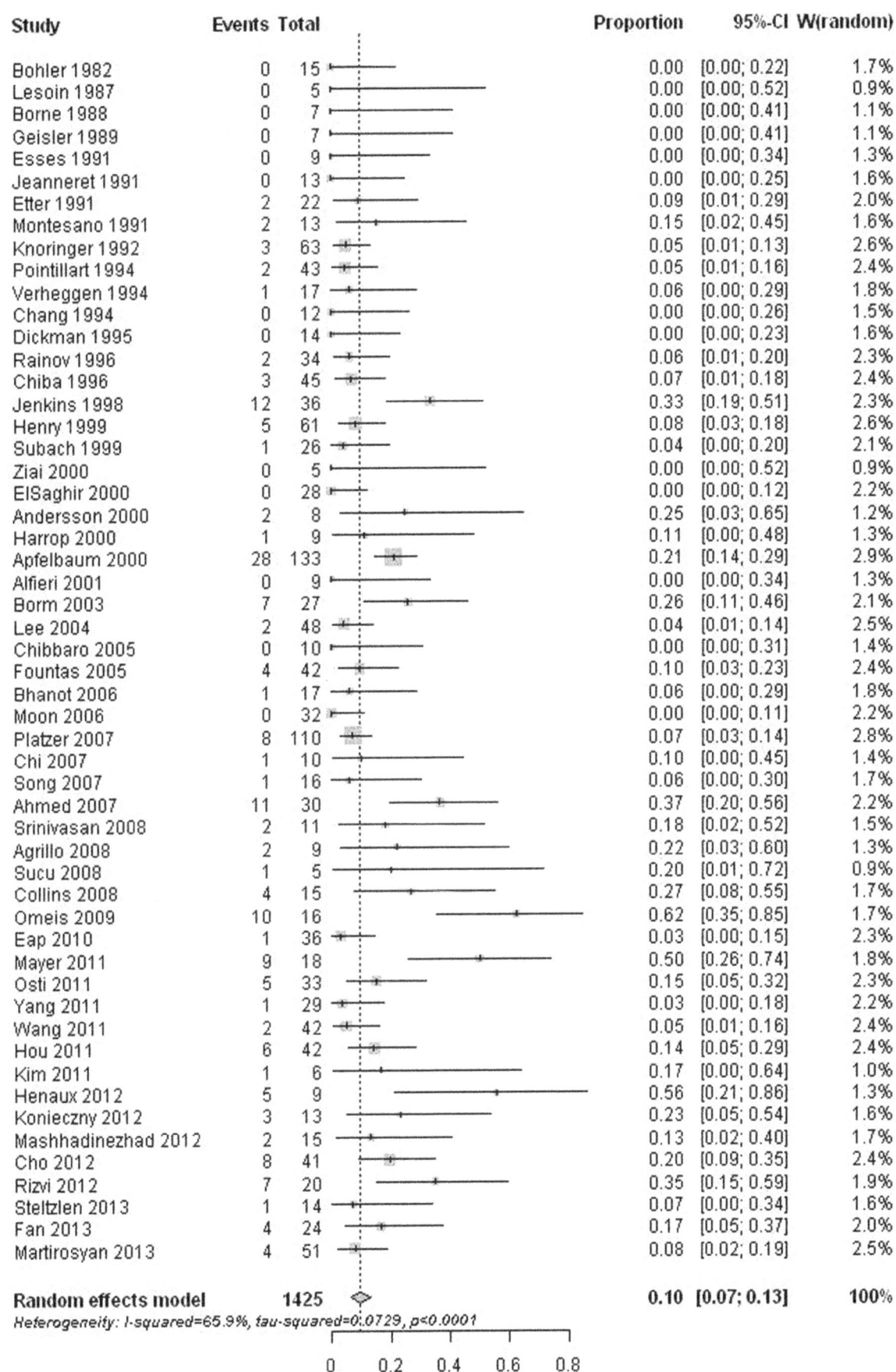

Figure 2. Forest plots showing the non-union rates (boxes) with 95% confidence of intervals (CIs; bars).

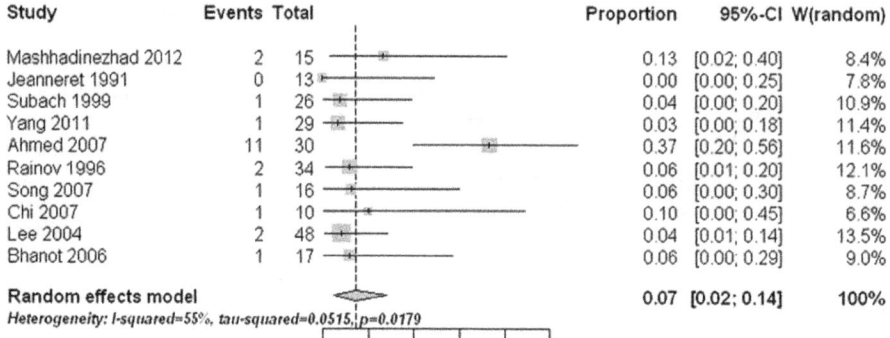

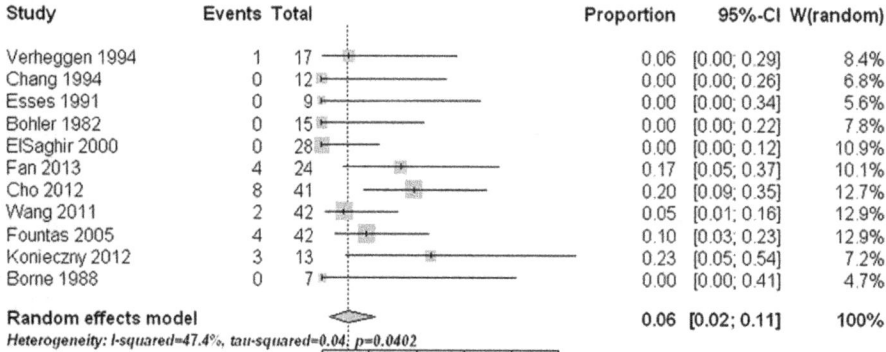

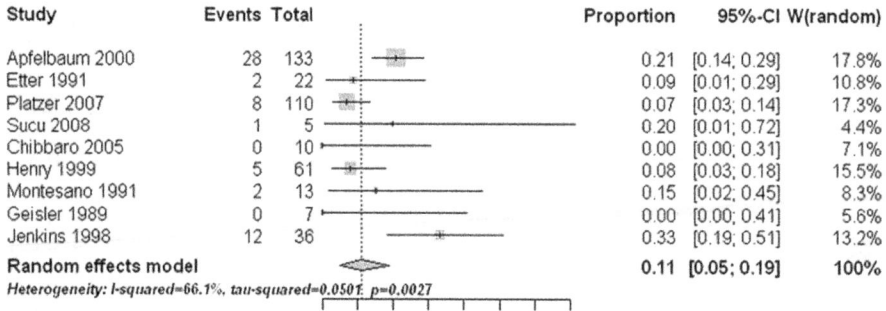

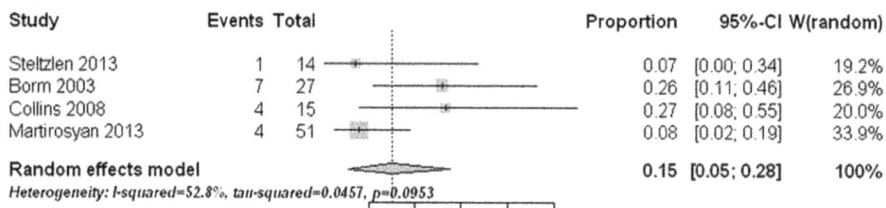

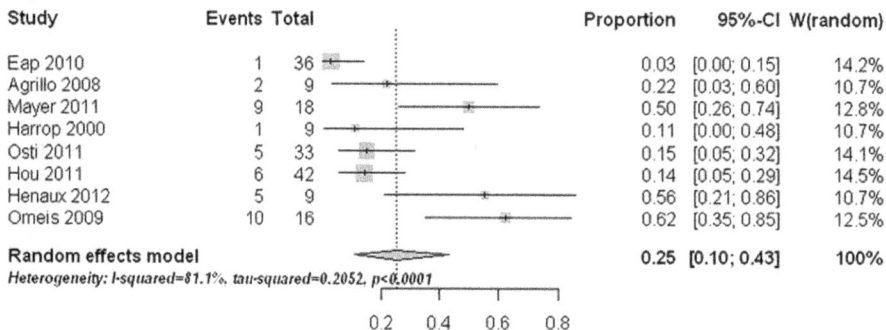

Figure 3. Forest plots showing the non-union rates (boxes) with 95% confidence of intervals (CIs; bars) in different age groups.

Study	Events	Total	Proportion	95%-CI	W(random)
Bohler 1982	1	15	0.07	[0.00; 0.32]	1.5%
Borne 1988	0	7	0.00	[0.00; 0.41]	0.8%
Geisler 1989	0	7	0.00	[0.00; 0.41]	0.8%
Jeanneret 1991	0	13	0.00	[0.00; 0.25]	1.3%
Etter 1991	3	22	0.14	[0.03; 0.35]	2.0%
Montesano 1991	3	13	0.23	[0.05; 0.54]	1.3%
Knoringer 1992	4	63	0.06	[0.02; 0.15]	3.8%
Verheggen 1994	2	17	0.12	[0.01; 0.36]	1.6%
Pointillart 1994	1	43	0.02	[0.00; 0.12]	3.1%
Chang 1994	0	12	0.00	[0.00; 0.26]	1.2%
Rainov 1996	3	34	0.09	[0.02; 0.24]	2.7%
Chiba 1996	1	45	0.02	[0.00; 0.12]	3.2%
Jenkins 1998	3	36	0.08	[0.02; 0.22]	2.8%
Morandi 1999	0	17	0.00	[0.00; 0.20]	1.6%
Henry 1999	2	61	0.03	[0.00; 0.11]	3.8%
Subach 1999	2	26	0.08	[0.01; 0.25]	2.2%
ElSaghir 2000	4	28	0.14	[0.04; 0.33]	2.4%
Apfelbaum 2000	10	133	0.08	[0.04; 0.13]	5.2%
Harrop 2000	1	9	0.11	[0.00; 0.48]	1.0%
Borm 2003	4	27	0.15	[0.04; 0.34]	2.3%
Lee 2004	4	48	0.08	[0.02; 0.20]	3.3%
Fountas 2005	1	42	0.02	[0.00; 0.13]	3.1%
Chibbaro 2005	0	10	0.00	[0.00; 0.31]	1.1%
Moon 2006	0	32	0.00	[0.00; 0.11]	2.6%
Bhanot 2006	1	17	0.06	[0.00; 0.29]	1.6%
Platzer 2007	8	110	0.07	[0.03; 0.14]	4.9%
Ahmed 2007	1	30	0.03	[0.00; 0.17]	2.5%
Chi 2007	0	10	0.00	[0.00; 0.31]	1.1%
Song 2007	1	16	0.06	[0.00; 0.30]	1.6%
Collins 2008	3	15	0.20	[0.04; 0.48]	1.5%
Srinivasan 2008	0	11	0.00	[0.00; 0.28]	1.2%
Sucu 2008	0	5	0.00	[0.00; 0.52]	0.6%
Agrillo 2008	1	9	0.11	[0.00; 0.48]	1.0%
Koller 2009	1	11	0.09	[0.00; 0.41]	1.2%
Omeis 2009	1	16	0.06	[0.00; 0.30]	1.6%
Eap 2010	1	36	0.03	[0.00; 0.15]	2.8%
Osti 2011	8	33	0.24	[0.11; 0.42]	2.6%
Yang 2011	0	29	0.00	[0.00; 0.12]	2.4%
Hou 2011	1	42	0.02	[0.00; 0.13]	3.1%
Kim 2011	1	6	0.17	[0.00; 0.64]	0.7%
Wang 2011	0	42	0.00	[0.00; 0.08]	3.1%
Cho 2012	5	41	0.12	[0.04; 0.26]	3.0%
Henaux 2012	0	9	0.00	[0.00; 0.34]	1.0%
Mashhadinezhad 2012	2	15	0.13	[0.02; 0.40]	1.5%
Kantelhardt 2012	1	6	0.17	[0.00; 0.64]	0.7%
Rizvi 2012	7	40	0.18	[0.07; 0.33]	3.0%
Konieczny 2012	3	13	0.23	[0.05; 0.54]	1.3%
Steltzlen 2013	2	14	0.14	[0.02; 0.43]	1.4%
Random effects model		**1336**	**0.05**	**[0.03; 0.07]**	**100%**

Heterogeneity: I-squared=29.8%, tau-squared=0.0152, p=0.0294

0   0.1   0.2   0.3   0.4   0.5   0.6

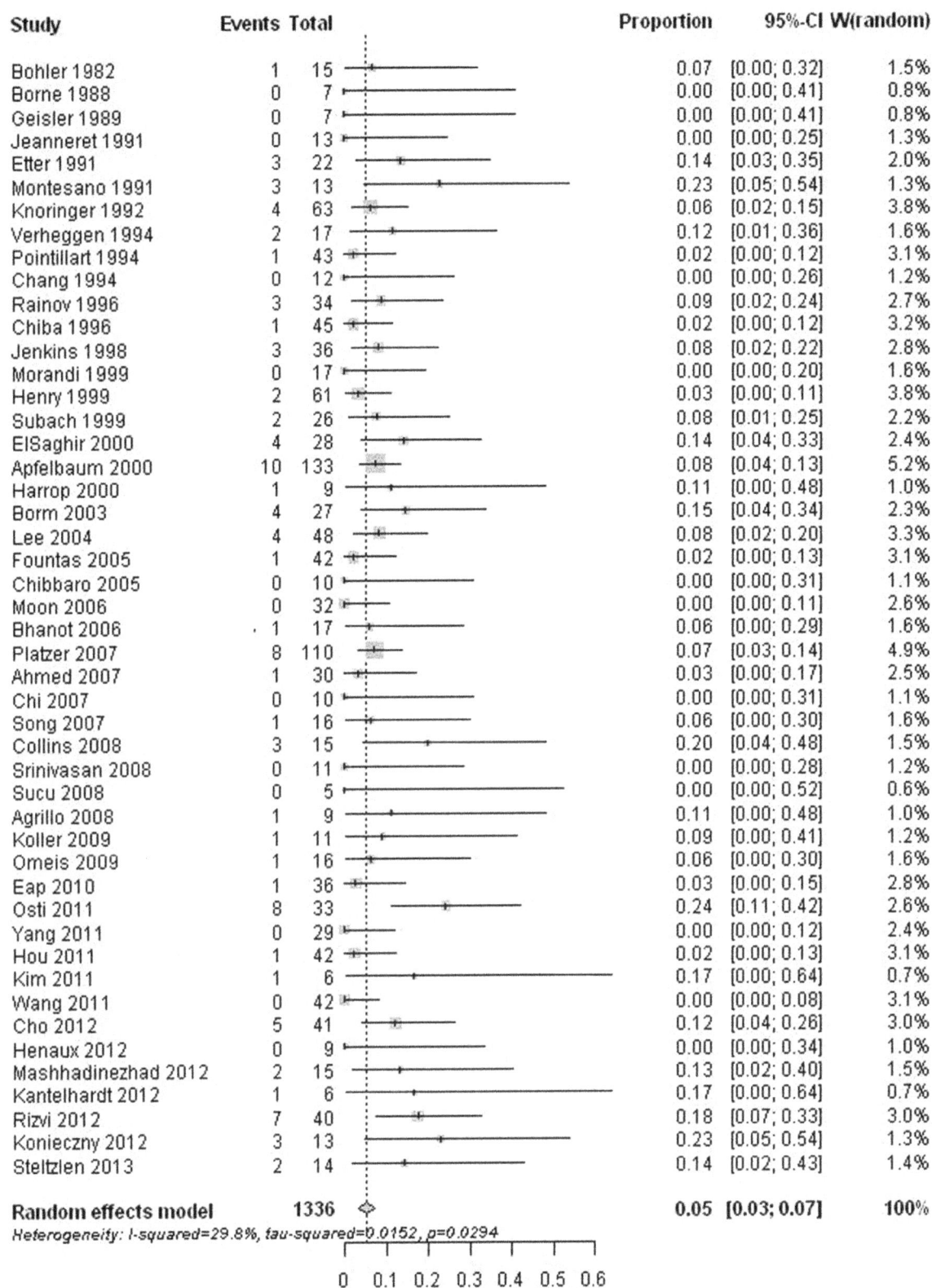

Figure 4. Forest plots showing the re-operation rates (boxes) with 95% confidence of intervals (CIs; bars).

analysis revealed that age had a significant effect on the estimate (p<0.0001). Subgroup comparisons indicated that the two old age groups (age 60 to <70 yrs and age ≥70 yrs) had significant higher dysphagia rates than those in the other three age groups (age ≤40, age 40 to <50, and age 50 to <60) (p<0.05). Pooled proportions for the other approach related complications like postoperative

Study	Events	Total		Proportion	95%-CI	W(fixed)
Geisler 1989	0	7		0.00	[0.00; 0.41]	1.3%
Montesano 1991	0	13		0.00	[0.00; 0.25]	2.4%
Chiba 1993	0	44		0.00	[0.00; 0.08]	7.8%
Verheggen 1994	1	17		0.06	[0.00; 0.29]	3.1%
Chang 1994	0	12		0.00	[0.00; 0.26]	2.2%
Subach 1999	0	26		0.00	[0.00; 0.13]	4.6%
ElSaghir 2000	0	29		0.00	[0.00; 0.12]	5.1%
Apfelbaum 2000	2	133		0.02	[0.00; 0.05]	23.3%
Fountas 2005	2	42		0.05	[0.01; 0.16]	7.4%
Chi 2007	0	10		0.00	[0.00; 0.31]	1.8%
Song 2007	0	16		0.00	[0.00; 0.21]	2.9%
Collins 2008	0	15		0.00	[0.00; 0.22]	2.7%
Srinivasan 2008	0	11		0.00	[0.00; 0.28]	2.0%
Yang 2011	1	29		0.03	[0.00; 0.18]	5.1%
Cho 2012	0	41		0.00	[0.00; 0.09]	7.2%
Mashhadinezhad 2012	0	15		0.00	[0.00; 0.22]	2.7%
Rizvi 2012	0	40		0.00	[0.00; 0.09]	7.1%
Aldrian 2012	1	25		0.04	[0.00; 0.20]	4.5%
Fan 2013	0	24		0.00	[0.00; 0.14]	4.3%
Steltzlen 2013	0	14		0.00	[0.00; 0.23]	2.5%
Fixed effect model		**563**		**0.00**	**[0.00; 0.01]**	**100%**

Heterogeneity: I-squared=0%, tau-squared=0, p=0.9877

```
0    0.1    0.2    0.3    0.4
```

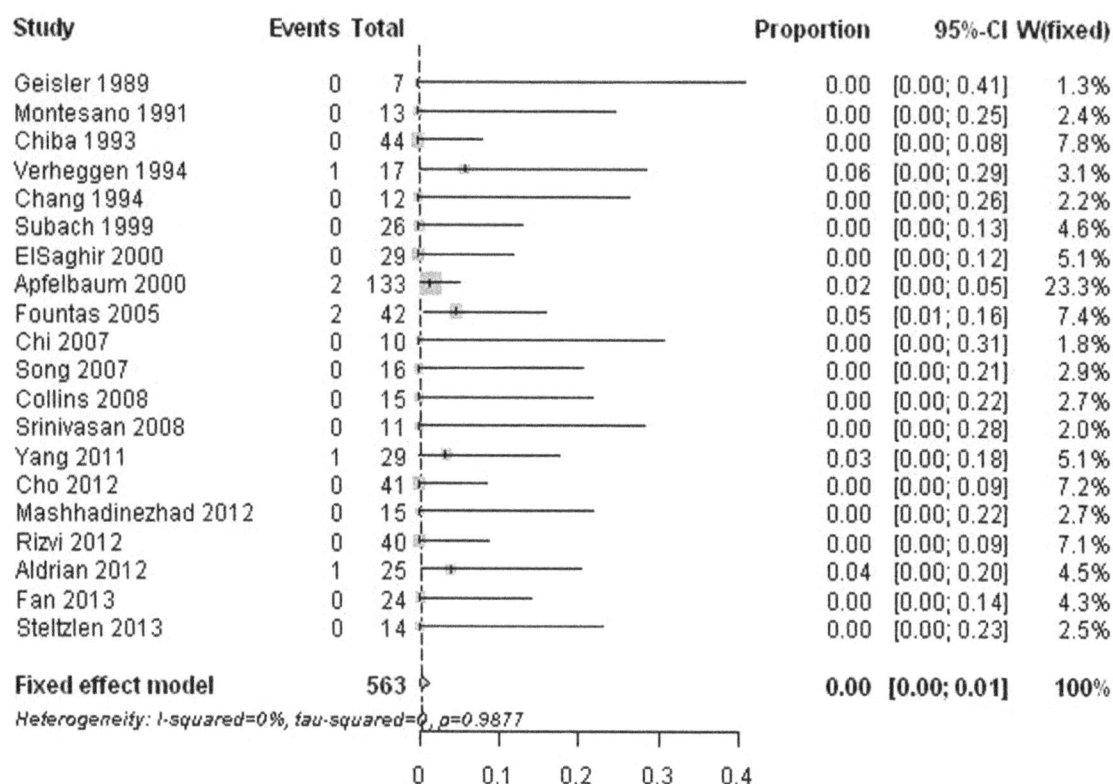

Figure 5. Forest plots showing the infection rates (boxes) with 95% confidence of intervals (CIs; bars).

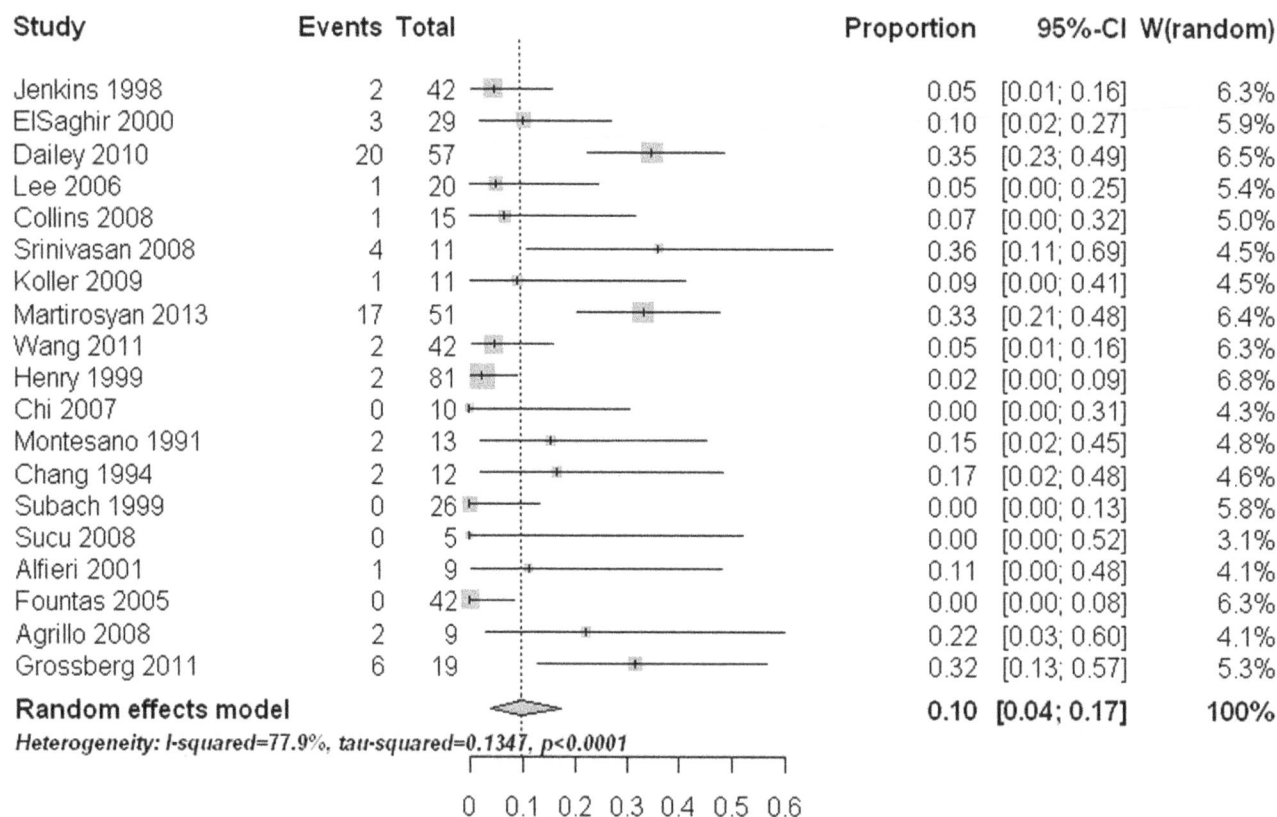

Study	Events	Total		Proportion	95%-CI	W(random)
Jenkins 1998	2	42		0.05	[0.01; 0.16]	6.3%
ElSaghir 2000	3	29		0.10	[0.02; 0.27]	5.9%
Dailey 2010	20	57		0.35	[0.23; 0.49]	6.5%
Lee 2006	1	20		0.05	[0.00; 0.25]	5.4%
Collins 2008	1	15		0.07	[0.00; 0.32]	5.0%
Srinivasan 2008	4	11		0.36	[0.11; 0.69]	4.5%
Koller 2009	1	11		0.09	[0.00; 0.41]	4.5%
Martirosyan 2013	17	51		0.33	[0.21; 0.48]	6.4%
Wang 2011	2	42		0.05	[0.01; 0.16]	6.3%
Henry 1999	2	81		0.02	[0.00; 0.09]	6.8%
Chi 2007	0	10		0.00	[0.00; 0.31]	4.3%
Montesano 1991	2	13		0.15	[0.02; 0.45]	4.8%
Chang 1994	2	12		0.17	[0.02; 0.48]	4.6%
Subach 1999	0	26		0.00	[0.00; 0.13]	5.8%
Sucu 2008	0	5		0.00	[0.00; 0.52]	3.1%
Alfieri 2001	1	9		0.11	[0.00; 0.48]	4.1%
Fountas 2005	0	42		0.00	[0.00; 0.08]	6.3%
Agrillo 2008	2	9		0.22	[0.03; 0.60]	4.1%
Grossberg 2011	6	19		0.32	[0.13; 0.57]	5.3%
Random effects model				**0.10**	**[0.04; 0.17]**	**100%**

Heterogeneity: I-squared=77.9%, tau-squared=0.1347, p<0.0001

```
0   0.1   0.2   0.3   0.4   0.5   0.6
```

Figure 6. Forest plots showing the rates of dysphagia (boxes) with 95% confidence of intervals (CIs; bars).

Study	Events	Total		Proportion	95%-CI	W(fixed)
Jenkins 1998	1	42		0.02	[0.00; 0.13]	16.7%
Borm 2003	1	27		0.04	[0.00; 0.19]	10.8%
Yang 2011	1	29		0.03	[0.00; 0.18]	11.6%
Fan 2013	0	24		0.00	[0.00; 0.14]	9.6%
Chi 2007	0	10		0.00	[0.00; 0.31]	4.1%
Montesano 1991	1	13		0.08	[0.00; 0.36]	5.3%
Chang 1994	3	12		0.25	[0.05; 0.57]	4.9%
Subach 1999	0	26		0.00	[0.00; 0.13]	10.4%
Sucu 2008	0	5		0.00	[0.00; 0.52]	2.2%
Fountas 2005	0	42		0.00	[0.00; 0.08]	16.7%
Grossberg 2011	1	19		0.05	[0.00; 0.26]	7.7%
Fixed effect model		249		0.01	[0.00; 0.04]	100%

Heterogeneity: I-squared=17.6%, tau-squared=0.0095, p=0.2759

```
   0   0.1  0.2  0.3  0.4  0.5
```

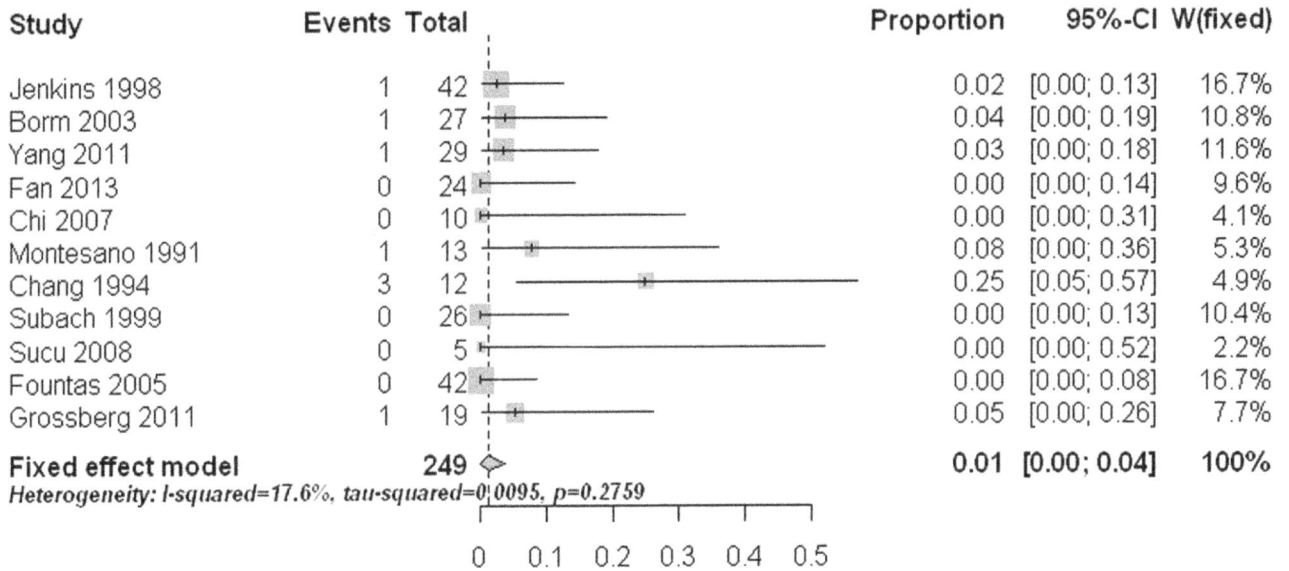

Figure 7. Forest plots showing the rates of hoarseness (boxes) with 95% confidence of intervals (CIs; bars).

hoarseness (1.2%, 95% CI: 0%–3.7%) (Figure 7), esophageal / retropharyngeal injury (0%, 95% CI: 0%–1.1%) (Figure 8), wound hematomas (0.2%, 95% CI: 0%–1.8%) (Figure 9), and spinal cord injury (0%, 95% CI: 0%–0.2%) (Figure 10) were very low. No significant publication bias was detected (p>0.1)

Discussion

We conducted this study to provide a better understanding of the frequency of non-union, infection, re-operation, and approach related complications after anterior screw fixation for type II and type III odontoid fractures. Non-union can be one of the most important outcomes, because it may lead to spinal cord injury due to atlantoaxial instability. Pooled analysis from our study showed that the non-union rate after AOSF was 10%. It seemed that the fusion rate of AOSF (90%) was better than that of the conservative treatment (60%–80%) [3], and was comparable to that of the posterior fixation (89%–100%) [5]. Therefore, AOSF might be a good choice for type II and type III odontoid fractures in selected patients. This study revealed that the re-operation rate was 5% after AOSF. The reasons for re-operation included non-union, screw failure, fracture re-dislocation, and occasionally hematoma. Since non-union accounted for fifty percent of the cases undergoing re-operation, obtaining bony fusion becomes the first priority in AOSF. Not all of the non-unions underwent second surgical interventions, because some of them (fibrous unions) were radiologically stable. For these cases, long term follow up was still essential. The infection rate in surgical site was very low with only seven cases identified during our review [24,33,41,60,61]. The pooled estimate was 0.2% without significant heterogeneity among the studies. All infection cases were superficial and were resolved without sequelae.

Our study revealed that age had a significant impact on the non-union rate. The non-union rate in patients younger than 50

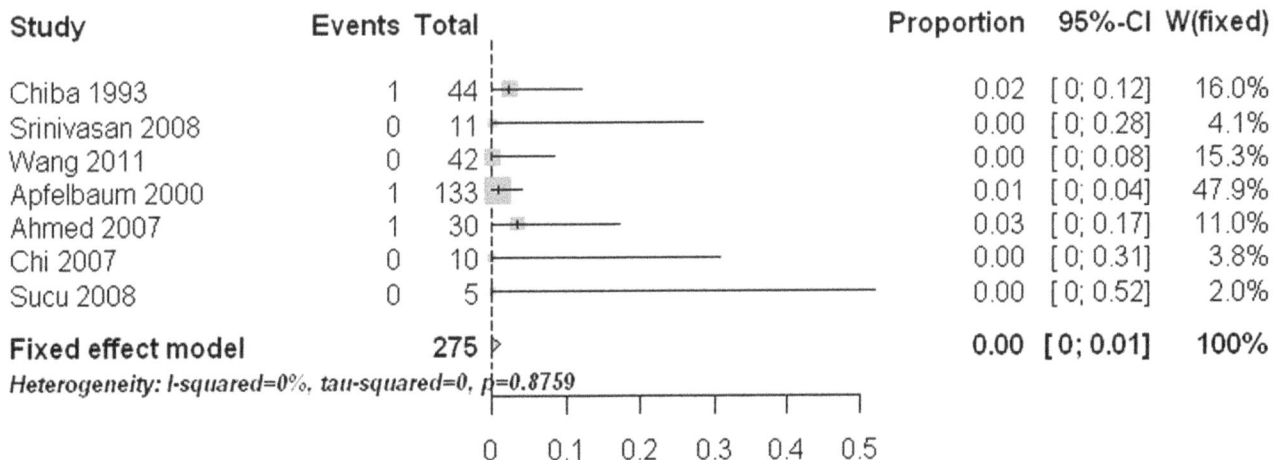

Study	Events	Total		Proportion	95%-CI	W(fixed)
Chiba 1993	1	44		0.02	[0; 0.12]	16.0%
Srinivasan 2008	0	11		0.00	[0; 0.28]	4.1%
Wang 2011	0	42		0.00	[0; 0.08]	15.3%
Apfelbaum 2000	1	133		0.01	[0; 0.04]	47.9%
Ahmed 2007	1	30		0.03	[0; 0.17]	11.0%
Chi 2007	0	10		0.00	[0; 0.31]	3.8%
Sucu 2008	0	5		0.00	[0; 0.52]	2.0%
Fixed effect model		275		0.00	[0; 0.01]	100%

Heterogeneity: I-squared=0%, tau-squared=0, p=0.8759

```
   0   0.1  0.2  0.3  0.4  0.5
```

Figure 8. Forest plots showing the rates of esophageal /retropharyngeal injury (boxes) with 95% confidence of intervals (CIs; bars).

Study	Events	Total		Proportion	95%-CI	W(fixed)
Lee 2006	0	20		0.00	[0.00; 0.17]	7.1%
Geisler 1989	0	7		0.00	[0.00; 0.41]	2.6%
Yang 2011	1	29		0.03	[0.00; 0.18]	10.2%
Etter 1991	2	23		0.09	[0.01; 0.28]	8.1%
Knoringer 1992	1	63		0.02	[0.00; 0.09]	21.9%
Chi 2007	0	10		0.00	[0.00; 0.31]	3.6%
Montesano 1991	0	13		0.00	[0.00; 0.25]	4.6%
Chang 1994	0	12		0.00	[0.00; 0.26]	4.3%
Subach 1999	0	26		0.00	[0.00; 0.13]	9.1%
Rizvi 2012	0	40		0.00	[0.00; 0.09]	13.9%
Fountas 2005	0	42		0.00	[0.00; 0.08]	14.6%
Fixed effect model		**285**		**0.00**	**[0.00; 0.02]**	**100%**

Heterogeneity: I-squared=0%, tau-squared=0, p=0.8366

0   0.1   0.2   0.3   0.4

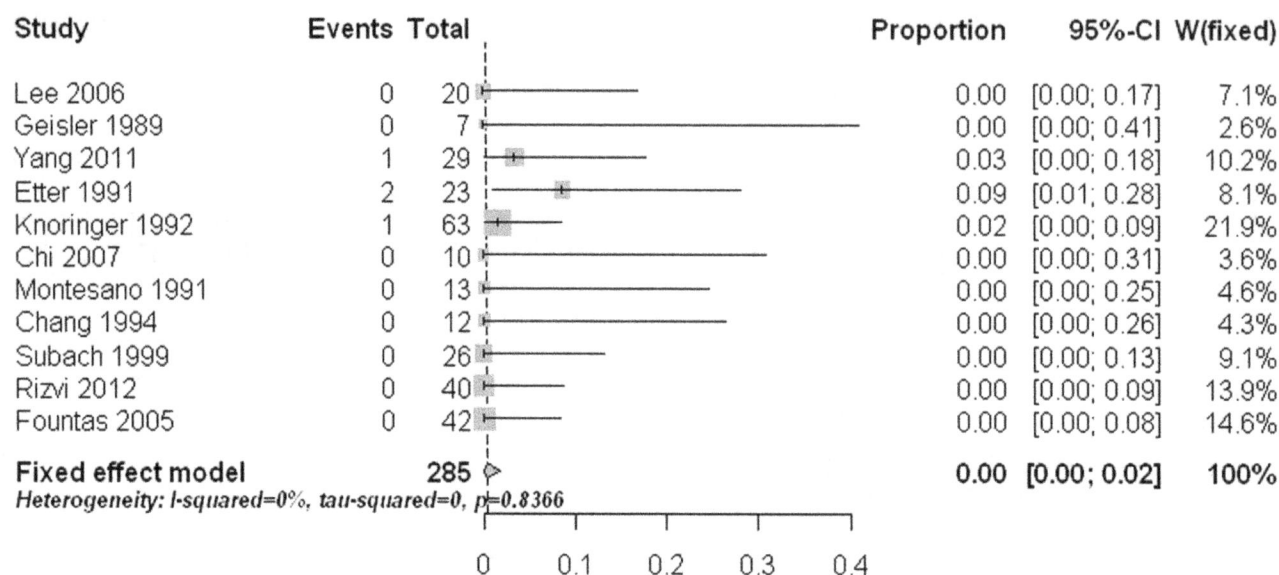

Figure 9. Forest plots showing the rates of wound hematomas (boxes) with 95% confidence of intervals (CIs; bars).

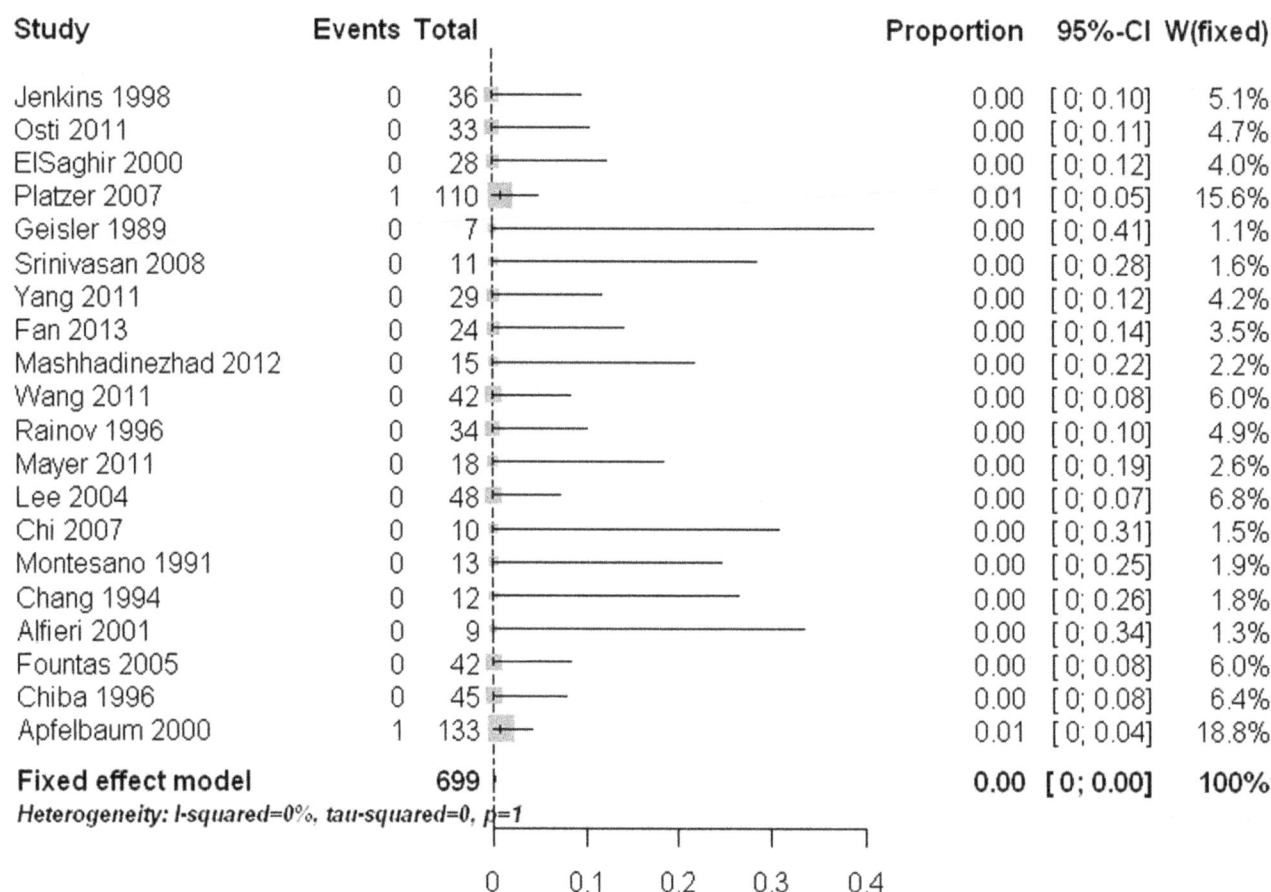

Study	Events	Total		Proportion	95%-CI	W(fixed)
Jenkins 1998	0	36		0.00	[0; 0.10]	5.1%
Osti 2011	0	33		0.00	[0; 0.11]	4.7%
ElSaghir 2000	0	28		0.00	[0; 0.12]	4.0%
Platzer 2007	1	110		0.01	[0; 0.05]	15.6%
Geisler 1989	0	7		0.00	[0; 0.41]	1.1%
Srinivasan 2008	0	11		0.00	[0; 0.28]	1.6%
Yang 2011	0	29		0.00	[0; 0.12]	4.2%
Fan 2013	0	24		0.00	[0; 0.14]	3.5%
Mashhadinezhad 2012	0	15		0.00	[0; 0.22]	2.2%
Wang 2011	0	42		0.00	[0; 0.08]	6.0%
Rainov 1996	0	34		0.00	[0; 0.10]	4.9%
Mayer 2011	0	18		0.00	[0; 0.19]	2.6%
Lee 2004	0	48		0.00	[0; 0.07]	6.8%
Chi 2007	0	10		0.00	[0; 0.31]	1.5%
Montesano 1991	0	13		0.00	[0; 0.25]	1.9%
Chang 1994	0	12		0.00	[0; 0.26]	1.8%
Alfieri 2001	0	9		0.00	[0; 0.34]	1.3%
Fountas 2005	0	42		0.00	[0; 0.08]	6.0%
Chiba 1996	0	45		0.00	[0; 0.08]	6.4%
Apfelbaum 2000	1	133		0.01	[0; 0.04]	18.8%
Fixed effect model		**699**		**0.00**	**[0; 0.00]**	**100%**

Heterogeneity: I-squared=0%, tau-squared=0, p=1

0   0.1   0.2   0.3   0.4

Figure 10. Forest plots showing the rates of spinal cord injury (boxes) with 95% confidence of intervals (CIs; bars).

years was 6%. Therefore, AOSF seems to be a good choice for young patients. Although the non-union rate reached 11% to 25% in patients aged 50 years or older, this rate was still acceptable as the non-union rate of conservative treatment for the elderly patients was very high (60% in Nourbakhsh' review [3], and 56%–72% in Huybregts' review [7]). Subgroup comparisons showed that age ≥70 had a significant higher non-union rate than the young had. Our findings were consistent with those reported by Platzer et al [46]. They observed that patients older than 65 years had a significantly higher non-union rate of 12% compared with that of 4% in younger individuals [46]. However, two other observational studies reported that age was not associated with fusion failure [38,62]. It was generally agreed that old patients had a higher chance to experience osteoporosis and diminished bone quality which might have an important effect on the fusion outcome. As none of the studies directly assessed osteoporosis of surgical patients, the bone quality information in different age groups was not clear. This could be one reason to explain the controversial results from different studies. Therefore, it is important for further studies to clarify the relationships among age, osteoporosis, and fusion outcomes after AOSF. Since elderly patients were more likely to experience non-unions, measures should be adopted to enhance the bony fusion in this population. Dailey et al [75] retrospectively analyzed the efficacy of AOSF in a group of patients with age over 70. They observed a significantly higher stabilization rate of 96% in patients when 2 screws were placed, compared with that of 56% in patients with only one screw used. However, in another group of relatively young patients, the difference became statistically insignificant [28]. Younger patients have better bone quality which could provide more stability at the surgical site. Thus, placing one screw may be sufficient. Nevertheless, the elderly patients might benefit from an additional screw which added rotational stability in the osteopenic bone [75].

Postoperative dysphagia was the main approach related complication after AOSF with pooled estimate of 10%, followed by postoperative hoarseness (1.2%). Esophageal /retropharyngeal injury, wound hematomas, and spinal cord injury were rare approach related complications. Noteworthy was that age also had a significant effect on postoperative dysphagia rate. Dysphagia is a known complication of anterior cervical spine surgery. A recent systematic review showed that female gender, advanced age, multilevel surgery, longer operating time and severe pre-operative neck pain may increase the risk of postoperative dysphagia after cervical spine surgery [79]. During our review, there was no study directly comparing the dysphagia rates among different age groups. Through this meta-analysis, we observed that age ≥60 had a significant higher dysphagia rate than the age <60 had. The possible reason for this fact was that the elderly patient's esophagus was less tolerant to retraction due to fibrosis [75]. Considering the relatively high dysphagia rate in the elderly after AOSF, strategies, such as using of perioperative methylprednisolone, monitoring of endotracheal tube cuff pressure, and preoperative tracheal/esophageal traction exercise, may be employed to reduce the risk of this complication [79].

There are some limitations existing in this study. First, this meta-analysis only focused on the rates of non-union, re-operation, infection, and approach related complications. We did not pool other outcomes like functional results and patient satisfactory outcome because they were not always reported or were reported in various forms. Even the outcomes we combined were not always available. Second, during the extraction of fusion data, we found the fusion status was assessed using different imaging modalities and non-union was defined according to different standards. Thus, pooling of relevant data might lead to bias even though we had predefined unified criteria for non-union. Third, extensive and significant heterogeneities were detected when we combined the rates of non-union, re-operation, and dysphagia. We had explored the heterogeneity through meta-regression analysis according to several study characteristics, but we only found age had a significant effect on the non-union and dysphagia rate. After subgroup analysis, we still observed heterogeneity in each age group, which meant there were potential other factors influencing the two outcomes. For re-operation, we failed to find potential factors which could explain the heterogeneity. The factors we analyzed represented the average value of each study, which could limit the exploration of the heterogeneity. Moreover, the heterogeneity might also be ascribed to various factors, such as other patient characteristics, fracture subtypes, and surgical techniques used. Lastly, the level of evidence of our analysis is low as none of the enrolled studies were randomized controlled trials. Despite these weaknesses, our study obtains some clinical significance since we pooled estimates based on a relatively large sample. This study provides a quantitative description of the frequencies of non-union, re-operation, infection, and approach related complications after AOSF for odontoid fractures. These data can be helpful in making informed surgical decisions. Further studies may be necessary to pool the functional outcomes of using this technique and to determine the factors affecting the efficacy.

Supporting Information

Table S1 Characteristics of the studies included for analyzing non-union, re-operation, and infection.

Table S2 Characteristics of the studies included for analyzing approach related complications.

Checklist S1 PRISMA Checklist.

Author Contributions

Conceived and designed the experiments: NFT FMM. Performed the experiments: NFT XQH LJW XLW. Analyzed the data: NFT XQH YSW XLZ YLC. Contributed reagents/materials/analysis tools: XYW FMM. Wrote the paper: NFT FMM.

References

1. Husby J, Sorensen KH (1974) Fracture of the odontoid process of the axis. Acta Orthop Scand 45: 182–192.
2. Maak TG, Grauer JN (2006) The contemporary treatment of odontoid injuries. Spine (Phila Pa 1976) 31: S53–60; discussion S61.
3. Nourbakhsh A, Shi R, Vannemreddy P, Nanda A (2009) Operative versus nonoperative management of acute odontoid Type II fractures: a meta-analysis. J Neurosurg Spine 11: 651–658.
4. Harrop JS, Hart R, Anderson PA (2010) Optimal treatment for odontoid fractures in the elderly. Spine (Phila Pa 1976) 35: S219–227.
5. Patel AA, Lindsey R, Bessey JT, Chapman J, Rampersaud R (2010) Surgical treatment of unstable type II odontoid fractures in skeletally mature individuals. Spine (Phila Pa 1976) 35: S209–218.
6. Pal D, Sell P, Grevitt M (2011) Type II odontoid fractures in the elderly: an evidence-based narrative review of management. Eur Spine J 20: 195–204.
7. Huybregts JG, Jacobs WC, Vleggeert-Lankamp CL (2013) The optimal treatment of type II and III odontoid fractures in the elderly: a systematic review. Eur Spine J 22: 1–13.
8. Anderson LD, D'Alonzo RT (1974) Fractures of the odontoid process of the axis. J Bone Joint Surg Am 56: 1663–1674.

156

New Frontiers in Geriatric Medicine

9. Brooks AL, Jenkins EB (1978) Atlanto-axial arthrodesis by the wedge compression method. J Bone Joint Surg Am 60: 279–284.
10. Grob D, Jeanneret B, Aebi M, Markwalder TM (1991) Atlanto-axial fusion with transarticular screw fixation. J Bone Joint Surg Br 73: 972–976.
11. Nakanishi T, Sasaki T, Tokita N, Hirabayashi K (1982) Internal fixation for the odontoid fracture. Orthop Trans 6: 176.
12. Bohler J (1982) Anterior stabilization for acute fractures and non-unions of the dens. J Bone Joint Surg Am 64: 18–27.
13. Lesoin F, Autricque A, Franz K, Villette L, Jomin M (1987) Transcervical approach and screw fixation for upper cervical spine pathology. Surg Neurol 27: 459–465.
14. Borne GM, Bedou GL, Pinaudeau M, Cristino G, Hussein A (1988) Odontoid process fracture osteosynthesis with a direct screw fixation technique in nine consecutive cases. J Neurosurg 68: 223–226.
15. Geisler FH, Cheng C, Poka A, Brumback RJ (1989) Anterior screw fixation of posteriorly displaced type II odontoid fractures. Neurosurgery 25: 30–37; discussion 37–38.
16. Esses SI, Bednar DA (1991) Screw fixation of odontoid fractures and nonunions. Spine (Phila Pa 1976) 16: S483–485.
17. Etter C, Coscia M, Jaberg H, Aebi M (1991) Direct anterior fixation of dens fractures with a cannulated screw system. Spine (Phila Pa 1976) 16: S25–32.
18. Jeanneret B, Vernet O, Frei S, Magerl F (1991) Atlantoaxial mobility after screw fixation of the odontoid: a computed tomographic study. J Spinal Disord 4: 203–211.
19. Montesano PX, Anderson PA, Schlehr F, Thalgott JS, Lowrey G (1991) Odontoid fractures treated by anterior odontoid screw fixation. Spine (Phila Pa 1976) 16: S33–37.
20. Knöringer P (1992) Internal fixation of dens fractures by double-threaded screws. Orthopedics and Traumatology: 231–245
21. Chiba K, Fujimura Y, Toyama Y, Takahata T, Nakanishi T, et al. (1993) Anterior screw fixation for odontoid fracture: clinical results in 45 cases. Eur Spine J 2: 76–81.
22. Chang KW, Liu YW, Cheng PG, Chang L, Suen KL, et al. (1994) One Herbert double-threaded compression screw fixation of displaced type II odontoid fractures. J Spinal Disord 7: 62–69.
23. Pointillart V, Orta AL, Freitas J, Vital JM, Senegas J (1994) Odontoid fractures. Review of 150 cases and practical application for treatment. Eur Spine J 3: 282–285.
24. Verheggen R, Jansen J (1994) Fractures of the odontoid process: analysis of the functional results after surgery. Eur Spine J 3: 146–150.
25. Dickman CA, Foley KT, Sonntag VK, Smith MM (1995) Cannulated screws for odontoid screw fixation and atlantoaxial transarticular screw fixation. Technical note. J Neurosurg 83: 1095–1100.
26. Chiba K, Fujimura Y, Toyama Y, Fujii E, Nakanishi T, et al. (1996) Treatment protocol for fractures of the odontoid process. J Spinal Disord 9: 267–276.
27. Rainov NG, Heidecke V, Burkert W (1996) Direct anterior fixation of odontoid fractures with a hollow spreading screw system. Acta Neurochir (Wien) 138: 146–153.
28. Jenkins JD, Coric D, Branch CL Jr (1998) A clinical comparison of one- and two-screw odontoid fixation. J Neurosurg 89: 366–370.
29. Henry AD, Bohly J, Grosse A (1999) Fixation of odontoid fractures by an anterior screw. J Bone Joint Surg Br 81: 472–477.
30. Morandi X, Hanna A, Hamlat A, Brassier G (1999) Anterior screw fixation of odontoid fractures. Surg Neurol 51: 236–240.
31. Subach BR, Morone MA, Haid RW Jr, McLaughlin MR, Rodts GR, et al. (1999) Management of acute odontoid fractures with single-screw anterior fixation. Neurosurgery 45: 812–819; discussion 819–820.
32. Andersson S, Rodrigues M, Olerud C (2000) Odontoid fractures: high complication rate associated with anterior screw fixation in the elderly. Eur Spine J 9: 56–59.
33. Apfelbaum RI, Lonser RR, Veres R, Casey A (2000) Direct anterior screw fixation for recent and remote odontoid fractures. J Neurosurg 93: 227–236.
34. ElSaghir H, Bohm H (2000) Anderson type II fracture of the odontoid process: results of anterior screw fixation. J Spinal Disord 13: 527–530; discussion 531.
35. Harrop JS, Przybylski GJ, Vaccaro AR, Yalamanchili K (2000) Efficacy of anterior odontoid screw fixation in elderly patients with Type II odontoid fractures. Neurosurg Focus 8: e6.
36. Ziai WC, Hurlbert RJ (2000) A six year review of odontoid fractures: the emerging role of surgical intervention. Can J Neurol Sci 27: 297–301.
37. Alfieri A (2001) Single-screw fixation for acute Type II odontoid fracture. J Neurosurg Sci 45: 15–18.
38. Borm W, Kast E, Richter HP, Mohr K (2003) Anterior screw fixation in type II odontoid fractures: is there a difference in outcome between age groups? Neurosurgery 52: 1089–1092; discussion 1092–1084.
39. Lee SC, Chen JF, Lee ST (2004) Management of acute odontoid fractures with single anterior screw fixation. J Clin Neurosci 11: 890–895.
40. Chibbaro S, Benvenuti L, Carnesecchi S, Marsella M, Serino D, et al. (2005) The use of virtual fluoroscopy in managing acute type II odontoid fracture with anterior single-screw fixation. A safe, effective, elegant and fast form of treatment. Acta Neurochir (Wien) 147: 735–739; discussion 739.
41. Fountas KN, Machinis TG, Kapsalaki EZ, Dimopoulos VG, Feltes CH, et al. (2005) Surgical treatment of acute type II and rostral type III odontoid fractures managed by anterior screw fixation. South Med J 98: 896–901.
42. Bhanot A, Sawhney G, Kaushal R, Aggarwal AK, Bahadur R (2006) Management of odontoid fractures with anterior screw fixation. J Surg Orthop Adv 15: 38–42.
43. Moon MS, Moon JL, Sun DH, Moon YW (2006) Treatment of dens fracture in adults: A report of thirty-two cases. Bull Hosp Jt Dis 63: 108–112.
44. Ahmed N, Loutfy M, Shershera W, Sleem A (2007) Fixation of Type II Odontoid Fractures with Anterior Single Screw. EJNS 22 137–146
45. Chi YL, Wang XY, Xu HZ, Lin Y, Huang QS, et al. (2007) Management of odontoid fractures with percutaneous anterior odontoid screw fixation. Eur Spine J 16: 1157–1164.
46. Platzer P, Thalhammer G, Ostermann R, Wieland T, Vecsei V, et al. (2007) Anterior screw fixation of odontoid fractures comparing younger and elderly patients. Spine (Phila Pa 1976) 32: 1714–1720.
47. Song KJ, Lee KB, Kim KN (2007) Treatment of odontoid fractures with single anterior screw fixation. J Clin Neurosci 14: 824–830.
48. Agrillo A, Russo N, Marotta N, Delfini R (2008) Treatment of remote type ii axis fractures in the elderly: feasibility of anterior odontoid screw fixation. Neurosurgery 63: 1145–1150; discussion 1150–1141.
49. Collins I, Min WK (2008) Anterior screw fixation of type II odontoid fractures in the elderly. J Trauma 65: 1083–1087.
50. Srinivasan U, Dhillon C, Mahesha K, Kumar P (2008) Anterior single lag screw fixation in type II Dens fracture—indian experience. Indian Journal of Neurotrauma 5: 87–91
51. Sucu HK, Akkol I, Minoglu M, Gelal F (2008) Percutaneous anterior odontoid screw fixation. Minim Invasive Neurosurg 51: 106–108.
52. Koller H, Acosta F, Forstner R, Zenner J, Resch H, et al. (2009) C2-fractures: part II. A morphometrical analysis of computerized atlantoaxial motion, anatomical alignment and related clinical outcomes. Eur Spine J 18: 1135–1153.
53. Omeis I, Duggal N, Rubano J, Cerabona F, Abrahams J, et al. (2009) Surgical treatment of C2 fractures in the elderly: a multicenter retrospective analysis. J Spinal Disord Tech 22: 91–95.
54. Eap C, Barresi L, Ohl X, Saddiki R, Mensa C, et al. (2010) Odontoid fractures anterior screw fixation: a continuous series of 36 cases. Orthop Traumatol Surg Res 96: 748–752.
55. Hou Y, Yuan W, Wang X (2011) Clinical evaluation of anterior screw fixation for elderly patients with type II odontoid fractures. J Spinal Disord Tech 24: E75–81.
56. Kim SK, Shin JJ, Kim TH, Shin HS, Hwang YS, et al. (2011) Clinical outcomes of halo-vest immobilization and surgical fusion of odontoid fractures. J Korean Neurosurg Soc 50: 17–22.
57. Mayer M, Zenner J, Auffarth A, Atzwanger J, Romeder F, et al. (2011) Efficacy of anterior odontoid screw fixation in the elderly patient: a CT-based biometrical analysis of odontoid fractures. Eur Spine J 20: 1441–1449.
58. Osti M, Philipp H, Meusburger B, Benedetto KP (2011) Analysis of failure following anterior screw fixation of Type II odontoid fractures in geriatric patients. Eur Spine J 20: 1915–1920.
59. Wang J, Zhou Y, Zhang ZF, Li CQ, Zheng WJ, et al. (2011) Comparison of percutaneous and open anterior screw fixation in the treatment of type II and rostral type III odontoid fractures. Spine (Phila Pa 1976) 36: 1459–1463.
60. Yang YL, Fu BS, Li RW, Smith PN, Mu WD, et al. (2011) Anterior single screw fixation of odontoid fracture with intraoperative Iso-C 3-dimensional imaging. Eur Spine J 20: 1899–1907.
61. Aldrian S, Erhart J, Schuster R, Wernhart S, Domaszewski F, et al. (2012) Surgical vs nonoperative treatment of Hadley type IIA odontoid fractures. Neurosurgery 70: 676–682; discussion 682–673.
62. Cho DC, Sung JK (2012) Analysis of risk factors associated with fusion failure after anterior odontoid screw fixation. Spine (Phila Pa 1976) 37: 30–34.
63. Henaux PL, Cueff F, Diabira S, Riffaud L, Hamlat A, et al. (2012) Anterior screw fixation of type IIB odontoid fractures in octogenarians. Eur Spine J 21: 335–339.
64. Kantelhardt SR, Keric N, Giese A (2012) Management of C2 fractures using Iso-C(3D) guidance: a single institution's experience. Acta Neurochir (Wien) 154: 1781–1787.
65. Konieczny MR, Gstrein A, Muller EJ (2012) Treatment algorithm for dens fractures: non-halo immobilization, anterior screw fixation, or posterior transarticular C1–C2 fixation. J Bone Joint Surg Am 94: e144(141–146).
66. Mashhadinezhad H, Samini F, Mashhadinezhad A, Birjandinejad A (2012) Clinical results of surgical management in type II odontoid fracture: a preliminary report. Turk Neurosurg 22: 583–587.
67. Rizvi SA, Fredo HL, Lied B, Nakstad PH, Ronning P, et al. (2012) Surgical management of acute odontoid fractures: surgery-related complications and long-term outcomes in a consecutive series of 97 patients. J Trauma Acute Care Surg 72: 682–690.
68. Martirosyan NL, Kalb S, Cavalcanti DD, Lochhead RA, Uschold TD, et al. (2013) Comparative Analysis of Isocentric 3-dimensional C-arm Fluoroscopy and Biplanar Fluoroscopy for Anterior Screw Fixation in Odontoid Fractures. J Spinal Disord Tech 26: 189–193.
69. Steltzlen C, Lazennec JY, Catonne Y, Rousseau MA (2013) Unstable odontoid fracture: Surgical strategy in a 22-case series, and literature review. Orthop Traumatol Surg Res. Epub ahead of print.
70. Fan K, Liao J, Niu C, Chen L, Chen W, et al. (2013) Anterior single-screw fixation in 24 patients with Type II odontoid fractures. Formosa n Journal of Musculosk eletal Disorde rs 4 26–31

71. Fujii E, Kobayashi K, Hirabayashi K (1988) Treatment in fractures of the odontoid process. Spine (Phila Pa 1976) 13: 604–609.
72. Berlemann U, Schwarzenbach O (1997) Dens fractures in the elderly. Results of anterior screw fixation in 19 elderly patients. Acta Orthop Scand 68: 319–324.
73. Fountas KN, Kapsalaki EZ, Karampelas I, Feltes CH, Dimopoulos VG, et al. (2005) Results of long-term follow-up in patients undergoing anterior screw fixation for type II and rostral type III odontoid fractures. Spine (Phila Pa 1976) 30: 661–669.
74. Lee SH, Sung JK (2006) Anterior odontoid fixation using a 4.5-mm Herbert screw: The first report of 20 consecutive cases with odontoid fracture. Surg Neurol 66: 361–366; discussion 366.
75. Dailey AT, Hart D, Finn MA, Schmidt MH, Apfelbaum RI (2010) Anterior fixation of odontoid fractures in an elderly population. J Neurosurg Spine 12: 1–8.

76. Cho DC, Sung JK (2011) Is All Anterior Oblique Fracture Orientation Really a Contraindication to Anterior Screw Fixation of Type II and Rostral Shallow Type III Odontoid Fractures? J Korean Neurosurg Soc 49: 345–350.
77. Grossberg J, Spader H, Belknap T, Oyelese A (2011) The use of the Mayfield Frame facilitates trajectory in anterior odontoid screw fixation. 27th annual meeting of the AANS/CNS section on disorder of the spine and peripheral nerves.
78. Wright JG, Swiontkowski MF, Heckman JD (2003) Introducing levels of evidence to the journal. J Bone Joint Surg Am 85-A: 1–3.
79. Cho SK, Lu Y, Lee DH (2013) Dysphagia following anterior cervical spinal surgery: a systematic review. Bone Joint J 95-B: 868–873

## 19

Functional Changes during Hospital Stay in Older Patients Admitted to an Acute Care Ward: A Multicenter Observational Study

Stefanie L. De Buyser[1]*, Mirko Petrovic[1], Youri E. Taes[2], Davide L. Vetrano[3], Andrea Corsonello[4], Stefano Volpato[5], Graziano Onder[3]

1 Department of Geriatrics, Ghent University Hospital, Ghent, Belgium, 2 Department of Endocrinology and Unit for Osteoporosis and Metabolic Bone Diseases, Ghent University Hospital, Ghent, Belgium, 3 Centro Medicina dell'Invecchiamento, Università Cattolica del Sacro Cuore, Rome, Italy, 4 Unit of Geriatric Pharmaco-epidemiology, IRCCS - Italian National Research Centre on Aging (INRCA), Cosenza, Italy, 5 Department of Medical Sciences, University of Ferrara, Ferrara, Italy

Abstract

Objectives: Changes in physical performance during hospital stay have rarely been evaluated. In this study, we examined functional changes during hospital stay by assessing both physical performance and activities of daily living. Additionally, we investigated characteristics of older patients associated with meaningful in-hospital improvement in physical performance.

Methods: The CRiteria to assess appropriate Medication use among Elderly complex patients project recruited 1123 patients aged ≥65 years, consecutively admitted to geriatric or internal medicine acute care wards of seven Italian hospitals. We analyzed data from 639 participating participants with a Mini Mental State Examination score ≥18/30. Physical performance was assessed by walking speed and grip strength, and functional status by activities of daily living at hospital admission and at discharge. Meaningful improvement was defined as a measured change of at least 1 standard deviation. Multivariable logistic regression models predicting meaningful improvement, included age, gender, type of admission (through emergency room or elective), and physical performance at admission.

Results: Mean age of the study participants was 79 years (range 65–98), 52% were female. Overall, mean walking speed and grip strength performance improved during hospital stay (walking speed improvement: 0.04±0.20 m/s, p<0.001; grip strength improvement: 0.43±5.66 kg, p=0.001), no significant change was observed in activities of daily living. Patients with poor physical performance at admission had higher odds for in-hospital improvement.

Conclusion: Overall, physical performance measurements show an improvement during hospital stay. The margin for meaningful functional improvement is larger in patients with poor physical function at admission. Nevertheless, most of these patients continue to have poor performance at discharge.

Editor: Heiner K. Berthold, Bielefeld Evangelical Hospital, Germany

Funding: This work was supported by the Italian Ministry of Labour, Health and Social Policy who funded the CRIME project (Bando Giovani Ricercatori 2007, convenzione no 4). Youri Taes is a Postdoctoral Fellow with the 'Fonds voor Wetenschappelijk Onderzoek – Vlaanderen' (FWO; Research Foundation – Flanders; http://www.fwo.be/Postdoctoraal-onderzoeker.aspx). The funders had no role in study design, data collection and analysis, decision to publish, or preparation of the manuscript.

Competing Interests: The authors have declared that no competing interests exist.

* E-mail: stefanie.debuyser@UGent.be

Introduction

Functional changes in older persons with an acute illness can be expected during hospital stay [1,2]. However, changes in physical performance during hospital stay have scarcely been evaluated. In the existing literature, in-hospital functional changes have been almost exclusively reported by changes in functional status [3–6], e.g. using the Barthel Index [7] and Katz's Activities of Daily Living (ADL) index [8]. Functional status measurements are self-reported and their accuracy can be affected by the complex circumstances of hospital stay. Sager *et al.* [9] found discrepancies between patient' assessments and performance-based measurements of the ability to do ADLs in a substantial proportion of hospitalised older persons. Bathing and dressing were the two activities in which agreement rates were the lowest. For example, patients who need help dressing because they are tethered to an intravenous pole, may have a clouded judgment about the ability to perform this ADL independently [5].

Alternatively, physical performance measurements (PPMs) can be used to assess physical function in older adults. PPMs can even identify more limitations in physical functioning than self-reported subjective measurements [10]. Furthermore, PPMs are more sensitive to change and might be more useful for longitudinal evaluations [11]. Finally, PPMs are more able to predict outcomes than self-reported measurements [12]. Results of functional change during hospital stay might be different for PPMs compared with ADL index [5,9].

Past studies have mainly focused on functional decline of acutely ill older patients during hospital stay [13–15]. Functional decline is strongly associated with nursing home admission [16] and 3-month mortality [6]. Nevertheless, functional improvement after hospital admission has also been reported [4–6].

This study had two objectives. The first objective was to examine functional changes during hospital stay in older patients admitted to geriatric or internal medicine acute care wards by assessing both physical performance and functional status. The second objective was to investigate which characteristics of older patients are associated with meaningful in-hospital improvement in physical performance.

Methods

Ethics statement

The study complies with the ethical rules for human experimentation that are stated in the Declaration of Helsinki. All participating hospitals (Gemelli Hospital, Università Cattolica del Sacro Cuore in Rome/University of Perugia/University of Ferrara/Italian National Research Center on Aging (INRCA) in Ancona/INRCA in Cosenza/INRCA in Fermo/INRCA in Rome) had obtained approval for the study from their ethical committee. Written, informed consent was obtained from all participants.

Data source & study population

Data from the CRiteria to assess appropriate Medication use among Elderly complex patients (CRIME) project were used. The CRIME project was initiated to assess prescribing patterns in older adults hospitalised across Italy and to produce recommendations for appropriate pharmacological prescribing in older complex patients. Details about the methodology of the CRIME project are reported elsewhere [17–19].

CRIME participants were patients aged 65 years or more, consecutively admitted to geriatric or internal medicine acute care wards of the seven above mentioned hospitals. Between June 2010 and May 2011, a total number of 1123 hospitalised older in-patients were enrolled in the CRIME project.

Data collection

A questionnaire was designed to assess the participants within 24 hours of admission and at daily intervals until discharge. Study researchers had received a two-day training course in which they were well-trained about how to correctly collect and report questionnaire data. The study researchers used a variety of information sources, including direct observation, clinical records, and interviews with the patients, family, friends or formal service providers. The questionnaire included demographics, type of admission (through emergency room or elective if planned previously), anthropometrics, socio-economics, cognitive status (30 items Mini-Mental State Examination (MMSE) [20]), psychological status (15 items Geriatric Depression Scale), drug use, medical diagnoses, and geriatric conditions (pain, falls, delirium, and pressure sores). Data on drug use, medical diagnoses and geriatric conditions were updated daily.

Physical function measurements

Physical function was assessed within the first 24 hours after hospital admission and the day of discharge by the study researchers. Walking speed (WS) was assessed by having the participant walk at his/her usual pace over a four-meter distance.

This test has shown a high test-retest reliability [12]. For the present study the fastest walk of two measurements was used in the analyses. Not all patients were ambulatory at admission. For this reason WS assessment was not performed in 228 patients.

Measurement of grip strength (GS) was performed using a North Coast Medical hand dynamometer. Patients were seated with the wrist in a neutral position and the elbow flexed 90°. In case a subject was unable to sit, GS was assessed lying at 30° in bed with the elbows supported. The highest value of two consecutive measurements obtained with the dominant hand was used in the analyses. A distinction was made between subjects unable to perform GS and subjects who did not execute the test despite being capable.

Dependency in ADLs (transferring, bathing, dressing, eating, bowel and bladder continence, and personal hygiene) was reported to assess functional status just before admission. Scores ranged from no to six dependencies.

Analytical approach

In order to exclude patients not able to complete the PPMs because of cognitive problems or inability to understand instructions, analyses were limited to patients with an MMSE score ≥18/30. This is in line with other projects focusing on physical performance in older persons [21]. Further, patients who died during hospital stay (N = 25) were excluded from the analyses. This left an analytical sample of 639 subjects. Various sub-analyses have been performed, for example, by excluding subjects unable to perform WS or GS at admission or by excluding subjects with high performance at admission (WS ≥0.8 m/s or GS ≥20 kg/30 kg for women/men).

Functional change was computed in the way that positive values indicate a functional improvement. In order to capture functional change in subjects unable to perform a test at admission or discharge, the value corresponding to the first percentile of admission performance of participants was assigned to these subjects and to those with a performance below the first percentile (WS: 0.23 m/s, GS: 5 kg). Subjects who did not perform GS despite being capable, were treated as missing variables (N = 4). Meaningful improvement in physical performance was defined as a measured change of at least 1 standard deviation (SD), this equals a 0.20 m/s increase in WS and 5 or 7 kg increase in GS for women or men, respectively. For functional status, change in the ability to do at least 1 ADL was considered meaningful.

To visualise the functional change according to admission performance, subjects were categorised into three groups according to physical performance at admission. WS categories were: unable to perform the test, less than 0.8 m/s, and at least 0.8 m/s [22]. GS categories were: unable to perform the test, less than 20 kg in women or 30 kg in men, and at least 20 kg in women or 30 kg in men [22].

Statistical methodology

Continuous variables were expressed as mean ± SD or median (first to third quartile), where appropriate. Countable variables were presented as absolute number and percentage (%) of the study population. In-hospital change in physical function was examined with paired samples T-tests or related-samples Wilcoxon signed rank test, where appropriate. Multivariable logistic regression was used to predict meaningful improvement in WS and GS. Regression models included age, gender, type of admission, and physical performance at admission (continuous variable). Additional analyses also included length of stay (days), MMSE score, comorbidity (sum), or number of drugs during stay. Hosmer-Lemeshow goodness-of-fit tests indicated no signs of a bad model fit. All analyses were performed using SPSS software, version 19.0 (SPSS Inc., Chicago, IL). Differences according to type of admission in ability to perform PPMs and in physical performance of participants were examined with Chi-square statistics and Independent-Samples T tests, respectively. The relationship between comorbidity and physical performance at admission was assessed using linear regression analyses. Statistical significance was indicated by a P value <0.05; all P values were two-tailed.

Results

Patient Characteristics

Age ranged between 65 and 98 years. Men and women were nearly equally represented (48% men). Slightly more than half of the patients were electively admitted (55%). Detailed characteristics of our sample are reported in Table 1. Most prevalent diseases were hypertension (N = 523, 82%), ischemic heart disease (N = 206, 32%), heart failure (N = 156, 25%), diabetes mellitus (N = 195, 31%), osteoarthritis (N = 239, 37%), chronic obstructive pulmonary disease (N = 237, 37%), and renal failure (N = 147, 23%).

Within patients admitted from the emergency room, 49% (N = 141) and 22% (N = 53) was unable to perform WS or GS, respectively. These proportions are substantially higher (P<0.001) than those in patients admitted electively (N = 87, 33% and N = 25, 8%). In patients able to perform, mean GS and WS performance did not significantly differ according to type of admission.

Changes during Hospital Stay in Physical Performance and Functional Status

Overall, mean WS and GS performance improved significantly during hospital stay (Table 2), but most patients had no meaningful change in WS (86%, N = 552) or GS (88%,

N = 558). Thirty-six% of subjects (N = 228) were unable to perform WS at admission, of these 23% (N = 52) regained their ability with a mean WS of 0.69±0.28 m/s at discharge. Twelve% was unable to perform GS at admission, of these 41% (N = 78) had regained function at discharge (mean GS = 17.48±10.61 kg). The mean and SD of GS change was larger in men than in women (1.02±6.65 kg vs. −0.12±4.50 kg). Table 2 provides more details concerning the changes in physical performance during hospital stay. Sub-analyses excluding subjects unable to perform WS or GS at admission led to similar mean changes.

Globally, functional status, expressed by ADL score, did not significantly change during hospital stay, only 38 subjects improved in ADL (P = 0.058). The great majority of the subjects (91%, N = 581) obtained the same score of admission at discharge (median admission score = 1 (0–2) dependencies).

Characteristics Associated with Meaningful Changes during Hospital Stay

As illustrated in Figure 1, in-hospital change in physical function varied according to admission performance. Subjects who were unable to perform WS at admission or with slow WS (<0.8 m/s) improved in mean WS performance during stay, but remained to have poor function at discharge. Similarly, subjects who were unable to perform GS or with weak GS at admission improved in mean GS performance during stay, but still performed poorly at discharge. Subjects with high GS performance at admission had a significant decline during hospital stay.

Table 3 shows the results from multivariable logistic regression analyses predicting meaningful improvement in WS or GS during hospital stay. These models illustrate an association of admission performance with functional improvement during hospital stay. The odds for in-hospital improvement decreased when patients were electively admitted and when they had higher performance at admission. Additionally, the odds for WS improvement during

Table 1. Characteristics of the study population (N = 639).

	Value
Age (years), mean ± SD	79.2±6.9
Gender (female), N (%)	331 (52)
Elective admission, N (%)	349 (55)
Walking speed category at admission, N (%)	
Unable to perform the test	228 (36)
<0.8 m/s	291 (46)
≥0.8 m/s	120 (19)
Grip strength category at admission, N (%)	
Unable to perform the test	78 (12)
<20 kg ♀/<30 kg ♂	368 (58)
≥20 kg ♀/≥30 kg ♂	189 (30)
ADL dependencies, median (IQR)	1 (0–2)
Length of stay (days), median (IQR)	9 (6–14)
MMSE, median (IQR)	25 (22–28)
Geriatric Depression Scale (15-items), median (IQR)*	4 (2–7)
Comorbidity sum, median (IQR)	4 (3–6)
N° drugs during stay, median (IQR)	9 (7–13)

*Geriatric Depression Scale data were missing for 48 subjects.
SD = standard deviation; ADL = Activities of Daily Living; IQR = interquartile range; MMSE = Mini-Mental State Examination.

Table 2. In-hospital change in physical performance.

	Admission Scores			In-hospital Change				
	N	mean	SD	mean	SD	% change vs. admission SD [a]	P	meaningful improvement % (N) [b]
Walking speed (m/s)	639	0.52	0.29	0.04	0.20	13.79	<0.001	10 (62)
Grip strength (kg)	635	19.16	10.36	0.43	5.66	4.15	0.001	7 (45)

[a]Percent change vs. standard deviation (SD) of the mean was calculated with the following formula: 100*mean change/SD of mean at admission.
[b]Meaningful improvement was defined as ≥0.20 m/s walking speed and ≥5 kg ♀/≥7 kg ♂ grip strength.
SD = standard deviation.

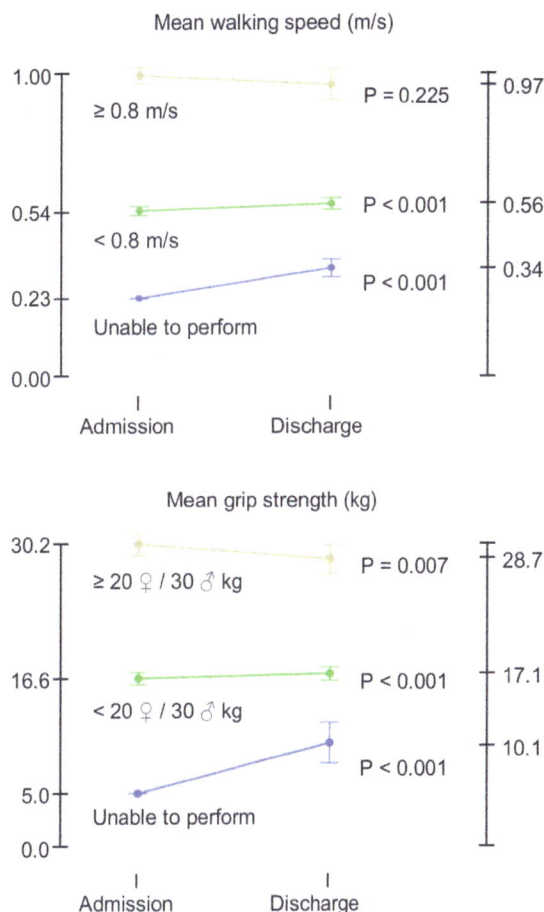

Figure 1. Change in physical performance measurements according to admission performance. Error bars represent 95% confidence intervals.

stay decreased with older age. Sub-analyses excluding subjects with high performance at admission led to similar results. Additional analyses including one extra covariate found length of stay (days), MMSE score, and number of drugs during stay not to be predictive of functional improvement. Higher comorbidity was associated with higher odds for meaningful improvement in GS (OR = 1.02, CI_{95} = 1.04–1.33, P = 0.009). Comorbidity sum was also significantly associated with GS performance at admission (β = −0.51, CI_{95} = −0.84−−0.19, P = 0.002).

Discussion

The *first* objective of this study was to examine functional changes during hospital stay in older patients admitted to acute care. Because functional change has scarcely been evaluated by PPMs, we have assessed both WS and GS performance at admission and at discharge.

PPMs have mostly been used in community-dwelling older persons, where a WS of 0.8 m/s has been accepted to define low WS [22]. Ostir *et al.* [23] assessed WS in acutely ill older patients admitted to acute care. They found 64% of patients could complete the WS test, with a mean performance of 0.53±0.25 m/s [23]. Their results are in perfect agreement with ours. Common gender-specific thresholds for GS to identify mobility limitations are 20 kg/30 kg [22] and 21 kg/37 kg [24] for women/men.

Table 3. Associations with meaningful improvement in physical performance during hospital stay.

	Walking speed improvement			Grip strength improvement		
	OR	CI_{95}	P	OR	CI_{95}	P
Age (years)	0.95	0.92–0.99	0.022	0.98	0.93–1.02	0.320
Gender (male)	1.48	0.87–2.55	0.148	1.70	0.89–3.26	0.110
Elective admission	0.42	0.24–0.74	0.003	0.46	0.23–0.93	0.030
Admission performance (m/s or kg)	0.19	0.06–0.57	0.003	0.86	0.82–0.91	<0.001

Data reported are from multivariable logistic regression models predicting improvement of ≥0.20 m/s in walking speed and improvement of ≥5 kg ♀/≥7 kg ♂ in grip strength.
OR = odds ratio; CI_{95} = 95% confidence interval.

Due to older inpatients' acute illness, high catabolism, bed rest, sleep deprivation, and polypharmacy, hospital stay is a risk factor for functional decline [1,2]. Nevertheless, we found an overall mean improvement in physical performance during hospital stay, while median functional status (ADL score) did not change significantly.

The detected improvement in physical performance might be part of a functional recovery trajectory, where functional improvement is preceded by functional decline before hospital admission as a consequence of the acute medical illness [4,5]. Stabilisation of the acute medical condition may outweigh the negative consequences of hospital stay on physical function [25].

The overall improvement in physical performance, observed in our study, is in line with the results of Volpato et al. [11] who reported in-hospital change in performance on the Short Physical Performance Battery [26] of 92 patients; 63% had better performance at hospital discharge. Similarly, Bodilsen et al. [25] reported an improvement during hospital stay in mean physical performance of 33 patients, quantified by the Timed Up and Go test. Furthermore, Purser et al. [27] reported a mean improvement in WS during stay of 0.03 m/s in frail older veterans.

Unlike two others studies [25,28], we could validate a significant improvement in mean GS performance during hospital stay. These other studies either excluded subjects unable to perform PPMs [25] or assessed changes after only one week of hospital stay [28]. In our study, subjects unable to perform had the greatest functional change and 65% of subjects stayed in hospital longer than seven days.

The *second* objective of this study was to investigate which patient characteristics are associated with meaningful in-hospital improvement. In our study, improvement in physical performance was related to admission performance, with poor performers experiencing meaningful improvements more frequently than good performers. These poor performers might have had a functional recovery trajectory with greater functional decline before admission. Since, in the study of Palleschi et al. [4], greater functional decline before hospital stay was a significant predictor of in-hospital functional improvement. In addition, a floor effect may clarify the observed improvement in poor performers, given that subjects unable to perform at admission could not further decline. When interpreting these results, one must consider that regression toward the mean might be responsible for improvement in poor performers and decline in good performers.

Older subjects had lower odds for WS improvement. Similarly, in the study of Covinsky et al. [5], older patients were more likely to fail to recover in ADL function during hospital stay.

Subjects who were electively admitted had lower odds to improve performance. Patients admitted from the emergency room often present with severe acute conditions, which may have led to a steep decline in physical performance before hospital admission. During hospital stay they can recover from the acute conditions and consequently improve their level of physical performance during stay. Patients admitted electively are less likely to present severe acute conditions. Therefore, they are less likely to improve during stay. Similarly, subjects with higher comorbidity might have a larger margin to recover from an acute condition than those with few diseases.

Performance-based versus patient-reported physical function

As reported in other studies, performance-based and patient-reported measurements of physical function appear to assess distinct and only partially overlapping domains of physical function [29,30]. Diehr et al. [31] found WS to be the most sensitive indicator of age-related decline in older adults. In our study, changes in WS and GS could be detected over the short period of time in hospital. On the contrary, the 6-item ADL scale did not seem suitable to assess in-hospital changes. Our results suggest that PPMs might be more sensitive to demonstrate functional changes during hospital stay, than self-reported functional status. Use of PPMs in the acute care setting should be encouraged, as PPMs may provide important clinical information in acutely ill older subjects. Multifaceted aspects of aging are integrated in physical functions measurements, including disease processes, nutritional status, and fitness [12]. In addition, low physical performance may reflect a state of frailty.

Limitations & Strengths

Our results have implications for the feasibility of PPMs in the acute care setting. We assigned a continuous value equivalent to the worst percentile of performance, to those patients who were unable to perform WS and GS. Just like Purser et al. [27], we found this to be a feasible way of tracking continuous improvement over time. Although this recoding may have introduced bias, we found that excluding those unable to perform led to similar mean changes. Unfortunately, the reason why subjects were unable to perform was not recorded. However, the exclusion of subjects with an MMSE below 18 removed patients not able to complete the test because of cognitive problems or inability to understand instructions. Therefore physical problems were the main reason why subjects were unable to perform PPMs.

An important variable not recorded is main reason of admission. The severity of the disease that led to hospital admission might very well be a confounding factor. However, we believe this factor is partially captured in the type of admission. Patients admitted from the emergency room often present with severe acute conditions, while patients admitted electively are less likely to present severe acute conditions. The high proportion of subjects unable to perform within patients admitted from the emergency room endorses this theory. Unfortunately, we do not have the data to fully explore these findings.

The percentage of subjects with meaningful change was relatively low. Our definitions of meaningful change (0.20 m/s WS and 5 or 7 kg GS women/men) seem roughly in line with those reported elsewhere [32–34]. Substantial meaningful change in 4-m WS observed in community-dwelling older adults was estimated at 0.10 m/s [32], while substantial meaningful improvement in WS observed during recovery from hip fracture was estimated between 0.17 to 0.26 m/s [33]. Estimates of meaningful change in WS may differ based on the direction of change or between patient populations [33]. Regarding GS, a change of more than 6 kg was suggested as necessary to detect a genuine change in GS 95% of the time [34]. It is conceivable that patients with relatively high performance on admission could not be able to demonstrate such meaningful improvement during hospital stay due to ceiling effects in PPMs. Sub-analyses have confirmed that predictive factors for functional change did not alter when subjects with high performance at admission were excluded.

Our study was restricted to functional changes from admission until discharge. Given the possibility that patients are admitted in the night, a 24-hour window was allowed to perform the first assessment. Medical therapy could have taken place between admission and assessment that could affect patients' physical performance. After hospital discharge, functional changes might still occur as part of the functional recovery trajectory. Volpato *et al.* [35] reported an improvement in 50% of patients in performance on the Short Physical Performance Battery [26] during the first month after discharge.

A strength of this study is the availability of comprehensive data. We present objective data in the clinical setting where PPMs have received little attention [35]. Our data demonstrate the feasibility of PPMs in acute care setting. Furthermore, we provide a better understanding of the dynamic nature of physical performance in older people with an acute illness during hospital stay. The multicentre design of the study improves generalisability of our results to acute care settings across Italy and Europe.

Further research

Both in community-dwelling and hospitalised older subjects, physical function measurements have shown their predictive value in terms of various adverse health-related outcomes, such as mortality, institutionalisation, and healthcare costs [36–38]. Our results suggest that the interpretation of physical performance at a single time point is not straightforward. More research is needed to determine how functional changes can add value to the prediction of hospital outcomes. Functional trajectories might even be more prognostic than single and static measurements of physical function [6].

Conclusions

This study was one of the few that observed in-hospital change in physical performance of older subjects. Overall, PPMs show an improvement during hospital stay. The margin for meaningful functional improvement is larger in patients with poor physical performance at admission. Nevertheless most of these patients continue to have poor performance at discharge.

Acknowledgments

The authors are grateful to Katrina Perehudoff for linguistic editing of the manuscript.

Author Contributions

Conceived and designed the experiments: GO AC SV. Performed the experiments: GO AC SV. Analyzed the data: SDB DV GO YT MP. Wrote the paper: SDB. Contributed to conception of the manuscript: SDB MP YT DV GO. Revised the manuscript critically: MP YT DV AC SV GO.

References

1. Hoenig H, Rubenstein L (1991) Hospital-associated deconditioning and dysfunction. J Am Geriatr Soc 39: 220–222.

2. Creditor MC (1993) Hazards of hospitalization of the elderly. Ann Intern Med 118: 219–223.

3. Landefeld C, Palmer R (1995) A randomized trial of care in a hospital medical unit especially designed to improve the functional outcomes of acutely ill older patients. N Engl J Med 332: 1338–1344.

4. Palleschi L, De Alfieri W, Salani B, Fimognari FL, Marsilii A, et al. (2011) Functional recovery of elderly patients hospitalized in geriatric and general medicine units. The progetto dimissioni in geriatria study. J Am Geriatr Soc 59: 193–199.

5. Covinsky KE, Palmer RM, Fortinsky RH, Counsell SR, Stewart AL, et al. (2003) Loss of independence in activities of daily living in older adults hospitalized with medical illnesses: increased vulnerability with age. J Am Geriatr Soc 51: 451–458.

6. Sleiman I, Rozzini R, Barbisoni P, Morandi A, Ricci A, et al. (2009) Functional trajectories during hospitalization: a prognostic sign for elderly patients. J Gerontol A Biol Sci Med Sci 64: 659–663.

7. Mahoney F, Barthel D (1965) Functional Evaluation: The Barthel Index. Maryl State Med J 14: 61–65.

8. Katz S, Ford AB, Moskowitz RW, Jackson BA, Jaffe MW (1963) Studies of illnes in the aged. The index of ADL: a standardized measure of biological and psychosocial function. JAMA 185: 914–919.

9. Sager M, Dunham N, Schwantes A, Mecum L, Halverson K, et al. (1992) Measurement of activities of daily living in hospitalized elderly: a comparison of self-report and performance-based methods. J Am Geriatr Soc 40: 457–462.

10. Guralnik J, Ferrucci L, Simonsick E, Salive M, Wallace R (1995) Lower-extremity function in persons over the age of 70 years as a predictor of subsequent disability. N Engl J Med 332: 556–561.

11. Volpato S, Cavalieri M, Guerra G, Sioulis F, Ranzini M, et al. (2008) Performance-based functional assessment in older hospitalized patients: feasibility and clinical correlates. J Gerontol A Biol Sci Med Sci 63: 1393–1398.

12. Studenski S, Perera S, Wallace D, Chandler JM, Duncan PW, et al. (2003) Physical performance measures in the clinical setting. J Am Geriatr Soc 51: 314–322.

13. Blè A, Volpato S, Pacetti M, Zuliani G (2003) Emotional vitality and change in lower extremity function after acute medical illness and hospitalization. J Am Geriatr Soc 51: 1814–1824.

14. Corsonello A, Pedone C, Lattanzio F, Lucchetti M, Garasto S, et al. (2009) Potentially inappropriate medications and functional decline in elderly hospitalized patients. J Am Geriatr Soc 57: 1007–1014.

15. Brown CJ, Friedkin RJ, Inouye SK (2004) Prevalence and outcomes of low mobility in hospitalized older patients. J Am Geriatr Soc 52: 1263–1270.

16. Fortinsky R, Covinsky KE, Palmer RM, Landefeld CS (1999) Effects of functional status changes before and during hospitalization on nursing home admission of older adults. J Gerontol A Biol Sci Med Sci 54: 521–526.

17. Fusco D, Lattanzio F, Tosato M, Corsonello A, Cherubini A, et al. (2009) Development of CRIteria to assess appropriate Medication use among Elderly complex patients (CRIME) project: rationale and methodology. Drugs Aging 26 Suppl 1: 3–13.

18. Tosato M, Settanni S, Antocicco M, Battaglia M, Corsonello A, et al. (2013) Pattern of Medication Use Among Older Inpatients in Seven Hospitals in Italy: Results from the Criteria to Assess Appropriate Medication Use Among Elderly Complex Patients (CRIME) Project. Curr Drug Saf 8: 98–103.

19. Vetrano DL, Landi F, De Buyser SL, Carfì A, Zuccalà G, et al. (2014) Predictors of length of hospital stay among older adults admitted to acute care wards: a multicentre observational study. Eur J Intern Med 25: 56–62.

20. Folstein M, Robins L, Helzer J (1983) The Mini-Mental State Examination. Arch Gen Psychiatry 40: 812.

21. Onder G, Penninx BWJH, Lapuerta P, Fried LP, Ostir G V, et al. (2002) Change in physical performance over time in older women: the Women's Health and Aging Study. J Gerontol A Biol Sci Med Sci 57: M289–93.

22. Lauretani F, Russo CR, Bandinelli S, Bartali B, Cavazzini C, et al. (2003) Age-associated changes in skeletal muscles and their effect on mobility: an operational diagnosis of sarcopenia. J Appl Physiol 95: 1851–1860.

23. Ostir G V, Berges I, Kuo Y-F, Goodwin JS, Ottenbacher KJ, et al. (2012) Assessing gait speed in acutely ill older patients admitted to an acute care for elders hospital unit. Arch Intern Med 172: 353–358.

24. Sallinen J, Stenholm S, Rantanen T, Heliövaara M, Sainio P, et al. (2010) Hand-grip strength cut points to screen older persons at risk for mobility limitation. J Am Geriatr Soc 58: 1721–1726.

25. Bodilsen AC, Pedersen MM, Petersen J, Beyer N, Andersen O, et al. (2013) Acute Hospitalization of the Older Patient: Changes in Muscle Strength and Functional Performance During Hospitalization and 30 Days After Discharge. Am J Phys Med Rehabil 92: 1–8.

26. Guralnik JM, Simonsick EM, Ferrucci L, Glynn RJ, Berkman LF, et al. (1994) A short physical performance battery assessing lower extremity function: association with self-reported disability and prediction of mortality and nursing home admission. J Gerontol 49: M85–94.

27. Purser JL, Weinberger M, Cohen HJ, Pieper CF, Morey MC, et al. (2005) Walking speed predicts health status and hospital costs for frail elderly male veterans. J Rehabil Res Dev 42: 535–546.

28. Bautmans I, Njemini R, Lambert M, Demanet C, Mets T (2005) Circulating acute phase mediators and skeletal muscle performance in hospitalized geriatric patients. J Gerontol A Biol Sci Med Sci 60: 361–367.

29. Bean JF, Olveczky DD, Kiely DK, LaRose SI, Jette AM (2011) Performance-based versus patient-reported physical function: what are the underlying predictors? Phys Ther 91: 1804–1811.

30. Wittink H, Rogers W, Sukiennik A, Carr DB (2003) Physical functioning: self-report and performance measures are related but distinct. Spine (Phila Pa 1976) 28: 2407–2413.

31. Diehr PH, Thielke SM, Newman AB, Hirsch C, Tracy R (2013) Decline in Health for Older Adults: Five-Year Change in 13 Key Measures of Standardized Health. J Gerontol A Biol Sci Med Sci 68: 1059–1067.

32. Perera S, Mody SH, Woodman RC, Studenski S a (2006) Meaningful change and responsiveness in common physical performance measures in older adults. J Am Geriatr Soc 54: 743–749.

33. Alley D, Hicks G, Shardell M, Hawkes W, Miller R, et al. (2011) Meaningful improvement in gait speed in hip fracture recovery. J Am Geriatr Soc 59: 1650–1657.

34. Nitschke J, McMeeken J, Burry H, Matyas T (1999) When is a change a genuine change? A clinically meaningful interpretation of grip strength measurements in healthy and disabled women. J Hand Ther 12: 25–30.

35. Volpato S, Cavalieri M, Sioulis F, Guerra G, Maraldi C, et al. (2011) Predictive value of the Short Physical Performance Battery following hospitalization in older patients. J Gerontol A Biol Sci Med Sci 66: 89–96.

36. Covinsky K, Justice A, Rosenthal GE, Palmer RM, Landefeld CS (1997) Measuring prognosis and case mix in hospitalized elders. J Gen Intern Med 12: 203–208.

37. Inouye SK, Peduzzi PN, Robison JT, Hughes JS, Horwitz RI, et al. (1998) Importance of functional measures in predicting mortality among older hospitalized patients. JAMA 279: 1187–1193.

38. De Buyser SL, Petrovic M, Taes YE, Toye KRC, Kaufman J-M, et al. (2013) Physical function measurements predict mortality in ambulatory older men. Eur J Clin Invest 43: 379–386.

## 20

Proteomics of Vitreous Humor of Patients with Exudative Age-Related Macular Degeneration

Michael Janusz Koss[1,2,3]*, **Janosch Hoffmann**[4], **Nauke Nguyen**[1], **Marcel Pfister**[2], **Harald Mischak**[4,5], **William Mullen**[5], **Holger Husi**[5], **Robert Rejdak**[6], **Frank Koch**[1], **Joachim Jankowski**[7], **Katharina Krueger**[7], **Thomas Bertelmann**[8], **Julie Klein**[4], **Joost P. Schanstra**[4,9,10], **Justyna Siwy**[4,7]

1 Department of Ophthalmology, Goethe University, Frankfurt am Main, Germany, 2 Doheny Eye Institute, Los Angeles, California, United States of America, 3 Department of Ophthalmology, Ruprecht Karls University, Heidelberg, Germany, 4 Mosaiques Diagnostics, Hannover, Germany, 5 BHF Glasgow Cardiovascular Research Centre, University of Glasgow, Glasgow, United Kingdom, 6 Department of General Ophthalmology, Lublin University, Poland, 7 Department of Nephrology, Endocrinology, and Transplantation Medicine Charité-Universitaetsmedizin, Berlin, Germany, 8 Department of Ophthalmology, Philipps University, Marburg, Germany, 9 Institut National de la Santé et de la Recherche Médicale (INSERM), U1048, Institut of Cardiovascular and Metabolic Disease, Toulouse, France, 10 Université Toulouse III Paul-Sabatier, Toulouse, France

Abstract

Background: There is absence of specific biomarkers and an incomplete understanding of the pathophysiology of exudative age-related macular degeneration (AMD).

Methods and Findings: Eighty-eight vitreous samples (73 from patients with treatment naïve AMD and 15 control samples from patients with idiopathic floaters) were analyzed with capillary electrophoresis coupled to mass spectrometry in this retrospective case series to define potential candidate protein markers of AMD. Nineteen proteins were found to be upregulated in vitreous of AMD patients. Most of the proteins were plasma derived and involved in biological (ion) transport, acute phase inflammatory reaction, and blood coagulation. A number of proteins have not been previously associated to AMD including alpha-1-antitrypsin, fibrinogen alpha chain and prostaglandin H2-D isomerase. Alpha-1-antitrypsin was validated in vitreous of an independent set of AMD patients using Western blot analysis. Further systems biology analysis of the data indicated that the observed proteomic changes may reflect upregulation of immune response and complement activity.

Conclusions: Proteome analysis of vitreous samples from patients with AMD, which underwent an intravitreal combination therapy including a core vitrectomy, steroids and bevacizumab, revealed apparent AMD-specific proteomic changes. The identified AMD-associated proteins provide some insight into the pathophysiological changes associated with AMD.

Editor: Sanjoy Bhattacharya, Bascom Palmer Eye Institute, University of Miami School of Medicine, United States of America

Funding: The study was financed in part by the Adolf Messer Stiftung in Königstein, Hessen, Germany; No additional external funding was received for this study. http://www.adolf-messer-stiftung.de/. The funders had no role in study design, data collection and analysis, decision to publish, or preparation of the manuscript.

Competing Interests: The authors have declared that no competing interests exist.

* E-mail: Michael.koss@me.com

Introduction

Age dependent alterations of the retinal pigment epithelium (RPE) and its basal membrane, called Bruchs membrane, are widely accepted as the main pathophysiological reason for age-related macular degeneration (AMD) and is thus the leading cause of blindness in people over the age of 60 years in industrialized countries [1]. The upregulation of vascular endothelial growth factor (VEGF) and the development of a choroidal neovascularization (CNV) are the blueprint for the conversion to the exudative or wet AMD form. Our understanding today of the disease and the interaction of intravitreal anti-VEGF treatment is thereby coined and determined by clinical diagnostics, mainly optical coherence tomography and fluorescein angiography. Since AMD is a pure retinochoroidal disease, circulating *in vivo* biomarkers such as HbA1c in the diagnosis and treatment of diabetes are still absent for AMD. Samples from the human vitreous might best

qualify as a source of biomarkers for AMD due to the proximity to the retina and the efflux of cytokines into the vitreous cavity [2]. However, most published protein analyses in exudative AMD derive from experimental animal models, *ex vivo* samples or *in vivo* from ocular anterior chamber aspirates (AC) with the incorporated flaws [3,4,5,6]. Ecker et al. demonstrated, that cytokine and growth factor levels from the AC do not reliably reflect those levels found in the vitreous and thus it is questionable to assess the activity of a purely retinochoroidal disease by examining an AC aspirate [2,7,8]. But results from vitreous samples in AMD are scarce and published data differs on patient selection, sampling technique and analysis method [7,9,10,11,12,13,14,15].

Proteome analysis allows the simultaneous assessment of a large number of proteins in a sample. Proteome analyses have been performed in a variety of ocular diseases, including primary open-angle glaucoma and cataract [16,17,18]. Further exploration of vitreous protein profiles was performed even tough clinical factors, like consistency of the vitreous, length of the eye, attachment of the posterior hyaloid are to date neglected in the literature [19]. Especially in the context of wet AMD the current proteomic data on vitreous or aqueous humor are incomplete.

Capillary electrophoresis coupled to mass spectrometry (CE-MS) is a powerful and very reproducible technology platform with known performance characteristics [20]. This automated, sensitive, fast proteome analysis technique [21] using CE as a front-end fractionation coupled to mass spectrometry, separates peptides and small proteins (<20 kDa) based on migration in the electrical field with high resolution in a single step. It enables analysis of thousands of peptides per sample using a sub-microliter sample volume and it has been used in numerous clinical biomarker studies, mostly examining urine as the specimen of interest [22,23].

In this pilot study, we performed a bottom-up analysis combing the reproducibility of CE-MS for selection of candidate marker proteins, and LC-MS/MS for sequence identification of these markers in vitreous of 73 AMD patients and controls. This led to the identification of a number of candidate proteins not previously shown to be involved in AMD. Systems biology analysis of the data suggested an increase in immune response, complement activation and protease activity to be involved in the pathophysiology of AMD.

Material and Methods

Sampling and patient characteristics

Vitreous samples were acquired at the beginning of an intravitreal combination treatment for wet AMD, which involved a 23-gauge core vitrectomy of at least 4 cc vitreous, before the application of bevacizumab, triamcinolone, and dexamethasone [22]. The same surgical technique was applied for the removal of idiopathic vitreous floaters, substituting balanced salt solution (BSS Plus, Alcon, Freiburg, Germany). This study adhered to the Declaration of Helsinki and was approved by the Investigational Review Board of the Goethe University. Written informed consent was obtained from all participants, explaining the risks and benefits of the treatment (the advantage of a combination treatment for wet AMD rather than with anti-VEGF monotherapy is summarized here [24,25,26]; the vitreous samples would otherwise have been disposed).

A total of 88 undiluted and previously untreated (any intraviteal drug application) samples were analyzed (**Table 1**). The 73 AMD samples came from 73 patients (50 women 23 men) with a mean age 77.8 ± 8.9 years (standard deviation). Sixteen of the 73 patients had a hemorrhagic CNV; 37 had an active CNV (10 with signs accompanying bleeding); 13 had a CNV and greater than 80% fibrous staining in the fluorescein angiography (FA); and 7 had a CNV-associated RPE detachment and no intraretinal fluid. These classifications were assigned after a complete ocular examination, which included a slit-lamp biomicroscopy, indirect ophthalmoscopy, color fundus photography, spectral domain optical coherence tomography (3D-OCT 2000, Topcon, Willich, Germany), and FA. Patients with previous intravitreal anti-VEGF treatment, including intraocular steroids, or systemic diabetes, nephropathy or uncontrolled hypertension were excluded. Patients with any other compromising ocular condition, such as diabetic retinopathy or uveitis, were also considered ineligible for this study.

All patients were recruited from the retina clinic of the department of ophthalmology from the Goethe University in Frankfurt am Main in Germany. Vitreous samples from 15 patients with idiopathic floaters (8 women, 7 men; mean age 60 ±

Table 1. Epidemiology of the samples.

		Number	Age (± SD)	Sex F	Sex M	Eye RE	Eye LE
AMD	Hemorrhagic CNV Bleeding	16	80.8 ± 9.0	15	1	6	10
	CNV With blood signs	10	77.7 ± 10.5	4	6	8	2
	Without blood signs	27	77.2 ± 7.4	17	10	12	15
	Fibrous	13	75.4 ± 8.1	9	4	8	5
	RPE-Detachment	7	78.3 ± 12.9	5	2	4	3
Control		15	60.0 ± 16.0	8	7	6	9

SD = standard deviation, F = female, M = male, RE/LE = right/left eye, CNV = choroidal neovascularization, AMD = age related macular degeneration, RPE = retinal pigment epithelium.

16 years) served as controls. All vitreous samples were stored at −80°C.

Tryptic digestion of vitreous

A 10-μL portion of the thawed sample was diluted with 90 μL 0.1% SDS, 20 mM DTT, and 0.1 M TrisHCl (pH = 7.6). The sample was sonicated at room temperature for 30 minutes to decrease viscosity and break up hyaluronic polymers contained in the vitreous humor. This was followed by denaturation at 95°C for 3 min. Samples were subsequently incubated with 80 mM Iodoacetamide at room temperature for 30 min in the absence of light, followed by the addition of ammonium bicarbonate buffer solution (300 μL, 50 mM) and applied to NAP-5 columns equilibrated in 50 mM ammonium bicarbonate buffer solution.

Twenty μg of Lyophilized trypsin was dissolved in 50 μL of buffer solution provided with the lypholized product. Two μL of this solution was added to the desalted sample. Trypsin digestion was carried out overnight at a temperature of 37°C. Subsequently the samples were lyophilized, stored at 4°C and resuspendend in HPLC-grade H_2O shortly before mass spectrometry analysis.

CE-MS analysis

CE-MS analysis was performed as described by Theodorescu et al [27]. A P/ACE MDQ capillary electrophoresis system (Beckman Coulter, Brea, CA) was linked online to a micro-TOF MS (Bruker Daltonik, Leipzig, Germany). The sprayer (Agilent Technologies, Santa Clara, CA) interfacing the CE and MS was grounded and the interface potential was adjusted to −4.5 kV. Signals were recorded at an m/z range of 350–3000. The detection limit of the TOF-Analyzer is in the range of 1 fmol [27].

Data processing

Analysis of raw CE-MS data was carried out using Mosaiques-Visu [28]. MosaiquesVisu uses isotope identification and conjugated mass detection for mass deconvolution. Signals with a signal-to-random noise ratio >4 and charge >1 were used. Mass spectral ion peaks from the same molecule at different charge states were deconvoluted into a single mass.

In total, 292 signals for mass and CE-time with a frequency ≥ 35% could be determined that served as reference signals for normalization of peptide CE-time and mass using linear regression. For signal intensity normalization, 22 internal standards were selected that were consistently detected in vitreous samples (average frequency 83%) and that did not appear to be significantly associated with the disease. This signal intensity normalization using internal standards has been shown to be a reliable method to address both analytical and biological variances in biological samples [29].

The normalized peptides were deposited, matched, and annotated in a Microsoft SQL database. Peptides were considered identical when deviation of mass was < ±50 ppm for an 800 Da peptide. The mass deviation was adjusted by an increase in size of up to ±75 ppm for 15 kDa. Peptides were considered identical if the CE-migration time window did not exceed 2–5%, continuously increasing between 19 and 50 min. A number of peptides were only sporadically observed. To eliminate such low relevance peptides, all peptides that appeared only once were removed and were not considered for further analysis.

Tandem mass spectrometry (MS/MS) sequencing

For MS/MS analysis five lyophilized, tryptic-digested randomly selected vitreous samples were dissolved in 15 μL distilled water. Fractionation was carried out according to Metzger et al. [30]

using a Dionex Ultimate 3000 Nano LC System (Dionex, Camberly, UK). After loading (5 μl) onto a Dionex 0.1×20 mm 5 μm C18 nano trap column at a flowrate of 5 μl/min in 98% 0.1% formic acid and 2% acetonitrile, sample was eluted onto an Acclaim PepMap C18 nano column 75 μm×15 cm, 2 μm 100 Å at a flow rate of 0.3 μl/min. The trap and nano flow column were maintained at 35°C. The samples were eluted with a gradient of solvent A:98% 0.1% formic acid, 2% acetonitrile verses solvent B: 80% acetonitrile, 20% 0.1% formic acid starting at 1% B for 5 minutes rising to 20% B after 90 min and finally to 40%B after 120 min. The column was then washed and re-equilibrated prior to the next injection. The eluant was ionized using a Proxeon nano spray ESI source operating in positive ion mode into an Orbitrap Velos FTMS (Thermo Finnigan, Bremen, Germany). Ionization voltage was 2.6 kV and the capillary temperature was 200°C. The mass spectrometer was operated in MS/MS mode scanning from 380 to 2000 amu. The top 20 multiply charged ions were selected from each scan for MS/MS analysis using HCD at 40% collision energy. The resolution of ions in MS1 was 60,000 and 7,500 for HCD MS2. The MS data and the human, non redundant database IPI were matched using the SEQUEST software. Trypsin was used as the enzyme while screening for proteins. Hydroxylated proline from collagen fragments and oxidation of methionine were accepted as variable modifications and carbamidomethylated cystein as fixed modification. A maximal mass deviation of 10 ppm for MS and 0.8 Da for MS/MS was accepted. Only proteins represented by a minimum two peptides were accepted in LC-MS/MS analysis. The sequences were matched to the detected CE-MS data as described by Zürbig et al [19]. Although in this matching procedure the LC retention time can not be used, CE-MS data generate an additional parameter that can be used in this matching procedure, which is the charge of the peptides (at low pH, the condition in which peptides are analysed by CE-MS). Therefore, even when having identical or very close masses in the LC-MS/MS analysis, discrimination between peptides with similar masses can be performed on the basis of their charge. This is due to the fact that the number of basic and neutral polar amino acids of peptide sequences distinctly correlates with their CE-MS migration time/molecular weight coordinates. In nearly all cases this allows linking a unique LC-MS/MS peptide to a CE-MS peptide as shown previously [19].

CE-MS peptides with sequencing information were combined for each protein. Protein abundance was calculated as the average of all normalized CE-MS peptide intensities for the given protein. Mean protein abundance in the case group was compared to the mean protein abundance in the control group. Protein entries were mapped to the SwissProt database using either the mapping service provided by UniProt or via Blast searching (web.expasy.org/blast/) and merged according to the SwissProt names.

Biomarker definition

Candidate AMD biomarkers were defined by examination of differences in frequency and signal intensity of the proteins between the AMD patients and controls. Mean CE-MS based protein signal intensity was used as a measure for relative abundance. Statistical analysis was performed using Graph Pad Prism 5.0 software. A F-test was performed to test for data distribution. When data were normally distributed, a parametric t-test was performed; otherwise, the statistical analysis was performed using a Mann-Whitney test or Wilcoxon signed rank test. Multiple hypotheses testing correction was performed using the Benjamini-Hochberg test for false discovery rate [31].

Bioinformatics analysis

Gene ontology (GO) keyword-cluster analysis was done using CytoScape (www.cytoscape.org) and the ClueGO plug-in, where statistically significant molecules with p-values of less than 0.05 were compared. The interactome analysis was performed using CytoScape and the Michigan Molecular Interactor plug-in (mimi.ncibi.org). Full interactome analysis was carried out by connecting molecules through neighboring proteins, whereas the condensed protein-protein interaction analysis was performed by searching for direct associations. The paradigm of this analysis is that molecules with similar cellular involvement tend to cluster together through physical interactions, such as molecular machines. The disease analysis is based on known or inferred genetic disorders associated with mutations of specific genes using the Online Mendelian Inheritance in Man database for data mining. An additional pathway analysis was carried out using the Kyoto encyclopedia of genes and genomes (KEGG) database, where KEGG accession numbers of the statistically significant molecules were used for mapping-queries. Additionally, disease-specific descriptions were retrieved from the Online Mendelian Inheritance in Man (OMIM) database as well as the UniProt database. Cellular expression data was also obtained from the latter resource.

Western blot analysis

To determine the protein levels of Transthyretin, Apolipoprotein A 1, Alpha-1 Antitrypsin, Serotransferrin and Retinol-binding protein 3 we obtained vitreous fluid as described above. The extracted proteins (20 μl/5 μg protein) were loaded and subjected to 12.5% sodium dodecyl sulfate-polyacrylamide gel electrophoresis (SDS-PAGE) for 30 min at 100 V and then 90 min at 150 V and subsequently transferred onto nitrocellulose membranes using Trans-Blot Turbo Transfer System (Bio-Rad, Hercules, CA, USA). The membranes were blocked for 1 h at room temperature in blocking buffer consisting of 5% BSA in PBS and 0.1% Tween. This was followed by a 4×5 min washing procedure in Wash Buffer (PBS + 0.1% Tween). Blots were incubated with primary antibodies (Santa Cruz Biotechnology) for 2 h at 4°C followed by incubation with secondary antibodies conjugated to horseradish peroxidase (Santa Cruz Biotechnology) for 2 h at 4°C. Blots were visualized with enhanced chemiluminescence (Amersham Biosciences, Piscataway, NJ, USA).

Results

Sequencing of tryptic peptides

Using LC-MS/MS, 622 of the tryptic peptides detected with CE-MS could be identified. The mass of sequenced peptides ranged between 804 and 3953 Da. These tryptic peptides corresponded to 97 different proteins in vitreous humor (**Table 2**).

Definition of AMD-specific proteins

Figure 1 is a descriptive presentation of the study setup and findings. All samples were analysed by CE-MS. Next, for statistical analysis, CE-MS detected tryptic peptides were matched to the sequences identified by LC-MS/MS. 622 of the CE-MS detected peptides could be identified by their amino acid sequence. These peptides were combined to 97 proteins as described [29] and this protein distribution was statistically analysed. 19 proteins displayed significant differential abundance in vitreous (**Table 3**). All proteins with a p-value of <0.05 were found to be upregulated in the AMD population.

Validation using Western blot analysis

Western blot analysis was used to verify the findings in **table 3** on 5 randomly selected proteins for which antibodies were readily available, using a new but small set of AMD and control samples (n = 4/group). Four out of the 5 proteins analyzed did not display a significant variation, but the fold increases for apolipoprotein A1 and transthyretin suggested increased expression in vitreous of AMD patients similarly to what observed in the intial CE-MS experiments. The absence of significance is most probably due to the small patient population used for in the validation experiments (**Table 4** and **Figure 2**). However, we validated increased alpha-1-antitrypsin abundance in vitreous of AMD patients (p = 0.02).

Gene enrichment and pathway analysis

The 19 proteins with differential abundance in AMD were analyzed for their biological process, molecular function and the cellular component. GO cluster analysis using ClueGO showed that these proteins are primarily involved in biological (ion) transport and secretion/exocytosis (platelet degranulation (ALB, TF, APOA1, SERPINA1, HRG, FGA) and fatty acid binding (RBP3, ALB, PTGDS)), protease inhibitor activity (ITIH1, SERPINA1, SERPINC1, HRG), and processes involving hydrogen peroxide (GPX3, HP). These molecules consist mostly of secreted proteins (**Figure 3A**).

A global interactome analysis of the statistically relevant proteins using the Michigan Molecular Interactor plug-in, which mines data from protein-protein, protein-gene, gene-gene, molecule-pathway, and molecule-keyword associations, resulted in a densely interconnected network (**Figure 3B**). This expanded network of 54 proteins, including molecules known to be associated with the query molecules, consists of an immunoglobulin-cluster and complement activation (containing IGHA1, IGKC, IGHG1, IGLC2, AHSG, ITIH1, and FGA), suggesting inflammation and acute phase response processes being activated in the original source tissue, and processes including cell adhesion, lipid metabolism (RBP3, PTGDS), transport (APOA1, ALB, TTR, TF), anti-apoptosis (GPX3), and proteolysis (proteases (HP) and protease inhibitors (HRG, SERPINA1 and SERPINC1)). Inter-linking molecules suggest an involvement of transcriptional elements such as ONECUT and HNF1A/4A, which are modulators of genes involved in lipid metabolic processes, blood coagulation

Analysis of the condensed network of direct interactions between the 19 proteins shows the immunoglobulin cluster containing IGLC2, IGKC, and IGHG1, binary interactions between ALB and ITIH1, and between HRG and FGA, as well as a binary cluster of APOA1 and TTR. The latter suggests that the peroxisome proliferator-activated receptor (PPAR) signaling pathway is perturbed in AMD through an association with TTR and fibrils (**Figure 3B**).

Data mining of the Online Mendelian Inheritance in Man database by associated disease clustering showed one relevant cluster consisting of APOA1 (cataract formation) and TTR (fibril formation (neurodegenerative)). The same components were also found by association using a similar approach to mine the disease entries in the KEGG database, where the common denominator was found as familial amyloidosis (KEGG disease entry H00845), linking it to the complement and coagulation cascade (**Figure 3C**). Furthermore KEGG pathway analysis also suggested an involvement of arachidonic acid metabolism to be modulated in AMD. Literature mining also revealed a semantic link between cataract formation and up-regulated levels of GPX3 in the lens.

Table 2. Proteins in vitreous humor detected by CE-MS and identified by LC-MS/MS analysis.

Protein	UniProt*	Peptide number**	Coverage*** (%)	Peptide number control****	Peptide number case****
Actin, aortic smooth muscle	P62736	1	3	0	1
Afamin	P43652	2	4	2	2
Angiotensinogen	P01019	1	2	1	1
Alpha-1-acid glycoprotein 1	P02763	7	27	7	7
Alpha-1-acid glycoprotein 2	P19652	3	15	3	3
Alpha-1-antitrypsin	P01009	20	52	20	20
Alpha-1B-glycoprotein	P04217	5	11	5	5
Alpha-2-HS-glycoprotein	P02765	4	16	4	4
Alpha-2-macroglobulin	P01023	13	10	9	13
Alpha-crystallin B chain	P02511	2	14	1	2
Amyloid-like protein 2	Q06481	2	4	2	2
Antithrombin-III	P01008	10	23	4	10
Apolipoprotein E	P02649	13	43	12	13
Apolipoprotein A-I	P02647	18	63	16	18
Apolipoprotein A-II	P02652	4	41	4	4
Apolipoprotein A-IV	P06727	10	30	5	10
Beta-2-microglobulin	P61769	2	17	1	2
Beta-crystallin B2	P43320	11	50	11	11
Chitinase-3-like protein 1	P36222	1	3	1	1
Ceruloplasmin	P00450	14	20	12	14
Clusterin	P10909	12	31	11	12
Collagen alpha-1(I) chain	P02452	2	1	2	2
Collagen alpha-1(II) chain	P02458	38	27	35	36
Collagen alpha-1(III) chain	P02461	1	2	1	1
Collagen alpha-1(IX) chain	P20849	5	9	4	5
Collagen alpha-1(V) chain	P20908	4	1	2	3
Collagen alpha-1(XI) chain	P12107	5	3	5	5
Collagen alpha-1(XII) chain	Q99715	1	1	1	1
Collagen alpha-1(XXII) chain	Q8NFW1	1	1	1	1
Collagen alpha-1(XXIII) chain	Q86Y22	1	3	1	1
Collagen alpha-1(XXVIII) chain	Q2UY09	1	2	0	1
Collagen alpha-2(IX) chain	Q14055	4	6	4	4
Collagen alpha-2(XI) chain	P13942	1	2	1	1
Collagen alpha-3(IX) chain	Q14050	5	7	5	5
Complement C3	P01024	32	23	23	32
Complement C4-B	P0C0L5	11	7	10	11
Complement factor B	P00751	5	7	3	5
Alpha-crystallin A chain	P02489	3	19	3	3
Cathepsin D	P07339	3	11	3	3
Cystatin-C	P01034	2	18	2	2
Dermcidin	P81605	3	23	1	3
Dickkopf-related protein 3	Q9UBP4	6	22	6	6
Double-strand break repair protein MRE11A	P49959	1	2	0	1
Fibrinogen alpha chain	P02671	4	6	3	4
Fibrinogen beta chain	P02675	1	3	1	1
Gelsolin	P06396	1	2	0	1
Glutathione peroxidase 3	P22352	4	23	3	4
Haptoglobin	P00738	13	24	10	13

Table 2. Cont.

Protein	UniProt*	Peptide number**	Coverage*** (%)	Peptide number control****	Peptide number case****
Hemoglobin subunit beta	P68871	1	9	1	1
Hemopexin	P02790	14	29	12	14
Heparin cofactor 2	P05546	1	2	1	1
Histidine-rich glycoprotein	P04196	2	4	2	2
Ig alpha-1 chain C region	P01876	3	8	3	3
Ig alpha-2 chain C region	P01877	4	8	2	2
Ig gamma-1 chain C region	P01857	11	37	11	11
Ig gamma-3 chain C region	P01860	4	12	3	4
Ig heavy chain V-III region GAL	P01781	2	8	1	2
Ig heavy chain V-III region TRO	P01762	1	6	1	1
Ig kappa chain V-I region EU	P01598	1	17	1	1
Ig kappa chain V-III region SIE	P01620	1	17	1	1
Ig kappa chain C region	P01834	5	80	4	5
Ig lambda-2 chain C regions	P0CG05	3	42	3	3
IgGFc-binding protein	Q9Y6R7	4	1	4	4
Immunoglobulin lambda-like polypeptide 5	B9A064	1	9	1	1
Inter-alpha-trypsin inhibitor heavy chain H1	P19827	3	4	3	3
Inter-alpha-trypsin inhibitor heavy chain H4	Q14624	2	2	1	2
Keratin, type I cytoskeletal 10	P13645	18	34	16	18
Keratin, type I cytoskeletal 14	P02533	3	7	2	3
Keratin, type I cytoskeletal 9	P35527	7	14	6	7
Keratin, type II cytoskeletal 1	P04264	18	26	17	17
Keratin, type II cytoskeletal 2 epidermal	P35908	3	6	3	3
Keratin, type II cytoskeletal 5	P13647	1	2	1	1
Keratin, type II cytoskeletal 6A	P02538	1	2	1	1
Keratin, type II cytoskeletal 6B	P04259	2	4	2	2
Kininogen-1	P01042	4	5	2	4
Leucine-rich alpha-2-glycoprotein	P02750	1	3	0	1
Opticin	Q9UBM4	3	9	2	3
Osteopontin	P10451	7	34	7	7
Pigment epithelium-derived factor	P36955	12	31	11	12
Plasminogen	P00747	1	1	0	1
Prostaglandin-H2 D-isomerase	P41222	4	21	4	4
Protein Jade-2	Q9NQC1	1	1	1	1
Protein S100-A7	P31151	1	11	1	1
Protein S100-A9	P06702	2	18	2	2
Prothrombin	P00734	2	4	2	2
Retinol-binding protein 3	P10745	15	18	14	15
Ig kappa chain V-III region VG	P04433	2	23	1	2
Plasma protease C1 inhibitor	P05155	5	12	5	5
Serotransferrin	P02787	44	55	43	44
Alpha-1-antichymotrypsin	P01011	15	36	12	15
Serum albumin	P02768	55	75	51	55
Complement C4-A	P0C0L4	1	1	1	1
Titin	Q8WZ42	1	0	0	1
Transthyretin	P02766	7	63	7	7
Vitamin D-binding protein	P02774	5	9	4	5
Vitronectin	P04004	3	9	2	3

Table 2. Cont.

Protein	UniProt*	Peptide number**	Coverage*** (%)	Peptide number control****	Peptide number case****
Zinc-alpha-2-glycoprotein	P25311	2	9	2	2

*Uniprot accession numbers that can be found on www.uniprot.org; ** Number of peptides observed by CE-MS analysis and sequenced by LC-MS/MS for each identified protein; *** Percentage of peptide coverage of the protein sequence; ****, Number of peptides observed by CE-MS and sequenced by LC-MS/MS in controls or cases.

Discussion

The aim of this pilot study was to test the hypothesis that specific proteins in vitreous samples of patients with exudative AMD are significantly associated with the disease and may lead to a better understanding of the pathophysiology of the disease.

We initially set out to analyze native peptides from vitreous (top-down strategy) with a mass of up to 20 kDa using CE-MS analysis. However, this strategy did not result in satisfactory data, as a result of high variability (Koss M et al. Proteomics in AMD; Poster 2927/A327 at the annual meeting of the Assiciation for Research in Vision and Ophtalmology (AVRO), Ft.Lauderdale, USA in 2012). A possible reason for the large variation between the measurements could be the presence of hyaluronic acid. Because of the highly negative charge of its monomers, hyaluronic acid reacts with positively charged proteins such as albumin to build up polyelectrolyte complexes displaying low solubility [32]. Since the top-down strategy failed to give the expected results, we changed the strategy and in the current study employed trypsin digested samples for proteome analysis of vitreous.

Using this bottom-up approach we could successfully analyze the vitreous humor samples with CE-MS, including fragments of proteins with molecular masses above 20 kDa. We identified a total of 97 proteins, 19 of those significantly increased in AMD patients. We selected 5 random proteins among these 19 for validation by Western blot analysis. One protein (alpha-1-antitrypsin) reached statistical significance while two others (transthyretin and apoliprotein A1) displayed a non-significant but increased abundance in AMD. The latter is most likely due to the low number of patients in the validation set (n = 4/group) and needs validation.

Most of the upregulated proteins in AMD patients are plasma proteins. Our findings therefore may, to some degree, be

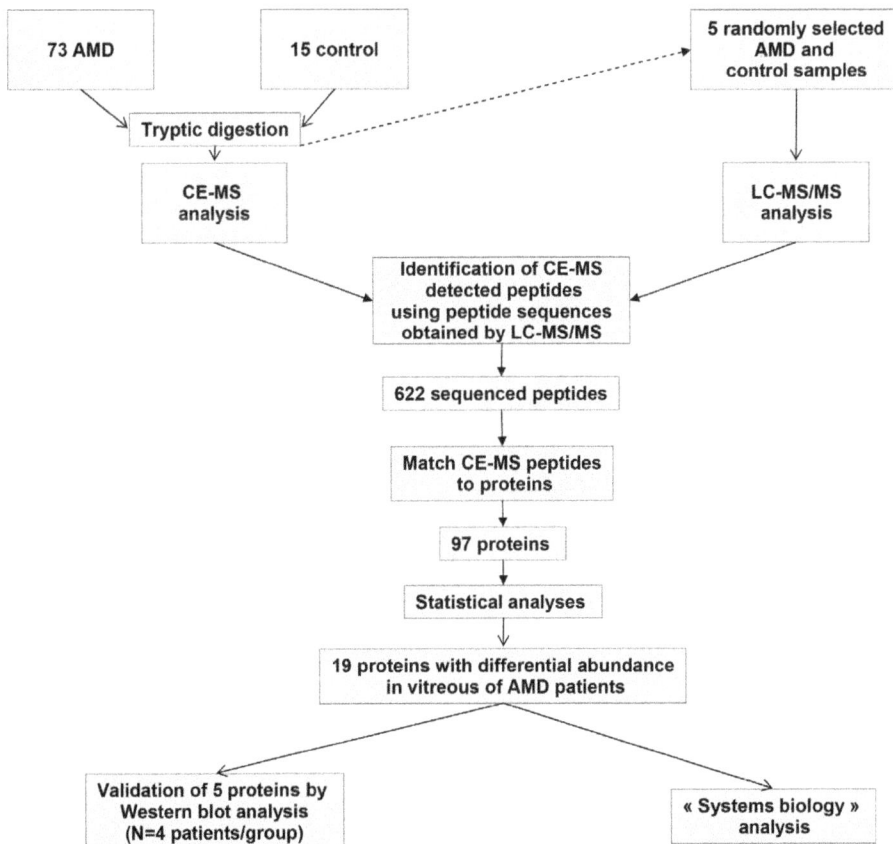

Figure 1. Study design and results.

Table 3. List of significant regulated proteins.

Protein name	Fold change AMD/ control	Standard deviation for fold change	p-value	adjusted p-value
Ig kappa/lambda chain C region	6.56	13.27	4.58E-06	4.45E-04
Serum albumin	1.91	1.49	3.27E-05	1.58E-03
Ig gamma-1 chain C region	3.14	4.70	6.54E-05	1.74E-03
Antithrombin-III	5.50	12.29	7.16E-05	1.74E-03
Ig lambda-2 chain C regions	4.55	9.94	1.30E-04	2.51E-03
Serotransferrin*	1.74	1.52	3.99E-04	6.45E-03
Afamin	3.28	6.58	1.93E-03	2.16E-02
Histidine-rich glycoprotein	10.85	49.18	2.45E-03	2.16E-02
Retinol-binding protein 3*	2.78	5.51	2.72E-03	2.20E-02
Apolipoprotein A-I*	2.30	3.62	3.88E-03	2.73E-02
Fibrinogen alpha chain	2.90	6.30	3.94E-03	2.73E-02
Ig alpha-1 chain C region	35.34	147.90	2.32E-03	2.16E-02
Alpha-2-HS-glycoprotein	2.58	5.78	1.55E-02	8.70E-02
Transthyretin*	1.74	2.11	1.61E-02	8.70E-02
Prostaglandin-H2 D-isomerase	1.65	1.97	2.33E-02	1.19E-01
Haptoglobin	2.92	7.89	3.34E-02	1.46E-01
Glutathione peroxidase 3	4.26	18.42	3.79E-02	1.51E-01
Alpha-1-antitrypsin*	1.73	2.56	4.04E-02	1.51E-01
Inter-alpha-trypsin inhibitor heavy chain H1	2.34	5.84	4.82E-02	1.67E-01

Legend: Fold change AMD/control. Fold increase or decrease observed in AMD patients compared to controls; p-value - unadjusted p-value (Wilcoxon signed-rank test); adjusted p-value - p-value corrected for multiple testing (Benjamini and Hochberg method) and expressed in bold, when statistically significant. * proteins selected for western-blot analysis.

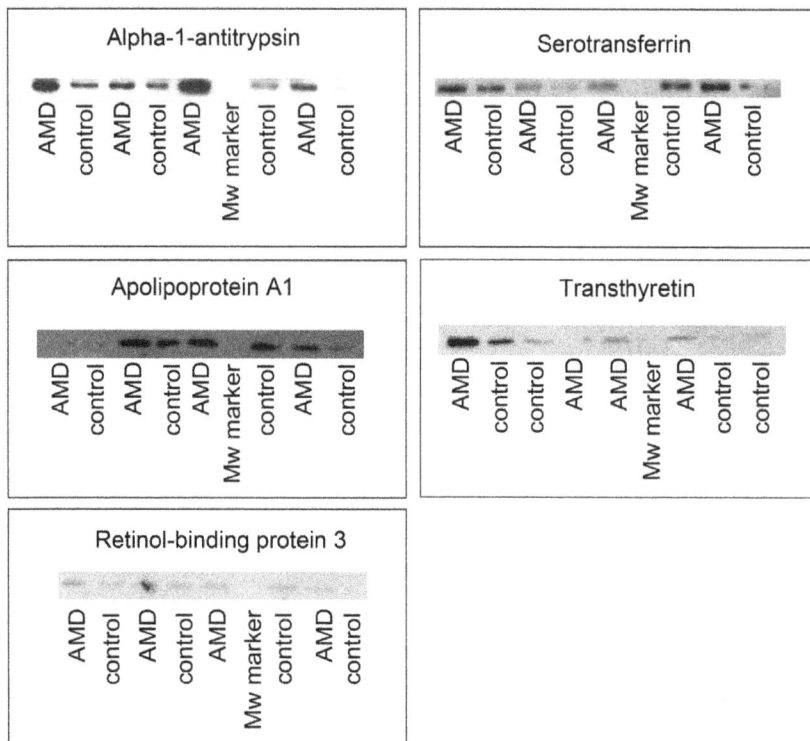

Figure 2. Western blot validation of candidate markers for AMD. Representative Western blots of analysis of expression of selected vitreous proteins.

Table 4. Western blot analysis of selected proteins found upregulated in vitreous of AMD patients by CE-MS.

Protein name	AMD	control	P-value	Fold change	Regulation in proteome analysis
Alpha-1-Antitrypsin	1618.6±610.2	689.5±174.1	p = 0.02	2.35	↑
Apolipoprotein A 1	1925.3±404.9	1463.2±360.4	p = 0.27	1.32	↑
Retinol-binding protein 3	471.9±50.9	427.3±53.9	p = 0.28	1.10	↑
Serotransferrin	1224.1±231.1	1059.6±247.7	p = 0.25	1.16	↑
Transthyretin	1169.8±592.8	747.4±143.8	p = 0.15	1.57	↑

Presented are the results of intensities measured by enhanced chemiluminescence from SDS PAGE Western blots. The mean ± standard deviation from 4 independent undiluted vitreous AMD and 4 independent undiluted vitreous control samples is given. P-values were calculated by the Mann-Whitney statistical test.

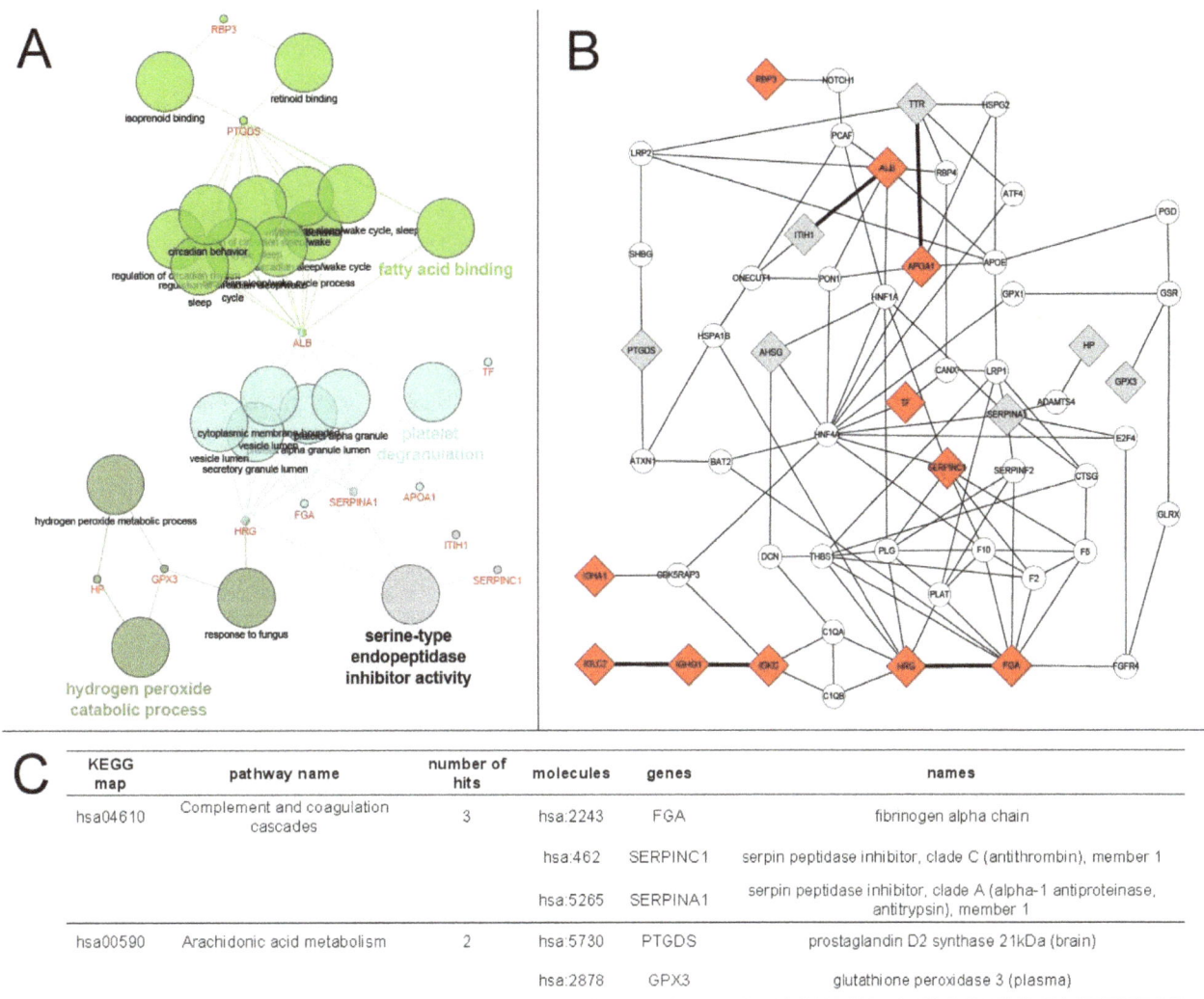

KEGG map	pathway name	number of hits	molecules	genes	names
hsa04610	Complement and coagulation cascades	3	hsa:2243	FGA	fibrinogen alpha chain
			hsa:462	SERPINC1	serpin peptidase inhibitor, clade C (antithrombin), member 1
			hsa:5265	SERPINA1	serpin peptidase inhibitor, clade A (alpha-1 antiproteinase, antitrypsin), member 1
hsa00590	Arachidonic acid metabolism	2	hsa:5730	PTGDS	prostaglandin D2 synthase 21kDa (brain)
			hsa:2878	GPX3	glutathione peroxidase 3 (plasma)

Figure 3. Bioinformatic analysis of identified biomarkers. A. Gene ontology analysis shows proteins involved in fatty acid binding. platelet degranulation. serine protease inhibitor activity and hydrogen peroxide catabolic processes. **B** Interaction network of identified biomarker candidates involving 18 out of the 19 proteins. Proteins involved in inflammation. acute phase response (including cellular adhesion). signaling via lipid-mediated pathways (including transport) and activation of proteolytic cascades. as well as transcriptional activity are indicated. Red diamonds indicate proteins which are significant after correction for multiple testing. and grey ones are the remainder of the query set. Circles indicate gap-fillers which were added to connect proteins via protein-protein interactions. Direct association between the significant biomarker set are indicated by a bold line. and relate to immune response (immunoglobulin cluster). protease inhibitor activity. and an activation of the peroxisome proliferator-activated receptor signaling pathway/CDC42 signal transduction pathway. as suggested through APOA1 interactions. **C.** Kyoto encyclopedia of genes and genomes pathway analysis. Statistically relevant biomarker proteins were mapped onto KEGG pathway maps and showed an involvement of fibril formation and inhibition of fibrinolysis in the coagulation cascade and association with arachidonic acid metabolism.

representative of the leakage from exudative CNV into the vitreous. Even though plasma proteins might not be responsible for the onset of an exudative AMD, their levels might be of diagnostic value for disease and represent the underlying pathophysiology of AMD. Future studies are important to identify which of these proteins are secreted from the abnormal CNV tissue.

The observed upregulation of a number of proteins in vitreous of AMD patients provides further insights into the pathophysiology of AMD:

Transport proteins

Upregulation of transport proteins such as albumin and serotransferrin in AMD patients confirms the findings from previous proteome analyses of anterior chamber fluids [5]. In addition, further transport proteins like transthyretin and apolipoprotein A-I were identified. All of these were upregulated in the AMD group; all are biologically essential for cell homeostasis (albumin) and are carriers of hormones like retinol (albumin and transthyretin) or ions (serotransferrin). It is important to stress that in chronic diseases, such as AMD, the dysregulation of these abundant proteins has been observed in serum [33,34], but so far, their presence in the vitreous has received little attention.

Inflammatory proteins

Immunoglobulin heavy chains and alpha-1-antitrypsin were upregulated in the AMD samples. Alpha-1-antitrypsin is an acute phase protein member of the serpin family that inhibits a wide variety of proteases and thereby protects tissues from enzymes of inflammatory cells, especially neutrophil elastase. This is the first time that increased alpha-1-antitrypsin abundance in vitreous has been associated with AMD. However alpha-1-antitrypsin does not seem specific for AMD since upregulation of alpha-1-antitrypsin was observed in both aqueous and blood of patients with glaucoma [35].

Mediators of coagulation

Fibrinogen is essential during coagulation as it is converted by plasmin into fibrin, and higher blood levels have been associated with AMD [36]. Rheopheresis, a treatment that microfilters fibrinogen from the blood of AMD patients, seems to be protective in the progression of AMD, however, the approach is controversial discussed [37]. In this study, we demonstrated that the fibrinogen alpha chain was upregulated in the AMD group. As for alpha-1-antitrypsin, although potentially involved in the pathophysiology of AMD, increased fibrinogen abundance in vitreous is not specific for AMD since such upregulation was previously also observed in vitreous samples of patients with diabetic retinopathy [38].

Specific ocular markers

In humans, prostaglandin H2-D isomerase catalyzes the conversion of prostaglandin H2 to prostaglandin D2, which functions as a neuromodulator and as a trophic factor in the central nervous system for fatty acid biosynthesis. Its occurrence has been described in proliferative diabetic retinopathy; but it has not been previously associated with AMD [39]. The inter-photoreceptor retinol binding protein is a large glycoprotein, located in the extracellular matrix between the RPE and the photoreceptors. It is known to bind retinoids and is thought to transport retinoids between the retinal pigment epithelium and the photoreceptors. Its potential involvement in AMD has recently been described based on the analysis of blood samples [40,41] and is confirmed by our findings.

The bioinformatic analyses using GO-term clustering, physical interaction module assembly, and KEGG pathway data mapping have shown an involvement of pathways consisting of fatty acid binding and transport, exocytosis, and protease inhibitory activity, which are also partially involved in Complement and coagulation cascades. However, more importantly is the notion that there appears to be an up-regulation of hydrogen peroxide catabolic processes, which suggest that oxidative stress is exerted in AMD.

The interactome analysis surprisingly showed a highly interconnected network of 18 of the 19 relevant proteins, where only 36 additional molecules were needed to generate a specific molecular network, suggesting that the up-regulated proteins form a potential dysregulated functional cluster encompassing immune responses and complement cascade proteins, protease cascades maybe linked to the membrane attack complex or possibly to counteract the enzymatic effect of up-regulated molecules such as GPX3, RBP3 and PTGDS, or as modulators of gene activation cascades. This unusually high selectivity also argues against the hypothesis that these proteins are observed in increased abundance merely as a result of unspecific leakage of plasma proteins, and support the hypothesis that the increase in these proteins is specifically linked to AMD.

The up-regulation of GPX3 is of particular interest, since it was shown previously that cataracts contain elevated levels of oxidants such as dehydroascorbic acid (DHA), indicative of oxidative stress, linked to a potentially elevated level of extracellular glutathione peroxidase GPX3 [42]. Mechanistically, the over-expression is suggested to result in accumulated oxidants in the glutathion/ascorbic acid homeostasis cycle, leading to DHA-polymer crystal formation in the lens as well as potentially toxic breakdown products of ascorbic acid.

In conclusion, in this study we could demonstrate that a bottom-up approach combining CE-MS (for protein selection) and LC-MS/MS (for protein identification) led to the identification of 19 candidate proteins in undiluted vitreous of AMD patients. Even with the limitations of this study (e.g., demographic matching, demand for validation in a larger cohort with a wider set of clinical parameters), the novel information gained from this study of a high number of undiluted vitreous samples provides additional insight into the pathophysiology of wet AMD.

Author Contributions

Conceived and designed the experiments: MK HM JH JPS FK. Performed the experiments: MK JH NN HM HH JJ FK. Analyzed the data: MK JH RR WM JK JS WM JPS. Contributed reagents/materials/analysis tools: JH MK NN JS KK HM JJ. Wrote the paper: MK JH TB JS MP JPS.

References

1. Evans JR (2001) Risk factors for age-related macular degeneration. Progress in retinal and eye research 20: 227–253.
2. Stefansson E (2009) Physiology of vitreous surgery. Graefes Arch Clin Exp Ophthalmol 247: 147–163.
3. Adamis AP, Shima DT, Tolentino MJ, Gragoudas ES, Ferrara N, et al. (1996) Inhibition of vascular endothelial growth factor prevents retinal ischemia-associated iris neovascularization in a nonhuman primate. Archives of ophthalmology 114: 66–71.
4. Funk M, Karl D, Georgopoulos M, Benesch T, Sacu S, et al. (2009) Neovascular age-related macular degeneration: intraocular cytokines and growth factors and the influence of therapy with ranibizumab. Ophthalmology 116: 2393–2399.
5. Grossniklaus HE, Green WR (2004) Choroidal neovascularization. Am J Ophthalmol 137: 496–503.
6. Kim TW, Kang JW, Ahn J, Lee EK, Cho KC, et al. (2012) Proteomic analysis of the aqueous humor in age-related macular degeneration (AMD) patients. Journal of proteome research 11: 4034–4043.

7. Ecker SM, Hines JC, Pfahler SM, Glaser BM (2011) Aqueous cytokine and growth factor levels do not reliably reflect those levels found in the vitreous. Molecular vision 17: 2856–2863.

8. Stefansson E, Loftsson T (2006) The Stokes-Einstein equation and the physiological effects of vitreous surgery. Acta Ophthalmol Scand 84: 718–719.

9. Angi M, Kalirai H, Coupland SE, Damato BE, Semeraro F, et al. (2012) Proteomic analyses of the vitreous humour. Mediators of inflammation 2012: 148039.

10. Ecker SM, Pfahler SM, Hines JC, Lovelace AS, Glaser BM (2012) Sequential in-office vitreous aspirates demonstrate vitreous matrix metalloproteinase 9 levels correlate with the amount of subretinal fluid in eyes with wet age-related macular degeneration. Molecular vision 18: 1658–1667.

11. Grus FH, Joachim SC, Pfeiffer N (2007) Proteomics in ocular fluids. Proteomics Clinical applications 1: 876–888.

12. Noma H, Funatsu H, Yamasaki M, Tsukamoto H, Mimura T, et al. (2008) Aqueous humour levels of cytokines are correlated to vitreous levels and severity of macular oedema in branch retinal vein occlusion. Eye 22: 42–48.

13. Pfister M, Koch FH, Cinatl J, Rothweiler F, Schubert R, et al. (2012) [Cytokine determination from vitreous samples in retinal vascular diseases.]. Der Ophthalmologe: Zeitschrift der Deutschen Ophthalmologischen Gesellschaft.

14. Walia S, Clermont AC, Gao BB, Aiello LP, Feener EP (2010) Vitreous proteomics and diabetic retinopathy. Seminars in ophthalmology 25: 289–294.

15. Yamane K, Minamoto A, Yamashita H, Takamura H, Miyamoto-Myoken Y, et al. (2003) Proteome analysis of human vitreous proteins. Molecular & cellular proteomics: MCP 2: 1177–1187.

16. Bennett KL, Funk M, Tschernutter M, Breitwieser FP, Planyavsky M, et al. (2011) Proteomic analysis of human cataract aqueous humour: Comparison of one-dimensional gel LCMS with two-dimensional LCMS of unlabelled and iTRAQ(R)-labelled specimens. Journal of proteomics 74: 151–166.

17. Chowdhury UR, Jea SY, Oh DJ, Rhee DJ, Fautsch MP (2011) Expression profile of the matricellular protein osteopontin in primary open-angle glaucoma and the normal human eye. Investigative ophthalmology & visual science 52: 6443–6451.

18. Cryan LM, O'Brien C (2008) Proteomics as a research tool in clinical and experimental ophthalmology. Proteomics Clinical applications 2: 762–775.

19. Zurbig P, Renfrow MB, Schiffer E, Novak J, Walden M, et al. (2006) Biomarker discovery by CE-MS enables sequence analysis via MS/MS with platform-independent separation. Electrophoresis 27: 2111–2125.

20. Mischak H, Vlahou A, Ioannidis JP (2013) Technical aspects and inter-laboratory variability in native peptide profiling: the CE-MS experience. Clinical biochemistry 46: 432–443.

21. Mischak H, Julian BA, Novak J (2007) High-resolution proteome/peptidome analysis of peptides and low-molecular-weight proteins in urine. Proteomics Clinical applications 1: 792.

22. Koss MJ, Scholtz S, Haeussler-Sinangin Y, Singh P, Koch FH (2009) Combined Intravitreal Pharmacosurgery in Patients with Occult Choroidal Neovascularization Secondary to Wet Age-Related Macular Degeneration. Ophthalmologica 224: 72–78.

23. Mischak H, Schanstra JP (2011) CE-MS in biomarker discovery, validation, and clinical application. Proteomics Clinical applications 5: 9–23.

24. Augustin AJ, Puls S, Offermann I (2007) Triple therapy for choroidal neovascularization due to age-related macular degeneration: verteporfin PDT, bevacizumab, and dexamethasone. Retina 27: 133–140.

25. Koch FH, Koss MJ (2011) Microincision vitrectomy procedure using Intrector technology. Archives of ophthalmology 129: 1599–1604.

26. Spaide RF (2006) Rationale for combination therapies for choroidal neovascularization. Am J Ophthalmol 141: 149–156.

27. Theodorescu D, Wittke S, Ross MM, Walden M, Conaway M, et al. (2006) Discovery and validation of new protein biomarkers for urothelial cancer: a prospective analysis. The lancet oncology 7: 230–240.

28. Neuhoff N, Kaiser T, Wittke S, Krebs R, Pitt A, et al. (2004) Mass spectrometry for the detection of differentially expressed proteins: a comparison of surface-enhanced laser desorption/ionization and capillary electrophoresis/mass spectrometry. Rapid communications in mass spectrometry: RCM 18: 149–156.

29. Jantos-Siwy J, Schiffer E, Brand K, Schumann G, Rossing K, et al. (2009) Quantitative urinary proteome analysis for biomarker evaluation in chronic kidney disease. Journal of proteome research 8: 268–281.

30. Metzger J, Negm AA, Plentz RR, Weismuller TJ, Wedemeyer J, et al. (2013) Urine proteomic analysis differentiates cholangiocarcinoma from primary sclerosing cholangitis and other benign biliary disorders. Gut 62: 122–130.

31. Benjamini Y, Hochberg Y (1995) Controlling the false discovery rate: a practical and powerful approach to multiple testing. J Royal Stat Soc B (Methodological): 125–133.

32. Wohlrab W, Neubert RRH, Wohlraub J (2004) Hyaluronsaeure und Haut. Aachen: Shaker. 384 p.

33. Chowers I, Wong R, Dentchev T, Farkas RH, Iacovelli J, et al. (2006) The iron carrier transferrin is upregulated in retinas from patients with age-related macular degeneration. Investigative ophthalmology & visual science 47: 2135–2140.

34. Wysokinski D, Danisz K, Blasiak J, Dorecka M, Romaniuk D, et al. (2013) An association of transferrin gene polymorphism and serum transferrin levels with age-related macular degeneration. Experimental eye research 1: 14–23.

35. Boehm N, Wolters D, Thiel U, Lossbrand U, Wiegel N, et al. (2012) New insights into autoantibody profiles from immune privileged sites in the eye: a glaucoma study. Brain, behavior, and immunity 26: 96–102.

36. Klingel R, Fassbender C, Fischer I, Hattenbach L, Gumbel H, et al. (2002) Rheopheresis for age-related macular degeneration: a novel indication for therapeutic apheresis in ophthalmology. Therapeutic apheresis: official journal of the International Society for Apheresis and the Japanese Society for Apheresis 6: 271–281.

37. Klingel R, Fassbender C, Heibges A, Koch F, Nasemann J, et al. (2010) RheoNet registry analysis of rheopheresis for microcirculatory disorders with a focus on age-related macular degeneration. Therapeutic apheresis and dialysis: official peer-reviewed journal of the International Society for Apheresis, the Japanese Society for Apheresis, the Japanese Society for Dialysis Therapy 14: 276–286.

38. Garcia-Ramirez M, Canals F, Hernandez C, Colome N, Ferrer C, et al. (2007) Proteomic analysis of human vitreous fluid by fluorescence-based difference gel electrophoresis (DIGE): a new strategy for identifying potential candidates in the pathogenesis of proliferative diabetic retinopathy. Diabetologia 50: 1294–1303.

39. Kim SJ, Kim S, Park J, Lee HK, Park KS, et al. (2006) Differential expression of vitreous proteins in proliferative diabetic retinopathy. Current eye research 31: 231–240.

40. Morohoshi K, Ohbayashi M, Patel N, Chong V, Bird AC, et al. (2012) Identification of anti-retinal antibodies in patients with age-related macular degeneration. Experimental and molecular pathology 93: 193–199.

41. Morohoshi K, Patel N, Ohbayashi M, Chong V, Grossniklaus HE, et al. (2012) Serum autoantibody biomarkers for age-related macular degeneration and possible regulators of neovascularization. Experimental and molecular pathology 92: 64–73.

42. Kisic B, Miric D, Zoric L, Ilic A, Dragojevic I (2012) Antioxidant capacity of lenses with age-related cataract. Oxidative medicine and cellular longevity 2012: 467130.

## 21

Obesity and Associated Lifestyle in a Large Sample of Multi-Morbid German Primary Care Attendees

Claudia Sikorski[1,2]*, Melanie Luppa[1], Siegfried Weyerer[3], Hans-Helmut König[4], Wolfgang Maier[5], Gerhard Schön[6], Juliana J. Petersen[7], Jochen Gensichen[8], Angela Fuchs[9], Horst Bickel[10], Birgitt Wiese[11], Heike Hansen[12], Hendrik van den Bussche[12], Martin Scherer[12], Steffi G. Riedel-Heller[1]

1 Institute of Social Medicine, Occupational Health and Public Health, University of Leipzig, Leipzig, Germany, 2 Leipzig University Medical Center, IFB AdiposityDiseases, Leipzig, Germany, 3 Central Institute of Mental Health, Medical Faculty Mannheim/Heidelberg University, Mannheim, Germany, 4 Department of Medical Sociology, Social Medicine and Health Economics, Hamburg-Eppendorf University Medical Center, Hamburg, Germany, 5 Department of Psychiatry and Psychotherapy, University of Bonn, Bonn, Germany, 6 Department of Medical Biometry and Epidemiology, Hamburg-Eppendorf University Medical Center, Hamburg, Germany, 7 Institute of General Practice, Goethe-University Frankfurt am Main, Frankfurt am Main, Germany, 8 Department of General Practice, Jena University Hospital, Jena, Germany, 9 Department of General Practice, Medical Faculty, University of Dusseldorf, Dusseldorf, Germany, 10 Department of Psychiatry, Technical University of Munich, München, Germany, 11 Institute for Biometry, Hannover Medical School, Hannover, Germany, 12 Department of Primary Medical Care, Hamburg-Eppendorf University Medical Center, Hamburg, Germany

Abstract

Background: Obesity and the accompanying increased morbidity and mortality risk is highly prevalent among older adults. As obese elderly might benefit from intentional weight reduction, it is necessary to determine associated and potentially modifiable factors on senior obesity. This cross-sectional study focuses on multi-morbid patients which make up the majority in primary care. It reports on the prevalence of senior obesity and its associations with lifestyle behaviors.

Methods: A total of 3,189 non-demented, multi-morbid participants aged 65–85 years were recruited in primary care within the German MultiCare-study. Physical activity, smoking, alcohol consumption and quantity and quality of nutritional intake were classified as relevant lifestyle factors. Body Mass Index (BMI, general obesity) and waist circumference (WC, abdominal obesity) were used as outcome measures and regression analyses were conducted.

Results: About one third of all patients were classified as obese according to BMI. The prevalence of abdominal obesity was 73.5%. Adjusted for socio-demographic variables and objective and subjective disease burden, participants with low physical activity had a 1.6 kg/m^2 higher BMI as well as a higher WC (4.9 cm, p<0.001). Current smoking and high alcohol consumption were associated with a lower BMI and WC. In multivariate logistic regression, using elevated WC and BMI as categorical outcomes, the same pattern in lifestyle factors was observed. Only for WC, not current but former smoking was associated with a higher probability for elevated WC. Dietary intake in quantity and quality was not associated with BMI or WC in either model.

Conclusions: Further research is needed to clarify if the huge prevalence discrepancy between BMI and WC also reflects a difference in obesity-related morbidity and mortality. Yet, age-specific thresholds for the BMI are needed likewise. Encouraging and promoting physical activity in older adults might a starting point for weight reduction efforts.

Editor: Heiner K. Berthold, Bielefeld Evangelical Hospital, Germany

Funding: The study is funded by the German Federal Ministry of Education and Research (grant numbers 01ET0725-31 and 01ET1006A-K). The authors acknowledge support from the German Research Foundation (DFG) and Leipzig University within the program of Open Access Publishing. The funding body had no further role in study design; in the collection, analysis and interpretation of data; in writing of the report; and the decision to submit the paper for publication.

Competing Interests: The authors have declared that no competing interests exist.

* Email: Claudia.Sikorski@medizin.uni-leipzig.de

Introduction

Obesity is recognized as a major health threat throughout the life-span. It is highly prevalent in older individuals. Currently, about one third of all US adults above the age of 60 must be considered obese [1] and a further rise can be expected as those generations age that contributed to rising obesity rates during the last years [2;3].

Obesity in older adults is associated with an elevated risk for cardiometabolic syndromes, physical disability, impaired quality of life, and even dementia [4] as well as substantial functional impairment [5]. Recent studies showed an increase in absolute mortality risk up to the age of 75 [6]. The obesity paradox that has been described, namely a survival benefit of overweight and obese elderly, may mainly be a result of a positive survival bias and unintended weight loss that may be linked to life-threatening illness [4]. Many questions, however, remain unanswered and need further investigation. One aspect would be to investigate the association of senior obesity with other accompanying factors, such as lifestyle behavior. In certain unhealthy lifestyle choices were highly prevalent in obese elderly, a truly protective effect of senior obesity may be even more in question.

An obesogenic environment accompanied by changes in lifestyle factors, such as unfavorable nutritional intake and low physical activity, accounts for parts of the obesity pandemic [7]. The influence of these lifestyle factors on senior obesity in a population of over 65-year-olds has hardly been investigated. A study in a sample including participants aged 75 and older, showed age-related differences in fat mass to be associated with lifestyle factors. Low physical activity and unfavorable nutritional intake was associated with obesity in younger and in older respondents [8]. As obese elderly benefit from intentional weight reduction, it is necessary to determine influential factors on senior obesity [9;10].

This is one of the first studies analyzing the association with specific lifestyle behaviors with obesity in the elderly. Since general practitioners (GPs) are the major health care provider for elderly individuals and the primary care level turned out to be the setting to address lifestyle pattern in those most in need, this study is based on a large sample of multi-morbid primary care attendees. This comprises a most relevant group of individuals with more than 3 chronic conditions, which make up to three quarters of patients in primary care [11]. Research has shown that this kind of at-risk population benefits from behavioral interventions as well but studies on obesity and lifestyle in this population are lacking up to this date [12].

This study therefore sought to firstly determine the prevalence of overweight and obesity in a multi-morbid sample of German elderly primary care attendees aged 65 and above. The application of less age-dependent measures than BMI for the assessment of senior obesity has been discussed. As waist circumference (WC) as a surrogate of fat distribution (e.g. abdominal obesity) has been shown to be a more adequate predictor of impaired outcomes and elevated mortality in obese elderly [13], both, BMI and WC, will be considered as indicators of obesity. The association of individual lifestyle factors on BMI and WC is investigated.

Methods

Sample

The data were derived from the German MultiCare1 study investigating patterns of multi-morbidity in primary health care. At baseline, 3,189 multi-morbid subjects aged 65 to 85 years were included in the sample (mean 74.4 years, 59.3% women). For inclusion criteria, multi-morbidity was defined as being diagnosed with at least three out of a list of 29 diseases and syndromes. The study design and sample characteristics have been described in detail elsewhere [14;15].

Data collection and assessment procedure

Between July 2008 and October 2009, participating GPs were interviewed regarding the patients' morbidity. All participating GPs received a thorough introduction to the study. Aside from the GP interview, GPs were asked to measure weight, height and waist circumference in each patient. Each questionnaire contained specific information where waist circumference was to be measured. WC was defined as the minimal circumference at the umbilicus in a standing patient.

Within the face-to-face patient interview with the participant, all relevant sociodemographic information was collected.

Dependent variables

Body Mass Index was calculated by dividing the measured body weight by the squared body height in meters. It was then categorized according to guidelines (underweight or normal weight ≤ 24.9 kg/m^2, overweight 24.9–29.9 kg/m^2 and obese ≥ 30 kg/m^2) [16]. Waist circumference was classified to be an indicator for abdominal obesity when it exceeded 102 cm for men and 88 cm for women [17]. These cut-points are associated with a significantly higher risk for metabolic and cardiovascular complications [18].

Independent variables

Four different lifestyle behaviors and their association with obesity were investigated. They were assessed by a variety of instruments.

Physical activity. The International Physical Activities Questionnaire (IPAQ-S7S) was used to rate the participants' level of activity [19]. Reliability of the IPAQ across different study populations ranged from Spearman's Rho = 0.66 to 0.88. For an elderly population the re-test reliability of this instrument was 0.65 and 0.57 for men and women aged 65 and older, but showed adequate validity [20]. All study participants were categorized as displaying low, moderate or high activity behavior. High activity behavior, for example, was defined in participants reporting vigorous-intensity activity on at least 3 days or a combination including vigorous-intensity activity on at least 7 days. Detailed information on the scoring procedure is provided by the IPAQ Research Committee [21].

Alcohol consumption. Alcohol consumption was determined by the AUDIT-C, a short screening test for alcohol disorders [22]. Alcohol consumption was classified according to gender-specific cut-off points. For men a score greater than 5 and for women a score greater than 2 was seen as high to risky alcohol consumption [23]. The AUDIT does not allow for a detailed analysis of alcohol units per week. One item asked the participants to state whether they never smoked, were former smokers or currently smoked.

Quality and quantity of food intake. Another lifestyle variable regarded food intake and nutritional behavior. A self-constructed scale consisting of 10 items was used to rate quantity of food (2 items: Meals per day and size of meal portions) and quality of food (8 items covering the different nutritional classes, such as dairy products, and their frequency of intake). Quantity of food was dichotomized – those that report to eat as proposed by the guidelines vs. those that eat too much (German Society for Nutrition) [24]. For each of the nine quality items, it was determined whether the amount of each nutritional class the participant consumed was guideline concordant (German Society for Nutrition) [24]. For example, participants were asked how many portions of dairy products they consumed during a day. The German Society for nutrition recommends three or more portions of dairy products. Respondents meeting that criterion scored one point on the self-constructed scale. A score ranging from 0 (not guideline concordant at all) to 8 (completely guideline concordant) was then dichotomized, including participants in the 75th percentile in a guideline concordant, healthy eating group. The 75th percentile started at a score of 4 points on the scale.

Confounding variables

Age, gender and education served as socio-demographic confounding variables. Age was introduced as a continuous variable. Education was classified according to the CASMIN classification (low, moderate, high attainment) [25]. Additionally, subjective and objective disease burden were introduced as confounding variables since these may influence the impact of life-style factors. Objective disease burden was calculated as a score that included the number of co-morbid conditions weighted by the severity of these conditions. As obesity is the outcome variable in this study, obesity was excluded from the count of co-morbidities. Current subjective disease burden was ranked on the visual analog scale (VAS) within EuroQol (EQ-5D) Scale with a scale from 0–100 [26]. Functional status was assessed by the Barthel index. Impaired activities of daily living (ADL) were used to determine physical impairment of the participant [27]. The index consists of 10 items that are scored in three categories (0 points = high level of impairment, 5 points = medium level of impairment, 10 points = unimpaired). Respondents with a total of 100 points were categorized as completely unimpaired, 85 to 95 points as somewhat in need for care, 35 to 80 points in need for care, and below 30 points participants were rated as highly in need for care [27].

Statistical analyses

In total, 3,127 participants (98%) had valid values for the BMI and were entered in cross-sectional analyses. Data on WC was available for 3,079 respondents (96%). In data cleansing, missing values were input for participants with extreme values (e.g. WC smaller than 50 or larger than 250 cm). Due to missing data on independent variables the number of complete cases for the full multivariate regression model amounts to 2,841 (89%).

All statistical analyses were performed using STATA 11.2 [28]. Chi-square test and oneway ANOVA and t-tests were used to test for significant proportion and mean differences, respectively. Different dependent variables (WC and BMI) were used as continuous variables in the linear regression models, adjusted for age, gender, education, objective and subjective disease burden as well as functional status. Margins were calculated from those models, representing the actual numerical difference in WC and BMI across different life-styles. Additionally, WC and BMI were used as categorical variables as described. For all analyses, "no response" codes were treated as missing values.

Ethics approval

The study is conducted in compliance with the Helsinki Declaration. The study protocol was approved by the Ethics Committee of the Medical Association of Hamburg in February 2008 and amended in November 2008 (Approval-No. 2881). Written informed consent was given by all participants prior to the interview.

Results

About one third of the participants (31.1%) were considered obese if BMI is taken into account. Women were more likely to be obese (34.0%) but less often overweight (38.3% compared to 51.1% in men). The mean BMI in men was 28.1 kg/m^2 and 28.3 kg/m^2 in women. Waist circumference categorization seemed more sensitive regarding abdominal obesity. Seventy-Three per cent of all participants had a waist circumference above the recommended level. An elevated WC was found in 79.4% of all women and 64.8% of all men. Men had a mean WC of 106.3 cm and women a mean WC of 98.4 cm. Almost all obese participants and even 62% of normal or underweight patients showed a waist circumference above the threshold (table 1).

Table 1 summarizes baseline characteristics of participants by general obesity status. Age, gender, educational attainment, mean lifestyle score, physical activity, smoking status, alcohol consumption and objective as well as subjective health perception were significantly associated with general obesity.

Baseline means of BMI and WC are reported in Table 2. In the analyses adjusted for potential confounders (e.g. age, gender and disease burden, model 2), subjects with a low level of physical activity had a higher BMI (+1.6 kg/m^2, p<0.001) and WC (+4.9 cm, p<0.001) compared to those with a high level of activity.

Participants with a high to risky alcohol consumption as well as current smokers showed lower BMI and WC compared to those that are abstinent from alcohol and tobacco. Eating behavior related variables were associated with neither BMI nor WC in the adjusted analyses.

In table 3 the full logistic models showing effects of differentiated health behaviors on categorical WC and BMI are displayed. Current smokers had lower probability of elevated BMI (OR = 0.377, p<0.001) but not WC (OR = 0.740, p = 0.060). Former smokers, however, displayed a higher WC (OR = 1.311, p = 0.009). High to risky alcohol consumption was associated with lower probabilities of obesity for both outcomes. Again, low physical activity was associated with a lower probability of elevated BMI and WC. Food quantity and quality remained without association. The models with individual health behaviors as independent variables accounted for 7.1% (BMI) and 6.0% (WC) of variance.

Discussion

This cross-sectional study set out to determine the prevalence of overweight and obesity assessed by different anthropometric measures in a multi-morbid sample of German elderly (65+) and to investigate factors associated with general and abdominal obesity with a special focus on lifestyle related behaviors. It finds differences in the prevalence of obesity according to BMI or waist circumference. Physical activity is clearly associated with a lower BMI and WC, even when controlling for disease burden and socio-demographic variables.

Three out of four participants within this study were affected by either overweight or obesity. A recent study was able to show similar prevalence rates. Our findings are almost an exact replication of the prevalence found in the elderly German population (National Nutrition Survey II, Nationale Verzehrsstudie II; 31% total prevalence of obesity, 43.5% overweight), although data was obtained in a multi-morbid sample [29]. The distinctiveness of multi-morbidity might be reflected in the high numbers of elevated waist circumference in our sample. In the general population only 44.5% (men, 60- to 69-years old) and 57% (70+) had a WC above the recommended threshold. In our sample that number was exceeded substantially (65%). About 50 to 60% of women in the general public had an elevated WC, compared to 80% in this sample. This is of special importance as it is known that women are prone to accumulate abdominal fat after menopause that may affect adverse outcomes, such as the incidence of diabetes [30–32].

WC might capture elevated risks of cardiovascular and metabolic conditions, which are known to be highly prevalent in multi-morbid samples [33], more adequately than BMI. Since the WC cut-offs, but not the BMI cut-offs, were set specifically at the point of elevated risk for these conditions, the higher prevalence of increased WC may not be surprising. These results go in line with a previous study, where the authors reported a prevalence of 47% for general obesity and 73% for abdominal obesity in a sample of multi-morbid participants [34]. This assumption is supported by a study of Spanish elderly of the general population (not specifically multi-morbid). There, prevalence numbers of central obesity are about the same as in our study, while abdominal obesity prevalence is higher (totaling 56%) but not to the extent as it was seen in the multi-morbid samples [35].

Alternatively, a measurement error in WC can be an explanation for the large deviance we find. WC is particular is not the easiest and most reliable measure of obesity, especially in the elderly. A recent study found that the point of measure

Table 1. Baseline characteristics according to weight status.

	Non-obese	Obese	p
Men, % (n)	43.0 (927)	35.2 (342)	<0.001[a]
Age, years ± SD	74.6±5.3	73.9±5.0	<0.001[b]
Waist circumference above recommended threshold, % (n)	62.0 (1.312)	98.7 (944)	<0.001[a]
Educational attainment, % (n)			<0.001[a]
Low	59.9 (1289)	68.4 (665)	
Middle	27.9 (601)	23.9 (232)	
High	12.1 (261)	7.7 (75)	
Objective disease burden[c], mean n ± SD	10.6±4.9	12.4±5.2	<0.001[b]
Subjective disease burden[d], mean ± SD	64.2±17.8	58.5±18.4	<0.001[b]
Lifestyle factors			
Quality of food % (n)			0.678[a]
High (>75th percentile)	43.4 (914)	42.6 (403)	
Low (< 75th percentile)	56.6 (1194)	57.4 (544)	
Quantity of food, guideline concordant, % (n)	83.6 (1795)	84.2 (815)	0.660[a]
Physical activity, % (n)			<0.001[a]
Low	27.7 (585)	44.3 (427)	
Moderate	45.0 (951)	36.6 (353)	
High	27.3 (576)	19.1 (184)	
Smoking status, % (n)			<0.001[a]
Never	46.5 (1001)	51.9 (504)	
Former	42.6 (916)	42.8 (416)	
Current	10.9 (234)	5.4 (52)	
Alcohol consumption, % (n)			<0.001[a]
Abstinent	22.2 (477)	30.7 (297)	
Low to Moderate	39.3 (844)	38.2 (370)	
High	38.5 (827)	31.3 (301)	

Weight status as determined by Body Mass Index (BMI ≥30);
[a]comparison between obese and non-obese based on chi-square test;
[b]comparison between obese and non-obese based t-test,
[c]number of diseases weighted by severity;
[d]visual analogue scale.

(narrowest point between the inferior rib border and the iliac crest) for WC may be difficult to find in the obese elderly which made up quite a proportion of this sample [36]. The measurement error can range from 0.7 cm to 15 cm [37] and this study lacks data for quality checks. Although WC measurement can therefore not be considered to detect small changes following interventions, its use can be valuable in epidemiological studies as this [38]. Furthermore, the lack of missing values as well as extreme outliers can be a potential indicator for valid data in this study.

Individual lifestyle choices have been shown to be significantly associated with the existence of obesity (e.g. [39]) and changing lifestyle patterns have shown to have effects on e.g. cognitive health [40]. This study therefore emphasizes the relevance of modifiable lifestyle factors in the development and maintenance of overweight and obesity. Although causal conclusions cannot be drawn from the cross-sectional study, controlling the effect of lifestyle factors for socio-demographic and disease related effects, eliminates some alternative explanations.

High to moderate physical activity was inversely associated with BMI and WC values. Obviously, a higher energy expenditure via physical activity balances out the energy homeostasis. This is of special importance since the resting metabolic rate is said to

decrease by 2–3% every life year [41], thus making physical activity crucial in maintaining a constant weight. A study was able to show that a diet accompanied by physical activity was most successful in weight loss efforts in a sample of 65-year-olds [42]. A review in adolescents suggests physical activity to act as a protective factor in obesity [43], but existent obesity might be a barrier to physical activity as well. A decrease in energy expenditure rather than an increase in energy intake is described to be responsible for the increase of total fat mass with age [41]. This decrease in energy expenditure is partly due to a decreased level of physical activity, suggesting that efforts to keep physical activity high even in older age might influence weight and fat mass [42]. Recent studies even show a beneficial effect of commenced physical activity in old age on the incidence of dementia, underlying the importance of physical activity [44;45].

It is difficult to understand the observed association between current smoking and lower BMI values. The present findings are in agreement with a previous report about Spanish elderly [34], but in contrast to what has been reported in Switzerland [46]. In current smokers, nicotine increases energy expenditure, but heavy smoking might also be associated with other obesogenic behaviors, suggesting an u-shaped association [46]. A prospective study

Table 2. Baseline Means of BMI and WC according to lifestyle factors.

	Bivariate Analyses		Model 1[a]		Model 2[b]	
	Mean (95% CIs)	p	Mean (95% CIs)	p	Mean (95% CIs)	p
BMI (kg/m^2)						
Quality of food						
High (>75th percentile)	28.1 [27.9 to 28.4]	0.413	28.2 [27.9 to 28.4]	0.621	28.2 [28.0 to 28.4]	0.933
Low (<75th percentile)	28.3 [28.1 to 28.5]		28.3 [28.0 to 28.5]		28.2 [27.8 to 28.5]	
Quantity of food						
Guideline concordant	28.2 [28.0 to 28.4]	0.742	28.1 [27.7 to 28.6]	0.703	28.2 [28.1 to 28.4]	0.564
Above guideline rec	28.2 [28.0 to 28.4].		28.2 [28.0 to 28.4]		28.1 [27.7 to 28.5]	
Physical activity						
Low	29.5 [29.2 to 29.8]	<0.001	29.6 [29.3 to 29.9]	<0.001	29.2 [28.9 to 29.5]	<0.001
Moderate	27.7 [27.5 to 28.0]	0.275	27.7 [27.5 to 28.0]	0.075	27.8 [27.6 to 28.1]	0.309
High	27.5 [27.1 to 27.8]		27.3 [27.0 to 27.7]		27.6 [27.3 to 28.0]	
Smoking status						
Never	28.4 [28.2 to 28.6]		28.4 [28.1 to 28.6]		28.4 [28.1 to 28.6]	
Former	28.4 [28.1 to 28.6]	0.883	28.4 [28.2 to 28.7]	0.902	28.4 [28.2 to 28.7]	0.801
Current	26.6 [26.0 to 27.1]	<0.001	26.4 [25.8 to 27.0]	<0.001	26.2 [25.7 to 26.8]	<0.001
Alcohol consumption						
Abstinent	28.9 [28.5 to 29.2]		28.8 [28.4 to 29.1]		28.5 [28.2 to 28.9]	
Low to Moderate	28.3 [28.0 to 28.6]	0.010	28.4 [28.2 to 28.7]	0.133	28.4 [28.1 to 28.7]	0.546
High	27.7 [27.4 to 28.0]	<0.001	27.6 [27.3 to 27.9]	<0.001	27.8 [27.6 to 28.1]	0.003
WC (cm)						
Quality of food						
High (>75th percentile)	100.8 [100.1 to 101.5]	0.006	101.2 [100.5 to 101.9]	0.201	101.7 [101.0 to 102.4]	0.858
Low (<75th percentile)	102.2 [101.5 to 102.8]		101.8 [101.2 to 102.4]		101.6 [101.0 to 102.2]	
Quantity of food						
Guideline concordant	103.2 [102.1 to 104.4]	0.002	101.7 [100.6 to 102.9]	0.757	101.6 [101.1 to 102.1]	0.891
Above guideline rec	101.3 [1000.7 to 101.8]		101.5 [101.0 to 102.0]		101.7 [100.6 to 102.8]	
Physical activity						
Low	105.1 [104.3 to 105.9]	<0.001	105.8 [105.0 to 106.6]	<0.001	104.7 [103.9 to 105.5]	<0.001
Moderate	100.0 [99.3 to 100.7]	0.652	100.0 [99.3 to 100.6]	0.069	100.4 [99.7 to 101.0]	0.322
High	99.8 [98.8 to 100.7]		98.9 [98.0 to 99.8]		99.8 [98.9 to 100.7]	
Smoking status						
Never	99.9 [99.2 to 100.5]		101.4 [100.7 to 102.0]		101.5 [100.8 to 102.2]	
Former	103.8 [103.1 to 104.5]	<0.001	102.4 [101.7 to 103.1]	0.054	102.4 [101.7 to 103.1]	0.097
Current	100.5 [98.9 to 102.0]	0.459	99.4 [97.9 to 100.9]	0.018	98.9 [97.4 to 100.4]	0.002
Alcohol consumption						
Abstinent	102.4 [101.4 to 103.3]		103.2 [102.3 to 104.1]		102.5 [101.6 to 103.4]	
Low to Moderate	103.6 [102.9 to 104.4]	0.041	101.8 [101.1 to 102.6]	0.027	101.8 [101.0 to 102.5]	0.239
High	98.8 [98.0 to 99.6]	<0.001	100.2 [99.4 to 101.0]	<0.001	100.9 [100.1 to 101.7]	0.008

Bivariate analyses and adjusted analyses for each lifestyle factor; BMI – Body Mass Index; WC – Waist circumference;
[a]adjusted for age, sex, educational attainment;
[b]adjusted for age, sex, educational attainment, subjective and objective disease burden and need for care.

showed that active smokers and quitting smokers had greater weight gains over a follow-up period of 50 months compared to those who did not smoke [47]. This fining in particular emphasizes the importance of attempt to reduce smoking at a population level as it seems to be a risk factor even for obesity. Current smoking may, via increased energy expenditure, positively influence weight status, but poses, in the long run, a risk factor.

The decrease in body size with increase of alcohol intake has been shown before, however, explanations are lacking [48]. This seems of special importance since this study used gender-specific cut-off values to determine high to risky consumption levels according to guidelines [23;49]. We were not able, however, to determine the kinds of drinks consumed which is one important factor discussed when evaluating the influence of alcohol consumption [48].

Table 3. Logistic regression BMI and WC with individual lifestyle behaviors[a].

Independent variables	Model 1 BMI obesity Odds Ratio	Model 2 WC obesity Odds Ratio
Level of activity (ref = high)		
Moderate activity	1.151	1.310
Low activity	1.988***	1.906***
Drinking behavior (ref = abstinent)		
Low to moderate consumption	0.894	0.860
High to risky consumption	0.699**	0.765**
Smoking status (ref = never)		
Former smoker	0.988	1.311**
Current smoker	0.377***	0.740
Quantity of food (ref = too little or guideline concordant)	0.973	0.988
Quality of food (score)	1.007	0.991
Constant	1.156	2.920***
Observations	2841	2802
Adjusted R^2	0.071	0.060

**p<0.01,
***p<0.001.
[a]adjusted for age, sex, educational attainment;
Abbreviations: BMI – Body Mass Index; WC – Waist circumference.

Dietary variables did not show significant effects on BMI or WC. Using a combined score to determine guideline concordant eating behavior may have resulted in a loss of relevant information, however, in post-hoc analyses, the individual influence of nutritional components (such as fruit and vegetable intake) was assessed, but did not yield clear associations either. For example, eating more portions of fruit every day, was associated with a lower likelihood of being abdominal obese (OR = 0.93, p = 0.040) but not general obese (OR = 0.96, p = 0.263). The effects vanish when controlling for educational attainment. This seems to support the assumption that individual eating choices are not as much of relevance as eating patterns, such as the Mediterranean Diet that has been shown to be associated with lower obesity prevalence [34]. Standardized scales to assess nutritional intake ought to be used. In depth investigation of the role of quality and quantity of food with objective assessment is obviously still needed.

Strengths and Limitations

This study has several strengths and limitations. It provides the first basis of data on obesity in multi-morbid senior citizens in German primary care. The large sample of participants increases likelihood of reliable results. Although the majority of GP patients in Germany can be considered multi-morbid, the selection of patients may have lead to a bias of the association between physical measures and health outcomes.

One important aspect that needs to be considered is the potentially limited validity of waist circumference measure in general practices. Although a specific instruction was in place and all GPs were thoroughly instructed, measurement errors cannot be ruled out. The kind of instruction that was used was easy to understand and was easily implemented. Previous research shows that the kind of protocol that is used has no influence on the prospective associations with mortality and morbidity [50].

The lifestyle factors that were included can be assessed easily which might be of importance when translating findings into prevention or intervention efforts. Obviously, a more in depth assessment of lifestyle factors might have contributed to a more detailed understanding of mechanisms. Furthermore, the self-report of e.g. food intake might be less reliable than an experimental assessment. There is no data available on the validity of the food scale that was used; however, it is closely related to previous food frequency questionnaires (FFQ). While the validity of these questionnaires declines with the length of the food list, this relatively short instrument may have an advantage. Coherence and grouping of the items fulfill criteria of valid FFQs [51]. Also, the IPAQ questionnaire has not been fully evaluated in elderly samples yet. Its moderate reliability will need further investigation; however, correlation with objective measures (accelerometer) was satisfactory in previous studies [20]. Also, retrospective data on weight course and nutrition especially during adulthood was not assessed. Because of the cross-sectional design of these analyses, causal relationships can only be hypothesized but not proven; however, longitudinal data from the same study will be available to enlighten open questions. These cross-sectional analyses provide first information and potentially associated variables that can now be investigated in follow-up studies.

Furthermore, the explained variance of the regression models was limited. Considering the complexity of BMI and WC determinants, however, we feel that it was sufficient. Obviously, including information on past weight, as well as genetic markers in the analyses would have further increased the level of explained variance.

Conclusions

Especially in multi-morbid patients, the prevalence of elevated waist circumference and obesity according to BMI differs substantially. Waist circumference might be an even more sensitive marker for obesity than the BMI. Age-specific thresholds for the

BMI are needed which can only be assessed through prospective studies. Of all lifestyle factors that were investigated, physical activity was the only one with a clear association to lower BMI and WC values. Motivating older adults to stay active seems crucial. In multi-morbid patients, one approach to achieve that goal may be through their general practitioner.

Acknowledgments

This article is on behalf of the MultiCare Cohort Study Group, which consists of Attila Altiner, Horst Bickel, Monika Bullinger, Hendrik van den Bussche, Anne Dahlhaus, Lena Ehreke, Michael Freitag, Angela Fuchs, Jochen Gensichen, Ferdinand Gerlach, Heike Hansen, Sven Heinrich, Susanne Höfels, Olaf von dem Knesebeck, Hans-Helmut König, Norbert Krause, Hanna Leicht, Margrit Löbner, Melanie Luppa, Wolfgang Maier, Christine Mellert, Anna Nützel, Juliana Petersen, Jana Prokein, Steffi Riedel-Heller, Ingmar Schäfer, Martin Scherer, Gerhard Schön, Susanne Steinmann, Sven Schulz, Karl Wegscheider, Jochen Werle, Siegfried Weyerer, and Birgitt Wiese.

We are grateful to the general practitioners in Bonn, Dusseldorf, Frankfurt/Main, Hamburg, Jena, Leipzig, Mannheim and Munich who supplied the clinical information on their patients, namely Theodor Alfen, Martina Amm, Katrin Ascher, Philipp Ascher, Heinz-Michael Assmann, Hubertus Axthelm, Leonhard Badmann, Horst Bauer, Veit-Harold Bauer, Sylvia Baumbach, Brigitte Behrend-Berdin, Rainer Bents, Werner Besier, Liv Betge, Arno Bewig, Hannes Blankenfeld, Harald Bohnau, Claudia Böhnke, Ulrike Börgerding, Gundula Bormann, Martin Braun, Inge Bürfent, Klaus Busch, Jürgen Claus, Peter Dick, Heide Dickenbrok, Wolfgang Dörr, Nadejda Dörrler-Naidenoff, Ralf Dumjahn, Norbert Eckhardt, Richard Ellersdorfer, Doris Fischer-Radizi, Martin Fleckenstein, Anna Frangoulis, Daniela Freise, Denise Fricke, Nicola Fritz, Sabine Füllgraf-Horst, Angelika Gabriel-Müller, Rainer Gareis, Benno Gelshorn, Maria Göbel-Schlatholt, Manuela Godorr, Jutta Goertz, Cornelia Gold, Stefanie Grabs, Hartmut Grella, Peter Gülle, Elisabeth Gummersbach, Heinz Gürster, Eva Hager, Wolfgang-Christoph Hager, Henning Harder, Matthias Harms, Dagmar Harnisch, Marie-Luise von der Heide, Katharina Hein, Ludger Helm, Silvia Helm, Udo Hilsmann, Claus W. Hinrichs, Bernhard Hoff, Karl-Friedrich Holtz, Wolf-Dietrich Honig, Christian Hottas, Helmut Ilstadt, Detmar Jobst, Gunter Kässner, Volker Kielstein, Gabriele Kirsch, Thomas Kochems, Martina Koch-Preißer, Andreas Koeppel, Almut Körner, Gabriele Krause, Jens Krautheim, Nicolas Kreff, Daniela Kreuzer, Franz Kreuzer, Judith Künstler, Christiane Kunz, Doris Kurzeja-Hüsch, Felizitas Leitner, Holger Liebermann, Ina Lipp, Thomas Lipp, Bernd Löbbert, Guido Marx, Stefan Maydl, Manfred Mayer, Stefan-Wolfgang Meier, Jürgen Meissner, Anne Meister, Ruth Möhrke, Christian Mörchen, Andrea Moritz, Ute Mühlmann, Gabi Müller, Sabine Müller, Karl-Christian Münter, Helga Nowak, Erwin Ottahal, Christina Panzer, Thomas Paschke, Helmut Perleberg, Eberhard Prechtel, Hubertus Protz, Sandra Quantz, Eva-Maria Rappen-Cremer, Thomas Reckers, Elke Reichert, Birgitt Richter-Polynice, Franz Roegele, Heinz-Peter Romberg, Anette Rommel, Michael Rothe, Uwe Rumbach, Michael Schilp, Franz Schlensog, Ina Schmalbruch, Angela Schmid, Holger Schmidt, Lothar Schmittdiel, Matthias Schneider, Ulrich Schott, Gerhard Schulze, Heribert Schützendorf, Harald Siegmund, Gerd Specht, Karsten Sperling, Meingard Staude, Hans-Günter Stieglitz, Martin Strickfaden, Hans-Christian Taut, Johann Thaller, Uwe Thürmer, Ljudmila Titova, Michael Traub, Martin Tschoke, Maya Tügel, Christian Uhle, Kristina Vogel, Florian Vorderwülbecke, Hella Voß, Christoph Weber, Klaus Weckbecker, Sebastian Weichert, Sabine Weidnitzer, Brigitte Weingärtner, Karl-Michael Werner, Hartmut Wetzel, Edgar Widmann, Alexander Winkler, Otto-Peter Witt, Martin Wolfrum, Rudolf Wolter, Armin Wunder, and Steffi Wünsch.

We also thank Corinna Contenius, Cornelia Eichhorn, Sarah Floehr, Vera Kleppel, Heidi Kubieziel, Rebekka Maier, Natascha Malukow, Karola Mergenthal, Christine Müller, Sandra Müller, Michaela Schwarzbach, Wibke Selbig, Astrid Steen, Miriam Steigerwald, and Meike Thiele for data collection as well as Ulrike Barth, Elena Hoffmann, Friederike Isensee, Leyla Kalaz, Heidi Kubieziel, Helga Mayer, Karine Mnatsakanyan, Michael Paulitsch, Merima Ramic, Sandra Rauck, Nico Schneider, Jakob Schroeber, Susann Schumann, and Daniel Steigerwald for data entry.

Author Contributions

Conceived and designed the experiments: CS ML BW SRH SW HHK WM GS JJP JG AF HB HH HvdB MS. Performed the experiments: ML BW SRH SW HHK WM GS JJP JG AF HB HH HvdB MS. Analyzed the data: CS ML SRH. Contributed reagents/materials/analysis tools: CS ML BW SRH SW HHK WM GS JJP JG AF HB HH HvdB MS. Wrote the paper: CS.

References

1. Freedman DS (2011) Obesity – United States, 1988–2008. Morb Mortal Wkly Rep Surveill Summ; 60: 73–77.
2. Flegal KM, Carroll MD, Ogden CL, Curtin LR (2010) Prevalence and Trends in Obesity Among US Adults, 1999–2008. JAMA; 303: 235–241.
3. Wang YC, McPherson K, Marsh T, Gortmaker SL, Brown M (2011) Health and economic burden of the projected obesity trends in the USA and the UK. Lancet; 378: 815–825.
4. Janssen I, Mark AE (2007) Elevated body mass index and mortality risk in the elderly. Obes Rev; 8: 41–59.
5. Jensen GL, Hsiao PY (2010) Obesity in older adults: relationship to functional limitation. Curr Opin Clin Nutr Metab Care; 13: 46–51.
6. Faeh D, Braun J, Tarnutzer S, Bopp M (2011) Obesity but not overweight is associated with increased mortality risk. Eur J Epidemiol.
7. Han JC, Lawlor DA, Kimm SY (2010) Childhood obesity. Lancet; 375: 1737–1748.
8. Atlantis E, Martin SA, Haren MT, Taylor AW, Wittert GA (2008) Lifestyle factors associated with age-related differences in body composition: the Florey Adelaide Male Aging Study. Am J Clin Nutr; 88: 95–104.
9. Lindstrom J, Neumann A, Sheppard KE, Gilis-Januszewska A, Greaves CJ, et al. (2010) Take action to prevent diabetes–the IMAGE toolkit for the prevention of type 2 diabetes in Europe. Horm Metab Res; 42 Suppl 1: S37–S55.
10. Paulweber B, Valensi P, Lindstrom J, Lalic NM, Greaves CJ, et al. (2010) A European evidence-based guideline for the prevention of type 2 diabetes. Horm Metab Res; 42 Suppl 1: S3–36.
11. Fortin M, Bravo G, Hudon C, Vanasse A, Lapointe L (2005) Prevalence of multimorbidity among adults seen in family practice. Ann Fam Med; 3: 223–228.
12. Dombrowski SU, Avenell A, Sniehott FF (2010) Behavioural interventions for obese adults with additional risk factors for morbidity: systematic review of effects on behaviour, weight and disease risk factors. Obes Facts; 3: 377–396.
13. Price GM, Uauy R, Breeze E, Bulpitt CJ, Fletcher AE (2006) Weight, shape, and mortality risk in older persons: elevated waist-hip ratio, not high body mass index, is associated with a greater risk of death. Am J Clin Nutr; 84: 449–460.
14. Schäfer I, Hansen H, Schon G, Maier W, Hofels S, et al. (2009) The German MultiCare-study: Patterns of multimorbidity in primary health care - protocol of a prospective cohort study. BMC Health Serv Res; 9: 145.
15. Schäfer I, Hansen H, Schön G, Höfels S, Altiner A, et al. (2011) The influence of age, gender and socio-economic status on multimorbidity patterns in primary care. First results from the MultiCare Cohort Study. Forthcoming 2011.
16. Benecke A, Vogel H [Overweight and obesity]. 16 edn. Robert Koch-Institut: Berlin, 2003.
17. National Institutes of Health (1998) Clinical guidelines on the identification, evaluation and treatment of overweight and obesity in adults - the evidence report. Obes Res; 6: 51S–209S.
18. World Health Organization (WHO) (2000) Obesity. Preventing and managing the global epidemic. WHO Technical Report Series; 894.
19. Craig CL, Marshall AL, Sjostrom M, Bauman AE, Booth ML, et al. (2003) International physical activity questionnaire: 12-country reliability and validity. Med Sci Sports Exerc; 35: 1381–1395.
20. Tomioka K, Iwamoto J, Saeki K, Okamoto N (2011) Reliability and validity of the International Physical Activity Questionnaire (IPAQ) in elderly adults: the Fujiwara-kyo Study. J Epidemiol; 21: 459–465.
21. IPAQ Research Committee (2005) Guidelines for Data Processing and Analysis of the International Physical Activity Questionnaire (IPAQ) – Short and Long Forms. Available: http://www.ipaq.ki.se/scoring.pdf Accessed 2013 Aug 21.
22. Bush K, Kivlahan DR, McDonell MB, Fihn SD, Bradley KA (1998) The AUDIT alcohol consumption questions (AUDIT-C): an effective brief screening test for problem drinking. Ambulatory Care Quality Improvement Project (ACQUIP). Alcohol Use Disorders Identification Test. Arch Intern Med; 158: 1789–1795.
23. Aertgeerts B, Buntinx F, Ansoms S, Fevery J (2001) Screening properties of questionnaires and laboratory tests for the detection of alcohol abuse or dependence in a general practice population. Br J Gen Pract; 51: 206–217.
24. Deutsche Gesellschaft für Ernährung (2011) [Nutritional guidelines]. Available: http://www.dge.de Accessed 2011 Aug 18.

25. Brauns H, Steinmann S (1999) Educational Reform in France, West-Germany and the United Kingdom: Updating the CASMIN Educational Classification. ZUMA-Nachrichten; 44: 7–45.
26. The EuroQol Group (1990) EuroQol - a new facility for the measurement of health related quality of life. Health Policy; 16: 199–208.
27. Collin C, Wade DT, Davies S, Horne V (1988) The Barthel ADL Index: a reliability study. Int Disabil Stud; 10: 61–63.
28. StataCorp (2009) Stata Statistical Software: Release 11. College Station. TX: StataCorp LP.
29. National Nutrition Survey II (2008) [Report of Results I]. Bundesforschungsinstitut für Ernährung und Lebensmittel. Available: http://www.was-esse-ich.de/uploads/media/NVS_II_Abschlussbericht_Teil_1_mit_Ergaenzungsbericht.pdf Accessed 2011 Sept 21.
30. Lovejoy JC (2003) The menopause and obesity. Prim Care; 30: 317–325.
31. Davis SR, Castelo-Branco C, Chedraui P, Lumsden MA, Nappi RE, et al. (2012) Understanding weight gain at menopause. Climacteric; 15: 419–429.
32. Maske UE, Scheidt-Nave C, Busch MA, Jacobi F, Weikert B, et al. (2014) [Comorbidity of Diabetes Mellitus and Depression in the General Population in Germany.]. Psychiatr Prax; May 23. [Epub ahead of print].
33. Marengoni A, Angleman S, Melis R, Mangialasche F, Karp A, et al. (2011) Aging with multimorbidity: a systematic review of the literature. Ageing Res Rev; 10: 430–439.
34. Bullo M, Garcia-Aloy M, Martinez-Gonzalez MA, Corella D, Fernandez-Ballart JD, et al. (2011) Association between a healthy lifestyle and general obesity and abdominal obesity in an elderly population at high cardiovascular risk. Prev Med; 53: 155–161.
35. Gomez-Cabello A, Pedrero-Chamizo R, Olivares PR, Luzardo L, Juez-Bengoechea A, et al. (2011) Prevalence of overweight and obesity in non-institutionalized people aged 65 or over from Spain: the elderly EXERNET multi-centre study. Obes Rev; 12: 583–592.
36. Gomez-Cabello A, Vicente-Rodriguez G, Albers U, Mata E, Rodriguez-Marroyo JA, et al. (2012) Harmonization process and reliability assessment of anthropometric measurements in the elderly EXERNET multi-centre study. PLoS One; 7: e41752.
37. Verweij LM, Terwee CB, Proper KI, Hulshof CT, van Mechelen W (2013) Measurement error of waist circumference: gaps in knowledge. Public Health Nutr; 16: 281–288.
38. Schunkert H, Moebus S, Hanisch J, Bramlage P, Steinhagen-Thiessen E, et al. (2008) The correlation between waist circumference and ESC cardiovascular risk score: data from the German metabolic and cardiovascular risk project (GEMCAS). Clin Res Cardiol; 97: 827–835.
39. Lahti-Koski M, Pietinen P, Heliovaara M, Vartiainen E (2002) Associations of body mass index and obesity with physical activity, food choices, alcohol intake, and smoking in the 1982-1997 FINRISK Studies. Am J Clin Nutr; 75: 809–817.
40. Merrill DA, Small GW (2011) Prevention in psychiatry: effects of healthy lifestyle on cognition. Psychiatr Clin North Am; 34: 249–261.
41. Villareal DT, Apovian CM, Kushner RF, Klein S (2005) Obesity in older adults: technical review and position statement of the American Society for Nutrition and NAASO, The Obesity Society. Am J Clin Nutr; 82: 923–934.
42. Villareal DT, Chode S, Parimi N, Sinacore DR, Hilton T, et al. (2011) Weight loss, exercise, or both and physical function in obese older adults. N Engl J Med; 364: 1218–1229.
43. Reichert FF, Baptista Menezes AM, Wells JC, Carvalho DS, Hallal PC (2009) Physical activity as a predictor of adolescent body fatness: a systematic review. Sports Med; 39: 279–294.
44. Sharma AM (2011) Physicians' calling patients on excess weight may provide reality check and increase desire to lose weight in overweight and obese individuals. Evid Based Med; Aug 18. [Epub ahead of print].
45. Post RE, Mainous AG III, Gregorie SH, Knoll ME, Diaz VA, et al. (2011) The influence of physician acknowledgment of patients' weight status on patient perceptions of overweight and obesity in the United States. Arch Intern Med; 171: 316–321.
46. Chiolero A, Jacot-Sadowski I, Faeh D, Paccaud F, Cornuz J (2007) Association of cigarettes smoked daily with obesity in a general adult population. Obesity (Silver Spring); 15: 1311–1318.
47. Basterra-Gortari FJ, Forga L, Bes-Rastrollo M, Toledo E, Martinez JA, et al. (2010) Effect of smoking on body weight: longitudinal analysis of the SUN cohort. Rev Esp Cardiol; 63: 20–27.
48. Yeomans MR (2010) Alcohol, appetite and energy balance: is alcohol intake a risk factor for obesity? Physiol Behav; 100: 82–89.
49. Bradley KA, Bush KR, Epler AJ, Dobie DJ, Davis TM, et al. (2003) Two brief alcohol-screening tests From the Alcohol Use Disorders Identification Test (AUDIT): validation in a female Veterans Affairs patient population. Arch Intern Med; 163: 821–829.
50. Ross R, Berentzen T, Bradshaw AJ, Janssen I, Kahn HS, et al. (2008) Does the relationship between waist circumference, morbidity and mortality depend on measurement protocol for waist circumference? Obes Rev; 9: 312–325.
51. Kristal, Alan R, Shattuk, Ann L, and Williams, Allen E (1992) Food Frequency Questionnaires for Diet Intervention Research. Available: http://www.nutrientdataconf.org/pastconf/ndbc17/5-5_kristal.pdf Accessed 2014 April 24.

## 22

Does Mortality Risk of Cigarette Smoking Depend on Serum Concentrations of Persistent Organic Pollutants? Prospective Investigation of the Vasculature in Uppsala Seniors (PIVUS) Study

Duk-Hee Lee[1,2], Lars Lind[3], David R. Jacobs Jr.[4,5], Samira Salihovic[6], Bert van Bavel[6], P. Monica Lind[7]*

1 Department of Preventive Medicine, School of Medicine, Kyungpook National University, Daegu, Korea, **2** BK21 Plus KNU Biomedical Convergence Program, Department of Biomedical Science, Kyungpook National University, Daegu, Korea, **3** Department of Medical Sciences, Cardiovascular Epidemiology, Uppsala University Hospital, Uppsala, Sweden, **4** Division of Epidemiology and Community Health, School of Public Health, University of Minnesota, Minneapolis, Minnesota, United States of America, **5** Department of Nutrition, University of Oslo, Oslo, Norway, **6** MTM Research Center, School of Science and Technology, Örebro University, Örebro, Sweden, **7** Department of Medical Sciences, Occupational and Environmental Medicine, Uppsala University, Uppsala, Sweden

Abstract

Cigarette smoking is an important cause of preventable death globally, but associations between smoking and mortality vary substantially across country and calendar time. Although methodological biases have been discussed, it is biologically plausible that persistent organic pollutants (POPs) like polychlorinated biphenyls (PCBs) and organochlorine (OC) pesticides can affect this association. This study was performed to evaluate if associations of cigarette smoking with mortality were modified by serum concentrations of PCBs and OC pesticides. We evaluated cigarette smoking in 111 total deaths among 986 men and women aged 70 years in the Prospective Investigation of the Vasculature in Uppsala Seniors (PIVUS) with mean follow-up for 7.7 years. The association between cigarette smoking and total mortality depended on serum concentration of PCBs and OC pesticides (P value for interaction = 0.02). Among participants in the highest tertile of the serum POPs summary score, former and current smokers had 3.7 (95% CI, 1.5–9.3) and 6.4 (95% CI, 2.3–17.7) times higher mortality hazard, respectively, than never smokers. In contrast, the association between cigarette smoking and total mortality among participants in the lowest tertile of the serum POPs summary score was much weaker and statistically non-significant. The strong smoking-mortality association observed among elderly people with high POPs was mainly driven by low risk of mortality among never smokers with high POPs. As smoking is increasing in many low-income and middle-income countries and POPs contamination is a continuing problem in these areas, the interactions between these two important health-related issues should be considered in future research.

Editor: Keitaro Matsuo, Kyushu University Faculty of Medical Science, Japan

Funding: This study was supported by the Swedish Research Council (VR) and the Swedish Research Council for Environment, Agricultural Sciences and Spatial Planning (FORMAS), Korea Health technology R&D Project, Ministry of Health & Welfare, Republic of Korea (A111716), and BK21 PLUS KNU Biomedical Convergence Program for Creative Talent. The funders had no role in study design, data collection and analysis, decision to publish, or preparation of the manuscript.

Competing Interests: The authors have declared that no competing interests exist.

* E-mail: monica.lind@medsci.uu.se

Introduction

Cigarette smoking, as a major risk factor for cancer, cardiovascular diseases, and pulmonary diseases, is an important cause of preventable death globally [1]. However, the magnitude of associations between cigarette smoking and mortality varies across countries and calendar time [2,3,4,5]. To date, this variation has been attributed mainly to methodological biases such as misclassification of smoking status, cohort effects, or random variation [2,3,4,5].

In our previous study [6], we formulated a novel hypothesis that persistent organic pollutants (POPs) modify the risk of cigarette smoking on death. POPs are lipophilic chemicals that accumulate in adipose tissue and are associated with the risk of various chronic diseases [7,8,9]. The biological plausibility for our hypothesis was

that experimental studies in mice reported that pretreatment with some POPs increased toxicity of important chemicals contained in cigarette smoke, like benzopyrene, dimethylnitrosamine, and N-nitrosodiethlyamine [10,11].

Supporting our prior hypothesis, we observed different associations between cigarette smoking and total mortality depending on serum concentrations of POPs among the elderly in the U.S. [6]. In that study, one surprising finding was that cigarette smoking did not increase the risk of mortality in the lowest category of POPs. Despite the possibility that smoking-related diseases risks are lower among the elderly than in younger persons due to selective survival [12], finding any subgroup with no association between cigarette smoking and mortality was unexpected.

Our earlier study is the only one published on this topic and the number of current smokers was too small [6]. Thus, we studied here whether the finding was replicable in another dataset. We evaluated if there are similar interactions of serum concentrations of POPs with cigarette smoking on the risk of mortality among men and women aged 70 years, living in the community of Uppsala, Sweden (Prospective Investigation of the Vasculature in Uppsala Seniors (PIVUS) study). Because our previous study found that, among various POPs, polychlorinated biphenyls (PCBs) or organochlorine (OC) pesticides showed clear interactions with cigarette smoking and mortality [6], we used POPs burden calculated based on serum concentrations of both OC pesticides and PCBs in this study.

Materials and Methods

Study subjects at baseline were 1,016 men and women, residents of Uppsala, Sweden and age 70 years at time of examination between April 2001 and June 2004. Among participants at baseline, 986 subjects had valid measurement of PCBs and OC pesticides at baseline. The study was approved by the Ethics Committee of the University of Uppsala. The participants gave written informed consent.

All subjects were investigated in the morning after an overnight fast, with no medication or smoking allowed after midnight. The participants were asked about their health behaviors, medical history, and regular medication. Body mass index (BMI) was derived from measured height and weight (kg/m^2). Serum cholesterol and triglyceride concentrations were determined in an enzymatic assay (Abbott, Abbott Park, IL, USA).

POPs were measured in stored plasma samples collected at baseline. Analyses of POPs were performed using a Micromass Autospec Ultima (Waters, Mildford, MA, USA) high resolution chromatography coupled to high resolution mass spectrometry (HRGC/HRMS) system based on the method by Sandau et al [13] with some modifications. All details of POPs analyses were provided elsewhere [14]. Among 16 PCB congeners and 5 OC pesticides, 2 OC pesticides (trans-chlordane and cis-chlordane) with detection rate <10% were not included in the final analyses. An established summation formula based on serum cholesterol and serum triglyceride concentrations was used to calculate the total amount of lipid in each plasma sample [15]. Thereafter the wet-weight concentrations of the POPs were divided by this lipid estimate to obtain lipid-normalized concentrations. As models based on wet-weight concentrations adjusted for serum cholesterol and triglyceride as covariates showed similar results, we presented the results based on lipid-normalized concentrations for the consistency of analytic strategy with the previous study [6].

The fact of death was ascertained through linkage to the Swedish Register of Death Causes at the National Board of Health and Welfare. Causes of death data were not available. Follow-up time for each person was calculated as the difference between the first examination date and the last known date alive or censored. Persons who survived the entire follow-up period were censored on Jan 1, 2012. Median follow-up time was 7.7 years (range 0.3–9.8 years) and we documented 111 deaths.

For the analysis, smoking status was expressed as never, former and current. First, we calculated the summary measure of 16 PCB congeners and 5 OC pesticides by summing the rank orders of the individual POPs for subjects with detectable values of each POP, assigning rank 0 to not detectable values. Three summary measures were made based on both PCBs and OC pesticides, PCBs only, and OC pesticides only.

Next, we checked if the associations between cigarette smoking and mortality differed by tertiles of the summary measures of POPs in predicting total mortality using Cox proportional hazard

models. P values for interaction were calculated based on three categories of each of POPs and cigarette smoking. Adjusting covariates were gender, physical activity (none, moderate, and vigorous), BMI (kg/m^2), and alcohol consumption (g/day). We further considered medication for diabetes or hypertension and history of myocardial infarction or stroke as possible confounders.

In addition to stratified analyses, adjusted HRs with the common reference group of never smokers within the 1st tertile of POPs were presented. Also, the same analyses were applied to the U.S. elderly within our previous study [6] because only results stratified analyses by POPs levels were previously reported in that study. Methodologic details have been presented [6]. All statistical analyses were performed with PC-SAS version 9.1.

Results

Baseline characteristics and history of chronic diseases according to cigarette smoking status were shown in Table 1. Compared to never or current smokers, former smokers tended to be men, more obese, alcohol drinkers, and more under diabetes medication. Current smokers were less obese and more physically inactive than never or former smokers. There were no statistical significant differences across smoking categories for prevalence of hypertension medication or history of myocardial infarction or stroke.

Table 2 indicates mean concentrations of individual POPs depending on cigarette smoking status. Among 16 PCBs, PCB074, PCB105, and PCB118 were statistically significant or marginally significantly lower in current vs. never smokers. These three PCBs have weak dioxin activity, however, other PCBs with dioxin activity like PCB126, PCB156, and PCB169 did not show any trend. On the contrary, among 3 OC pesticides, p,p'-DDE had higher levels among current than never smokers.

When POPs were not considered in analyses, adjusted hazard ratios (HRs) for all-cause mortality were 1.3 for former smokers and 2.1 (95% CI: 1.2–3.7) for current smokers, compared with never smokers. However, the associations were substantially different depending on summary measures of POPs (Table 3). Compared with 70 year old people within the 1st or 2nd tertiles of summary measures of PCBs and OC pesticides, those within the 3rd tertile showed strong associations between cigarette smoking and total mortality. Adjusted HRs were 3.7 (1.5–9.3) for former smokers and 6.4 (2.3–17.7) for current smokers. Further adjustment for medication for diabetes or hypertension and history of myocardial infarction or stroke did not change the result. Summary measures calculated from PCBs or OC pesticides separately showed similar associations (Table S1).

Figure 1 shows adjusted HRs when never smokers within the 1st tertile of PCBs and OC pesticides were used as the common reference group. Never smokers within the 3rd tertile of PCBs and OC pesticides showed a statistically significantly lower risk of mortality with adjusted HR of 0.3 (0.1–0.9) while current smokers with the same levels of POPs concentrations had a statistically significantly higher risk of mortality with adjusted HR of 2.3 (1.0–5.0). When we applied the same analyses to the U.S. elderly who were included in our previous study, patterns were similar to those in the current study, although no individual HR reached statistical significance (Figure S1). In that study, the summary measures for PCBs and for OC pesticides were separate because PCB vs OC pesticide measurements were performed in different participants.

To better understand possible confounding, Table 4 compared baseline characteristics of 4 subgroups (never smokers & low POPs, current smokers & high POPs, never smokers & low POPs, and current smokers & high POPs), in particular focusing on never smokers with high POPs who had the lowest mortality. Compared

Table 1. Baseline characteristics according to the status of cigarette smoking among 986 elderly aged 70, Prospective Investigation of the Vasculature in Uppsala Seniors (PIVUS) study.

Characteristics	Status of cigarette smoking			p value
	Never smokers (N = 471)	Former smokers (N = 410)	Current smokers (N = 105)	
Men (%)	44.4	57.6	47.6	0.01
BMI (kg/m², %)				<0.01
<25	34.4	26.6	51.4	
25-<30	44.8	48.1	34.3	
≥30	20.8	25.4	14.3	
Exercise (%)				0.01
No	8.5	11.7	18.1	
Mild	64.1	63.4	66.7	
Moderate or vigorous	27.4	24.9	15.2	
Alcohol consumption (g/day, %)				<0.01
0	17.2	11.5	14.3	
1–14	75.2	74.8	80.0	
≥15	7.6	13.7	5.7	
Diabetes medication (%)	4.7	8.8	4.8	0.03
Hypertension medication (%)	29.5	33.4	27.6	0.34
History of myocardial infarction (%)	5.7	8.3	10.7	0.13
History of stroke (%)	3.2	3.9	4.8	0.69

to other subgroups, 70 year old participants within the never smokers & high POPs group were the most physically active and had the lowest prevalence of history of myocardial infarction.

Discussion

Generally, the present study replicated our report in a U.S. elderly population [6]. The association between cigarette smoking and total mortality depended on serum concentration of summary scores reflecting the background mixture of PCBs and/or OC pesticides. When POPs were not considered in the analyses, the risk of mortality among current-smokers was about two times higher than never smokers. However, among elderly with relatively high POPs, former or current smokers had about 4 to 7 times higher mortality than never smokers while the association between cigarette smoking and total mortality much weaker and statistically non-significant among elderly with relatively low serum concentrations of POPs. In addition to the main results, a subsidiary finding of lower concentrations of dioxin-like PCBs among smokers than never smokers was also similar to finding in the previous study [6].

These findings suggested that different concentrations of POPs among populations may partly explain variability in smoking-related total mortality association across previous epidemiological studies [2,3,4,5]. More importantly, the similar weak association between cigarette smoking and mortality among the elderly people in the lowest category of POPs from these two studies could indicate that the presence of certain levels POPs is a necessary factor for cigarette smoking to increase the risk of death in the elderly.

At first, we had expected the interaction between these two factors to be driven by the high risk of death among current smokers with high POPs. However, these two studies showed that

the strong association between cigarette smoking and mortality among the elderly with high POPs had a strong component of low mortality in never smokers as well as of high mortality in former or current smokers.

The very low mortality among the 150 never smokers in PIVUS with high POPs is a provocative finding. A similar pattern of reduced mortality was apparent in the National Health and Nutrition Examination Survey (NHANES) (Figure S1), suggesting that this finding is not simply bias or chance. An ecologic finding in the cohort study of male British doctors may be viewed as concordant. In that study, the excess mortality associated with smoking was greater during the second half of follow-up (1971~1991) than the first half (1951~1971) [2], largely because the mortality rate among non-smokers had decreased substantially over time while the mortality rate among smokers had remained about constant [2]. Historically, PCBs and OC pesticides were widely used after World War II and periods with the highest body burden of POPs were 1960s and 1970s [16]. Therefore, any effect due to high POPs may be more strongly reflected in the latter part of cohort study.

It is difficult to explain very low mortality among never smokers with high POPs. One possible explanation is survival bias. However, for survival bias to explain this finding, never smokers with high POPs must have had a higher death rate before reaching age 70 than other subgroups like active smokers with high POP, leaving healthier survivors to participate in the PIVUS and NHANES studies. This would be an odd pattern. Also, compared to other subgroups, the elderly never smokers with high POPs were the most physically active and had the lowest prevalence of history of myocardial infarction, both of which might predispose to reduced mortality rate. Therefore, this type of survival bias would seem to be unlikely even though we cannot totally exclude it.

Table 2. Adjusted* serum concentrations (geometric means, ng/g lipid) of individual polychlorinated biphenyls (PCBs) or organochlorine (OC) pesticides according to the status of cigarette smoking, Prospective Investigation of the Vasculature in Uppsala Seniors (PIVUS) study.

Analytes	Status of cigarette smoking			p for trend
	Never smokers (N = 471)	Former smokers (N = 410)	Current smokers (N = 105)	
Polychlorinated biphenyls (PCBs)				
PCB074[†]	14.1	13.6	12.9	0.09
PCB099	13.4	13.7	14.3	0.38
PCB105[†]	5.0	5.0	4.1	0.02
PCB118[†]	31.0	30.7	25.0	<0.01
PCB126[†]	5.9	5.9	6.5	0.44
PCB138	123.7	124.5	135.4	0.15
PCB153	213.7	216.5	228.3	0.19
PCB156[†]	23.7	23.1	24.7	0.78
PCB157	4.4	4.3	4.5	0.70
PCB169[†]	25.8	25.9	26.7	0.52
PCB170	75.5	75.3	80.1	0.30
PCB180	177.6	177.3	187.1	0.37
PCB189	3.2	3.2	2.9	0.34
PCB194	16.0	15.2	17.2	0.88
PCB206	4.2	3.9	4.1	0.23
PCB209	4.0	3.8	4.0	0.36
Organochlorines pesticides (OCPs)				
p,p'-DDE	270.1	296.4	322.4	0.04
Trans-nonachlor	20.6	21.9	21.8	0.14
Hexachlorobenzene	40.1	39.1	39.5	0.46

*Adjusted for gender, BMI, exercise, and alcohol consumption.
[†]POPs with dioxin activity.

Table 3. Adjusted hazard ratios (HRs)* and 95% confidence intervals (CIs) for all-cause mortality rate by summary measures[†] of polychlorinated biphenyls (PCBs) or organochlorine (OC) pesticides, Prospective Investigation of the Vasculature in Uppsala Seniors (PIVUS) study.

		Status of cigarette smoking			p for trend	p for interaction
		Never smokers	Former smokers	Current smokers		
All subjects						
	Cases/No	40/471	50/410	21/105		
	Adjusted HR(95%CI)	Referent	1.3(0.9–2.0)	2.1(1.2–3.7)	<0.01	
Summary measure of 16 PCBs and 3 OC pesticides						
1st tertile	Cases/No	16/160	19/138	5/30		
	Adjusted HR(95%CI)	Referent	1.2 (0.6–2.4)	1.4 (0.5–4.0)	0.46	0.02
2nd tertile	Cases/No	18/161	10/134	5/34		
	Adjusted HR(95%CI)	Referent	0.7 (0.3–1.6)	1.2 (0.5–3.4)	0.97	
3rd tertile	Cases/No	6/150	21/138	11/41		
	Adjusted HR(95%CI)	Referent	3.7 (1.5–9.3)	6.4 (2.3–17.7)	<0.01	

*Hazard Ratios (HRs) adjusted for gender, BMI, exercise, and alcohol consumption.
[†]Values of compounds belonging to in each summary measure were individually ranked; the rank orders of the individual POPs were summed to calculate summary measures and the summaries were divided into tertiles.

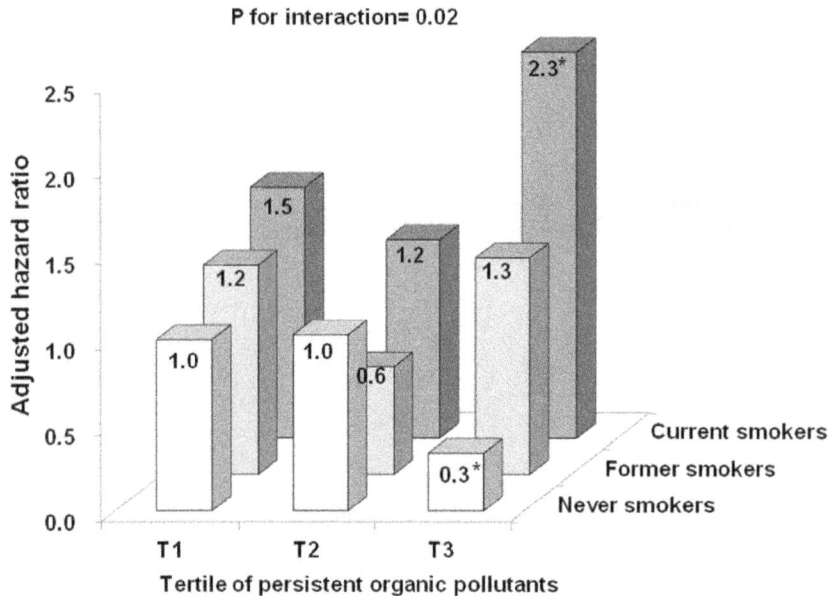

Figure 1. Interactions of cigarette smoking with summary measure of polychlorinated biphenyls (PCBs) and organochlorines (OC) pesticides on mortality. Hazard ratios (HRs) were estimated using a common reference group (never smokers & T1), adjusted for gender, BMI, exercise, and alcohol consumption. T1, first tertile; T2, second tertile; T3, third tertile, Prospective Investigation of the Vasculature in Uppsala Seniors (PIVUS) study.

In addition, low mortality in relation to high POPs is biologically plausible under some conditions, a case in point relating to associations between POPs and telomeres. Telomere length has been proposed as a marker of mitotic cell age and as a general index of human aging [17]. In our previous cross-sectional study among apparently healthy Koreans [18], telomere length was increasing across serum concentrations of POPs within the lower range of POPs. In that study, the interpretation was that low dose POPs may act as a tumor promoter in carcinogenesis based on experimental findings on arsenic. For example, low concentrations of arsenic relevant to current human exposure elongated telomeres in vitro and increased *myc* and *ras* oncogenes while high concentrations of arsenic decreased telomere length [19]. As *myc* oncogene can activate telomerase [20], the authors interpreted these experimental findings on arsenic as a role of tumor promoter of low dose arsenic in human.

However, an opposite interpretation of how POPs relate to telomere length is also possible. It is well-known that shorter telomere length is associated with higher risk of early death [21]. There is a higher mortality rate, especially from heart disease and infectious disease, among elderly people who have shorter telomeres in blood DNA [22]. Therefore, in PIVUS and NHANES persons with relatively high serum POPs concentrations within background exposure levels may have had a longer survival than persons with lower serum POPs concentrations. As cigarette smoking is reported to decrease telomere length [23], longer survival with higher POPs could be observed only in never smokers, as we observed in these two studies.

Although molecular mechanisms for low dose POPs to increase telomere length have not been studied, one speculation is that certain levels of POPs might excite production of cytoprotective and restorative proteins including growth factors, phase II and antioxidant enzymes, and protein chaperones, known as hormetic effects [24]. Increased telomerase activity or slow-down of age-dependent telomere shortening has been regarded as one marker of activation of cytoprotective and restorative proteins [25]. Some

previous human and experimental studies support possible beneficial effects of certain levels of POPs. For example, decreased risk of soft tissue sarcoma was reported with increased concentrations of dioxins or PCBs with dioxin activity in the general population[26]. Also, in some animal studies of low doses of TCDD or DDT, there was a tendency towards fewer tumors or altered hepatic foci than in controls, indicating an anti-carcinogenic process [27,28]. Furthermore, decreased lipid peroxidation level in rats treated with low dose DDT was reported, compared to control rats [29].

Studies of the levels of POPs in the global environment show that emission sources of a number of POPs in the last 20 years have shifted from industrialized countries of the Northern Hemisphere to less developing countries in tropical and subtropical regions [30]. This is due to a late production ban on OC pesticides: some OC pesticides are still being used in agriculture and for the control of diseases, such as malaria [31]. Also, there is another active exposure source of PCBs through e-waste recycling in these countries [32]. Although the burden of cigarette smoking use is currently greatest in high-income countries, rates of smoking are increasing in many low-income and middle-income countries. Therefore, the interaction between these two important health-related issues, POPs and cigarette smoking, should be further studied from a variety of viewpoints including molecular mechanisms.

The strengths of our study include the homogenous age and community-based sampling of study subjects. There were some limitations to our study. Due to a limited sample size, we could not consider more detailed information on cigarette smoking like total pack-years or duration of smoking cessation in analyses. In addition, analyses focusing on cause-specific mortality were not possible as cause of death information was not available. Finally, even though the consistency of findings across two studies lends credence to our findings and seems to reduce the likelihood that our finding is explainable by chance or bias, our findings still require replication by other cohort studies.

Table 4. Comparison of baseline characteristics among 4 subgroups, Prospective Investigation of the Vasculature in Uppsala Seniors (PIVUS) study.

	Low POPs		High POPs		
	Never smokers (N = 160)	Current smokers (N = 30)	Never smokers (N = 150)	Current smokers (N = 41)	p value
Dead (%)	10.0	16.7	4.0	26.8	<0.01
Men (%)	31.9	40.0	56.0	53.7	<0.01
BMI (kg/m², %)					<0.01
<25	26.3	46.7	36.0	48.8	
25-<30	40.6	36.7	51.3	46.3	
≥30	33.1	16.7	12.7	4.9	
Moderate or vigorous exercise (%)					<0.01
No	10.0	10.0	10.7	26.8	
Mild	63.8	80.0	58.7	61.0	
Moderate or vigorous	26.3	10.0	30.7	12.0	
Alcohol consumption (g/day, %)					0.03
0	20.6	20.0	14.0	7.3	
1–14	76.3	76.7	74.0	85.4	
≥15	3.1	3.3	12.0	7.3	
Diabetes medication (%)	3.8	0%	7.3	9.8	0.17
Hypertension medication (%)	31.3	30.0	31.3	22.0	0.68
History of myocardial infarction (%)	6.9	13.8	4.0	15.0	0.05
History of stroke (%)	1.9	6.7	5.3	4.9	0.35

This study has confirmed a strong association between cigarette smoking and mortality among elderly people with relatively high POPs, but a much weaker and not statistically significant smoking-mortality association among those with relatively low POPs. However, the observation that the lowest mortality was seen among never smokers with high POPs is provocative and requires further studies on the role of POPs in longevity. In addition more prospective studies in human, in-vitro and in-vivo experimental studies would help to elucidate potential molecular mechanisms.

Supporting Information

Figure S1 Interactions of cigarette smoking with summary measure of polychlorinated biphenyls (PCB) or organochlorine (OC) pesticides predicting mortality in the U.S. general population (reanalyses of published results using the same National Health and Nutrition Examination Survey (NHANES) datasets (Lee, 2013). Number of study subjects and deaths were 610 and 142 for

PCB analyses and 702 and 157 for OC pesticide analyses. Hazard ratios (HRs) were estimated using a common reference group (never smokers & T1), adjusted for gender, BMI, exercise, and alcohol consumption. T1, first tertile; T2, second tertile; T3, third tertile. Although none of the HRs was statistically significantly different from the reference group, as previously reported, interaction p-values were 0.008 for PCBs and 0.024 for OC pesticides.

Table S1

Author Contributions

Conceived and designed the experiments: DHL LL PML. Performed the experiments: DHL LL PML. Analyzed the data: DHL. Contributed reagents/materials/analysis tools: SS BB. Wrote the paper: DHL LL DRJ SS BB PML.

References

1. Murray CJ, Lopez AD (1997) Mortality by cause for eight regions of the world: Global Burden of Disease Study. Lancet 349: 1269–1276.
2. Doll R, Peto R, Wheatley K, Gray R, Sutherland I (1994) Mortality in relation to smoking: 40 years' observations on male British doctors. Bmj 309: 901–911.
3. Hunt D, Blakely T, Woodward A, Wilson N (2005) The smoking-mortality association varies over time and by ethnicity in New Zealand. Int J Epidemiol 34: 1020–1028.
4. Jacobs DR Jr, Adachi H, Mulder I, Kromhout D, Menotti A, et al. (1999) Cigarette smoking and mortality risk: twenty-five-year follow-up of the Seven Countries Study. Arch Intern Med 159: 733–740.
5. van de Mheen PJ, Gunning-Schepers IJ (1996) Differences between studies in reported relative risks associated with smoking: an overview. Public Health Rep 111: 420–426; discussion 427.
6. Lee YM, Bae SG, Lee SH, Jacobs DR, Lee DH (2013) Associations between cigarette smoking and total mortality differ depending on serum concentrations

of persistent organic pollutants among the elderly. J Korean Med Sci 28: 1122–1128.
7. Carpenter DO (2011) Health effects of persistent organic pollutants: the challenge for the Pacific Basin and for the world. Rev Environ Health 26: 61–69.
8. Ha MH, Lee DH, Jacobs DR (2007) Association between serum concentrations of persistent organic pollutants and self-reported cardiovascular disease prevalence: results from the National Health and Nutrition Examination Survey, 1999–2002. Environ Health Perspect 115: 1204–1209.
9. Lee DH, Lee IK, Song K, Steffes M, Toscano W, et al. (2006) A strong dose-response relation between serum concentrations of persistent organic pollutants and diabetes: results from the National Health and Examination Survey 1999–2002. Diabetes Care 29: 1638–1644.
10. Diwan BA, Ward JM, Kurata Y, Rice JM (1994) Dissimilar frequency of hepatoblastomas and hepatic cystadenomas and adenocarcinomas arising in hepatocellular neoplasms of D2B6F1 mice initiated with N-nitrosodiethylamine

and subsequently given Aroclor-1254, dichlorodiphenyltrichloroethane, or phenobarbital. Toxicol Pathol 22: 430–439.

11. Hutton JJ, Meier J, Hackney C (1979) Comparison of the in vitro mutagenicity and metabolism of dimethylnitrosamine and benzo[a]pyrene in tissues from inbred mice treated with phenobarbital, 3-methylcholanthrene or polychlorinated biphenyls. Mutat Res 66: 75–94.

12. Psaty BM, Koepsell TD, Manolio TA, Longstreth WT Jr, Wagner EH, et al. (1990) Risk ratios and risk differences in estimating the effect of risk factors for cardiovascular disease in the elderly. J Clin Epidemiol 43: 961–970.

13. Sandau CD, Sjodin A, Davis MD, Barr JR, Maggio VL, et al. (2003) Comprehensive solid-phase extraction method for persistent organic pollutants. Validation and application to the analysis of persistent chlorinated pesticides. Anal Chem 75: 71–77.

14. Salihovic S, Lampa E, Lindstrom G, Lind L, Lind PM, et al. (2012) Circulating levels of persistent organic pollutants (POPs) among elderly men and women from Sweden: results from the Prospective Investigation of the Vasculature in Uppsala Seniors (PIVUS). Environ Int 44: 59–67.

15. Phillips DL, Pirkle JL, Burse VW, Bernert JT Jr, Henderson LO, et al. (1989) Chlorinated hydrocarbon levels in human serum: effects of fasting and feeding. Arch Environ Contam Toxicol 18: 495–500.

16. Solomon GM, Weiss PM (2002) Chemical contaminants in breast milk: time trends and regional variability. Environ Health Perspect 110: A339–347.

17. Blackburn EH (2005) Telomeres and telomerase: their mechanisms of action and the effects of altering their functions. FEBS Lett 579: 859–862.

18. Shin JY, Choi YY, Jeon HS, Hwang JH, Kim SA, et al. (2010) Low-dose persistent organic pollutants increased telomere length in peripheral leukocytes of healthy Koreans. Mutagenesis 25: 511–516.

19. Zhang TC, Schmitt MT, Mumford JL (2003) Effects of arsenic on telomerase and telomeres in relation to cell proliferation and apoptosis in human keratinocytes and leukemia cells in vitro. Carcinogenesis 24: 1811–1817.

20. Wu KJ, Grandori C, Amacker M, Simon-Vermot N, Polack A, et al. (1999) Direct activation of TERT transcription by c-MYC. Nat Genet 21: 220–224.

21. Bakaysa SL, Mucci LA, Slagboom PE, Boomsma DI, McClearn GE, et al. (2007) Telomere length predicts survival independent of genetic influences. Aging Cell 6: 769–774.

22. Cawthon RM, Smith KR, O'Brien E, Sivatchenko A, Kerber RA (2003) Association between telomere length in blood and mortality in people aged 60 years or older. Lancet 361: 393–395.

23. Valdes AM, Andrew T, Gardner JP, Kimura M, Oelsner E, et al. (2005) Obesity, cigarette smoking, and telomere length in women. Lancet 366: 662–664.

24. Mattson MP (2008) Hormesis defined. Ageing Res Rev 7: 1–7.

25. Yokoo S, Furumoto K, Hiyama E, Miwa N (2004) Slow-down of age-dependent telomere shortening is executed in human skin keratinocytes by hormesis-like-effects of trace hydrogen peroxide or by anti-oxidative effects of pro-vitamin C in common concurrently with reduction of intracellular oxidative stress. J Cell Biochem 93: 588–597.

26. Tuomisto J, Pekkanen J, Kiviranta H, Tukiainen E, Vartiainen T, et al. (2005) Dioxin cancer risk—example of hormesis? Dose Response 3: 332–341.

27. Sukata T, Uwagawa S, Ozaki K, Ogawa M, Nishikawa T, et al. (2002) Detailed low-dose study of 1,1-bis(p-chlorophenyl)-2,2,2- trichloroethane carcinogenesis suggests the possibility of a hormetic effect. Int J Cancer 99: 112–118.

28. Viluksela M, Bager Y, Tuomisto JT, Scheu G, Unkila M, et al. (2000) Liver tumor-promoting activity of 2,3,7,8-tetrachlorodibenzo-p-dioxin (TCDD) in TCDD-sensitive and TCDD-resistant rat strains. Cancer Res 60: 6911–6920.

29. Shutoh Y, Takeda M, Ohtsuka R, Haishima A, Yamaguchi S, et al. (2009) Low dose effects of dichlorodiphenyltrichloroethane (DDT) on gene transcription and DNA methylation in the hypothalamus of young male rats: implication of hormesis-like effects. J Toxicol Sci 34: 469–482.

30. Tanabe S, Minh TB (2010) Dioxins and organohalogen contaminants in the Asia-Pacific region. Ecotoxicology 19: 463–478.

31. Wong MH, Leung AO, Chan JK, Choi MP (2005) A review on the usage of POP pesticides in China, with emphasis on DDT loadings in human milk. Chemosphere 60: 740–752.

32. Someya M, Ohtake M, Kunisue T, Subramanian A, Takahashi S, et al. (2010) Persistent organic pollutants in breast milk of mothers residing around an open dumping site in Kolkata, India: specific dioxin-like PCB levels and fish as a potential source. Environ Int 36: 27–35.

## 23

Incidence and Predictors of Multimorbidity in the Elderly: A Population-Based Longitudinal Study

René Melis[1], Alessandra Marengoni[2,3], Sara Angleman[3], Laura Fratiglioni[3,4]*

1 Department of Geriatric Medicine/Nijmegen Alzheimer Centre 925, Radboud University Nijmegen Medical Centre, Nijmegen, The Netherlands, 2 Geriatric Unit, Department of Clinical and Experimental Science, University of Brescia, Brescia, Italy, 3 Aging Research Center (ARC), Karolinska Institutet (Neurobiology, Care Science and Society Department) and Stockholm University, Stockholm, Sweden, 4 Stockholm Gerontology Research Center, Stockholm, Sweden

Abstract

Background: We aimed to calculate 3-year incidence of multimorbidity, defined as the development of two or more chronic diseases in a population of older people free from multimorbidity at baseline. Secondly, we aimed to identify predictors of incident multimorbidity amongst life-style related indicators, medical conditions and biomarkers.

Methods: Data were gathered from 418 participants in the first follow up of the Kungsholmen Project (Stockholm, Sweden, 1991–1993, 78+ years old) who were not affected by multimorbidity (149 had none disease and 269 one disease), including a social interview, a neuropsychological battery and a medical examination.

Results: After 3 years, 33.6% of participants who were without disease and 66.4% of those with one disease at baseline, developed multimorbidity: the incidence rate was 12.6 per 100 person-years (95% CI: 9.2–16.7) and 32.9 per 100 person-years (95% CI: 28.1–38.3), respectively. After adjustments, worse cognitive function (OR, 95% CI, for 1 point lower Mini-Mental State Examination: 1.22, 1.00–1.48) was associated with increased risk of multimorbidity among subjects with no disease at baseline. Higher age was the only predictor of multimorbidity in persons with one disease at baseline.

Conclusions: Multimorbidity has a high incidence at old age. Mental health-related symptoms are likely predictors of multimorbidity, suggesting a strong impact of mental disorders on the health of older people.

Editor: Angelo Scuteri, INRCA, Italy

Funding: This study was funded by research grants from the Swedish Council for Working Life and Social Research. The funders had no role in study design, data collection and analysis, decision to publish, or preparation of the manuscript.

Competing Interests: The authors have declared that no competing interests exist.

* Email: alessandra.marengoni@ki.se

Introduction

During the last two decades, research on multimorbidity, defined as the coexistence of a number of chronic diseases in the same individual, has rapidly increased. As chronic conditions are strongly related to aging, the majority of studies focused on the elderly population. However, since now, only selected aspects of multimorbidity were investigated, such as prevalence and consequences of co-existing diseases [1]. These previous reports have clearly shown that multimorbidity affects a large proportion of older persons ranging from 55 to 98% across studies depending on definition, age of the population and data source [2,3]. It has been established that there is a clear association between increasing number of chronic diseases and disability [4–6], poor quality of life [6,7] and high health care utilization [8,9].

Development of multimorbidity and identification of possible predictors of multimorbidity has been explored in few studies, which showed that 1-year incidence of multimorbidity (defined as 2 or more new diseases) was 1.3% in the whole population including all ages [10]. A few possible risk factors for multimorbidity were identified, such as increasing age [10] and a low socioeconomic status [10–12], whereas a large social network seemed to play a protective role [13]. Recently, the mediating role

of smoking and body mass index (BMI) on the educational effect was detected in a German population [11].

In the current study, we aimed to estimate the incidence of multimorbidity, and to identify possible predictors for multimorbidity. Several factors were evaluated, including life-style related factors, medical conditions and biomarkers. As the effect of these factors may depend on the health status of a person, we stratified participants at baseline according to presence or absence of one chronic disease.

Methods

Study design and participants

This study gathered data from the Kungsholmen Project (KP), which is a cohort study on aging and dementia carried out in Stockholm, Sweden, in a population of 75 years and older subjects (n = 2368) [14]. The KP was approved by the ethics committee of the Karolinska Institute. Each participant signed a written informed consent. The current study used as sample the 418 participants in the first KP follow up (1991–1993) who were living independently and were not affected by multimorbidity. Among them, 149 did not have any chronic disease and 269 were affected by only one chronic disease. After 3-year follow-up, 28 participants refused to be re-assessed; thus complete data on 390 persons were available for analysis (140 without any chronic disease and 250 with one disease).

Data collection

At all examinations in the KP the data were collected following the same standardized protocols, including a social interview, a neuropsychological battery and a medical examination [14]. Blood samples were obtained for several laboratory tests. The elderly and their next-of-kin were interviewed by trained nurses using a structured questionnaire on living conditions and social status.

Chronic diseases

A disease was classified as chronic if it satisfied one of the following criteria: 1. being permanent, 2. caused by non-reversible pathological alteration, 3. requiring rehabilitation, or 4. requiring a long period of care. Chronic conditions were assessed using multiple sources [2]: the diagnoses made by the physicians at each assessment in the KP assessments using data from medical history and medication use, clinical examination, and laboratory testing, and the computerized Stockholm Inpatient Registry. The inpatient registry encompasses all hospitals in the Stockholm area since 1969, and records up to six diagnoses at discharge. To increase completeness of the data on the presence or absence of each disease, in addition to this information we used the ATC [18] coded medication data to establish the presence of cancer, depression, diabetes, hypertension, Parkinson's disease, and thyroid disease from the use of medication only prescribed for these specific conditions. Also, we used the laboratory data on hemoglobin to establish the presence of anemia using an algorithm classifying males with Hb of <13 g/l and females with Hb of <12 g/l as anemic according to WHO criteria [19]. Dementia diagnoses were made using the DSMIII-R criteria by a senior neurologist, and the diagnosis of a major depression by a psychiatrist according to DSM-IV [20,21]. The list of chronic diseases included in the calculation of multimorbidity is shown in (Table S1).

Of the 390 study participants included in these analyses, 86 persons (20 of 149 without disease and 66 of 269 with one disease at baseline) died before the follow-up assessment and for these individuals the presence of multimorbidity was calculated on the basis of the inpatient registry data only.

Incident multimorbidity

Multimorbidity was the primary outcome measure in this study and was defined as any co-occurrence of two or more chronic conditions in the same individual, whether coincidental or not [10]. Incident cases were defined as subjects with no or only one chronic disorder at baseline who developed at least another chronic disease during the 3-year follow-up.

Possible predictors of multimorbidity

We examined the following variables:

- Social demographic measures: age (years), sex, living situation, living arrangement, and education. Education was measured by the maximum years of formal schooling, and this variable was dichotomized (≥ 8 versus <8 years) according to our previous study [2]. Living arrangement was dichotomized into living alone or living with others.

Lifestyle related factors: physical activity, smoking, and alcohol drinking. Physical activity was assessed approximately three years before the baseline of the current study, and was dichotomized in the analyses into 'no physical activity' and 'at least weekly physical activity'. Smoking was operationalized in the analyses in three classes. Alcohol drinking was operationalized in the analyses as 'less than 1 unit per week', 'between 1 and 7 units per week', and '7 or more units per week'.

- Physical examination variables: Body Mass Index (BMI, kg/m^2), heart rate (beats/min), blood pressure (mmHg), and the six Katz items on Activities of Daily Living [15];
- Laboratory findings: hemoglobin (Hb, g/l), albumin (Alb, g/l), erythrocyte sedimentation rate (ESR, mm/hour), and white blood cell count (WBC, $*10^9$ leukocytes/l);
- Affective and cognitive scales: the Comprehensive Psychopathological Rating Severity scale for mood related and motivation related symptoms of depression (CPRS, range 0-48, where higher score indicates more symptoms; [16]); global cognition using the Mini Mental State Examination (MMSE, range 0-30, where higher score indicate better cognition; [17]). CPRS is a structured psychiatric interview with both directed questions and observations. The CPRS severity subscale for mood-related symptoms assesses the following four symptoms on a scale from 0-6: dysphoria, appetite disturbance, feelings of guilt, and thoughts of death. The severity subscale for motivation-related symptoms assesses: lack of interest, psychomotor change, loss of energy, and concentration difficulties, again scoring 0-6 per item. If the participant was not able to answer the questions reliably, an informant was contacted.

Statistical analysis

Using descriptive statistics the baseline characteristics were presented grouping the participants according to the presence of no or one chronic disease. Cumulative incidence for multimorbidity was calculated by the number of new cases of multimorbidity during the follow-up period divided by the number of subjects at risk in the population at the beginning of the study and not lost to follow up due to withdrawal of informed consent; 95% confidence intervals were calculated according to the binomial distribution. Multimorbidity incidence rates were calculated as the number of new cases of multimorbidity divided by the total person-time observed between the two assessments or until date of death. Exact Poisson rate 95% confidence intervals were calculated. Logistic regression analysis was used to study the effect of the possible predictors of multimorbidity, starting with univariate analyses checking the effect of each variable separately, followed by bivariate analyses taking into account the effect of the presence of one disease at baseline and next by adding an interaction term between the predictor of interest and the presence of one disease. Since the interaction analyses showed that the presence of disease at baseline was likely an effect modifier, the multivariate analyses were stratified for the presence or absence of disease at baseline. All missing values in the variables that were used in the analyses for this study – potential predictors as well as the dependent variables – were imputed twenty times assuming a multivariate normal distribution of the data using SAS Proc MI and SAS Proc MIANALYZE to calculate measures of precision. All results reported in this paper are based on the imputed datasets. A series of sensitivity analyses were run.

Results

At baseline 418 participants were living independently and were not affected by multimorbidity. As 28 subjects refused the follow-up assessment, 390 participants were included in the analysis: of these, 140 participants had no disease and 250 participants had one disease at the baseline (Table 1). After three years, among the 140 participants who were without any chronic disease at baseline 50 (35.7%; 95% CI = 27.8–43.7) still were without disease, 43 (30.7%; 95% CI = 23.1–38.4) had one disease and 47 (33.6%; 95% CI = 25.8–41.4) developed multimorbidity. The 3-year cumulative incidence for multimorbidity in this group was 33.6%. In the subgroup of the 250 participants with one disease at baseline, 22 (8.8%; 95% CI = 5.3–12.3) were without morbidity, 62 (24.8%; 95% CI = 19.5–30.2) still have one disease and 166 (66.4%; 95% CI = 60.5–72.3) developed multimorbidity. The 3-year cumulative incidence for multimorbidity in this group was 66.4%. The incidence rate was 12.6 per 100 person-years (95% CI: 9.2–16.7) and 32.9 per 100 person-years (95% CI: 28.1–38.3), respectively. Further, we calculated the incidence rates separately for the two subgroups (subjects with one or no chronic disease at baseline), and stratified by gender and age. Results are reported in Figure 1. The risk of developing multimorbidity was higher among subjects with one disease and older people; no substantial gender differences were detected.

In the univariate models several factors were associated with an increased relative odd of incident multimorbidity at follow up in the whole group of 390 participants (Table 2). As already said in the methods, the interaction between potential predictors of incident multimorbidity and the presence of one disease at baseline was statistically significant for almost all variables. Thus, all analyses were run after stratification for absence or presence of one disease at baseline.

The multivariate models combined potential predictors, and confounders as they were derived from the univariate analyses and the analyses were stratified for the presence or absence of one disease at baseline (Table 3). In the final multivariate adjusted model for persons without any disease at baseline, global cognition (MMSE) was significantly (OR 1.22, 95% confidence interval 1.00–1.48, p = 0.05) related to multimorbidity occurrence and mood (CPRS) almost (OR 1.18, 95%-CI 0.99–1.40, p = 0.06). In the multivariate adjusted model for persons with already one disease at baseline, only higher age was significantly related to multimorbidity incidence at follow up (table 3; OR 1.09, 1.01–1.17, p = 0.03). No further statistically significant predictors of multimorbidity incidence were identified in this stratum, however, drinking less than 1 unit of alcohol per week was associated with an OR of 1.87 (0.98–3.58) at p = 0.06.

Sensitivity analysis

As global cognition (MMSE) and mood (CPRS) turned out to be likely predictors of multimorbidity, we reran the analyses with dementia and depression not counted for the incidence of multimorbidity at follow up in order to rule out the effect of these two predictors. The results showed that the correlations of MMSE and CPRS score with multimorbidity were comparable. The association with MMSE diminished slightly to OR 1.15 (0.93–1.41, p = 0.19). The association with CPRS increased slightly: OR 1.20 (1.00–1.44, p = 0.05). Further, we calculated the associations of MMSE quartile scores as categorical variable with multimorbidity occurrence (best performing quartile as the reference group) for the two subgroups with and without morbidity at baseline. These results suggest that it is perhaps the two lowest quartiles (an MMSE below 27) that have the strongest association with multimorbidity occurrence in the group without disease at baseline (Table S2).

Discussion

A systematic review of the literature on multimorbidity [1] identified very few prospective studies which evaluated incidence and predictors of multimorbidity. In the present study, we used data on the older population enrolled in the Kungsholmen Project to quantify the incidence of multimorbidity over a period of three years. In this 78+ year-old population, multimorbidity had a high incidence as it developed with a rate of approximately 12 per 100 person-years in people not affected by any chronic disorders and 33 per 100 person-years in those with already one disease at baseline. Secondly, among the few factors identified as possible predictors of multimorbidity onset, clinical symptoms related to mental disorders emerged as the most important factors to identify people at risk to develop multimorbidity among subjects without any disease. Lower cognitive abilities and perhaps also increasing number of depression-related symptoms predicted the development of multimorbidity in persons with no disease at baseline. Among participants with already one disease, only age was a predictor of multimorbidity incidence.

In 1998, van den Akker and colleagues reported that cumulative incidence of multimorbidity, defined as 2 or more new diagnoses during one year, was 1.3% in the general population (all ages) but >5% in those aged 80 and older [10]. However, the authors did not select persons according to the presence of none or one plus disease at baseline. In our study, the cumulative incidence of multimorbidity in very old elderly differed depending on the absence or presence of one disease at baseline. In fact, two third of participants affected by already one disease became multimorbid after only 3 years compared to one third of those without any disease. Anyhow even taking into account this last group, the estimates of annual cumulative incidence and the incidence rates were double higher than those reported by van den Akker [10]. Dissimilarities in the diagnoses recording (van den Akker evaluated multimorbidity in a general practice setting) may explain this difference.

Despite the fact than more than 50% of 75+ old subjects are affected by multimorbidity, little research has focused on risk factors and predictors of this syndrome. A couple of papers focused on the impact of socioeconomic status on the development of multimorbidity [11,22]. Childhood financial hardship and lifetime earnings were associated with multimorbidity being the latter a protective factor [22] and lower education was associated with multimorbidity [11]. In this study using data from the Kungsholmen population that is over age 75 we found that education, which is a good indicator of SES, education was positively associated with incident multimorbidity, although without reaching statistical significance, especially in participants with no disease at baseline. In the Kungsholmen Project, data on another indicator of SES were collected, e.g. lifetime occupation. Due to the high correlation between occupation-based SES and education in this population we did not use the occupation variable in the present study. In fact, previous analyses on prevalent multimorbidity in the Kungsholmen Project showed that occupation-based SES had a crude association with multimorbidity, but not when adjusted for education. Besides, low education showed a strong association with multimorbidity independent of high or low occupation-based SES [2].

We found that at higher age cognition and depressive symptoms were possible predictors of multimorbidity onset in people who were without significant chronic morbidity at baseline. In the older population, depressive symptoms are commonly associated with chronic medical conditions. The finding was confirmed – even strengthened slightly – when we excluded depression diagnosis

1

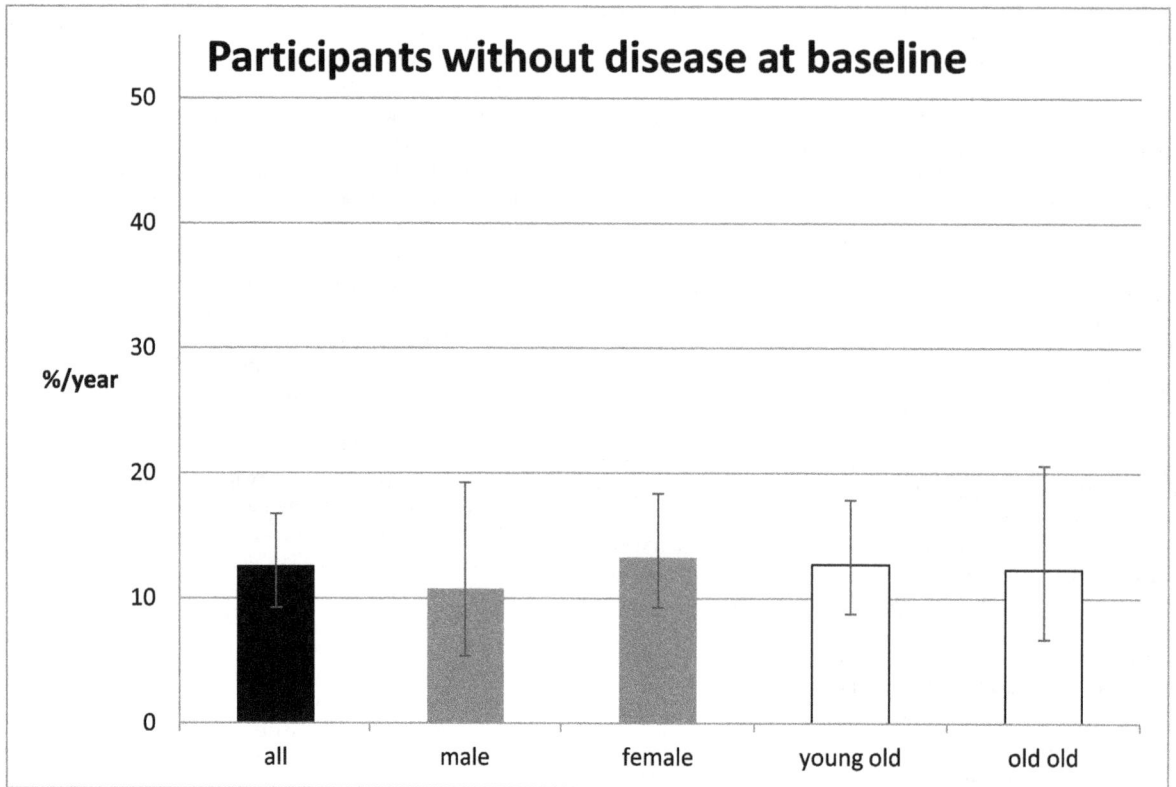

2

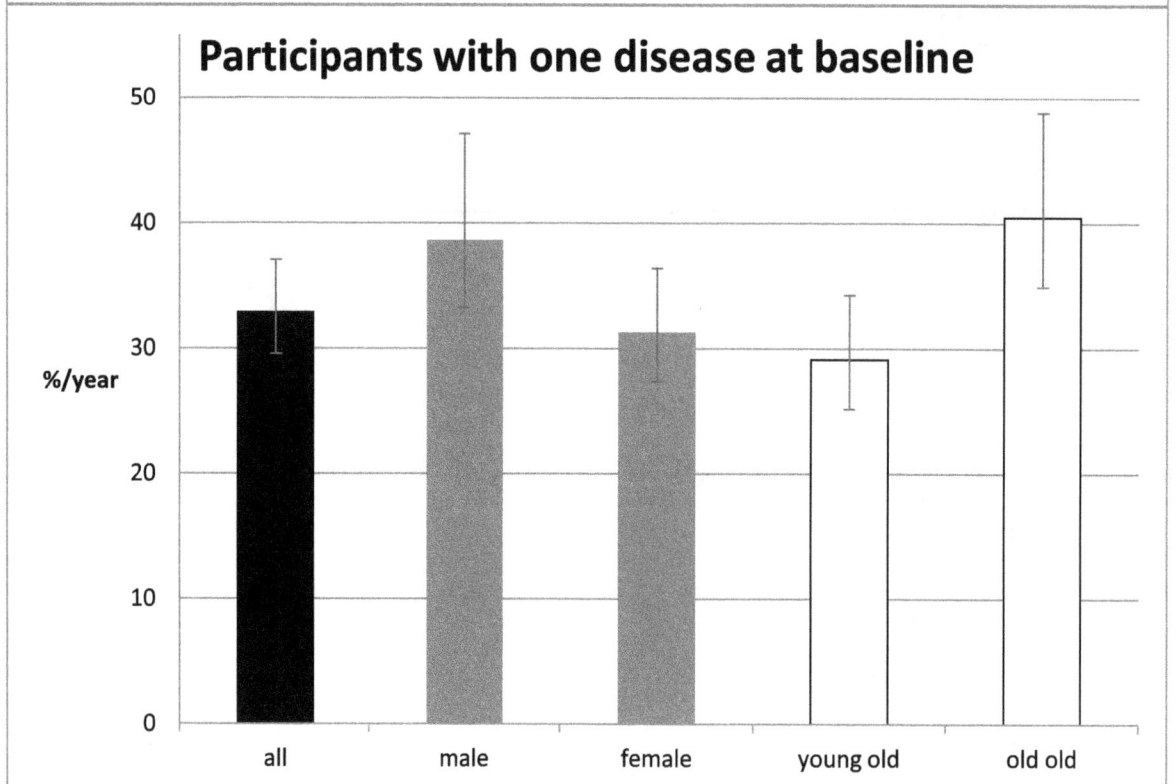

3

4

Figure 1. Multimorbidity (two or more diseases) incidence rates (95% confidence intervals) for participants without and with one disease at baseline (black) and by sex (grey) and age category (young old: <85 years and old old: ≥85 years, white).

Table 1. Baseline characteristics of the participants according to the presence/absence of one chronic disease.

	No chronic disease n = 140	One chronic disease N = 250
Age (year), mean (sd)	83.3 (3.7)	84.2 (4.2)
Female, n (%)	102 (73)	190 (76)
Low education (<8 years), n (%)	58 (42)	110 (44)
MMSE, mean (sd)	27 (2)	26 (4)
Living alone*, n (%)	102 (73)	179 (72)
At least one ADL disability, n (%)	21 (15)	58 (23)
Physically active, n (%)	30 (21)	28 (11)
Smoking, n (%)		
Non-smoker	83 (61)	141 (62)
Former smoker	24 (18)	59 (26)
Current smoker	29 (21)	27 (12)
Alcohol drinking, n (%)		
<1 unit/week	88 (63)	165 (69)
1–6 units/week	48 (35)	66 (28)
≥7 units/week	4 (3)	7 (3)
Body Mass Index, n (%)		
<18.5 kg/m^2	6 (5)	16 (8)
18.5–25 kg/m^2	93 (75)	127 (64)
>25 kg/m^2	25 (20)	57 (29)
Heart rate, n (%)		
≤60 bpm	20 (14)	26 (11)
61–100 bpm	115 (83)	214 (87)
≥100 bpm	3 (2)	6 (2)
Diastolic blood pressure (mmHg), mean (sd)	80 (11)	81 (11)
Systolic blood pressure (mmHg), mean (sd)	158 (20)	160 (21)
CPRS, mean (sd)	2.1 (2.4)	2.1 (2.8)
Hemoglobin (g/l), mean (sd)	138 (9)	137 (13)
WBC (*10^9 leucocytes/l), mean (sd)	6.5 (1.5)	6.9 (2.1)
ESR (mm/hour), mean (sd)	16 (14)	19 (15)
Albumin (g/l), mean (sd)	42.2 (2.3)	42.3 (2.8)

*As opposed to living independently but with others.
ADL, Activities of Daily Living (measured with Katz ADL, 0–6, higher score indicates worse function).
CPRS, Comprehensive Psychopathological Rating Severity (0–48, higher score indicates more depressive symptoms).
ESR, Erythrocyte Sedimentation Rate.
MMSE, Mini-Mental State Examination (0–30, higher score indicates better function).
WBC, white blood cell.

from the multimorbidity definition. Depression can delay diagnosis of other diseases and negatively affect medication adherence and healthy behaviors to prevent other clinical conditions [23]. Moreover, depressive symptoms may lead to social isolation. Van den Akker and colleagues found that living in a family compared to living alone and a large social network were protective factors for multimorbidity occurrence [13]. This result is consistent with previous studies showing that older age depression was associated with several adverse outcomes if not adequately treated, such as increased risk of disability, poor quality of life and mortality [24,25]. On the other hand, chronic diseases increase the risk of depression, with the prevalence of depression being up to five times higher in persons with chronic medical conditions [26]. This strong association can be explained by the presence of disability, pain and polypharmacy in the elderly affected by multiple diseases. In this study, depressive symptoms

were measured three years before the diagnosis of multimorbidity, thus the possibility of such reverse causation seems unlikely. Finally, the mechanism linking depressive symptoms to incident multimorbidity may be chronic inflammation. In fact, several studies have shown higher circulating pro-inflammatory cytokines levels in depressive disorders [27]. Unfortunately, in the Kungsholmen Project such markers of inflammation were not available.

Further, a worse MMSE was a predictor of the occurrence of multimorbidity in those participants free from any disease. So far, cognitive impairment has mainly been studied as a consequence of several chronic diseases and also of multimorbidity [28]. Previous cross-sectional and longitudinal studies reported a positive association between poor health and multimorbidity and cognitive complaints or impairment [29,30]. In our study, worse cognition measured three years before the multimorbidity assessment was associated with the development of multimorbidity. It is possible

Table 2. The crude odds ratios (OR) and 95% confidence intervals (95% CI) of potential predictors for multimorbidity separately for the two subgroups of people with no or one disease at baseline.

Predictor of interest	No chronic disease at baseline (n = 140)	One chronic disease at baseline (n = 250)
	OR (95% CI)*	OR (95% CI)*
Age (years, continuous)	1.00 (0.91–1.10)	1.08 (1.01–1.16)**
Sex (female *vs* male)	1.34 (0.60–3.01)	0.73 (0.38–1.37)
Education (low *vs* high education)	1.81 (0.89–3.69)	1.22 (0.72–2.08)
Living alone *vs* living with other	1.34 (0.60–3.01)	1.06 (0.59–1.90)
Katz ADL (number of disabilities, continuous)	0.76 (0.27–2.11)	1.29 (0.85–1.94)
Hemoglobin (g/l, continuous)	0.97 (0.93–1.01)	1.00 (0.98–1.02)
ESR (mm/hour, continuous)	1.05 (1.01–1.08)**	1.01 (0.99–1.03)
WBC* (10^9 leucocytes/l, continuous)	1.18 (0.92–1.51)	1.08 (0.94–1.25)
Albumin (g/l, continuous)	1.05 (0.90–1.21)	0.97 (0.88–1.07)
Heart rate		
≤60 *vs* 60–99 bpm	1.81 (0.69–4.75)	0.97 (0.41–2.28)
≥100 *vs* 60–99 bpm	4.18 (0.37–47.66)	1.07 (0.19–5.98)
Diastolic blood pressure (increase of 10 mmHg)	0.71 (0.49–1.03)***	0.91 (0.72–1.16)
Systolic blood pressure (increase of 10 mmHg)	0.92 (0.77–1.11)	0.99 (0.88–1.12)
Physical activity (yes *vs* no)	0.42 (0.16–1.11)***	1.30 (0.55–3.09)
Depressive symptoms (CPRS, continuous)	1.16 (1.00–1.35)**	1.04 (0.94–1.15)
Worse cognitive abilities (MMSE, continuous)	1.25 (1.06–1.48)**	1.06 (0.99–1.14)***
Smoking (3 categories: never, former, current, continuous)	0.92 (0.59–1.43)	1.14 (0.77–1.70)
Alcohol drinking		
<1 unit/week *vs* 1–6 units/week	1.02 (0.48–2.17)	1.89 (1.05–3.40)**
≥7 units/week *vs* 1–6 units/week	19.44 (0.70–538.9)***	3.85 (0.52–28.4)
BMI		
<18.5 *vs* 18.5–25 kg/m²	1.07 (0.20–5. 78)	0.93 (0.31–2.76)
>25 *vs* 18.5–25 kg/m²	1.26 (0.49–3.25)	1.26 (0.69–2.38)

*the odd ratios presented are for the continuous and ordinal variables the odds ratio for an increase of one unit/level unless stated otherwise and for the dichotomized variables for presented dichotomy.
**$p < 0.05$.
***$p < 0.10$.
ADL, activities of daily living (0–6, higher score indicates worse function).
CPRS, Comprehensive Psychopathological Rating Severity (0–48, higher score indicates more depressive symptoms).
BMI, Body Mass Index.
ESR, erythrocyte sedimentation rate.
MMSE, mini-mental state examination (0–30, higher score indicates better function).
WBC, white blood count.

that cognitive decline is a manifestation of a latent and still undiagnosed chronic disease such as low oxygen levels in chronic respiratory diseases, insulin imbalance in diabetes, and thyroid hormone deficiency or excess in thyroid dysfunction may have already affected the brain [31]. Silent brain infarction may also be present. Another explanation is that cytokine activated immune system dysregulation as well as chronic stress, both frequent in the elderly, may affect first the brain and secondly the body through the imbalance of the adrenocortico axis [32]. Finally, the same disease pathology or risk factors may lead to both cognitive impairment and specific chronic disease; for example estrogen deficiency may be associated with both cognitive impairment and osteoporosis.

Among characteristics that we did not find associated with incident multimorbidity, there were some life-style factors usually correlated with chronic diseases, such as smoking and alcohol. Indeed, the leading chronic-disease causes of death can be attributed to tobacco use and alcohol consumption beyond

physical inactivity [33]. Our findings may be due to a survival effect. In fact, subjects who are continuous smokers have a high mortality risk and many of them probably died before the enrolment in the present study. The lack of the expected association of alcohol intake with multimorbidity can be also being due to the common underrating of alcohol intake in interviews. Remarkably, in people who had one disease at baseline already, drinking less than one unit of alcohol per week was associated with an increased occurrence of multimorbidity three years later as compared to moderate drinkers. We want to be cautious interpreting this finding, however, it could be that non-drinkers actually stopped drinking due to their health condition. Thus, they might be at higher risk for increasing disease burden than moderate drinkers. It has been suggested that moderate "alcohol consumption may represent a marker of higher social level [and] superior health status" [34].

Table 3. Association between potential predictors and the incidence of multimorbidity in persons with and without one chronic disease at baseline.

Predictors of interest	No chronic disease at baseline (n = 140)	One chronic disease at baseline (n = 250)
	OR (95% CI)*	OR (95% CI)*
Age (years, continuous)	0.99 (0.89–1.11)	1.09 (1.01–1.17)**
Sex (female vs male)	0.87 (0.30–2.52)	0.88 (0.42–1.87)
Education (low vs high education)	1.36 (0.56–3.32)	0.94 (0.51–1.75)
Katz ADL (number of disabilities, continuous)	0.80 (0.25–2.60)	1.01 (0.64–1.60)
Hemoglobin (g/l, continuous)	0.98 (0.93–1.03)	1.01 (0.99–1.04)
ESR (mm/hour, continuous)	1.02 (0.99–1.06)	1.02 (0.99–1.04)
WBC (*10^9 leucocytes/l, continuous)	1.19 (0.89–1.58)	1.06 (0.92–1.22)
Diastolic blood pressure (increase of 10 mmHg)	0.98 (0.94–1.01)	0.99 (0.96–1.02)
Physical activity (yes vs no)	0.44 (0.15–1.28)	1.55 (0.61–3.92)
Depressive symptoms (CPRS, continuous)	1.18 (0.99–1.40)***	1.03 (0.93–1.14)
Worse cognitive abilities (MMSE, continuous)	1.22 (1.00–1.48)**	1.04 (0.96–1.12)
Smoking (3 categories: never, former, current, continuous)	0.86 (0.49–1.52)	1.29 (0.80–2.07)
Alcohol drinking		
<1 unit/week vs 1–6 units/week	0.90 (0.36–2.22)	1.87 (0.98–3.58)***
≥7 units/week vs 1–6 units/week	11.43 (0.37–348.43)	2.89 (0.36–22.97)
BMI		
<18.5 kg/m² vs 18.5–25 kg/m²	1.30 (0.11–7.98)	0.95 (0.30–3.03)
>25 kg/m² vs 18.5–25 kg/m²	1.48 (0.47–4.71)	1.33 (0.68–2.60)

Odds Ratio (OR) and 95% confidence intervals (95% CI) from multivariate logistic regression models.
*the odd ratios presented are for the continuous and ordinal variables the odds ratio for an increase of one unit/level unless stated otherwise and for the dichotomized variables for presented dichotomy.
**p<0.05.
***p<0.10.
ADL, activities of daily living (0–6, higher score indicates worse function).
BMI, Body Mass Index.
CPRS, Comprehensive Psychopathological Rating Severity (0–48, higher score indicates more depressive symptoms).
ESR, erythrocyte sedimentation rate.
MMSE, mini-mental state examination (0–30, higher score indicates better function).
WBC, white blood count.

Limitations

Because of the study design, characteristics of the patients were assessed only in a single measurement at baseline. Some factors, such as physical activity, are considered relatively stable, but they can change over time, especially as a result of a disease. In line with previous studies [12,35], a follow-up time of three years was chosen for the calculation of incident cases. In fact, distribution of diseases is not random in time, but disease susceptibility is markedly different according to the duration of the follow-up interval, and the stability of several individual characteristics over time is not known [12]. Second, we pre-selected a list of 39 chronic diseases, thus automatically excluding some others (although rare); moreover, for a number of participants we had to rely only on hospital registry information, which may differ in some way from those who were seen by the study physician for a second time, although this is also a strength for those who died in between intervals and could still be included thanks to the registry information.

Conclusions

Multimorbidity has a high incidence in the elderly, especially in those with already one disease at baseline. Worse cognition and low mood emerged as possible predictors of development of multimorbidity, suggesting a strong influence of mental disorders on the health of older people. Due to increasing life expectancy, prevalence of chronic diseases is expected to increase in the near future [36]. The coexistence of multiple chronic diseases has been found to be associated with several adverse outcomes as well as high medical care costs. Identifying at risk subjects to develop multimorbidity may help to implement prevention strategies among older people.

Supporting Information

Table S1 List of chronic diseases included in the calculation of multimorbidity (chronic diseases present at least once in the complete KP cohort of participants who participated in the first follow up).

Table S2 The crude odds ratios (OR) and 95% confidence intervals (95% CI) of MMSE quartile scores for multimorbidity separately for the two subgroups of people with no or one disease at baseline with the people in Q1 (MMSE 29–30) as reference category (on unimputed dataset, because there were no missings for the variables involved).

Author Contributions

Conceived and designed the experiments: RM AM SA LF. Analyzed the data: RM AM. Wrote the paper: RM AM. Critically reviewed the manuscript: SA LF.

References

1. Marengoni A, Angleman S, Melis R, Mangialasche F, Karp A, et al (2011) Ageing with multimorbidity: a systematic review of the literature. Ageing Res Rev 10: 430–439.
2. Marengoni A, Winblad B, Karp A, Fratiglioni L (2008) Prevalence of chronic diseases and multimorbidity among the elderly population in Sweden. Am J Public Health 98: 1198–1200.
3. Fortin M, Stewart M, Poitras ME, Almirall J, Maddocks H (2012) A systematic review of prevalence studies on multimorbidity: toward a more uniform methodology. Ann Fam Med 10: 142–151.
4. Bayliss EA, Bayliss MS, Ware JE Jr, Steiner JF (2004) Predicting declines in physical function in persons with multiple chronic medical conditions: What we can learn from the medical problem list. Health and Quality of Life Outcomes 2: 47.
5. Marengoni A, von Strass E, Rizzato D, Winblad B, Fratiglioni L (2009) The impact of chronic multimorbidity and disability on functional decline and survival in elderly persons. A community-based, longitudinal study. J Intern Med 265; 288–295.
6. Loza E, Jover JA, Rodriguez L, Carmona L; EPISER Study Group (2009) Multimorbidity: prevalence, effect on quality of life and daily functioning, and variation of this effect when one condition is a rheumatic disease. Semin Arthritis Rheum 38: 312–319.
7. Byles JE, D'Este C, Parkinson L, O'Connell R, Treloar C (2005) Single index of multimorbidity did not predict multiple outcomes. J Clin Epidemiol 58: 997–1005.
8. Wolff JL, Starfield B, Anderson G (2002) Prevalence, expenditures, and complications of multiple chronic conditions in the elderly. Arch Intern Med 162: 2269–2276.
9. Schneider KM, O'Donnel BE, Dean D (2009) Prevalence of multiple chronic conditions in the United States' Medicare population. Health and Quality of Life Outcomes 7: 82.
10. van den Akker M, Buntinx F, Metsemakers JF, Roos S, Knottnerus JA (1998) Multimorbidity in general practice: prevalence, incidence, and determinants of co-occurring chronic and recurrent diseases. J Clin Epidemiol 51: 367–375.
11. Nagel G, Peter R, Braig S, Hermann S, Rohrmann S, Linseisen J (2008) The impact of education on risk factors and the occurrence of multimorbidity in the EPIC-Heidelberg cohort. BMC Public Health 8: 384.
12. van den Akker M, Buntinx F, Metsemakers JF, Knottnerus JA (2000) Marginal impact of psychosocial factors on multimorbidity: results of an explorative nested case-control study. Soc Sci Med 50: 1679–1693.
13. van den Akker M, Buntinx F, Metsemakers JF, van der Aa M, Knottnerus JA (2001) Psychosocial patient characteristics and GP-registered chronic morbidity: a prospective study. J Psychosom Res 50: 95–102.
14. Fratiglioni L, Viitanen M, Backman L, Sandman PO, Winblad B (1992) Occurrence of dementia in advanced age: the study design of the Kungsholmen Project. Neuroepidemiology 11 Suppl 1: 29–36.
15. Katz A, Ford AB, Moskowitz RW (1963) Studies of illness in the aged. The index of ADL: a standardized measure of biological and psychological function. JAMA 185: 914–919.
16. Åsberg M, Montgomery SA, Perris C, Schalling D, Sedvall G (1978) A Comprehensive Psychopathological Rating Scale. Acta Psychiatr Scand 271: 5–27.
17. Folstein MF, Folstein SE, McHugh PR (1975) The Mini-Mental State. A practical method of grading the cognitive state of patients for the clinician. J Psychiatric Res 12: 189–198.
18. World Health Organization (1990) Guidelines for ATC Classification. WHO Collaborating Centre for Drug Statistics Methodology, Norway and Nordic Councils on Medicines, Sweden.
19. World Health Organization (1968) Nutritional anemias. Report of a WHO scientific group. Geneva, Switzerland; Technical Report Series No. 405.
20. Fratiglioni L, Grut M, Forsell Y, Viitanen M, Winblad B (1992) Clinical diagnosis of Alzheimer's disease and other dementias in a population survey. Agreement and causes of disagreement in applying Diagnostic and Statistical Manual of Mental Disorders, Revised Third Edition, Criteria. Arch Neurol 49: 927–932.
21. American Psychiatric Association (1994) *Diagnostic and Statistical Manual of Mental Disorders*, Fourth Edition (DSM-IV). Washington, DC: American Psychiatric Association.
22. Tucker-Seeley RD, Li Y, Sorensen G, Subramanian SV (2011) Lifecourse socioeconomic circumstances and multimorbidity among older adults. BMC Public Health 14; 11: 313.
23. Prince M, Patel V, Saxena S, Maj M, Maselko J, et al (2007) No health without mental health. Lancet 370; 859–877.
24. Covinsky KE, Kahana E, Chin MH, Palmer RM, Fortinsky RH, et al (1999) Depressive symptoms and 3-year mortality in older hospitalized medical patients. Ann Intern Med 130: 563–569.
25. Koenig HG, George LK (1998) Depression and physical disability outcomes in depressed medically ill hospitalized older adults. Am J Geriatr Psychiatry 6: 230–247.
26. Moussavi S, Chatterji S, Verdes E, Tandon A, Patel V, et al (2007) Depression, chronic diseases, and decrements in health: results from the World Health Surveys. Lancet 370: 851–858.
27. Raedler TJ (2011) Inflammatory mechanisms in major depressive disorder. Curr Opin Psychiatry 24: 519–525.
28. Melis RJ, Marengoni A, Rizzuto D, Teerenstra S, Kivipelto M, et al (2013) The influence of multimorbidity on clinical progression of dementia in a population-based cohort. PloS One 8: e84014.
29. Lyketsos CG, Toone L, Tschanz J, Rabins PV, Steinberg M, et al, Cache County Study Group (2005) Population-based study of medical comorbidity in early dementia and "cognitive impairment, no dementia (CIND)": Association with functional and cognitive impairment: The Cache County Study. Am J Geriatr Psychiatry 577; 13: 656–664.
30. Aarts S, van den Akker M, Hajema KJ, van Ingen AM, Metsemakers JF, et al (2011) Multimorbidity and its relation to subjective memory complaints in a large general population of older adults. Int Psychogeriatr 23: 632 624.
31. Gasquoine PG (2011) Cognitive impairment in common, non-central nervous system medical conditions of adults and the elderly. J Clin Exp Neuropsychol 33: 486–496.
32. Peavy GM, Salmon DP, Jacobson MW, Hervey A, Gamst AC, et al (2009) Effects of chronic stress on memory decline in cognitively normal and mildly impaired older adults. Am J Psychiatry 166: 1384–1391.
33. Mokdad AH, Marks JS, Stroup DF, Gerberding JL (2004) Actual causes of death in the United States, 2000. JAMA 291: 1238–1245.
34. Hansel B, Thomas F, Pannier B, Bean K, Kontush A, et al (2010) Relationship between alcohol intake, health and social status and cardiovascular risk factors in the Urban Paris-Ile-de-France Cohort: is the cardioprotective action of alcohol a myth? Eur J Clin Nutr 64: 561–568.
35. Seeman T, Guralnik JM, Kaplan GA, Knudsen L, Cohen R (1989) The health consequences of multiple morbidity in the elderly: the Alameda County Study. J Aging Health 1: 50–66.
36. Uijen AA, van de Lisdonk EH (2008) Multimorbidity in primary care: prevalence and trend over the last 20 years. Eur J Gen Pract 14 Suppl 1: 28–32.

## 24

Trends in Inequalities in Health, Risk and Preventive Behaviour among the Advanced-Age Population in Austria

Johanna Muckenhuber[1]*, Karina Fernandez[2], Nathalie T. Burkert[1], Franziska Großschädl[1], Wolfgang Freidl[1], Éva Rásky[1]

1 Department of Social Medicine and Epidemiology, Medical University Graz, Graz, Austria, 2 Department of business education and development, Karl-Franzens-University Graz, Graz, Austria

Abstract

Background: Although a number of previous research studies have focused on the long-term analysis of the health and health behaviour of the elderly, there is still a shortage of information in relation to the long-term trends regarding health or risk and preventive behaviour in the elderly population taking into account gender differences and differences in educational level.

Methods: The database comprised subsamples of the Austrian Micro-Census, including individuals aged 65 years and older, for the years 1983, 1991, 1999, and subsamples of the ATHIS (Austrian Health Interview Survey) 2007. A trend analysis was conducted for four health-related variables with the year of the survey and education as predictors. The analysis was stratified by sex.

Results: We found a general trend towards better self-rated health, better preventive and less risk behaviour among the elderly, while the body mass index has been increasing over the years. There are indeed gender differences regarding the trend in smoking behaviour. While the prevalence of male smoking has been steadily decreasing, female smoking prevalence has not changed. At all points in time, individuals with higher education had significantly better self-rated health than those with lower education but the association between education and preventive behaviour significantly decreased over the years.

Conclusion: We agree with previous research in concluding that preventive action and health promotion should aim in particular to support older women and men with lower education.

Editor: Gianluigi Forloni, "Mario Negri" Institute for Pharmacological Research, Italy

Funding: The authors have no support or funding to report.

Competing Interests: The authors have declared that no competing interests exist.

* E-mail: johanna.muckenhuber@medunigraz.at

Introduction

Compressing morbidity and maintaining health in the older population will be important challenges for public health activities during the next decades. Knowledge about trends in health, in preventive and in risk behaviour of older persons will be helpful in taking preventive action in order to improve health and decrease the prevalence of risk behaviour [1].

There is contradictory evidence regarding Fries' theory of compression of morbidity [2]. Empirical findings do not support recent compression of morbidity for the United States [3]. For the Austrian population Fries's theory has been confirmed and it has been argued that social changes and preventive efforts of the last decades have led to the compression of morbidity in late(r) life [4].

Research has found growing percentages of older people showing better preventive behaviour [5] and decreasing percentages for risk behaviour such as smoking [1]. By contrast, long-term trends of an increasing body mass index (BMI) have been observed

[6,7]. It has been shown, that disability-free life expectancy has increased for more severe levels of disability or activity restrictions over the last decades [8].

Persons with low socio-economic status (SES) have poorer health than those with high SES [9]. This association is even stronger in the older than in the younger population [10].

Although a number of previous research studies have focused on the long-term analysis of the health and health behaviour of the elderly, there is still a shortage of information in relation to the long-term trends regarding health or risk and preventive behaviour in the elderly population taking into account gender differences and differences in educational level. In particular, there is a lack of knowledge concerning long-term trends in the association between educational level and self-rated health among the older population.

The aim of our study, therefore, was to investigate the long-term changes in self-rated health, in the prevalence of preventive and health behaviour, and in the strength of the association between educational level and self-rated health, while also taking gender differences into account.

Data and Methods

The study was carried out in compliance with the declaration of Helsinki. The ethics committee of the Medical University of Graz approved this study

The database comprised two subsamples of the Austrian Micro-Census including i) individuals aged 75 years or older, and ii) individuals aged 65 years or older, for the years 1983 (N (65+) = 9217 (38.1% male)), 1991 (N (65+) = 8782 (36.7% male)), 1999 (N (65+) = 9416 (39.1% male)) plus two corresponding subsamples of the ATHIS (Austrian Health Interview Survey) 2007 (N (65+) = 3564 (41.5% male)). Face to face questionnaire interviews were conducted. Data was collected and provided by the Austrian Statistical Agency (Statistics Austria, 2011). The sample was representative for the Austrian population of the respective age-group.

Multivariate regression analyses were conducted concerning four health-related variables:
- Self-rated health (1 = very good, to 5 = very bad health)
- Vaccination against influenza (yes/no)
- Smoking habits (smoking yes/no) and
- Self-reported body mass index (bmi = kg/m^2).

We applied 4 models with linear regression analysis and 4 models with logistic regression analysis. In doing so, we used centred variables in order to avoid the common problem of multicollinearity, which can occur in regression models with interaction terms [11].

The year of the survey was integrated as dummy variable, with 1983 as category of reference.

In order to investigate the changing influence of "educational level" over time, we integrated the educational level and calculated interaction effects between the level of education and the year each survey was conducted. The level of education differentiated between compulsory education (nine years of schooling) and higher education. The analysis was stratified by sex.

Results

Our decision to analyse two subsamples came up during the study. At first we were mainly interested in persons of higher age (75 years or older). However, the subsample for this age group was rather small, so we decided to also include the subsample of 65 years and older, and to compare the results of the two age groups. We thus chose to describe the results for the group 75 years or older (see Table 1), and in cases of differing results to also describe results for the subsample of 65 years and older (see Table 2).

Trends in health and in male vs. female health behaviour

As shown in Figure 1 and in Tables 1 and 2, covering the years 1983 to 2007, we found a trend towards better self-rated health and improved health behaviour but also a higher BMI among older people for this period.

There was a continuous trend towards better self-rated health, with the best rating in 2007 for both older men (mean value (m): 2.72) and older women (m: 2.79) and the worst rating in 1983 (men, m: 2.99, women, m: 3.06). There was one exception, for men the difference in self-rated health between 1983 and 1999 is not significant.

The BMI increased significantly from 1983 (men, m: 24.35, women, m: 24.26) to 2007 (men, m: 25.55, women, m: 25.91). This increase was significant for men as well as for women, with

Table 1. Long-term-trends of health and health behaviour in persons 75 years and older (% yes, N, Mean Scores with SD, tests on significant differences between educational levels: Chi^2 and ANOVA) and trend in association (Spearman correlation rs and level of significance) between educational level and self-rated health.

| | Men: Logistic regression | | Men: Linear regression | | Women: logistic regression | | Women: logistic regression | |
| | Vaccination | Smoking | BMI | health | Vaccination | Smoking | BMI | health |
	Exp(B)	Exp(B)	stand Beta	stand Beta	Exp(B)	Exp(B)	stand Beta	stand Beta
Level of Education	,523(,000/−1,80E+253)	1,517**(1,180/1,951)	−,039(−,575/,007)	−,145***(−,365/−,209)	,659(0,000/−1,80E+253)	,388***(,275/,546)	−,084***(−1,179/−,589)	−,147***(−,404/−,275)
Year 1983: category of reference								
Year_1991	,000(,000/−1,80E+253)	1,835***(1,362/2,472)	,051*(,038/,761)	−,080**(−,265/−,071)	,000(0,000/−1,80E+253)	,923(,594/1,434)	−,008(−,437/,288)	−,043*(−,165/−,007)
Year_1999	,254***(,194/,333)	2,201***(1,661/2,917)	,166***(,940/1,625)	−,012(−,117/,067)	,322***(,263/,392)	,747(,500/1,115)	,107***(,638/1,284)	−,036*(−,142/−,001)
Year_2006	,161***(,121/,216)	3,524***(2,338/5,310)	,136***(,889/1,701)	−,065**(−,277/−,059)	,198***(,160/,245)	1,254(,757/2,079)	,171***(1,561/2,288)	−,083***(−,287/−,127)
Year_1991*Edu	3,328(,000/−1,80E+253)	,889(,444/1,782)	,006(−,730/,929)	−,031(−,367/,079)	2,504(0,000//−1,80E+253)	,771(,284/2,094)	−,010(−1,078/,641)	−,019(−,274/,101)
Year_1999*Edu	1,535(,884/2,664)	1,260(,679/2,338)	,044(−,033/1,449)	−,014(−,259/,140)	1,799*(1,151/2,810)	,494(,205/1,191)	,032(−,116/1,381)	−,008(−,201/,126)
Year_2006*Edu	2,571**(1,429/4,628)	,463(,207/1,038)	,059*(,218/,227)	,000(−,226/,227)	2,036**(1,269/3,268)	,748(,257/2,178)	,021(−,328/1,324)	−,002(−,190/,172)

Results of the four regression models, individuals 75 years old or older.
* p< = 0.05; ** p< = 0.005; *** p< = 0.001.

Table 2. Long-term-trends of health and health behaviour in persons 65 years and older (% yes, N, Mean Scores with SD, tests on significant differences between educational levels: Chi² and ANOVA) and trend in association (Spearman correlation rs and level of significance) between educational level and self-rated health.

	Vaccination	Smoking	BMI	health	Vaccination	Smoking	BMI	health
	Men: Logistic regression		Men: Linear regression		Women: logistic regression		Women: logistic regression	
	Exp(B)	Exp(B)	stand Beta	stand Beta	Exp(B)	Exp(B)	stand Beta	stand Beta
Level of Education	,622(0,000/−1,80E+253)	1,444***(1,263/1,650)	−,008(−,238/,114)	−,167***(−,365/−,275)	,705(0,000/−1,80E+253)	,412***(,348/,488)	−,079***(−1,006/−,635)	−,160***(−,384/−,308)
Year 1983: category of reference								
Year_1991	,000(0,000/−1,80E+253)	1,533***(1,304/1,802)	,052***(,206/,644)	−,064***(−,188/−,077)	,000(0,000/−1,80E+253)	,871(,703/1,079)	,040**(,142/,594)	−,057***(−,156/−,063)
Year_1999	,308***(,261/,363)1,7977E	1,671***(1,434/1,946)	,152***(,990/1,410)	−,007(−,068/,039)	,332***(,292/,378)	,865(,704/1,063)	,113***(,835/1,256)	−,037**(−,114/−,028)
Year_2006	,177***(,148/,213)	2,585***(2,079/3,214)	,150***(1,263/1,781)	−,043**(−,177/−,045)	,233***(,202/,268)	1,197(,916/1,563)	,141***(1,496/1,991)	−,064***(−,218/−,115)
Year_1991*Edu	2,427(0,000/−1,80E+253)	,864(,594/1,257)	−,013(−,735/,260)	−,011(−,179/,074)	2,012(0,000/−1,80E+253)	1,012(,629/1,629)	,003(−,458/,603)	−,015(−,176/,043)
Year_1999*Edu	1,418*(1,011/1,989)	,808(,581/1,123)	,036*(,133/1,026)	,019(−,035/,192)	1,423*(1,066/1,900)	,784(,504/1,219)	,019(−,097/,866)	,007(−,069/,130)
Year_2006*Edu	1,845**(1,280/2,660)	,604*(,391/,931)	,014(−,252/,798)	,008(−,094/,174)	1,641**(1,199/2,248)	1,155(,664/2,011)	,009(−,326/,773)	−,009(−,163/,064)

Results of the four regression models, individuals 65 years old or older.
* $p \leq 0.05$; ** $p \leq 0.005$; *** $p \leq 0.001$.

one exception. For the subsample of women 75 years or older, no significant increase in BMI between 1983 and 1991 was found; however, a significant increase in BMI appeared when comparing the year 2007 to the years 1991 and 1999.

The percentage of men and women vaccinated against influenza was significantly higher in 1999 (men: 30.6%, women: 26.9%) and in 2007 (men 38.8%, women 37.8%) when compared to 1983 (men: 7.2%, women: 8.3%). Such a significant increase was not found between 1983 and 1991, neither for men nor for women.

For men, we observed a significant decrease in the percentage of smokers, with the highest percentage in 1983 (23.3%) and the lowest percentage in 2007 (7.7%). For women, by contrast, we found neither increase nor decrease in smoking behaviour over the years (2.8% smokers in 1983, 2.7% in 2007).

Differences according to educational level

Table 1 shows that, consistently over the years, both men and women with high levels of education reported significantly better self-rated health than people with low levels of education.

Consistently over the years, women with low levels of education had a significantly higher BMI than women with higher levels of education. Leaving interaction effects aside, no such educational difference was found in men.

Setting interaction effects aside between the level of education and the year of the survey, significantly more older men with a low level of education were smokers compared to those with a high level of education. On the other hand, significantly more older women with high levels of education were smokers compared to those with a low level of education.

Changes over the years in the association between educational level and self-rated health

As shown in Figure 1, the relationship between the level of education and the percentage of men and women vaccinated against influenza changed significantly over the years. For both men and women, the educational difference played no significant role in 2007 when compared to 1983. For women, this also applies to the comparison between 1999 and 1983. In men, however, no such continuous pattern was found: the educational difference in respect of those being vaccinated against influenza was greater in 1999 than in 1983.

No significant interaction effects were found between the year of the survey and the educational effect on self-rated health and on the BMI. Consistently over the years, individuals with higher education had significantly better self-rated health than those with lower education, and also consistently over the years, women with a low level of education had a higher BMI than those with a high level of education.

Discussion

In accordance with previous research [2,4], our analyses have shown a trend towards better health among the older population. In line with other studies [9,12], our analyses have shown individuals with higher education to have better self-reported health than those with lower education. In accordance with some [12] though in contrast to other results [13], educational differences in self-rated health remained consistent over the years.

The persisting association between educational level and health among the older population might have two major causes. On the one hand, a low educational level is still associated with poor living standards [14]. Furthermore, with higher age, individuals have fewer possibilities to compensate for difficult living conditions such

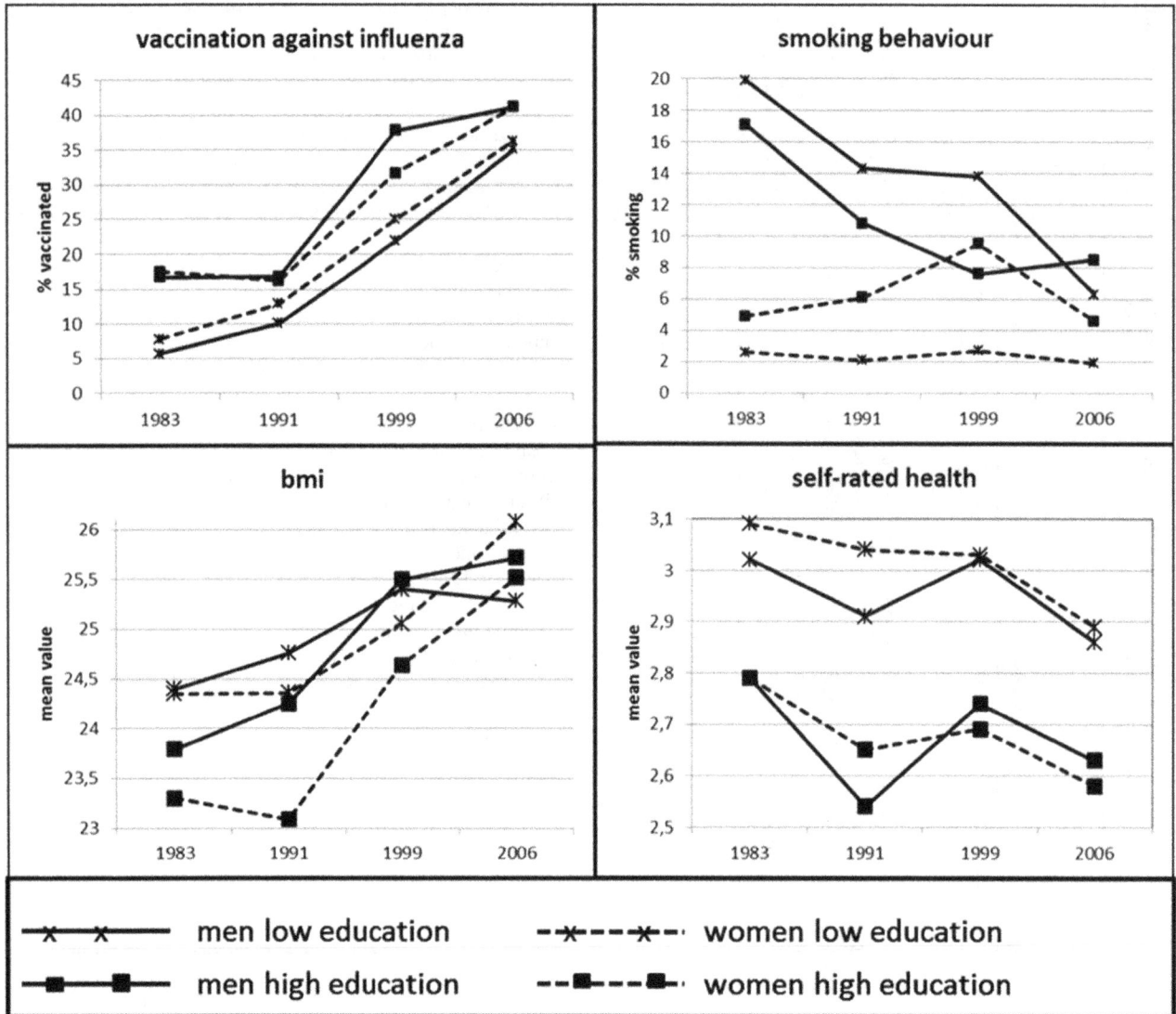

Figure 1. Long-term-trends of health and of health- and risk behaviour in persons 75 years and older.

as insufficient heating etc. On the other hand, we have observed an increasing prevalence of preventive behaviour during the last decades. Even though we found the educational gap regarding preventive behaviour to have decreased over the years, preventive measures still reach population groups with higher education more easily and better than groups with lower education [15]. This might also have contributed to the persisting educational gap in health.

In line with some previous research [5,16,17] but in contrast to other research [18–20], we found increasing influenza vaccination coverage over the years. Regarding the case of Austria, we found very high rates of influenza vaccination within the older population as opposed to the general population. In contrast to previous research focussing on the general population [21], we found a steady increase in the proportion of older people vaccinated. In addition, we found decreasing educational differences over the years. These results might be explained by the fact that influenza vaccination is promoted by general practitioners in particular among the older population. Since older individuals with both higher and lower levels of education regularly see a G.P.,

this direct way of promoting the vaccination might have a particularly marked effect on the lower educated.

In accordance with some previous research on the general population [22,23] but in contrast to other studies focussing on older people [24], we found a trend toward increasing BMI among the older population.

In accordance with previous results, we found smoking prevalence in men to decline over the years [25,26] but no such decline can be reported for older women. This might be an effect of the age cohort with constantly low smoking prevalence (under 10%) in older women.

In contrast to previous research reporting lower percentages of smokers amongst both men and women with higher levels of education compared to those with lower levels of education [27–29], our study found a higher percentage of older women smoking within the higher educational level group compared to the lower educational level group. This might also be an effect of the age cohort. We assume that in the older female population smoking might be more readily accepted among the higher educated than among the lower educated women, since in the past smoking was culturally less readily accepted for women than for men and even less accepted for women with a low level of education. We found different trends in smoking behaviour for men. In contrast to previous research showing greater declines in smoking among the higher educated than among the lower educated [29,30], our results show a greater decline in smoking prevalence for men with lower education than for men with higher education. This could be due to existing differences in the extent of smoking. Literature has shown heavy smoking to be more frequent among men with lower education than among men with higher education [31]. Possibly heavy smokers are more willing to stop smoking at a higher age than smokers who perceive themselves as light smokers.

Strengths and limitations

Strengths.   Among the strengths of the study are the relatively high number of individuals included for analysis, the high data quality and the representative sample, the long time span analysed and the analysis of trends in differences regarding the educational level.

Limitations.   One limitation of the study is that only a limited number of variables could be used for analysis and compared over the years because of the differing measures for health and for preventive and risk behaviour in the four data sets.

Another limitation is the measurement of "educational level". We had to divide education into basic low education and the wide category of high education, since there are very few women with higher education, in particular in the first years surveyed. When splitting the educational level into a greater number of categories, the number of older women with higher education turned out to be too small to perform a statistical analysis.

Conclusions.   Our analysis has shown the enduring importance of the educational level for self-rated health over the years, so we agree with previous research [32] in concluding that preventive action and health promotion should in particular aim to support older women and men with lower education.

Author Contributions

Analyzed the data: JM KF NB FG WF ER. Wrote the paper: JM.

References

1. Marques-Vidal P, Cerveira J, Paccaud F, Cornuz J (2011) Smoking trends in Switzerland, 1992-2007: a time for optimism? J Epidemiol Community Health 65: 281–286.
2. Fries JF (1989) The compression of morbidity: Near or far? Milbank Memorial Foundation Quaterly/Health and Society 67: 208–232.
3. Crimmins EM, Beltran-Sanchez H (2011) Mortality and Morbidity Trends: Is There Compression of Morbidity? J Gerontol Ser B-Psychol Sci Soc Sci 66: 75–86. doi:10.1093/geronb/gbq088.
4. Doblhammer G, Kytir J (2001) Compression or expansion of morbidity? Trends in healthy-life expectancy in the elderly Austrian population between 1978 and 1998. Social Science and Medicine 52: 385–391.
5. Lu P, Singleton J, Rangel M, Wortley P, Bridges C (2005) Influenza vaccination trends among 65 years or older in the United States, 1989-202. Archives of internal Medicine 165: 1849–1856.
6. Grossschaedl F, Stronegger WJ (2013) Long-term trends in obesity among Austrian adults and its relation with the social gradient: 1973-2007. Eur J Public Health 23: 306–312. doi:10.1093/eurpub/cks033.
7. Staub K, Ruhli F, Woitek U, Pfister C (2010) BMI distribution/social stratification in Swiss conscripts from 1875 to present. European Journal of Clinical Nutrition 64: 335–340.
8. Cambois E, Clavel A, Romieu I, Robine J-M (2008) Trends in disability-free life expectancy at age 65 in France: consistent and diverging patterns according to the underlying disability measure. Eur J Ageing 5: 287–298. doi:10.1007/s10433-008-0097-1.
9. Freidl W, Stronegger W, Rasky E, Neuhold C (2001) Associations of income with self-reported ill-health and health resources in a rural community sample of Austria. Sozial- und Präventivmedizin 46: 106–114.
10. Chandola T, Ferrie J, Sacker A, Marmot M (2007) Social inequalities in self-reported health in early old age: follow-up of prospective cohort study. British Medical Journal 334: 990–993B.
11. Aiken L, West S (1991) Multiple Regression: Testing and interpreting interactions. Newbury Park, London, Delhi: Sage Publications.
12. Krokstad S, Kunst A, Westin S (2002) Trends in health inequalities by educational level in a Norwegian total population study. J Epidemiol Community Health 56: 375–380.
13. Dalstra J, Kunst A, Geurts J, Frenken F, Mackenbach J (2002) Trends in socioeconomic health inequalities in the Netherlands, 1981–1999. J Epidemiol Community Health 56: 927–934.
14. WHO Comission on Social Determinants of Health (CSDH) (2008) Closing the gap in a generation. Health equity through action on the social determinants of health. Final Report.
15. Stronegger W, Freidl W, Rasky E, Berghold A (1998) Educational status and resources for child care as predictors of TBE vaccination coverage in schoolchildren of an endemic area in Austria. Zentralblatt für Hygiene und Umweltmedizin 201: 437–445.
16. Kwong JC, Rosella LC, Johansen H (2007) Trends in influenza vaccination in Canada, 1996/1997 to 2005. Health reports/Statistics Canada, Canadian Centre for Health Information = Rapports sur la sante/Statistique Canada, Centre canadien d'information sur la sante 18.
17. Rodriguez de Azero M (2008) Trends in seasonal influenza vaccine distribution in the European Union: 2003-4 to 2007-8. Euro surveillance: bulletin Europeen sur les maladies transmissibles = European communicable disease bulletin 13.
18. Blank PR, Freiburghaus AU, Ruf BR, Schwenkglenks MM, Szucs TD (2008) Trends in Influenza Vaccination Coverage Rates in Germany over Six Seasons from 2001/02 to 2006/07. Med Klin 103: 761–768. doi:10.1007/s00063-008-1121-0.
19. Castilla J, Martinez-Baz I, Godoy P, Toledo D, Astray J, et al. (2013) Trends in influenza vaccine coverage among primary healthcare workers in Spain, 2008-2011. Prev Med 57: 206–211. doi:10.1016/j.ypmed.2013.05.021.
20. Jimenez-Trujillo I, Lopez-de Andres A, Hernandez-Barrera V, Carrasco-Garrido P, Santos-Sancho JM, et al. (2013) Influenza vaccination coverage rates among diabetes sufferers, predictors of adherence and time trends from 2003 to 2010 in Spain. Human vaccines & immunotherapeutics 9. doi:10.4161/hv.23926.
21. Kunze U, Bohm G, Groman E (2013) Influenza vaccination in Austria from 1982 to 2011: A country resistant to influenza prevention and control. Vaccine 31. doi:10.1016/j.vaccine.2013.08.050.
22. Loranta V, Tongletb R (2010) Obesity: trend in inequality. J Epidemiol Community Health 54: 637–638.
23. Zaninotto P, Head J, Stamatakis E, Wardle H, Midell J (2009) Trends in obesity among adults in England from 1993 to 2004 by age and social class and projections of prevalence to 2012. J Epidemiol Community Health 63: 140–146.
24. Kahn H, Cheng Y (2008) Longitudinal changes in BMI and in an index estimating excess lipids among white and black adults in the United States. International Journal of Obesity 32: 136–143.
25. Regidor E, De Mateo S, Ronda E, Sánchez-Payá J, Gutiérrez-Fisac J, et al. (2010) Heterogeneous trend in smoking prevalence by sex and age group following the implementation of a national smoke-free law. J Epidemiol Community Health online 2010.
26. Sardu C, Mereu A, Pitzalis G, Minerba L, Contu P (2006) Smoking trends in Italy from 1950 to 2000. J Epidemiol Community Health 60: 799–803.
27. Johnson W, Kyvik KO, Mortensen EL, Skytthe A, Batty GD, et al. (2011) Does Education Confer a Culture of Healthy Behavior? Smoking and Drinking Patterns in Danish Twins. Am J Epidemiol 173: 55–63. doi:10.1093/aje/kwq333.
28. Panasiuk L, Mierzecki A, Wdowiak L, Paprzycki P, Lukas W, et al. (2010) Prevalence of Cigarette Smoking among Adult Population in Eastern Poland. Annals of agricultural and environmental medicine 17: 133–138.
29. Smith P, Frank J, Mustard C (2009) Trends in educational inequalities in smoking and physical activity in Canada: 1974–2005. J Epidemiol Community Health 63: 317–323.
30. Giskes K, Kunst A, Benach J, Borrell C, Costa G, et al. (2005) Trends in smoking behaviour between 1985 and 2000 in nine European countries by education. J Epidemiol Community Health 59: 395–401.
31. Baumert J, Ladwig K-H, Ruf E, Meisinger C, Doering A, et al. (2010) Determinants of Heavy Cigarette Smoking: Are There Differences in Men and Women? Results From the Population-Based MONICA/KORA Augsburg Surveys. Nicotine Tob Res 12: 1220–1227. doi:10.1093/ntr/ntq172.
32. Stafford M, Nazroo J, Popay J, Whitehead M (2008) Tackling inequalities in health: evaluating the New Deal for Communities initiative. Journal of Epidemiology and Community Health 62: 298–304.

## 25

Evaluation of the Accuracy of Anthropometric Clinical Indicators of Visceral Fat in Adults and Elderly

Anna Karla Carneiro Roriz[1,2]*, Luiz Carlos Santana Passos[1,3], Carolina Cunha de Oliveira[1,4], Michaela Eickemberg[5,6], Pricilla de Almeida Moreira[2], Lílian Ramos Sampaio[2,7]

1 Postgraduation Program of Medicine and Health, Federal University of Bahia, Salvador, Bahia, Brazil, 2 School of Nutrition, Nutrition Science Department, Federal University of Bahia, Salvador, Bahia, Brazil, 3 Faculty of Medicine, Department of Medicine, Federal University of Bahia, Salvador, Bahia, Brazil, 4 Nutrition Department, Federal University of Sergipe, Lagarto, Sergipe, Brazil, 5 Institute of Collective Health, Federal University of Bahia, Salvador, Bahia, Brazil, 6 Bahiana School of Medicine and Public Health, Salvador, Bahia, Brazil, 7 Postgraduation Program in Food and Nutrition, Federal University of Bahia, Salvador, Bahia, Brazil

Abstract

Background: Visceral obesity is associated with higher occurrence of cardiovascular events. There are few studies about the accuracy of anthropometric clinical indicators, using Computed Tomography (CT) as the gold standard. We aimed to determine the accuracy of anthropometric clinical indicators for discrimination of visceral obesity.

Methods: Cross-sectional study with 191 adults and elderly of both sexes. Variables: area of visceral adipose tissue (VAT) identified by CT, Waist-to-Height Ratio (WHtR), Conicity index (C index), Lipid Accumulation Product (LAP) and Visceral Adiposity Index (VAI). ROC analyzes.

Results: There were a strong correlation between adiposity indicators and VAT area. Higher accuracy of C index and WHtR (AUC≥0.81) than the LAP and the VAI was observed. The higher AUC of LAP and VAI were observed among elderly with areas of 0.88 (CI: 0.766–0.944) and 0.83 (CI: 0.705–0.955) in men and 0.80 (CI: 0.672–0.930) and 0.71 (CI: 0.566–0.856) in women, respectively. The cutoffs of C index were 1.30 in elderly, in both sexes, with sensitivity ≥92%, the LAP ranged from 26.4 to 37.4 in men and from 40.6 to 44.0 in women and the VAI was 1.24 to 1.45 (sens≥76.9%) in men and 1.46 to 1.84 in women.

Conclusion: Both the anthropometric indicators, C Index and WHtR, as well as LAP and VAI had high accuracy in visceral obesity discrimination. So, they are effective in cardiovascular risk assessment and in the follow-up for individual and collective clinical practice.

Editor: Stephen L. Atkin, Weill Cornell Medical College Qatar, Qatar

Funding: This study was funded by the Brazilian National Council for Scientific and Technological Development and by Foundation Coordination of Improvement of Higher Education Personnel by Ministry of Education through research scholarship to AKCR. The funding source had no role in study design, data collection and analysis, decision to publish, or preparation of the manuscript.

Competing Interests: The authors have declared that no competing interests exist.

* Email: karlaroriz@hotmail.com

Introduction

Visceral obesity is associated to higher incidence of type 2 diabetes, dyslipidemia, insulin resistance, hypertension, particularly cardiovascular disease (CVD) that are considered as important causes of mortality and high costs in the world [1,2].

The quantification of visceral obesity is best determined by imaging exams such as Computed Tomography (CT), that is the gold standard method, but it requires high cost, difficult operation and radiation exposure. On the other hand, anthropometric clinical indicators are easily obtained and, if accurate, they offer diagnosis possibility in primary care and in the follow-up without any of the CT inconveniences. Currently few studies are available with data from adult and elderly subjects divided by sex to evaluate the accuracy of indicators in the prediction of visceral fat.

Recently, Lipid Accumulation Product (LAP) and Visceral Adiposity Index (VAI) have been proposed as alternative assessment parameters of the excessive lipids accumulation. The LAP expresses a continuous risk and it is a predictor of cardiovascular disease and mortality [3] and the VAI expresses the visceral fat function associated with cardiometabolic risk [4] and it also evaluates the risk of complications related to visceral obesity [4,5]. Both have not been explored yet in regard to their ability to discriminate excess of visceral fat, measured by CT, as well as the Conicity Index (C Index) and Waist-to-Height Ratio (WHtR). In addition, there are few studies that evaluated the accuracy these indicators of visceral fat between adults and elderly individuals, in both sexes.

There are evidences that anthropometric indicators of abdominal obesity are good predictors of cardiovascular risk and mortality [6–10], but there are few studies that compare these indicators in relation to the LAP and the VAI as this study intended to do. The aim of this study was to determine the accuracy of anthropometric clinical indicators for discrimination of visceral obesity.

Table 1. Descriptive analysis of the anthropometric clinical indicators and visceral adipose tissue area, and the mean comparison of these variables, by sex and age group.

	Men			Women		
	20–59 years (n = 49)	60 years (n = 45)	p	20–59 years (n = 49)	60 years (n = 45)	p
WHtR	0.51 (0.07)	0.57 (0.07)	0.001**	0.53 (0.07)	0.59 (0.07)	0.001**
C Index	1.23 (0.09)	1.31 (0.08)	0.001**	1.21 (0.08)	1.29 (0.09)	0.001**
VAI	1.57 (0.98)	1.73 (1.08)	0.470	1.67 (1.33)	2.15 (1.44)	0.090
LAP	35.66 (31.07)	43.27 (30.64)	0.240	34.12 (27.66)	47.60 (26.98)	0.020*
VAT	94.18 (58.74)	157.80 (86.08)	0.001**	72.20 (43.88)	122.53 (48.94)	0.001**

Data are mean_S.D.
Abbreviations: WHtR: Waist-to-height ratio; C Index: Conicity Index; VAI: Visceral adipose index; LAP: Lipid accumulation product; VAT: Visceral adipose tissue area (cm^2).
*p≤0.05;
**p≤0.01.

Methods and Materials

Study design and data collection

The transversal study was performed in the University Hospital and at the School of Nutrition of the Federal University of Bahia (UFBA), during the first trimester of 2009, conducted by the team of the Center of Studies and Intervention in Aging Area of UFBA in Salvador, the third largest city in Brazil. Two-hundred individuals from the outpatient clinic and the community were alocated by convenience for equitable stratification of variables: sex, age and body mass, the latter one determined by Body Mass Index (BMI), dividing patient weight in kilograms by the square of patient height in meters, specific for each age group.

The sample size was defined according to the possibilities of human and material resources, as well as the analysis of the sample size of previous studies [11–13] and the careful sample stratification. Individuals were selected following the same ratio between adults and elderly, men and women, presence and absence of excess body mass in order to achieve greater representativeness of the groups equally in terms of the amount of visceral fat, since the presence/absence of comorbidities has an influence in this amount of fat.

Exclusion criteria. individuals under twenty years old, Body Mass Index >40 kg/m^2, patients with severe malnutrition and severe neurological and muscular disorders, pregnant and breastfeeding women, individuals that recently suffered abdominal surgery (<6 months) or had tumor, hepatomegaly, splenomegaly and/or ascites or any problem that compromises the recommended techniques for anthropometric and visceral fat measurement by computed tomography.

Anthropometric clinical indicators

All clinical, anthropometric, laboratory and imaging by computed tomography evaluations were standardized and measured by a properly trained staff. Measurements of weight and height were obtained according to the techniques proposed by Lohman et al (1988) [14]. We directly measured weight in kilograms using a Portable, digital scale (Filizola, São Paulo, Brazil) with capacity up to 150 Kg and a precision of 100 g. The Height was measured in centimeters with a portable stadiometer (Seca, TBW Importing *Ltda.*). Waist Circumference (WC) was measured at the midpoint between the lower costal margin and the iliac crest, we used an inelastic measuring tape of 1 mm precision.

Measurements were obtained in duplicate and their averages were used for the analyzes. The WHtR was calculated by the WC (cm) divided by the height (cm). The Conicity index was obtained by the formula proposed by Valdez (1991) [15]:

$$C\,Index = \frac{WC\,(cm)}{0.109\;X\;\sqrt{Weight\,(Kg)/Height\,(m)}}$$

Table 2. Correlation coefficient between visceral adipose tissue area and the indicators of adiposity in both sexes according to age group.

	Visceral Adipose Tissue Area			
	Men		Women	
	20–59 years	≥60 years	20–59 years	≥60 years
WHtR	0.79**	0.80**	0.73**	0.64**
C Index	0.68**	0.82[1]**	0.72**	0.47**
VAI	0.50[1]**	0.56[1]**	0.38**	0.47**
LAP	0.70[1]**	0.73[1]**	0.61**	0.60**

Abbreviations: WHtR: Waist-to-height ratio; C Index: Conicity Index; VAI: Visceral adipose index; LAP: Lipid accumulation product.
**p≤0.01.
[1]Spearman's correlation coefficient.

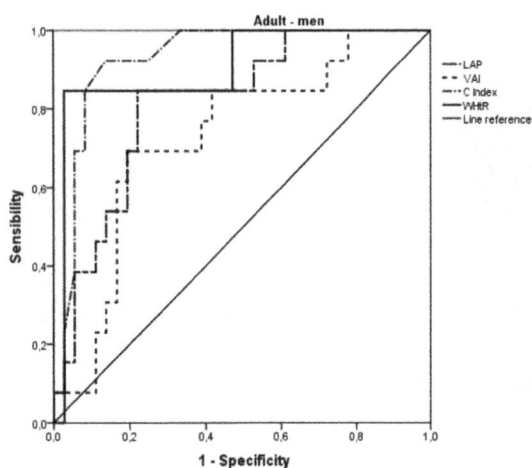

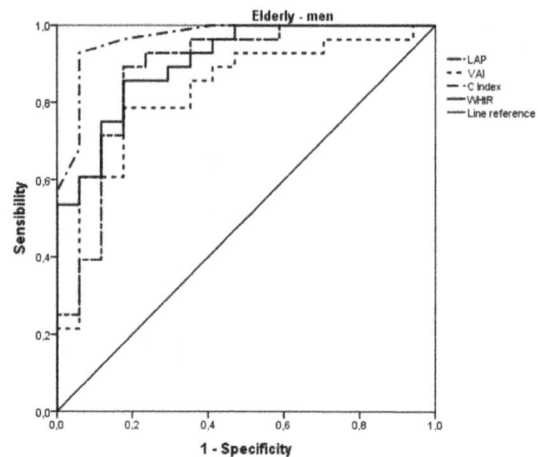

AUC– LAP: 0.81* (CI: 0.686–0.942); VAI: 0.73* (CI: 0.571–0.886); C Index: 0.93* (CI: 0.854–1.003); WHtR: 0.91* (CI: 0.799–1.009)

AUC–LAP: 0.88** (CI:0.766–0.944); VAI: 0.83**(CI: 0.705–0.955); C Index: 0.97** (CI: 0.918–1.017); WHtR: 0.90** (CI: 0.820–0.991)

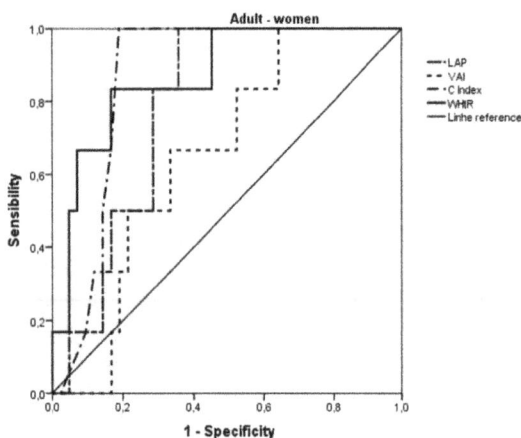

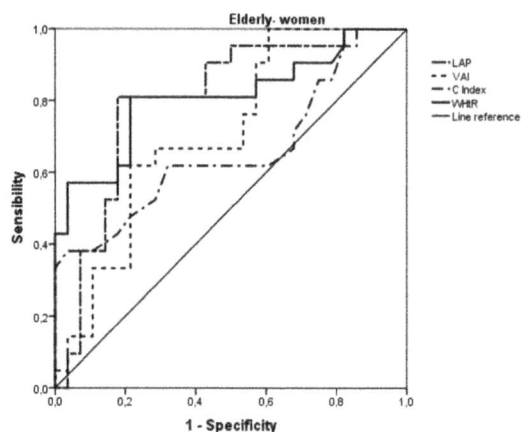

AUC– LAP: 0.78* (CI: 0.652–0.919); VAI: 0.65 (CI: 0.472–0.838); C Index: 0.86** (CI: 0.762–0.964); WHtR: 0.87** (CI: 0.730–1.008)

AUC–LAP: 0.80** (CI:0.672–0.930); VAI: 0.71* (CI: 0.566–0.856); C Index: 0.66 (CI: 0.496–0.822); WHtR: 0.81** (CI: 0.678–0.939)

Figure 1. ROC analysis with Areas Under the Curve (AUC) of indicators of adiposity in predicting visceral obesity (TAV area >130 cm²). In this Figure are presented the areas under the ROC curves of anthropometric clinical indicators, classified by sex and age groups. In both sexes the majority of indicators had strong predictive ability to detect the presence of visceral obesity, i.e., AUC above 0.80. Abbreviations: AUC: Areas under the ROC curves, CI: Confidence Interval; LAP: Lipid accumulation product; VAI: Visceral adipose index; C Index: Conicity Index; WHtR: Waist-to-height ratio. *p≤0.05; **p≤0.01.

All individuals were submitted to a blood sample collection. They had fasted for 12 hours. The blood samples were used to measure the high-density lipoprotein (HDL) and triglycerides (TG) levels. They were quantified using a colorimetric system, dry chemistry method, with kits manufactured by Ortho-Clinical

Diagnostics, Rochester, NY. For conversion between units, mg/dl to mmol/L, it was multiplied by 0.0113.

The VAI was obtained by the formulas proposed by Amato et al (2010) [4]: for males, $VAI = (WC/36.58 + (1.89 \times BMI)) \times (TG/0.81) \times (1.52/HDL)$ and females, $VAI = (WC/39.68 + (1.88 \times BMI)) \times (TG/1.03) \times (1.31/HDL)$. The LAP was obtained

Table 3. ROC analysis with Cutoff points, sensitivity and specificity of indicators of adiposity that correspond to VAT area of $\geq$ 130 cm^2 for men and women according to age group.

	20–59 years			≥60 years		
	Cutoff	Sens. (PPV)	Spec. (NPV)	Cutoff	Sens. (PPV)	Spec. (NPV)
MEN						
WHtR	0.54	84.6 (68.7)	86.1 (93.9)	0.55	85.7 (88.9)	82.4 (77.8)
C Index	1.26	92.3 (70.5)	86.1 (96.9)	1.30	92.9 (91.6)	94.1 (89.0)
VAI	1.45	76.9 (41.6)	61.1 (88.0)	1.24	78.6 (84.6)	76.5 (68.5)
LAP	37.4	84.6 (57.9)	77.8 (93.3)	26.4	92.9 (94.7)	76.5 (86.7)
WOMEN						
WHtR	0.59	83.3 (41.6)	83.3 (97.2)	0.58	81.0 (74.0)	78.6 (84.6)
C Index	1.25	100 (42.9)	81.0 (100)	1.30	61.9 (59.2)	67.9 (70.3)
VAI	1.46	66.7 (22.2)	66.7 (93.3)	1.84	66.7 (60.9)	67.9 (73.1)
LAP	40.6	83.3 (29.4)	71.4 (96.8)	44.0	81.0 (77.3)	82.1 (85.2)

Abbreviations: Sens: Sensitivity; Spec: Specificity; PPV: Positive predictive value; NPV: Negative predictive value; WHtR: Waist-to-height ratio; CI: Conicity Index; VAI: Visceral adipose index; LAP: Lipid accumulation product.

by the formulas proposed by Kahn et al (2005) [3]. For males, LAP = (WC [cm]–65)×(triglyceride concentration [mmol/L]) and females, LAP = (WC [cm]–58)×/triglyceride concentration [mmol/L]).

Tomographic image of Visceral Adipose Tissue area (VAT)

The area of Visceral Adipose Tissue was measured by computed tomography obtained by the CT Spirit Siemens of the Radiology Service from the University Hospital of UFBA and analyzed by a single specialized technician. The examination was performed in complete fast of 4 hours without administration of barium or organic iodinated contrast, with the patient in supine position and the arms extended overhead. The area was obtained from a single axial CT slice at the level of L4–L5, with a slice thickness of 10 mm and an exposure time of three seconds, according to a technique proposed by Seidell et al (1987) [16]. The VAT area was described in square centimeters.

The tomographic program was used with x-ray CT scanner parameters of 140 kV and 45 mA, being employed the density of −50 and −150 Hounsfield units for the identification of fat tissue. Visceral obesity was identified by the VAT area above 130 cm^2 [17].

Statistical Analyzes

For descriptive analysis it was used the means, standard deviations, as well as the Kolmogorov-Smirnov test and the histogram to assess the distribution of the variables. In adittion, we used Student t-test and the Wilcoxon test to compare the mean of the variables of normal and non-normal distribution, respectively. The coefficient of variation was calculated to assess the inter and intra examiner variability of the anthropometric measures. The correlations by the Pearson's and Spearman's correlation coefficient according to the variables linearity.

The areas under the ROC curves (Receiver Operating Characteristic) (AUC) were calculated by adiposity indicators in the identification of discriminatory power for visceral obesity. The area under ROC curve value equal 1 means perfect accuracy of diagnosis and the closer to this value and greater than 0.75, it is, it has a precision sensibility [18]. Sensibility, specificity, positive predictive value (PPV) and negative predictive value (NPV), and

their respective cutoffs with more appropriate balance between them were examined. A confidence interval (CI) of 95% was adopted. The significance level was set at p<0.05. For the analyzes it was used the statistical program SPSS; version 16.0 (SPSS Inc., Chicago, IL, EUA).

Ethics Statement

This study was approved by the Ethics Committee in Research of the School of Nutrition (license numbers: 01/09), Federal University of Bahia, in Salvador, Brazil. All participants agreed in participating in this research by signing a written informed consent. The study did not involve procedures of high risk for the individuals and all received the test results, and they were seen at nutrition clinics of the University Hospital and referred for health follow-up, where necessary.

Results

Two-hundred individuals were evaluated, from whom 9 were excluded (TG values >400 mg/dl and outliers of the visceral fat), totaling 191 participants in this study. The anthropometric data obtained correlation coefficient of intra and inter evaluator exceeding 0.90 confirming the reliability of the measures collection. In Table 1, the mean WHtR was 0.57 and 0.59 in elderly men and elderly women, respectively. The mean C Index was higher in the elderly group of both sexes. It was verified that the LAP and VAI had higher means in elderly comparing with group of adults, in both sexes, however this difference did not have statistical significant, except the mean of the LAP in women. The average area of VAT was over 130 cm^2 only in elderly men (p<0.05) (Table 1).

In both sexes it was found that anthropometric indicators had strong correlations with the VAT area, increasing from the group of adults to the one of older men and in women the inverse was observed. The LAP showed strong correlation with VAT area, r$\geq$ 0.70 (p$\leq$0.01) and r$\geq$0.60 (p$\leq$0.01) respectively in men and women. The strongest correlation of the VAI was r = 0.56 (p$\leq$ 0.01) in elderly men, while in elderly women the correlation was moderate (Table 2).

In Figure 1 and Table 3, the analyzes of the ROC curves of anthropometric clinical indicators are presented. In both sexes the WHtR and C Index showed a higher area under the ROC curve than the LAP and the VAI, i.e., AUC≥0.90 in men and AUC≥0.86 in women, except in elder women. The VAI had larger areas in elderly, with AUC = 0.83 (CI: 0.705–0.955) in men and AUC = 0.71 (CI: 0.566–0.856) in women. Regarding other indicators, the VAI had the lower discriminatory power (Figure 1).

It is observed in Table 3 that the cutoffs of WHtR were similar between age groups, in both sexes, with sensibility and specificity above 81.0% and 78.6%, respectively. Regarding C Index, elderly had cutoffs of 1.30, with sensibility and specificity of 92.9% and 94.1% in men and 61.9% and 67.9% in women, respectively (Table 3).

The LAP cutoffs ranged from 26.4 to 37.4 in men, reaching a PPV of 94.7% with sensibility and specificity of 92.9% and 76.5% respectively, in the men older than sixty years while in women the LAP ranged from 40.6 to 44.0, with sensibility and specificity of 81.0% and 82.1%, respectively in elderly women. The VAI cutoffs were 1.45 (sens: 76.9%; spec: 61.1%) and 1.24 (sens: 78.6%; spec: 76.5%) in adults and elderly men, respectively. Among women the cutoffs were 1.46 in adults and 1.84 in elderly with sensitivity and specificity above 66.7% (Table 3).

Discussion

The present study showed that the clinical anthropometric indicators had strong correlations with visceral fat and most of the areas under the ROC curve gained predictive power with the increasing of age, being more expressive, especially in men. This is the first study that evaluates the accuracy of the LAP and the VAI compared to anthropometric indicators for the detection of visceral obesity as measured by computed tomography in both sexes.

In this study, the WHtR and C Index evaluated well the visceral obesity. The C Index incorporates three very instructive measures, including the WC, which is common to the other indicators here evaluated. The C Index proved to be one of the most accurate in the discrimination of the visceral obesity, especially in men. It detects the changes in fat distribution, allowing comparisons between individuals that had different measurements of body weight and height [19]. Studies show that C Index has been a good predictor of high coronary risk [20] with AUC of 0.80 (95% CI: 0.74–0.85) and cardiovascular risk [21], as well as the WHtR [22].

The WHtR allows identifying the waist circumference of the risk to an individual's height and was better than the C Index only in the older women in this study. A systematic review showed that the WHtR was better than WC and BMI in predicting CVD in 86% of studies in men and in 91% in women [23].

Regarding the LAP, there was an increase of accuracy comparing younger and elderly individuals in both sexes in this study. The LAP estimates the over-accumulation of lipids, rising more quickly with the age for men than for women, which may contribute to the increasing in cardiovascular events in younger men [3]. In this study, the LAP and the WHtR had similar accuracy (AUC = 0.80) to identify visceral obesity in older women. Studies showed the discriminatory power of the LAP for other events, such as the incidence of diabetes that was similar to waist to hip ratio and WHtR [24] and in the prediction of metabolic syndrome where there was superiority of the LAP in relation to WHtR [25–27].

In this study, despite the VAI having positive correlation with visceral fat, it had shown lower accuracy compared to other indicators, in both sexes, however there was good accuracy in the elderly. In the same way as the LAP, the VAI has been reported to predict other events resulting from excess of visceral fat [28–30] not of visceral obesity itself, as in the present study.

Overall, the most indicators of this study demonstrated that elderly men had better correlation and accuracy in discrimination of the excess of visceral fat than adults men. The inverse was observed to women, possibly because of the physical and hormonal changes that happen to women in the postmenopausal. However, this more detailed investigation wasn't the goal of this study. Furthermore, the LAP and the VAI showed lower accuracy comparing to the WHtR and the C Index because of bioquimics tests (TG, HDL), which constitute their respective equations and have weaker correlations with visceral fat than the anthropometry [31].

The cutoff points of the indicators evaluated in this study to identify the visceral obesity are still a gap in the literature. The values for the elderly, who have not been previously identified are of particular interest. For the WHtR, the cutoffs were similar to those found in other studies to identify high coronary risk [32,33] and to discriminate diabetes, hypertension and dyslipidemia [34]. However, we didn't find other studies about the discrimination of visceral obesity, which showed the cutoff of anthropometric clinical indicators, as this study does. Therefore, it is recommended to consider that the waist should not be greater than half of the height of a particular individual as this would indicate a health risk.

The theoretical range of the C Index is between 1.00 and 1.73 and this ratio increases with the accumulation of abdominal fat, already taking into account its height and weight, increasing the risk of diseases [35]. In this study the C Index was able to detect more cases of visceral obesity in men than in women, with values from 1.26 to 1.30 in adults and elderly respectively. Studies have suggested cutoffs of the C Index in order to identify high coronary risk and hypertension [9,36], however, they were assessed only in adults and not in the elderly.

For the LAP, this study identified values above 26.4 and 40.6 in men and women respectively, i.e., values for women were superior than for men to detect visceral obesity. There is information about the LAP cutoffs to detect other events, among them, a study with spanish adults [26] identified the LAP value above 48.9 in men and 31.7 in women to detect metabolic syndrome. In relation to the VAI, cutoffs were similar among adults, while among the elderly, men had a value of 1.24, being lower than that of women that was 1.84. The results presented here show that values above those cutoffs allow to estimate visceral obesity and underscore the importance of obtaining and using specific cutoffs points for each population.

The scarcity of studies about this subject and which evaluated anthropometry with the LAP and the VAI, using this imaging method restricted the comparison of results between the tested age groups. As shown in most studies [2], the measurement of single computed tomography scan, especially at L4–L5 position minimizes radiation exposure of the individual and reduces cost. This way we have chosen this position this study. Further studies are needed, with larger samples, allowing generalizations and comparisons among different populations.

This study reinforces that individuals should be assessed early and periodically, through accurate methods, considering its ease of use in large scale and low cost, especially those one that replace the CT, such as WHtR, C Index, LAP and VAI, enabling a better nutritional clinical evaluation in elderly and adults able to intervene effectively for the prevention and/or treatment of visceral obesity related to cardiovascular risk.

In conclusion, visceral obesity, considered a large spectrum of cardiovascular risk, was highly discriminated by both anthropometric indicators, C Index and WHtR, as well as by the LAP and the VAI. Therefore, these methods are effective tools in cardiovascular risk assessment and in the follow-up for individual and collective clinical practice.

Acknowledgments

Disclaimer: The authors had full access to all data and accept full responsibility for the content of this report.

The authors are grateful to all participants and technical staff that were involved in data collection procedures.

Author Contributions

Conceived and designed the experiments: AKR LCP CCO ME PAM LRS. Performed the experiments: AKR CCO ME PAM LRS. Analyzed the data: AKR CCO. Wrote the paper: AKR LCP CCO LRS. Reviewed and approved the final version of the manuscript: AKR LCP CCO ME PAM LRS. Author proofing: AKR.

References

1. Poirier P, Giles TD, Bray GA, Hong Y, Stern JS, et al. (2006) Obesity and cardiovascular disease: pathophysiology, evaluation, and effect of weight loss an update of the 1997 American Heart Association Scientific Statement on Obesity and Heart Disease From the Obesity Committee of the Council on Nutrition, Physical Activity, and Metabolism. Circulation 113: 898–918.

2. Tchernof A, Despres JP (2013) Pathophysiology of human visceral obesity: an update. Physiological Reviews 93(1): 359–404.

3. Kahn H (2005) The "lipid accumulation product" performs better than the body mass index for recognizing cardiovascular risk: a population-based comparison. BMC Cardiovascular Disorders 5: 26.

4. Amato MC, Giordano C, Galia M, Criscimanna A, Vitabile S, et al. (2010) Visceral Adiposity Index: a reliable indicator of visceral fat function associated with cardiometabolic risk. Diabetes Care 33: 920–922.

5. Amato MC, Giordano C, Pitrone P, Galluzzo A (2011) Cut-off points of the visceral adiposity index (VAI) identifying a visceral adipose dysfunction associated with cardiometabolic risk in a Caucasian Sicilian population. Lipids in Health and Disease 10: 183.

6. Savva SC, Lamnisos D, Kafatos AG (2013) Predicting cardiometabolic risk: waist-to-height ratio or BMI. A meta-analysis. Diabetes, Metabolic Syndrome and Obesity: Targets and Therapy 6: 403–419.

7. Schneider HJ, Friedrich N, Klotsche J, Pieper L, Nauck M, et al. (2010) The predictive value of different measures of obesity for incident cardiovascular events and mortality. J Clin Endocrinol Metab 95: 1777–1785.

8. Guasch-Ferré M, Bulló M, Martínez-González MÁ, Corella D, Estruch R, et al. (2012) Waist-to-height ratio and cardiovascular risk factors in elderly individuals at high cardiovascular risk. PLoS ONE 7(8): e43275.

9. Pitanga FJG (2011) Anthropometry for the assessment of abdominal obesity and coronary risk. Rev Bras Cineantropom Desempenho Hum 13(3): 238–241.

10. Lee CM, Huxley RR, Wildman RP, Woodward M (2008) Indices of abdominal obesity are better discriminators of cardiovascular risk factors than BMI: a meta-analysis. J Clin Epidemiol 61: 646–653.

11. Sampaio LR, Simões EJ, Assis AMO, Ramos LR (2007) Validity and Reliability of the Sagittal Abdominal Diameter as a Predictor of Visceral Abdominal Fat. Arq Bras Endocrinol Metab; 51: 980–986.

12. Demura S, Sato S (2007) Prediction of visceral fat area in Japanese adults: proposal of prediction method applicable in a field setting. Eur J Clin Nutr.; 61(6): 727–35.

13. Bouza A, Bellido D, Rodríguez B, Pita S, Carreira J (2008) Estimacíon de la grasa abdominal visceral y subcutánea en pacientes obesos a través de ecuaciones de regressíon antropométricas. Revista Española de Obesidade; 6(3): 153–162.

14. Lohman TG; Roche AF; Martorell R (1988) Anthropometric standardization reference manual. Illinois: Human Kinetics Books; p.177.

15. Valdez R (1991) A simple model-based index of abdominal adiposity. J Clin Epidemiol 44(9): 955–6.

16. Seidell JC, Oosterlee A, Thijssen MAO, Burema J (1987) Assessment of intra-abdominal and subcutaneous abdominal fat: relation between anthropometry and computed tomography. Am. J. Clin. Nutr. 45: 7–13.

17. Hunter GR, Snyder SW, Kekes-Szabo T, Nicholson C, Berland L (1994) Intra-abdominal adipose tissue values associated with risk of possessing elevated blood lipids and blood pressure. Obes Res 2: 563–568.

18. Perkins NJ, Schisterman EF (2006) The inconsistency of "optimal" cutpoints obtained using two criteria based on the receiver operating characteristic curve. Am J Epidemiol 163: 670–675.

19. Almeida RT, Almeida MMG, Araújo TM (2009) Abdominal obesity and cardiovascular risk: performance of anthropometric indexes in women. Arq Bras Cardiol. 92(5): 375–80.

20. Pitanga FJG, Lessa I (2005) Anthropometric indexes of obesity as an instrument of screening for high coronary risk in adults in the city of Salvador - Bahia. Arq. Bras. Cardiol. 85(1): 26–31.

21. Vidigal FC, Rosado LEFPL, Rosado GP, Ribeiro RCL, Franceschini SCC, et al. (2013) Predictive ability of the anthropometric and body composition indicators for detecting changes in inflammatory biomarkers. Nutr Hosp. 28(5): 1639–1645.

22. Ashwell M, Gunn P, Gibson S (2012) Waist-to-height ratio is a better screening tool than waist circumference and BMI for adult cardiometabolic risk factors: systematic review and meta-analysis. Obes Rev 13: 275–286.

23. Browning LM, Hsieh SD, Ashwell M (2010) A systematic review of waist-to-height ratio as a screening tool for the prediction of cardiovascular disease and diabetes: 0.5 could be a suitable global boundary value. Nutr Res Rev 23: 247–269.

24. Bozorgmanesh M, Hadaegh F, Azizi F (2010) Diabetes prediction, lipid accumulation product, and adiposity measures; 6-year follow-up: Tehran lipid and glucose study. Lipids in Health and Disease, 9: 45.

25. Chiang JK, Koo M (2012) Lipid accumulation product: a simple and accurate index for predicting metabolic syndrome in Taiwanese people aged 50 and over. BMC Cardiovascular Disorders 12: 78.

26. Tellechea ML, Aranguren F, Martínez-Larrad MT, Serrano-Ríos M, Taverna MJ, et al. (2009) Ability of Lipid Accumulation Product to Identify Metabolic Syndrome in Healthy Men From Buenos Aires. Diabetes Care 32: 7.

27. Taverna MJ, Martinez-Larrad MT, Frechtel GD, Serrano-Rios M (2011) Lipid accumulation product: a powerful marker of metabolic syndrome in healthy population. Eur J Endocrinol. 164, 559–567.

28. Knowles M, Paiva LL, Sanchez SE, Revilla L, Lopez T, et al. (2011) Waist Circumference, Body Mass Index, and Other Measures of Adiposity in Predicting Cardiovascular Disease Risk Factors among Peruvian Adults. Int. J Hypertens 1–10.

29. Bozorgmanesh M, Farzad H, Davoud K, Fereidoun A (2012) Prognostic significance of the Complex "Visceral Adiposity Index" vs. simple anthropometric measures: Tehran lipid and glucose study. Cardiovascular Diabetology 11: 20.

30. Elisha B, Messier V, Karelis A, Coderre L, Bernard S, et al. (2013) The Visceral Adiposity Index: Relationship with cardiometabolic risk factors in obese and overweight postmenopausal women - A MONET group study. Applied Physiology, Nutrition, and Metabolism 38(8): 892–899.

31. Roriz AKC, Mello AL, Guimarães JF, Santos FC, Medeiros JMB, et al. (2010) Imaging assessment of visceral adipose tissue and its correlations with metabolic alterations. Arq Bras Cardiol 95(6), 698–704.

32. Pitanga FJG, Lessa Ines (2006) Razão cintura-estatura como discriminador do risco coronariano de adultos. Rev Assoc Med Bras 52(3), 157–161.

33. Haun DR, Pitanga FJG, Lessa I (2009) Waist/height ratio compared with other anthropometric indicators of obesity as a predictor of high coronary risk. Rev Assoc Med Bras 55(6): 705–11.

34. Berber A, Gómez-Santos R, Fanghänel G, Sánchez-Reyes L (2001) Anthropometric indexes in the prediction of type 2 diabetes mellitus, hypertension and dyslipidaemia in a Mexican population. Int J Obes Relat Metab Disord 25: 1794–1799.

35. Valdez R, Seidell JC, Ahn YI, Weiss KM (1993) A new index of abdominal adiposity as an indicator of risk for cardiovascular disease. A cross-population study. Int J Obes Relat Metab Disord 17: 77–82.

36. Silva DAS, Petroski EL, Peres MA (2013) Accuracy and measures of association of anthropometric indexes of obesity to identify the presence of hypertension in adults: a population-based study in Southern Brazil. Eur J Nutr 52: 237–246.

Permissions

All chapters in this book were first published in PLOS ONE, by The Public Library of Science; hereby published with permission under the Creative Commons Attribution License or equivalent. Every chapter published in this book has been scrutinized by our experts. Their significance has been extensively debated. The topics covered herein carry significant findings which will fuel the growth of the discipline. They may even be implemented as practical applications or may be referred to as a beginning point for another development.

The contributors of this book come from diverse backgrounds, making this book a truly international effort. This book will bring forth new frontiers with its revolutionizing research information and detailed analysis of the nascent developments around the world.

We would like to thank all the contributing authors for lending their expertise to make the book truly unique. They have played a crucial role in the development of this book. Without their invaluable contributions this book wouldn't have been possible. They have made vital efforts to compile up to date information on the varied aspects of this subject to make this book a valuable addition to the collection of many professionals and students.

This book was conceptualized with the vision of imparting up-to-date information and advanced data in this field. To ensure the same, a matchless editorial board was set up. Every individual on the board went through rigorous rounds of assessment to prove their worth. After which they invested a large part of their time researching and compiling the most relevant data for our readers.

The editorial board has been involved in producing this book since its inception. They have spent rigorous hours researching and exploring the diverse topics which have resulted in the successful publishing of this book. They have passed on their knowledge of decades through this book. To expedite this challenging task, the publisher supported the team at every step. A small team of assistant editors was also appointed to further simplify the editing procedure and attain best results for the readers.

Apart from the editorial board, the designing team has also invested a significant amount of their time in understanding the subject and creating the most relevant covers. They scrutinized every image to scout for the most suitable representation of the subject and create an appropriate cover for the book.

The publishing team has been an ardent support to the editorial, designing and production team. Their endless efforts to recruit the best for this project, has resulted in the accomplishment of this book. They are a veteran in the field of academics and their pool of knowledge is as vast as their experience in printing. Their expertise and guidance has proved useful at every step. Their uncompromising quality standards have made this book an exceptional effort. Their encouragement from time to time has been an inspiration for everyone.

The publisher and the editorial board hope that this book will prove to be a valuable piece of knowledge for researchers, students, practitioners and scholars across the globe.

List of Contributors

Ramit Ravona-Springer and Keren Koifman
Memory clinic, Sheba Medical Center, Tel Hashomer, Ramat Gan, Israel

Anthony Heymann
Department of Family Medicine, University of Tel Aviv, Tel Aviv, Israel

James Schmeidler, Mary Sano and Jeremy M. Silverman
Department of Psychiatry, Icahn School of Medicine at Mount Sinai, New York, United States of America

Erin Moshier and James Godbold
Department of Preventive Medicine, Icahn School of Medicine at Mount Sinai, New York, United States of America

Derek Leroith
Department of Medicine, Icahn School of Medicine at Mount Sinai, New York, United States of America

Sterling Johnson
Geriatric Research Education and Clinical Center, Madison VA Hospital and Alzheimer's Disease Research Center, Department of Medicine, University of Wisconsin, WI, United States of America

Rachel Preiss and Hadas Hoffman
Maccabi Health Services, Tel Aviv, Israel

Michal Schnaider Beeri
Department of Psychiatry, Icahn School of Medicine at Mount Sinai, New York, United States of America
The Joseph Sagol Neuroscience Center, Sheba Medical Center, Ramat Gan, Israel

Cong-Zhi Wang
Paul C. Lauterbur Research Center for Biomedical Imaging, Institute of Biomedical and Health Engineering, Shenzhen Institutes of Advanced Technology, Chinese Academy of Sciences, Shenzhen, China
Interdisciplinary Division of Biomedical Engineering, the Hong Kong Polytechnic University, Hong Kong, China
Beijing Center for Mathematics and Information Interdisciplinary Sciences, Beijing, China

Tian-Jie Li and Yong-Ping Zheng
Interdisciplinary Division of Biomedical Engineering, the Hong Kong Polytechnic University, Hong Kong, China

Richard A. I. Bethlehem
Experimental Psychology, Helmholtz Institute, Utrecht University, Utrecht, The Netherlands
Autism Research Centre, Department of Psychiatry, University of Cambridge, Cambridge, United Kingdom

Serge O. Dumoulin, Edwin S. Dalmaijer and Stefan Van der Stigchel
Experimental Psychology, Helmholtz Institute, Utrecht University, Utrecht, The Netherlands

Miranda Smit and Tanja C. W. Nijboer
Experimental Psychology, Helmholtz Institute, Utrecht University, Utrecht, The Netherlands
Rudolf Magnus Institute of Neuroscience and Centre of Excellence for Rehabilitation Medicine, University Medical Centre Utrecht and Rehabilitation Centre De Hoogstraat, Utrecht, The Netherlands

Tos T. J. M. Berendschot
University Eye Clinic Maastricht, Maastricht, The Netherlands

Danjun Feng
School of Nursing, Shandong University, Jinan, China

Linqin Ji
School of Psychology, Shandong Normal University, Jinan, China

Lingzhong Xu
Department of Health Services Management and Maternal & Child Healthcare, Shandong University, Jinan, China

Ta-Chien Chan
Research Center for Humanities and Social Sciences, Academia Sinica, Taipei, Taiwan, Republic of China

Yang-chih Fu
Institute of Sociology, Academia Sinica, Taipei, Taiwan, Republic of China

Da-Wei Wang
Institute of Information Science, Academia Sinica, Taipei, Taiwan, Republic of China

Jen-Hsiang Chuang
Deputy Director-General's Office, Centers for Disease Control, Taipei, Taiwan, Republic of China
Institute of Public Health, National Yang-Ming University, Taipei, Taiwan, Republic of China

Pallavi Banjare, Jalandhar Pradhan
Department of Humanities & Social Sciences, National Institute of Technology (NIT), Rourkela, Odisha, India

Tonje H. Stwea, Ken J. Hetlelid, Hilde Lohne-Seiler, Svanhild Ådnanes, Thomas Bjørnsen, Svein Salvesen and Sveinung Berntsen
Department of Public Health, Sport and Nutrition, University of Agder, Kristiansand, Norway

Lene F. Andersen
Department of Nutrition, Institute of Basic Medical Sciences, University of Oslo, Oslo, Norway

Gøran Paulsen
Department of Physical Performance, Norwegian School of Sport Sciences, Oslo, Norway

Paul Mitchell and Elena Rochtchina
Department of Ophthalmology and Westmead Millennium Institute, University of Sydney, Westmead, New South Wales, Australia

Neil Bressler
Wilmer Eye Institute, Johns Hopkins University, Baltimore, Maryland, United States of America

Quan V. Doan and Mark Danese
Outcomes Insights, Inc., Westlake Village, California, United States of America

Chantal Dolan
CMD Consulting, Inc., Sandy, Utah, United States of America

Alberto Ferreira and Aaron Osborne
Novartis, Basel, Switzerland

Shoshana Colman
Genentech, Inc., South San Francisco, California, United States of America

Tien Y. Wong
Singapore Eye Research Institute, National University of Singapore, Singapore, Singapore
Centre for Eye Research Australia, University of Melbourne, Parkville, Victoria, Australia

Yuan-Chi Shen
Department of Urology, Kaohsiung Chang Gung Memorial Hospital, Kaohsiung, Taiwan
Cheng Shiu University, Kaohsiung, Taiwan

Shih-Feng Weng
Department of Medical Research, Chi Mei Medical Center, Tainan, Taiwan
Department of Hospital and Health Care Administration, Chia Nan University of Pharmacy and Science, Tainan, Taiwan

Jhi-Joung Wang
Department of Medical Research, Chi Mei Medical Center, Tainan, Taiwan

Kai-Jen Tien
Division of Endocrinology and Metabolism, Department of Internal Medicine, Chi Mei Medical Center, Tainan, Taiwan
The Center of General Education, Chia Nan University of Pharmacy and Science, Tainan, Taiwan

Giuseppe Grosso, Sabrina Castellano, Fabio Galvano, Claudio Bucolo and Filippo Drago
Department of Clinical and Molecular Biomedicine, Section of Pharmacology and Biochemistry, University of Catania, Catania, Italy

Andrzej Pajak
Department of Epidemiology and Population Studies, Jagiellonian University Medical College, Krakow, Poland

Stefano Marventano
Department "G.F. Ingrassia", Section of Hygiene and Public Health, University of Catania, Catania, Italy

Filippo Caraci
Department of Educational Sciences, University of Catania, Catania, Italy
IRCCS Associazione Oasi Maria S.S. – Institute for Research on Mental Retardation and Brain Aging, Troina, Enna, Italy

Wei-Ting Chang and Ping-Yen Liu
Division of Cardiology, Internal Medicine, National Cheng Kung University Hospital, Tainan, Taiwan Institute of Clinical Medicine, National Cheng Kung University, Tainan, Taiwan

Jung-San Chen, Yung-Kung Hung and Jer-Nan Juang
Department of Engineering Science, National Cheng Kung University, Tainan, Taiwan

Wei-Chuan Tsai
Division of Cardiology, Internal Medicine, National Cheng Kung University Hospital, Tainan, Taiwan

Bum-Joo Cho, Jang Won Heo and Hum Chung
Department of Ophthalmology, Seoul National University College of Medicine, Seoul, Korea
Department of Ophthalmology, Seoul National University Hospital, Seoul, Korea

Jae Pil Shin
Department of Ophthalmology, Kyungpook National University School of Medicine, Daegu, Korea

Jeeyun Ahn and Tae Wan Kim
Department of Ophthalmology, Seoul National University College of Medicine, Seoul, Korea
Department of Ophthalmology, Seoul Metropolitan Government Seoul National University Boramae Medical Center, Seoul, Korea

Olivier Beauchet and Christine Merjagnan
Department of Neuroscience, Angers University Hospital, Angers, France Biomathics, Paris, France

Cyrille P. Launay and Anastasiia Kabeshova
Department of Neuroscience, Angers University Hospital, Angers, France

Cédric Annweiler
Department of Neuroscience, Angers University Hospital, Angers, France
Department of Medical Biophysics, the University of Western Ontario, London, Canada

Korinna Karampampa, Anders Ahlbom and Karin Modig
Institute of Environmental Medicine, Unit of Epidemiology, Karolinska Institutet, Stockholm, Sweden

Tomas Andersson
Institute of Environmental Medicine, Unit of Epidemiology, Karolinska Institutet, Stockholm, Sweden
Centre for Occupational and Environmental Medicine, Stockholm County Council, Stockholm, Sweden

Sven Drefahl
Institute of Environmental Medicine, Unit of Epidemiology, Karolinska Institutet, Stockholm, Sweden
Department of Sociology, Demography Unit, Stockholm University, Stockholm, Sweden

Matteo Cesari
Institut du Vieillissement, Gérontopôle, Centre Hospitalier Universitaire de Toulouse, Toulouse, France
Inserm UMR1027, Université de Toulouse III Paul Sabatier, Toulouse, France

Laurent Demougeot, Henri Boccalon and Sophie Guyonnet
Institut du Vieillissement, Gérontopôle, Centre Hospitalier Universitaire de Toulouse, Toulouse, France

Gabor Abellan Van Kan, Bruno Vellas and Sandrine Andrieu
Institut du Vieillissement, Gérontopôle, Centre Hospitalier Universitaire de Toulouse, Toulouse, France
Inserm UMR1027, Université de Toulouse III Paul Sabatier, Toulouse, France

Anna K. Stuck, Marie Méan, Nicolas Rodondi and Drahomir Aujesky
Division of General Internal Medicine, Bern University Hospital, Bern, Switzerland

Andreas Limacher
CTU Bern, Department of Clinical Research, and Institute of Social and Preventive Medicine, University of Bern, Bern, Switzerland

Marc Righini
Division of Angiology and Hemostasis, Geneva University Hospital, Geneva, Switzerland

Kurt Jaeger
Division of Angiology, Basel University Hospital, Basel, Switzerland

Hans-Jürg Beer
Cantonal Hospital of Baden, Baden, Switzerland

Joseph Osterwalder
Emergency Department, Cantonal Hospital of St. Gallen, St. Gallen, Switzerland

Beat Frauchiger
Department of Internal Medicine, Cantonal Hospital of Frauenfeld, Frauenfeld, Switzerland

Christian M. Matter
Cardiovascular Research, Institute of Physiology, Zurich Center for Integrative Human Physiology, University of Zurich, Zurich, Switzerland
Division of Cardiology, Zurich University Hospital, Zurich, Switzerland

Nils Kucher
Division of Angiology, Bern University Hospital, Bern, Switzerland

Michael Egloff
Division of Diabetology, Geneva University Hospital, Geneva, Switzerland

Markus Aschwanden
Division of Angiology, Basel University Hospital, Basel, Switzerland

Marc Husmann
Clinic of Angiology, Zurich University Hospital, Zurich, Switzerland

Anne Angelillo-Scherrer
University Clinic of Hematology and Hematology Central Laboratory, Bern University Hospital, Bern, Switzerland

Fabiana Di Marco, Mattia Di Paolo, Stefania Romeo, Linda Colecchi and Lavinia Fiorani
Department of Biotechnology and Applied Clinical Science, University of L'Aquila, L'Aquila, Italy

Sharon Spana
Discipline of Physiology and Bosch Institute, University of Sydney, Sydney, New South Wales, Australia

Jonathan Stone
Discipline of Physiology and Bosch Institute, University of Sydney, Sydney, New South Wales, Australia

Silvia Bisti
Department of Biotechnology and Applied Clinical Science, University of L'Aquila, L'Aquila, Italy
ARC Centre of Excellence in Vision Science, The Australian National University, Canberra, Australia

Nai-Feng Tian, Xu-Qi Hu, Xiang-Yang Wang, Yong-Long Chi and Fang-Min Mao
Department of Orthopaedic Surgery, Second Affiliated Hospital of Wenzhou Medical University, Wenzhou, Zhejiang, China

Li-Jun Wu and Xin-Lei Wu,
Institute of Digitized Medicine, Wenzhou Medical University, Wenzhou, Zhejiang, China

Yao-Sen Wu
Department of Orthopaedics, Second Affiliated Hospital, School of Medicine, Zhejiang University, Hangzhou, Zhejiang, China

Xiao-Lei Zhang
Department of Orthopaedic Surgery, Second Affiliated Hospital of Wenzhou Medical University, Wenzhou, Zhejiang, China
Center for Stem Cells and Tissue Engineering, School of Medicine, Zhejiang University, Hangzhou, Zhejiang, China

Stefanie L. De Buyser and Mirko Petrovic
Department of Geriatrics, Ghent University Hospital, Ghent, Belgium

Youri E. Taes
Department of Endocrinology and Unit for Osteoporosis and Metabolic Bone Diseases, Ghent University Hospital, Ghent, Belgium

Davide L. Vetrano and Graziano Onder
Centro Medicina dell'Invecchiamento, Università Cattolica del Sacro Cuore, Rome, Italy

Andrea Corsonello
Unit of Geriatric Pharmaco-epidemiology, IRCCS - Italian National Research Centre on Aging (INRCA), Cosenza, Italy

Stefano Volpato
Department of Medical Sciences, University of Ferrara, Ferrara, Italy

Michael Janusz Koss
Department of Ophthalmology, Goethe University, Frankfurt am Main, Germany

Doheny Eye Institute, Los Angeles, California, United States of America
Department of Ophthalmology, Ruprecht Karls University, Heidelberg, Germany

Janosch Hoffmann
Mosaiques Diagnostics, Hannover, Germany

Nauke Nguyen
Department of Ophthalmology, Goethe University, Frankfurt am Main, Germany

Marcel Pfister
Doheny Eye Institute, Los Angeles, California, United States of America

Harald Mischak
Mosaiques Diagnostics, Hannover, Germany
BHF Glasgow Cardiovascular Research Centre, University of Glasgow, Glasgow, United Kingdom

William Mullen and Holger Husi
BHF Glasgow Cardiovascular Research Centre, University of Glasgow, Glasgow, United Kingdom

Robert Rejdak
Department of General Ophthalmology, Lublin University, Poland

Frank Koch
Department of Ophthalmology, Goethe University, Frankfurt am Main, Germany

Joachim Jankowski and Katharina Krueger
Department of Nephrology, Endocrinology, and Transplantation Medicine Charité-Universitaetsmedizin, Berlin, Germany

Thomas Bertelmann
Department of Ophthalmology, Philipps University, Marburg, Germany

Julie Klein
Mosaiques Diagnostics, Hannover, Germany

Joost P. Schanstra
Mosaiques Diagnostics, Hannover, Germany
Institut National de la Santé et de la Recherche Médicale (INSERM), U1048, Institut of Cardiovascular and Metabolic Disease, Toulouse, France
Universite´ Toulouse III Paul-Sabatier, Toulouse, France

Justyna Siwy
Mosaiques Diagnostics, Hannover, Germany
Department of Nephrology, Endocrinology, and Transplantation Medicine Charité-Universitaetsmedizin, Berlin, Germany

Claudia Sikorski
Institute of Social Medicine, Occupational Health and Public Health, University of Leipzig, Leipzig, Germany
Leipzig University Medical Center, IFB AdiposityDiseases, Leipzig, Germany

Melanie Luppa and Steffi G. Riedel-Heller
Institute of Social Medicine, Occupational Health and Public Health, University of Leipzig, Leipzig, Germany

Siegfried Weyerer
Central Institute of Mental Health, Medical Faculty Mannheim/Heidelberg University, Mannheim, Germany

Hans-Helmut König
Department of Medical Sociology, Social Medicine and Health Economics, Hamburg-Eppendorf University Medical Center, Hamburg, Germany

Wolfgang Maier
Department of Psychiatry and Psychotherapy, University of Bonn, Bonn, Germany

Gerhard Schön
Department of Medical Biometry and Epidemiology, Hamburg-Eppendorf University Medical Center, Hamburg, Germany

Juliana J. Petersen
Institute of General Practice, Goethe-University Frankfurt am Main, Frankfurt am Main, Germany

Jochen Gensichen
Department of General Practice, Jena University Hospital, Jena, Germany

Angela Fuchs
Department of General Practice, Medical Faculty, University of Dusseldorf, Dusseldorf, Germany

Horst Bickel
Department of Psychiatry, Technical University of Munich, München, Germany

Birgitt Wiese
Institute for Biometry, Hannover Medical School, Hannover, Germany

Heike Hansen, Hendrik van den Bussche and Martin Scherer
Department of Primary Medical Care, Hamburg-Eppendorf University Medical Center, Hamburg, Germany

Duk-Hee Lee
Department of Preventive Medicine, School of Medicine, Kyungpook National University, Daegu, Korea,
BK21 Plus KNU Biomedical Convergence Program, Department of Biomedical Science, Kyungpook National University, Daegu, Korea

Lars Lind

Department of Medical Sciences, Cardiovascular Epidemiology, Uppsala University Hospital, Uppsala, Sweden

David R. Jacobs Jr.
Division of Epidemiology and Community Health, School of Public Health, University of Minnesota, Minneapolis, Minnesota, United States of America
Department of Nutrition, University of Oslo, Oslo, Norway

Samira Salihovic and Bert van Bavel
MTM Research Center, School of Science and Technology,Örebro University,Örebro, Sweden

P. Monica Lind
Department of Medical Sciences, Occupational and Environmental Medicine, Uppsala University, Uppsala, Sweden

René Melis
Department of Geriatric Medicine/Nijmegen Alzheimer Centre 925, Radboud University Nijmegen Medical Centre, Nijmegen, The Netherlands

Alessandra Marengoni
Geriatric Unit, Department of Clinical and Experimental Science, University of Brescia, Brescia, Italy

Aging Research Center (ARC), Karolinska Institutet (Neurobiology, Care Science and Society Department) and Stockholm University, Stockholm, Sweden

Sara Angleman
Aging Research Center (ARC), Karolinska Institutet (Neurobiology, Care Science and Society Department) and Stockholm University, Stockholm, Sweden

Laura Fratiglioni
Aging Research Center (ARC), Karolinska Institutet (Neurobiology, Care Science and Society Department) and Stockholm University, Stockholm, Sweden
Stockholm Gerontology Research Center, Stockholm, Sweden

Johanna Muckenhuber, Nathalie T. Burkert, Franziska Großschädl, Wolfgang Freidl and Éva Rásky
Department of Social Medicine and Epidemiology, Medical University Graz, Graz, Austria

Karina Fernandez
Department of business education and development, Karl-Franzens- University Graz, Graz, Austria

Anna Karla Carneiro Roriz
Postgraduation Program of Medicine and Health, Federal University of Bahia, Salvador, Bahia, Brazil
School of Nutrition, Nutrition Science Department, Federal University of Bahia, Salvador, Bahia, Brazil

Luiz Carlos Santana Passos
Postgraduation Program of Medicine and Health, Federal University of Bahia, Salvador, Bahia, Brazil
Faculty of Medicine, Department of Medicine, Federal University of Bahia, Salvador, Bahia, Brazil

Carolina Cunha de Oliveira
Postgraduation Program of Medicine and Health, Federal University of Bahia, Salvador, Bahia, Brazil
Nutrition Department, Federal University of Sergipe, Lagarto, Sergipe, Brazil

Michaela Eickemberg
Institute of Collective Health, Federal University of Bahia, Salvador, Bahia, Brazil
Bahiana School of Medicine and Public Health, Salvador, Bahia, Brazil

Pricilla de Almeida Moreira
School of Nutrition, Nutrition Science Department, Federal University of Bahia, Salvador, Bahia, Brazil

Lílian Ramos Sampaio
School of Nutrition, Nutrition Science Department, Federal University of Bahia, Salvador, Bahia, Brazil
Postgraduation Program in Food and Nutrition, Federal University of Bahia, Salvador, Bahia, Brazil

Index

www.ingramcontent.com/pod-product-compliance
Lightning Source LLC
Chambersburg PA
CBHW082045190326
41458CB00010B/3467